Development of Formulas of Chinese Medicine

方 剂 学 发 挥

Editor-in-Chief   Liu Gongwang
Translator-in-Chief   Liu Changlin
English Editor   Donald P. Lauda
Translation Reviser   Shuji Goto   Liu Gongwang

Huaxia Publishing House

Editor-in-chief

Liu Gongwang

Associate Editor-in-chief

Akira Hyodo   Hiromichi Yasui   Jiao Miao

Editors

Li Qinghe   Nian Li   Wang Yuxing
Takasi Izimi   Wang Xiuyun   Ma Zuoying
Shang Xiukui   Xiao Xuefeng   Meng Xiangwen
Dong Hongying   Liu Enshun   Kan Xiangling

Translator-in-chief

Liu Changlin

Translators

Ma Zuoying   Yang Zheng   Tu Jinli

English Editor

Donald P. Lauda

Translation Reviser

Shuji Goto   Liu Gongwang

Illustrator

Gong Baoxi

Supervisors

Shuji Goto   Dai Ximeng   Donald P. Lauda

A Guide to the Reader

1. This book is intended mainly for the physicians and dedicated medical students who need to design a formula in terms of the principles of determination for treatment based on differentiation of syndromes in the clinic. Thus, the dosages of all selected formulas in this book, exclusive of those not fit for decoction, are only for decoction use.

2. The dosages marked in each formula in this book are the common dosages. In the clinic, they may be modified appropriately according to the patient's condition and physician's experience.

3. Since the components, dosages and processing methods of the proprietary Chinese medicines relate to special techniques of modern processing industry of Chinese medicinal herbs, they are left out in this book. The emphasis is laid on their composition, action and application.

4. Since some banned drugs such as rhinoceros horn and tiger bone are included in certain ancient prescriptions, they are replaced with other drugs in this book, For instance, rhinoceros horn is substituted with water buffalo horn and tiger bone with antler.

5. As for the dosages and administration of the proprietary Chinese medicines, since they are varied owing to the different manufacturers, they are not marked in this book. When these medicines are administered, the patients may refer to the manufacturer's drug specification or the doctor's advice.

6. In this book, each formula follows an image that illustrates the indicated syndromes of the formula. Of the images, most are made by ourselves but some are referred to those recorded in the Japanese book "Illustrated Survey of Abdominal Syndromes" published by Public House of Japanese Medical Way, for which we are greatly indebted.

7. The item of "Applied Syndrome" listed in each formula refers to the differentiation or diagnosis of TCM syndromes. The "Indications" refer to the diagnosis of a disease by means of western medicine. In the clinic, they should be referred to with each other by combining disease differentiation with syndrome differentiation.

8. The item of "Points in Constitution" listed in each formula is the essence in drug composition and core in designing a formula.

9. The prescriptions listed in "Associated Formulas" for each formula have the characteristic of being similar in components or in effects. The purpose of doing so is to help widen the train of thoughts and explore its source, which will surely benefit us in differentiating the syndrome and designing a formula.

Preface

The basic content of this "*Clinical Essentials of Contemporary Series Chinese Medine*" initially came from my lecture notes on Traditional Chinese Medicine prepared for Gero Missoni, an Austrian physician, and other doctors in 1989. The notes were supplemented during the next two years when I lectured at the Toulouse University in France. Later, this material was enhanced and became especially valuable when I began to work with the Goto College of Medical Arts and Sciences in Japan in 1996 to train postgraduate students in a master's degree course in TCM. Since then, the material has been continually revised in my annual lectures in Japan and has gradually been put into book form and translated into Japanese and English.

This series consists of three books: *Chinese Herbal Medicine*, *Fundamentals of Formulas of Chinese Medicine* and *Clinical Chinese Medicine*. They are not alike the basic textbooks of TCM nor the general books of clinical treatment. The aim of compiling this series is to integrate the knowledge of the ancient and the present, emphasize the main points, use succinct language and retain the essence and depth of TCM simply and easily. When reading, the readers may move from one subject to the other and from the rudimentary to the advanced to guide their clinical practice. This series is designed mainly for clinical physicians and foreign scholars who have some understanding of TCM.

The book *Fundamentals of Formulas of Chinese Medicine* includes two volumes. Volume One is mainly comprised of representative or classic prescriptions and those that are of guiding significance in the establishment of therapy and designing of formulas. Volume Two mainly consists of the famous prescriptions handed down from physicians in the successive dynasties. Besides, it also includes the *kanpo* created by the Japanese physicians. Thus, Volume One may be regarded as the basis of formula-ology of Traditional Chinese Medicine and Volume Two as the elaboration of it.

There are ten chapters altogether in Volume One, which includes the formulas for six channel syndromes of exogenous febrile disease and those for syndromes of Weifen, Qifen, Yingfen and Xuefen in epidemic febrile diseases. These are placed first as the formulas for six channel syndromes of exogenous febrile diseases designed by Zhang Zhongjing, a famous physician in the Han Dynasty who was honored by later physicians as "the father of classic formulas". When they are integrated with the formulas for syndrome of Weifen, Qifen, Yingfen and Xuefen in epidemic diseases, a general idea can be easily given in the treatment of febrile diseases. The other formulas are sorted out according to the theory of five zang-organs of the heart, liver, spleen, lung and kidney. In addition, formulas for women diseases, external diseases and other diseases are also embodied in it. By doing so, it is hoped that readers can gain a thorough understanding of prescriptions through mastery of basic theory and therapy of TCM. The contents of these chapters are indispensable knowledge in learning the formulas of TCM.

Volume Two contains 14 chapters. They are classified, based on modern medical systems, as formulas for the respiratory, circulatory, digestive, urinary and reproductive and metabolic system, for gynecological, pediatric, surgical, orthopadic and dermatic disease as well as for diseases of five sense organs, disease of eyes, tumors and external use so as to be applied easily in treating patients. When this volume is used with reference to Volume One, it is easy to understand the source of formula-designing and principle of formula-modifying, gaining the effect of bringing out the best in each other.

In this book each formula is described in terms of its source, composition, action, applied syndrome, application, caution and associated formulas with the view of comprehensively introducing the formula to have the learners master well the application of the formulas in the clinic. In order to make it easy to understand, analyze and memorize the formulas, an analytic illustration is given for each formula. For those that are not expounded, extra notes are included to make a further explanation.

Following the way in which the Japanese medical book *Brief Survey of Abdominal Syndromes* is written, each formula listed in Volume One has a diagram and image designed to leave a deep impression on the reader so as to memorize the formula easily.

During the last ten years, parts of it were used by many practitioners. With the encouragement and support of Dai Ximeng, the president of Tianjin College of TCM and Dr. Shuji Goto, the president of Japanese Goto College of Medical Arts and Sciences, I was determined to have it published to share it with more people. Acknowledgement should be presented to Professor Hiromitsi Yasui and Akira Hyodo from Japan and my colleagues from China for their concerned assistance and constant hard work. Through their efforts it has become possible to publish this book after several revisions of the original materials.

Chinese Medical Formula-ology is the pivot of the four processes of the basic theory, establishment of therapy, prescription of formulas and choice of herbs in the diagnosis and treatment based on differentiation of syndromes. Formulas consisting of herbs equally depend on the therapy selected. They are the sign of ancient people's valuable experience and the precious jewel of TCM. Ancient physicians often said that "imitating teacher's designing of formulas but never the formula itself", which means that most of the ancient therapies were embodied in the formula, especially in Zhang Zhongjing's formulas. That is also the essential reason why Zhang Zhongjing is known as "father of Classic formulas".

Just like the Chinese saying of "waiting by the stump of a tree for the appearance of hares rather than hunting for them", using a fixed formula to treat varied diseases is the characteristic of treatment in TCM. There are countless prescriptions, but Chinese medical therapies can be established in number. In this volume the author, by improving and developing Cheng's eight therapeutic methods, subdivides the eight therapies into 64 methods and places them firstly in the General Introduction of the book with the purpose of dominating the variety of formulas from the angle of the establishment of therapy.

In ancient times there was a saying that "it is easy to find 1,000 formulas but hard to find a single satisfactory solution". This has often encouraged me to make very careful observations in my clinical practice. During my 30 years teaching and practicing, I have explored the great mystery of Traditional Chinese Medicine and have tried to perfect my practice. But I very much approves of the wisdom found within the book *"Posthumous Works of Various Physicians"* which points out that frequent practical use of one's knowledge and scrupulous diagnostic practice can give rise to creative new clinical applications. I also think this is the way forward for the development of TCM formulas in the future.

Professor Liu Gongwang
June 6, 2002

Contents

Chapter One

Formulas for Diseases of the Respiratory System ································ (1)
  1. Cough-Stopping Powder (止嗽散, zhi suo san) ···························· (1)
  2. Mystery Decoction (神秘汤, shen mi tang) ································ (4)
  3. Tendrilleaf Fritillary Bulb and Snakegourd Fruit Powder
    (贝母瓜蒌散, bei mu gua lou san) ·· (6)
  4. Lung-Clearing Decoction (清肺汤, qing fei tang) ······················· (8)
  5. Yin-Nourishing and Fire-Eliminating Decoction
    (滋阴降火汤, zi yin jiang huo tang) ······································· (10)
  6. Yin-Nourishing Real Treasure Decoction (滋阴至宝汤, zi yin zhi bao tang) ········· (12)
  7. Lil y Metal-Consolidating Decoction (百合固金汤, bai he gu jin tang) ········· (14)
  8. Harmony-Preserving Decoction (保和汤, bao he tang) ················ (17)
  9. Lunar Corona Pill (月华丸, yue hua wan) ································ (20)
  10. Ten Charred Herbs Powder (十灰散, shi hui san) ···················· (23)
  11. Divaricate Saposhnikovia Miraculous Powder
     (防风通圣散, fang feng tong sheng san) ································· (25)
  12. Five Retentions Powder (五积散, wu ji san) ··························· (27)

Additional Formulas ··· (31)
  Qi-Dispersing and Lung-Regulating Pill (通宣理肺丸, tong xuan li fei wan) ········· (31)
  Pleurisy Decoction Number One (胸膜炎汤Ⅰ号, xiong mo yan tang yi hao) ········· (33)
  Pleurisy Decoction Number Two (胸膜炎汤Ⅱ号, xiong mo yan tang er hao) ········· (35)

Chapter Two

Formulas for Diseases of the Circulatory System ···························· (38)
  1. Liver-Subduing and Wind-Stopping Decoction
    (镇肝熄风汤, zhen gan xi feng tang) ······································· (38)
  2. Sweeping Down Decoction for Tension Hypertension (建瓴汤, jian ling tang) ······· (41)
  3. Gambirplant Hooked Stem and Branch Powder (钩藤散, gou teng san) ········· (43)
  4. Chinese Angelica, Gentian and Aloes Pill
    (当归龙荟丸, dang gui long hui wan) ······································ (45)

Additional Formulas ··· (48)
  Yang Hyperactivity-Checking Decoction with Seven Drugs

　　　　（七物降下汤, qi wu jiang xia tang） ································· (48)
　Blood Pressure-Reducing Decoction(降压汤, jiang ya tang) ················ (49)
　Qi-Replenishing and Yin-Nourishing Decoction(益气养阴汤, yi qi yang yin tang) ······ (51)
　Lipide-Lowering and Vessels-Dredging Decoction
　　　　（降脂通脉饮, jiang zhi tong mai yin） ······················· (53)
　Coronary Heart Disease Tablet Number Two 冠心Ⅱ号(guan xin er hao)
　　　　〔Coronary Heart Disease Tablet(冠心片, guan xin pian)〕 ············ (56)
　Heart-Stimulating Decoctio(强心饮, qiang xin yin) ······················· (59)
　Heart Failure Mixture(心衰合剂, xin shuai he ji) ························ (60)
　Heart Rhythm-Adjusting Mixture(整律合剂, zheng lu he ji) ··············· (63)
　Palpitation-Relieving Decoction(宁心汤, ning xin tang) ··················· (65)

Chapter Three

Formulas for Diseases of the Digestive System ································ (67)
　1. Middle-Jiao-Calming Powder(安中散, an zhong san) ···················· (67)
　2. Chinese Angelica Decoction (当归汤, dang gui tang) ··················· (70)
　3. Dan-Shen Decoction (丹参饮, dan shen yin) ··························· (72)
　4. Immortal Viscera-Nourishing Decoction
　　　　（真人养脏汤, zhen ren yang zang tang） ······················ (74)
　5. Common Aucklandia and Areca Seed Pill
　　　　（木香槟榔丸, mu xiang bing lang wan） ······················· (76)
　6. Immature Bitter Orange Stagnation-Dispelling Pill
　　　　（枳实导滞丸, zhi shi dao zhi wan） ·························· (79)
　7. Spleen-Warming Decoction(温脾汤, wen pi tang) ······················· (82)
　8. Intestines-Moistening Pill (润肠丸, run chang wan) ···················· (84)
　9. Coptis Decoction(黄连汤, huang lian tang) ···························· (86)
　10. Dysentery-Stopping Pill(驻车丸, zhu che wan) ························ (88)
　11. "B" Character Decoction(乙字汤, yi zi tang) ························· (91)
　12. Yang-Lifting and Stomach-Benefiting Decoction
　　　　（升阳益胃汤, sheng yang yi wei tang） ······················· (92)
　13. Common Burreed and Kwangsi Turmeric Decoction
　　　　（荆蓬煎丸, ji peng jian wan） ································ (94)
Additional Formulas ··· (97)
　Heat-Removing Decoction for Acute Pancreatitis
　　　　（胰腺清化汤, yi xian qing hua tang） ························ (97)
　Blood Stasis-Removing Decoction for Acute Appendicitis
　　　　（阑尾化瘀汤, lan wei hua yu tang） ·························· (99)
　Gallstones-Removing Decoction(胆道排石汤, dan dao pai shi tang) ········· (101)
　Liver-Soothing Decoction(舒肝饮, shu gan yin) ·························· (104)

Liver-Recuperating Pill(复肝丸, fu gan wan) ·· (107)

Esophagitis Pill (食道炎丸, shi dao yan wan) ·· (111)

Dryness-Moistening and Stomach-Nourishing Decoction
　(润燥养胃汤, run zao yang wei tang) ·· (113)

Chapter Four

Formulas for Diseases of the Urogenital System ·································· (116)

　1. Field Thistle Decoction(小蓟饮子, xiao ji yin zi) ································ (116)

　2. Powder for Five Kinds of Stranguria(五淋散, wu lin san) ····················· (118)

　3. Sevenlobed Yam Decoction for Clearing Turbid Urine
　　(萆薢分清饮, bi xie fen qing yin) ·· (120)

　4. Heart-Clearing Lotus Seed Decoction(清心莲子饮, qing xin lian zi yin) ······ (122)

　5. Lung-Clearing Decoction(清肺饮, qing fei yin) ···································· (123)

　6. Chinese Eaglewood Wood Powder (沉香散, chen xiang san) ····················· (125)

　7. Decoction for Diuresis (疏凿饮子, shu zao yin zi) ································ (127)

　8. Spleen-Reinforcing Decoction(实脾饮, shi pi yin) ································ (129)

　9. Water Retention-Removing Decoction(分消汤, fen xiao tang) ··················· (132)

　10. Golden Lock Pill for Solidating Essence (金锁固精丸, jin shuo gu jing wan) ······ (134)

　11. Kidney Yang-Strengthening Pill(壮阳丹, zhang yang dan) ······················· (136)

　12. Liver-Warming Decoction(暖肝煎, nuan gan jian) ································ (138)

　13. Tangerine Pit Pill (橘核丸, ju he wan) ·· (140)

　14. Bank-Consolidating Pill(巩堤丸, gong di wan) ···································· (142)

　15. Three Talents Marrow-Preserving Pill (三才封髓丹, san cai feng sui dan) ······ (144)

Additional Formulas ·· (146)

　Pilose Asiabell, Membranous Milkvetch Decoction for Stranguria due to Overstrain
　　(参芪劳淋汤, shen qi lao lin tang) ·· (146)

　Effective Formula for Kidney Recuperation(肾康灵, shen kang ling) ············· (148)

　Nephritis Decoction(肾炎汤, shen yang tang) ·· (151)

　Aconite and Rhubarb Decoction(附子大黄汤, fu zi da huang tang) ················ (153)

　Powder for Urine Retention(癃闭散, long bi san) ···································· (155)

　Renal Colic Decoction(肾绞痛汤, shen jiao tong tang) ······························· (157)

　Effective Formula for Impotence (亢痿灵, kang wei ling) ·························· (159)

　Essence-Supplementing, Kidney-Invigorating and Breeding Decoction
　　(填精补肾育种汤, tian jing bu shen yu zhong tang) ································ (162)

　Formula for Immune Infertility Number One
　　(免疫性不育Ⅰ号方, mian yi xing bu yu yi hao fang) ······························· (165)

Chapter Five

Formulas for the Nervous and Psychogenic Diseases ······ (167)
  1. Head-Clearing and Pain-Alleviating Decoction
    (清上蠲痛汤, qing shang juan tong tang) ······ (167)
  2. Tea-Blended Szechwan Lovage Powder
    (川芎茶调散, chuan xiong cha tiao san) ······ (169)
  3. Gallbladder-Warming Decoction(温胆汤, wen dan tang) ······ (171)
  4. Bamboo Shavings Gallbladder-Warming Decoction
    (竹茹温胆汤, zhu ru wen dan tang) ······ (174)
  5. Liver-Inhibiting Powder(抑肝散, yi gan san) ······ (176)
  6. Miraculous Musk Powder(妙香散, miao xiang san) ······ (178)
  7. Heart-Washing Decoction(洗心汤, xi xin tang) ······ (180)
  8. Lucid Yang-Generating Decoction(滋生清阳汤, zi sheng qing yang tang) ······ (182)
  9. Magnetite and Cinnabar Pill(磁朱丸, ci zhu wan) ······ (185)
  10. Face Distortion-Treating Powder(牵正散, qian zheng san) ······ (187)
  11. Minor Life-prolonging Decoction(小续命汤, xiao xu ming tang) ······ (188)
  12. Iron Scales Decoction(生铁落饮, sheng tie luo yin) ······ (190)

Additional Formulas ······ (193)
  Dawn Formula for Vascular Headache
    (曙光血管头痛方, shu guang xue guan tou tong fang) ······ (193)
  Brain-Benefiting and Blood-Activating Formula
    (益脑活血方, yi nao huo xue fang) ······ (195)

Chapter Six

Formulas for Endocrine and Metabolic Diseases ······ (198)
  1. Jade Liquid Decoction (Yuye Decoction, 玉液汤, yu ye tang) ······ (198)
  2. Seaweed Jade Kettle Decoction(海藻玉壶汤, hai zao yu hu tang) ······ (200)
  3. Internally Scrofula-Eliminating Pill(内消瘰疬丸, nei xiao lei li wan) ······ (202)
  4. Ten Strong Tonic Herbs Decoction(十全大补丸, shi quan da bu wan) ······ (204)
  5. Ginseng Nutrition Decoction(人参养荣汤, ren shen yang rong tang) ······ (206)

Additional Formulas ······ (210)
  Blood Sugar-Reducing Decoction(降糖汤, jian tang tang) ······ (210)
  Goiter-Curing Decoction(平甲汤, ping jia tang) ······ (212)
  An Obesity-Reducing Formula(轻身一方, qing shen yi fang) ······ (214)
  Hemocyte-Increasing Mixture(升血合剂, sheng xue he ji) ······ (217)
  Qi-Replenishing and Rash-Dissipating Decoction
    (益气化斑汤, yi qi hua ban tang) ······ (220)

Chapter Seven

Formulas for Gynecological Diseases ································· (223)
  1. Szechwan Lovage and Chinese Angelica Decoction for Regulating Blood Flow
    （芎归调血饮，xiong gui tiao xue yin）····························· (223)
  2. Zhechong Decoction（折冲饮，zhe chong yin）······················ (225)
  3. Liver-Clearing and Depression-Alleviating Decoction
    （清肝达郁饮，qing gan da yu yin）································ (228)
  4. Motherwort Gold-Exceeding Pill（益母胜金丹，yi mu sheng jin dan）····· (230)
  5. Menstruation-Normalizing Decoction（顺经汤，shun jing tang）······ (232)
  6. Pregnancy-Promoting Pearl（毓麟珠，yu lin zhu）·················· (234)
  7. Miscarriage-Preventing Pill（寿胎丸，shou tai wan）··············· (236)
  8. Taishan Rock Powder（泰山磐石散，tai shan pan shi san）········· (239)
  9. Blood Stasis-Removing Decoction（通瘀煎，tong yu jian）·········· (241)
  10. Liver-Clearing and Stranguria-Treating Decoction
    （清肝止淋汤，qin gan zhi lin tang）······························· (243)
  11. Postmenopausal Bleeding-Preventing Decoction（安老汤，an lao tang）····· (244)
  12. Springing like Lactation-Promoting Powder
    （下乳涌泉散，xia ru yong quan san）····························· (247)

Additional Formulas ··· (250)
  Charred Fortune Windmillpalm Petiole and Charred Cattail Pollen Powder
    （棕蒲散，zong pu san）··· (250)
  Formula for Exfetation Number Two（宫外孕Ⅱ号，gong wai yun er hao）··· (252)
  Two Immortals Powder（二仙汤，er xian tang）······················ (254)

Chapter Eight

Formulas for Pediatric Diseases ·· (256)
  1. Spleen-Invigorating Pill（启脾丸，qi pi wan）······················· (256)
  2. Largehead Atractylodes Powder with Seven Herbs
    （七味白术散，qi wei bai zhu san）································ (258)
  3. Cold-Expelling and Convulsion-Relieving Decoction
    （逐寒荡惊汤，zhu han dang jing tang）···························· (260)
  4. Viscera-Benefiting and Consciousness-Restoring Decoction
    （可保立苏汤，ke bao li su tang）·································· (261)
  5. Primary Qi-Regulating Powder（调元散，tiao yuan san）············ (263)
  6. Silk Pouch Pill（布袋丸，bu dai wan）····························· (265)
  7. Shen's Pill for Decreasing Urination（沈氏闷泉丸，shen shi men quan wan）······ (267)
  8. Hang Xie Pellet（沆瀣丹，hang xie dan）··························· (268)

Additional Formulas ··· (271)
   Infantile Convulsion-Relieving Pill(小儿回春丹, xiao er hui chun dan)······ (271)
   Cormorant Saliva Pill(鸬鹚涎丸, lu ci xian wan) ························ (273)
   Infantile Four Symptoms Pill(小儿四症丸, xiao er si zhen wan)············· (275)
   Lower-Warming and Upper-Clearing Decoction
     (温下清上汤, wen xia qing shang tang)······························· (278)
   Caloglossa Leprieurii Decoction(鹧鸪菜汤, zhe gu cai tang) ··············· (279)

Chapter Nine

Formulas for Orthopaedic and Surgical Diseases ······················· (281)
  1. Notopterygium Dampness-Expelling Decoction
    (羌活胜湿汤, jiang huo sheng shi tang) ······························ (281)
  2. Major Divaricate Saposhuikovia Decoction(大防风汤, dan fang feng tang) ··· (283)
  3. Coix Seed Decoction(薏苡仁汤, yi yi ren tang) ························ (286)
  4. Cassia Twig, White Peony and Common Anemarrhena Decoction
    (桂枝芍药知母汤, gui zhi shao yao zhi mu tang) ······················ (289)
  5. Doubleteeth Pubescent Angelica and Chinese Taxillus Twig Decoction
    (独活寄生汤, du huo ji sheng tang) ································· (292)
  6. Channels-Dredging and Blood-Activating Decoction
    (疏经活血汤, shu jing huo xue tang) ································ (295)
  7. Dreging and Dissipating Powder(通导散, tong dao san) ················· (298)
  8. Miraculous Collateral-Activating Pill(活络效灵丹, huo luo xiao ling dan) ······ (300)
  9. Anti-Bruise Powder(七厘散, qi li san) ································ (302)
  10. Blood-Activating and Hardness-Removing Decoction
     (活血化坚汤, huo xue hua jian tang) ······························ (304)
  11. Four Powerful Herbs Decoction(四妙勇安汤, si miao yong an tang) ······ (306)
  12. Snakegourd and Great Burdock Achene Decoction
     (瓜蒌牛蒡汤, gua lou niu bang tang) ······························· (308)
Additional Formula ·· (311)
   Formula for Craniocerebral Contusion Number Two
     (头伤Ⅱ号, tou shang er hao)·· (311)

Chapter Ten

Formulas for Dermatose ··· (313)
  1. Bupleurum Liver-Clearing Decoction(柴胡清肝饮, chai hu qing gan yin) ······ (313)
  2. Head-Clearing Divaricate Saposhnikovia Decoction
    (清上防风汤, qing shang fang feng tang) ····························· (315)
  3. Major Weeping Forsythia Capsule Decoction (大连翘汤, da lian qiao tang) ······ (317)

4. Cow Bezoar Toxin-Removing and Swelling-Reducing Pill
   (牛黄醒消丸, niu huang xin xiao wan) ·· (319)
5. Sevenlobed Yam Diuresis-Inducing Decoction
   (萆薢渗湿汤, bi xie shen shi tang) ·· (321)
6. Chinese Angelica Decoction(当归饮子, dang gui yin zi) ·················· (322)
7. Lung-Clearing Loquat Leaf Powder (清肺枇杷散, qing fei pi pa san) ······ (325)
8. Great Burdock Achene Muscles-Relieving Decoction
   (牛蒡解肌汤, niu bang jie ji tang) ·· (327)

Additional Formulas ··· (329)
  Ten Herbs Antiphlogistic Decoction(十味败毒汤, shi wei bai du tang) ··········· (329)
  Schizonepeta and Forsythia Decoction(荆芥连翘汤, jing jie lian qiao tang) ····· (331)
  Pueraria and Safflower Decoction(葛根红花汤, ge gen hong hua tang) ·········· (333)
  Prescription for Treating Head Boils(治头疮一方, zhi tou chuang yi fang) ······ (334)
  Five Herbs Detoxicating Powder(五物解毒散, wu wu jie du san) ················· (336)
  Prescription for Treating Alopecia Areata(治斑秃方, zhi ban tu fang) ············ (337)
  Verruca-Removing Decoction(除疣汤, chu you tang) ································ (340)

Chapter Eleven

Formulas for Otorhinolaryngologic Diseases ··································· (343)
1. Miraculous Pill with Six Drugs(六神丸, liu shen wan) ······················ (343)
2. Hoarseness-Relieving and Aphonia-Treating Pills
   (响声破笛丸, xiang sheng po di wan) ·· (345)
3. Wind-Dispelling and Toxin-Removing Decoction
   (驱风解毒汤, qu feng jie du tang) ··· (346)
4. Magnolia Lung-Clearing Decoction(辛夷清肺汤, xin yi qing fei tang) ······ (348)
5. Lung-Warming and Running-Stopping Decocting
   (温肺止流汤, wen fei zhi liu tang) ·· (349)

Additional Formulas ··· (352)
  Minor Bupleurum Decoction Plus Balloonflower and Gypsum
    (小柴胡桔梗石膏汤, xiao chai hu jie gen shi gao tang) ··························· (352)
  Szechwan Lovage And Magnolia plus Pueraria Decoction
    (葛根汤加川芎辛夷汤, ge gen tang jia chuan xiong xin yi tang) ················ (353)
  Hoarseness-Relieving and Aphonia-Healing Tablet(清音片, qing yin pian) ······ (355)

Chapter Twelve

Formulas for Ophthalmopathy ··· (357)
1. Four Herbs and Five Kernals Pill(四物五子丸, si wu wu zi wan) ············ (357)
2. Dendrobium Eyesight-Improving Pill(石斛夜光丸, shi hu yie guang wan) ··· (360)

3. Yingzhong Powder(应钟散, ying zhong san) ···················· (364)
  4. Vision Acuity-Improving Pill(驻景丸, zhu jing wan) ············· (366)
  5. Qi-Replenishing, Hearing-improving and Eyesight-Acuminating Decoction
     (益气聪明汤, yi qi cong ming tang) ······················· (367)
Additional Formula ·· (370)
  Liver-Clearing and Kidney-Nourishing Decoction
     (清肝养肾汤, qing gan yang shen tang) ····················· (370)

Chapter Thirteen

Formulas for Cancer and AIDS ·· (374)
  1. Asiatic Rhinoceros Bezoar Pill(犀黄丸, xi huang wan) ············ (374)
  2. Minor Panacea Pellet(小金丹, xiao jin dan) ····················· (376)
  3. Liver-Clearing and Stagnation-Removing Decocting
     (清肝解郁汤, qing gan jie yu tang) ························ (378)
Additional Formulas ··· (381)
  Lung-Strengthening and Cancer-Resisting Decoction
     (固金抗癌汤, gu jin kang ai tang) ·························· (381)
  Jinyan Pill(金岩丸, jin yan wan) ··· (382)
  Dwarf Lilyturf, Cochinchinese Asparagus and Tonkin Sophora Decoction
     (双冬豆根汤, shuang dong dou gen tang) ····················· (384)
  Silkworm with Batrytis Larva and Wasps Nest Decoction
     (僵蚕蜂房汤, jiang can feng fang tang) ······················ (386)
  Dysphagia-Treating Powder(治膈散, zhi ge san) ···················· (388)
  Liver-Recuperating Prescription(肝复方, gan fu fang) ··············· (390)
  Modified Tuckahoe Powder With Five Herbs(加味五苓散, jia wei wu ling san) ····· (392)
  Pilose Asiabell, Membranous Milkvetch, Desertliving Cistanche and
     Shorthorned Epimedium Decoction(参芪蓉仙汤, shen qi rong xian tang) ····· (394)
  Modified Toxin-Removing Fairy Decoction
     (解毒玉女煎加减方, jie du yu nu jian jia jian fang) ············· (397)
  Pathogen-Clearing and Mass-Resolving Decoction(清消汤, qing xiao tang) ········ (399)
  Jackinthepulpit, Pinellia, Common Selfheal Fruit-Spike, Grassleaf Sweetflag
     and Two Pieces of Centipedes Decoction
     (星夏草菖双龙汤, xing xia cao chang shuang long tang) ········· (401)
  Bupleurum, Snakegourd Fruit and Appendiculate Cremastra Pseudobulb Decoction
     (柴胡蒌姑汤, chai hu lou gu tang) ·························· (403)
  Prescription for Ovarian Cancer(治卵巢癌方, zhi luan chao ai fang) ····· (405)
  Compound Jade Spring Pill(复方玉泉丸, fu fang yu quan wan) ········· (407)

Chapter Fourteen

Formulas for External Use and Others ·· (409)
  1. Golden Powder(金黄散, jin huang san)··· (409)
  2. Yang-Harmonizing and Stagnation-Removing Plaster
     (阳和解凝膏, yang he jie ning gao) ·· (410)
  3. Sores-Treating Medicated Thread(三品一条枪, san pin yi tiao qiang) ············ (412)
  4. Nine to One Powder(九一丹, jiu yi dan) ·· (413)
  5. Yuhong Ointment for Promoting Tissue Regeneration
     (生肌玉红膏, sheng ji yu hong gao) ·· (414)
  6. Itching-Alleviating Decoction(塌痒汤, ta yang tang) ····························· (415)
  7. Common Cnidium Powder(蛇床子散, she chuang zi san) ······················· (417)
  8. Borneol and Borax Powder(冰硼散, bing peng san) ···························· (418)
  9. Instant Effective Powder(立效散, li xiao san) ·································· (420)

Additional Formulas ·· (422)
  Zhonghuang Ointment(中黄膏, zhong huang gao) ··································· (422)
  Sovereign Wart-Eliminating Liniment(疣灵搽剂, you ling cha ji) ····················· (423)
  Three Huang Lotion(三黄洗剂, san huang xi ji) ······································ (425)
  Pain-Alleviating and Swelling-Reducing Plaster
    (镇痛消肿膏, zhen tong xiao zhong gao) ··· (426)
  Centipede Powder(蜈蚣粉, wu gong fen) ·· (428)

Chapter One
Formulas for Diseases of the Respiratory System

Chinese drugs and prescriptions have good effects on diseases of the respiratory system by anti-infection, anti-inflammation, expelling the phlegm, relieving cough and asthma. Though respiratory diseases are closely related to the spleen and kidney, most of them result from the problem of the lung. They are mainly caused by pathogenic wind-cold or wind-heat according to differentiation. The pathogenesis is usually abnormal rising of lung-qi and accumulation of phlegm-dampness in the lung. The prescriptions for the respiratory tract infection, pneumonia, acute trachitis, chronic trachitis, bronchial asthma and pneumonectasis are widely used in clinic.

1. Cough-Stopping Powder (止嗽散, zhi suo san)

Source: *Comprehension of Medicine* 《医学心悟》
Composition: Tatarian Arster Root (紫菀, Ziyuan)6g
Willowleaf Swallowwort Rhizome (白前, Baiqian)6g
Sessile Stemona Root (百部, Baibu)6g
Balloonflower Root (桔梗, Jiegeng)6g
Tangerine Peel (橘皮, Jupi)6g
Fineleaf Schizonepeta Herb (荆芥, Jingjie)6g
Licorice Root (甘草, Gancao)6g
Actions: Stopping cough and resolving phlegm, relieving the exterior syndrome and dispersing the lung.
Applied Syndrome: Cough due to exterior wind attacking the lung manifested as cough, itching in the throat, difficult expectoration, or accompanied with low fever and slight aversion to cold, thin and white tongue coating with floating pulse.
Points in Constitution: It is said in *Comprehension of Medicine* 《医学心悟》 that "The property of this formula is warm, moist and medium. It can promote the dispersing function of the lung to expel pathogens without side effects. The function of the lung-qi will return to normal as soon as the pathogen is eliminated." This formula is characterized by warming, moistening and moderation. It is most suitable for unceasing cough due to dysfunction of lung-qi with incomplete elimination of external pathogen. In clinic, it can be modified to treat various cough due to the different syndromes such as exterior syndrome, interior syndrome, heat syndrome, cold syndrome, deficient syndrome and excessive syndrome.
Indications:
1. Acute bronchitis

Cough-Stopping Powder
(Lung-Dispersing and Cough-Stopping Method)

Ingredients	Effects	Combined Effects	Syndrome	Chief Symptoms
Tatarian Aster Root (紫菀, Ziyuan)6g Willowleaf Swallowwort Rhizome (白前, Baiqian)6g Sessile Stemona Root (百部, Baibu)6g Balloonflower Root (桔梗, Jiegeng)6g	Stopping cough and resolving phlegm	Stopping cough and resolving phlegm, relieving the exterior syndrome and dispersing the lung	Cough due to exterior evil (failure of lung qi in dispersion and descent as the result of wind attacking the lung)	Cough, difficult expectoration, low fever and slight aversion to cold, thin and white tongue coating with floating pulse
Tangerine Peel (橘皮, Jupi)6g	Dispersing the lung and regulating qi, stopping cough and resolving phlegm			
Fineleaf Schizonepeta Herb (荆芥, Jingjie)6g	Expelling wind and relieving the exterior syndrome			
Licorice Root (甘草, Gancao)6g	Coordinating the actions of the above herbs			

2. Upper respiratory tract infection
3. Whooping cough

Precaution: This formula emphasizies the cough-stopping and phlegm-resolving actions, so it has not obvious wind-dispelling and exterior-relieving actions. For the patient with definite exterior syndrome, appropriate amount of exterior-relieving drugs should be added.

Associated Formulas:

1. Cough-Relieving and Phlegm-Resolving Decoction (宁嗽化痰汤, ning sou hua tan tang) *Standard for Diagnosis and Treatment* 《证治准绳》

This is comprised of Balloonflower Root (桔梗, Jiegeng), Bitter Orange (枳壳, Zhiqiao), Pinellia Rhizome (半夏, Banxia), Tangerine Peel (橘皮, Jupi), Whiteflower Hogfennel Root (前胡, Qianhu), Lobed Kudzuvine Root (葛根, Gegen), Tuckahoe (茯苓, Fuling), White Mulberry Root-Bark (桑白皮, Sangbaipi), Fried Apricot Seed (炒杏仁, Chao Xingren), Ephedra (麻黄, Mahuang)(take large dose in winter and small dose in summer), Perilla Leaf (紫苏, Zisu), Licorice Root (甘草, Gancao) and Fresh Ginger (生姜, Shengjiang). Its actions are promoting the dispersing function of the lung and relieving the exterior syndrome, relieving cough and removing phlegm. It is indicated for cold with cough and stuffiness of the nose due to wind-cold.

2. Cough-Relieving Decoction (宁嗽汤, ning sou tang) *Source and Cause of Miscellaneous Diseases* 《杂病源流犀烛》

This is comprised of Balloonflower Root (桔梗, Jiegeng), Bitter Orange (枳壳, Zhiqiao), Pinellia Rhizome (半夏, Banxia), Tangerine Peel (橘皮, Jupi), Whiteflower Hogfennel Root (前胡, Qianhu), Lobed Kudzuvine Root (葛根, Gegen), Tuckahoe (茯苓, Fuling), White Mulberry Root-Bark (桑白皮, Sangbaipi), Perilla Leaf (紫苏, Zisu), Apricot Seed (杏仁, Xingren), Licorice root (甘草, Gancao) and Fresh Ginger (生姜, Shengjiang). Its actions are promoting the dispersing function of the lung, relieving cough and removing phlegm. It is indicated for cough due to exterior evils.

3. Modified Decoction of Three Miraculous Drugs(加减三奇汤, jia jian san qi tang) *Invention of Medicine* 《医学发明》

This is comprised of Balloonflower Root (桔梗, Jiegeng), Pinellia Rhizome (半夏, Banxia), Tangerine Peel (橘皮, Jupi), Green Tangerine Peel (青皮, Qingpi), Ginseng (人参, Renshen), White Mulberry Root-Bark (桑白皮, Sangbaipi), Apricot Seed (杏仁, Xingren), Perilla Leaf (紫苏, Zisu) and Chinese Magnoliavine Fruit (五味子, Wuweizi). Its actions are regulating qi, relieving cough and removing phlegm. It is indicated for cough caused by adverse rising of lung qi, asthma with profuse expectoration and chest disorder.

4. Decoction with Ginseng for Lung Disorders and Puerperal Blood Stasis(加参安肺生化汤, jia shen an fei sheng hua tang) *Fu Qingzhu's Obstetrics and Gynecology* 《傅青主女科》

This is comprised of Szechwan Lovage Rhizome (川芎, Chuanxiong), Balloonflower Root (桔梗, Jiegeng), Pinellia Rhizome (半夏, Banxia), Tangerine Peel (橘红, Juhong), Ginseng (人参, Renshen), Common Anemarrhena Rhizome (知母, Zhimu), White Mulberry Root-Bark (桑白皮, Sangbaipi), Apricot Seed (杏仁, Xingren), Chinese Angelica Root (当归, Danggui) and Licorice Root (甘草, Gancao). Its actions are replenishing qi, relieving cough and removing phlegm. It is indicated for puerperal cough, profuse expectoration, fever, excessive sweat due to weakness and exterior wind attack.

5. Pill for Clearing Away Heat at Qifen and Resolving Phlegm (清气化痰丸, qing qi hua tan wan) *Verification on Medical Prescriptions* 《医方考》

This is comprised of Snakegourd Seed (瓜蒌仁, Gualouren), Prepared Pinellia Rhizome (制半夏, Zhi Banxia), Tangerine Peel (橘皮, Jupi), Baikal Skullcap Root (黄芩, Huangqin), Apricot Seed (杏仁, Xingren), Immature Bitter Orange (枳实, Zhishi), Tuckahoe (茯苓, Fuling), Arisaema with Bile (胆南星, Dannanxing) and Fresh Ginger Juice (生姜汁, Shengjiangzhi). Its actions are clearing away heat and removing phlegm, regulating qi and relieving cough. It is indicated for cough and asthma due to heat-phlegm.

6. Mulbery and Chrysanthemum Decoction (桑菊饮, sang ju yin) *Detailed Analysis of Epidemic Febrile Diseases* 《温病条辨》

This is comprised of Mulberry Leaf (桑叶, Sangye), Chrysanthemum Flower (菊花, Juhua), Reed Rhizome (芦根, Lugen), Balloonflower Root (桔梗, Jiegeng), Apricot Seed (杏仁, Xingren), Bitter Orange (枳壳, Zhiqiao), Licorice Root (甘草, Gancao) and Wild Mint Herb (薄

荷，Bohe). Its actions are expelling wind and clearing away heat, promoting the dispersing function of the lung and relieving cough. It is indicated for cough due to attack of exogenous wind-heat.

7. General Recipe for Treating Cough（咳嗽统治方，kou sou tong zhi fang） *Author's Experienced Prescription*（笔者经验方）

This is composed of Arctium Fruit（牛蒡子，Niubangzi）, Common Yam（山药，Shanyao）, Whiteflower Hogfennel root（前胡，Qianhu）, Stemona（百部，Baibu）, Ballonflower root（桔梗，Jiegeng）, Immature Bitter Orange（枳壳，Zhiqiao) and Licorice Root（甘草，Gancao）. Its actions are stopping cough and removing phlegm. It is indicated for lingering cough due to exopathy and internal injury without other symptoms.

2. Mystery Decoction（神秘汤，shen mi tang）

Source: *The Medical Secrets of An Official*《外台秘要》
Composition: Ephedra（麻黄，Mahuang）6g
Perilla Leaf（紫苏叶，Zisuye）6g
Tangerine Peel（橘皮，Jupi）6g
Chinese Thorowax Root（柴胡，Chaihu）6g
Apricot Seed（杏仁，Xingren）9g
Officinal Magnolia Bark（厚朴，Houpo）6g
Licorice Root（甘草，Gancao）6g

Actions: Dispersing the lung and arresting asthmMedicala, relieving the exterior syndrome and regulating flow of qi.

Applied Syndrome: Attack on the exterior of the body by the wind-cold and failure of lung-qi in dispersion, manifested as feeling of fullness and stuffiness in the chest and hypochondria, asthma and cough, inability to lie flat, profuse and white expectoration, occasional chills and fever, thin, white and greasy tongue coating, floating and wiry pulse.

Points in Constitution: In this formula, the three ingredients [Ephedra（麻黄，Mahuang）], Apricot Seed（杏仁，Xingren）and Licorice Root（甘草，Gancao）of the Three Drugs Decoction（三拗汤，san ao tang）are used to disperse the function of the lung to alleviate asthma. The use of Officinal Magnolia Bark（厚朴，Houpo）and Tangerine Peel（橘皮，Jupi）is to regulate the flow of qi to relieve the depressed liver-qi. The application of Chinese Thorowax Root（柴胡，Chaihu）and Perilla Leaf（紫苏，Zisu）is to relieve the exterior syndrome and also to sooth the liver and regulate the flow of qi. The composition of this formula shows that qi must be regulated in order to relieve asthma and expel phlegm.

Indications:
1. Bronchitis asthma
2. Cold due to wind cold with a severe feeling of chest oppression

Precaution: It is not suitable for cough and asthma due to yin and qi deficiency.

Mystery Decoction
(Lung-Dispersing and Asthma-Arresting Method)

Ingredients	Effects	Combined Effects	Syndrome	Chief Symptoms
Ephedra (麻黄, Mahuang)6g Apricot Seed (杏仁, Xingren)9g Licorice Root (甘草, Gancao)6g	Dispersing the lung and relieving asthma	Dispersing the lung and relieving the exterior syndrome, regulating flow of qi and arresting asthma	Asthma and cough due to wind-cold attacking the lung	Cough and asthma, inability to lie flat, white and profuse expectoration, feeling of fullness and stuffiness over the chest and hypochondria, occasional chills and fever, thin and white greasy coating, floating. and wiry pulse
Officinal Magnolia Bark (厚朴, Houpo)6g Tangerine Peel (橘皮, Jupi)6g	Activating flow of qi and resolving phlegm			
Perilla Leaf (紫苏叶, Zisuye)6g	Relieving the exterior syndrome and regulating flow of qi			
Chinese Thorowax Root (柴胡, Chaihu)6g	Harmonizing functions of the Shaoyang system and reducing fever			

Associated Formulas:

1. Perilla Decoction for Keeping Qi Downward (苏子降气汤, su zi jiang qi tang) *Prescriptions of Taiping Benevolent Despensary*《和剂局方》

This is composed of Perilla Seed (苏子, Suzi), Pinellia Rhizome (半夏, Banxia), Whiteflower Hogfennel Root (前胡, Qianhu), Officinal Magnolia Bark (厚朴, Houpo), Cassia Bark (肉桂, Rougui), Chinese Angelica Root (当归, Danggui) and Prepared Licorice Root (炙甘草, Zhi Gancao). Its actions are warming and removing cold phlegm, descending qi and relieving asthma. It is indicated for cough and asthma due to insufficiency of kidney-yang and accumulation of phlegm in the lung characterized by deficiency in the lower jiao and excess in the upper jiao.

2. General Recipe for Treating Asthma(哮喘统治方, xiao chuan tong zhi fang) *Author's Experienced Prescription*(笔者经验方)

This consists of Ephedra(麻黄,Mahuang), Earthworm(地龙,Dilong), Batryticated Silkworm (白僵蚕,Baijiangcan), Belamcanda Rhizome(射干,Shegan), Asarum Herb(细辛, Xixin), Dried Ginger(干姜, Ganjiang), Schisandra Fruit(五味子,Wuweizi) and Prepared Licorice Root(炙甘草,Zhigancao). Its actions are relieving asthma and arresting cough. It is indicated for asthma and asthmatic bronchitis. If the case is accompanied with excessive heat, Gypsum(石膏,Shigao) and Houttuynia(鱼腥草,Yuxingcao) are added.

3. Tendrilleaf Fritillary Bulb and Snakegourd Fruit Powder （贝母瓜蒌散, bei mu gua lou san）

Source: *Comprehension of Medicine*《医学心悟》
Composition: Snakegourd Fruit（瓜蒌, Gualou）9g
Tendrilleaf Fritillary Bulb（贝母, Beimu）9g
Snakegourd Root（天花粉, Tianhuafen）6g
Tuckahoe（茯苓, Fuling）6g
Tangerine Peel（橘皮, Jupi）6g
Balloonflower Root（桔梗, Jiegeng）6g
Actions: Moistening the lung and clearing away heat, resolving phlegm and regulating flow of qi.
Applied Syndrome: Cough with sticky sputum due to dryness and yin deficiency of the lung or abnormal accumulation and consumption of body fluid by deficient fire. This is manifested as dry cough or cough with sticky sputum, dry throat and mouth, white and dry or yellow tongue coating, thin and slippery pulse.

Tendrilleaf Fritillary Bulb and Snakegourd Fruit Powder
（Dryness-Removing and Phlegm-Resolving Method）

Ingredients	Effects	Combined Effects	Syndrome	Chief Symptoms
Snakegourd Fruit（瓜蒌, Gualou）9g Tendrilleaf Fritillary Bulb（贝母, Beimu）9g	Resolving dry phlegm, moistening the lung and stopping cough	Clearing away heat and moistening the lung, regulating flow of qi and removing phlegm	Cough with sticky sputum	Dry cough, difficult expectoration, dry throat and mouth, white and dry or yellow tongue coating, thin and smooth pulse
Snakegourd Root（天花粉, Tianhuafen）6g	Clearing away heat and dryness, promoting the production of body fluid			
Tuckahoe（茯苓, Fuling）6g Tangerine Peel（橘皮, Jupi）6g	Invigorating the spleen and inducing diuresis, regulating flow of qi and removing phlegm			
Balloonflower Root（桔梗, Jiegeng）6g	Dispersing the lung and relieving cough			

Points in Constitution: The combination of Snakegourd Fruit（瓜蒌, Gualou）, Tendrilleaf Fritillary Bulb（贝母, Beimu）and Snakegourd Root（天花粉, Tianhuafen）can not only clear away heat, promote the production of body fluid, but also moisten the lung and eliminate phlegm. They are the key drugs for cough with heat-phlegm or sticky sputum due to dryness of the lung and deficiency of yin.

Indications:

1. Acute and chronic bronchitis
2. Pleurisy
3. Pneumonia
4. Aspiration pulmonary abscess

Precautions:

1. It is not suitable for dry cough, hemoptysis, hectic fever, night sweating, red tongue with less coating, thin and rapid pulse simply due to yin deficiency of the lung and kidney.
2. It should be used cautiously for cough due to damp-phlegm.

Associated Formulas:

1. Perilla Seed and Apricot Seed Decoction（苏子杏汤, su zi xing tang）*Syndrome-Cause-Pulse-Treatment*《症因脉治》

This consists of Perilla Seed（苏子, Suzi）, Apricot Seed（杏仁, Xingren）, Balloonflower Root（桔梗, Jiegeng）, Bitter Orange（枳壳, Zhiqiao）, Divaricate Saposhnikovia Root（防风, Fangfeng）, Pinellia Rhizome（半夏, Banxia）and Snakegourd Fruit（瓜蒌, Gualou）. Its actions are regulating qi, resolving phlegm and relieving cough. It is mainly indicated for constant cough with difficult expectoration..

2. Tendrilleaf Fritillary Bulb Powder（贝母散, bei mu san）*Standard for Diagnosis and Treatment*《证治准绳》

This is comprised of Tendrilleaf Fritillary Bulb（贝母, Beimu）, Apricot Seed（杏仁, Xingren）, White Mulberry Root-Bark（桑白皮, Sangbaipi）, Chinese Magnoliavine Fruit（五味子, Wuweizi）, Common Anemarrhena Rhizome（知母, Zhimu）, Licorice Root（甘草, Gancao）, Common Coltsfoot Flower（款冬花, Kuandonghua）and Fresh Ginger（生姜, Shengjiang）. Its actions are astringing the lung, relieving cough and removing phlegm. It is mainly indicated for acute cough which can not be cured over a long time.

3. Infantile Cough-Relieving Pallet（小儿止咳金丹, xiao er zhi ke jin dan）*Collection of Prescriptions of National Chinese Patent Medicine*《全国中成药处方集》(Tianjin Volume 天津方)

This is comprised of Tendrilleaf Fritillary Bulb（川贝母, Chuan Beimu）, Figwort Root（玄参, Xuanshen）, Dwarf Lilyturf Root（麦门冬, Maimendong）, Apricot Seed（杏仁, Xingren）, Arisaema with Bile（胆南星, Dannanxing）, Charred Areca Seed（焦槟榔, Jiao Binlang）, White Mulberry Root-Bark（桑白皮, Sangbaipi）, Balloonflower Root（桔梗, Jiegeng）, Bamboo Shavings（竹茹, Zhuru）, Snakegourd Root（天花粉, Tianhuafen）, Snakegourd Seed（瓜蒌仁, Gualouren）, Licorice Root（甘草, Gancao）, Perilla Seed（苏子, Suzi）, Common Anemarrhena Rhizome（知母, Zhimu）and Perilla Leaf（紫苏, Zisu）. Its actions are clearing away heat and moistening the lung, removing phlegm and relieving cough. It is indicated chiefly for cough due to wind attack, fever, yellowish aputum, dry mouth and tongue, abdominal fullness and constipation.

4. Cochinchinese Asparagus Decoction (门冬饮子, men dong yin zi) *Syndrome-Cause-Pulse-Treatment* 《症因脉治》

This is comprised of Cochinchinese Asparagus Root (天门冬, Tianmendong), Dwarf Lilyturf Root (麦门冬, Maimendong), White Mulberry Root-Bark (桑白皮, Sangbaipi), Bitter Orange (枳壳, Zhiqiao), Balloonflower Root (桔梗, Jiegeng), Fineleaf Schizonepeta Herb (荆芥, Jingjie) and Licorice Root (甘草, Gancao). Its actions are clearing away lung heat, moistening dryness, regulating qi and resolving phlegm. It is indicated for cough, thirst, dysphoria and a smothery sensation with desire to drink and difficult expectoration due to impairment of the lung by dryness.

5. Snake Gallbladder and Tendrilleaf Fritillary Bulb Powder (蛇胆川贝散, she dan chuan bei san) *Chinese Pharmacopoeia* 《中国药典》

This is comprised of Snake Gallbladder Juice (蛇胆汁, Shedanzhi) and Tendrilleaf Fritillary Bulb (川贝母, Chuan Beimu). Its actions are clearing away heat and moistening the lung, removing phlegm and relieving cough. It is indicated for cough with yellow and profuse sputum, bitter taste in the mouth and stuffiness in the chest due to phlegm-heat.

4. Lung-Clearing Decoction (清肺汤, qing fei tang)

Source: *Curative Measures for Diseases* 《万病回春》
Composition: Baikal Skullcap Root (黄芩, Huangqin) 6g
Balloonflower Root (桔梗, Jiegeng) 6g
Tangerine Peel (橘皮, Jupi) 6g
Tuckahoe (茯苓, Fuling) 6g
Apricot Seed (杏仁, Xingren) 6g
Chinese Angelica Root (当归, Danggui) 6g
Licorice Root (甘草, Gancao) 3g
Tendrilleaf Fritillary Bulb (贝母, Beimu) 3g
White Mulberry Root-bark (桑白皮, Sangbaipi) 6g
Cochinchinese Asparagus Root (天门冬, Tianmendong) 9g
Cape Jasmine Fruit (山栀子, Shanzhizi) 3g
Dwarf Lilyturf Root (麦门冬, Maimendong) 9g
Chinese Magnoliavine Fruit (五味子, Wuweizi) 6g
Fresh Ginger (生姜, Shengjiang) 3g
Chinese Date (大枣, Dazao) 3g

Actions: Nourishing yin and clearing away lung-heat, regulating flow of qi and resolving phlegm.

Applied Syndrome: Cough due to lung heat manifested as cough with profuse and sticky sputum, dryness of mouth and throat, hoarse sound and sore throat, or bloody sputum, night sweating, feverish sensation in the five centers, red tongue with little coating, thin and rapid pulse.

Lung-Clearing Decoction
(Lung-Clearing and Phlegm-Resolving Method)

Ingredients	Effects	Combined Effects	Syndrome	Chief Symptoms
White Mulberry Root-Bark (桑白皮, Sangbaipi)6g Cape Jasmine Fruit (山栀子, Shanzhizi)3g Baikal Skullcap Root (黄芩, Huangqin)6g	Clearing away lung heat and resolving phlegm	Clearing away lung heat and resolving phlegm, nourishing yin and removing dryness	Dry cough due to lung heat	Cough with profuse and sticky sputum, or bloody sputum, dry mouth and throat, sore throat, feverish sensation in the five centers, red tongue with little coating, thin and rapid pulse
Balloonflower Root (桔梗, Jiegeng)6g Tangerine Peel (橘皮, Jupi)6g Tuckahoe (茯苓, Fuling)6g Apricot Seed (杏仁, Xingren)6g Tendrilleaf Fritillary Bulb (贝母, Beimu)3g	Relieving cough and eliminating phlegm			
Dwarf Lilyturf Root (麦门冬, Maimendong)9g Cochinchinese Asparagus Root (天门冬, Tianmendong)9g Chinese Magnoliavine Fruit (五味子, Wuweizi)6g	Nourishing lung-yin			
Chinese Angelica Root (当归, Danggui)6g	Warming and activating blood flow to prevent blood stasis			
Licorice Root (甘草, Gancao)3g Fresh Ginger (生姜, Shengjiang)3g Chinese Date (大枣, Dazao)3g	Regulating *yingfen* and *weifen*			

Points in Constitution: This formula has united with all the functions of clearing away heat, eliminating phlegm, regulating the flow of qi to relieve cough and nourishing yin to moisten the lung and it is applied for irritating dry cough due to yin deficiency and the lung-heat. Its composition is moderate and can conveniently be modified in accordance with different symptoms.

Indications:
1. Acute bronchitis
2. Chronic bronchitis

Precaution: This formula also has the functions of clearing away heat, removing phlegm and regulating qi, but its heat-clearing action is comparatively weak. For those with excessive fire, it is better to use Qi-Clearing and Phlegm-Resolving Pill(清气化痰丸, qing qi hua tan wan).

Associated Formulas:

1. Qi-Clearing and Phlegm-Resolving Pill(清气化痰丸, qing qi hua tan wan) *Verification on Medical Prescriptions*《医方考》

This is comprised of Snakegourd Seed(瓜蒌仁, Gualouren), Prepared Pinellia Rhizome(制半夏, Zhi Banxia), Tangerine Peel(橘皮, Jupi), Baikal Skullcap Root(黄芩, Huangqin), Apricot Seed(杏仁, Xingren), Immature Bitter Orange(枳实, Zhishi), Tuckahoe(茯苓, Fuling), Arisaema with Bile(胆南星, Dannanxing) and Fresh Ginger Juice(生姜汁, Shengjiangzhi). Its actions are clearing away heat and eliminating fire, removing phlegm and regulating qi. It is indicated for cough and expectoration of phlegm due to accumulation of phlegm and fire in the interior.

2. Lung-Clearing and Phlegm-Resolving Decoction(清金化痰汤, qing jin hua tan tang) *General Guiding Prescriptions*《统旨方》

This is comprised of Baikal Skullcap Root(黄芩, Huangqin), Cape Jasmine Fruit(山栀子, Shanzhizi), Common Anemarrhena Rhizome(知母, Zhimu), White Mulberry Root-Bark(桑白皮, Sangbaipi), Snakegourd Seed(瓜蒌仁, Gualouren), Tendrilleaf Fritillary Bulb(贝母, Beimu), Dwarf Lilyturf Root(麦门冬, Maimendong), Tuckahoe(茯苓, Fuling), Tangerine Peel(橘皮, Jupi), Balloonflower Root(桔梗, Jiegeng) and Licorice Root(甘草, Gancao). Its actions are moistening dryness and removing phlegm. It is indicated for cough due to accumulation of heat and phlegm in the lung.

5. Yin-Nourishing and Fire-Eliminating Decoction
(滋阴降火汤, zi yin jiang huo tang)

Source: *Curative Measures for Diseases*《万病回春》
Composition: Chinese Angelica Root(当归, Danggui)6g
White Peony Root(白芍药, Baishaoyao)9g
Dried Rehmannia Root(生地黄, Shengdihuang)6g
Prepared Rehmannia Root(熟地黄, Shudihuang)6g
Dwarf Lilyturf Root(麦门冬, Maimendong)9g
Cochinchinese Asparagus Root(天门冬, Tianmendong)9g
Common Anemarrhena Rhizome(知母, Zhimu)6g
Chinese Corktree Bark(黄柏, Huangbai)6g
Largehead Atractylodes Rhizome(白术, Baizhu)6g
Tangerine Peel(橘皮, Jupi)6g
Prepared Licorice Root(炙甘草, Zhi Gancao)6g
Fresh Ginger(生姜, Shengjiang)3g
Chinese Date(大枣, Dazao)6g
Actions: Nourishing yin and eliminating fire.
Applied Syndrome: Syndrome of yin deficiency with hyperactivity of fire due to yin deficiency

of both the lung and kidney. It is manifested as dry cough with scanty sputum, hectic fever and night sweating, dry mouth and irritability, dry skin, red tongue and less coating, thin and rapid pulse.

Yin-Nourishing and Fire-Eliminating Decoction
(Yin-Nourishing and Fire-Eliminating Method)

Ingredients	Effects	Combined Effects	Syndrome	Chief Symptoms
Chinese Angelica Root (当归, Danggui)6g White Peony Root (白芍药, Baishaoyao)9g Dried Rehmannia Root (生地黄, Shengdihuang)6g Prepared Rehmannia Root (熟地黄, Shudihuang)6g Dwarf Lilyturf Root (麦门冬, Maimendong)9g Cochinchinese Asparagus Root (天门冬, Tianmendong)9g	Nourishing yin and enriching blood	Nourishing yin and eliminating fire	Yin deficiency and hyperactivity of fire	Dry cough with scanty sputum, hectic fever and night sweating, dry mouth and irritability, dry skin, red tongue with littlle coating, thin and rapid pulse
Common Anemarrhena Rhizome (知母, Zhimu)6g Chinese Corktree Bark (黄柏, Huangbai)6g	Eliminating fire and reduce fever of deficient type			
Largehead Atractylodes Rhizome (白术, Baizhu)6g Tangerine Peel (橘皮, Jupi)6g	Invigorating the spleen and regulating flow of qi			
Prepared Licorice Root (炙甘草, Zhi Gancao)6g Fresh Ginger (生姜, Shengjiang)3g Chinese Date (大枣, Dazao)6g	Coordinating *yingfen* and *weifen*			

Points in Constitution: This formula, in fact, is the Four Herbs Decoction (四物汤, si wu tang) by removing Szechwan Lovage Rhizome (川芎, Chuanxiong) but adding Dwarf Lilyturf Root (麦冬, Maidong) and Cochinchinese Asparagus Root (天冬, Tiandong) to nourish yin and enrich blood, Common Anemarrhena Rhizome (知母, Zhimu) and Chinese Corktree Bark (黄柏, Huangbai) to clear away heat and to retain yin, and Tangerine Peel (陈皮, Chenpi) and Largehead Atractylodes Rhizome (白术, Baizhu) to invigorate the spleen, protect the stomach and to benefit the lung. The characteristic of this formula is nourishing yin to reduce pathogenic fire without harming the Middle-jiao. The effect of this formula is better than that of Major Yin-Nourishing Pill (大补阴丸, da bu yin wan), which is the origination of this formula.

Indications:
1. Vegetative nerve functional disturbance
2. Restoration stage of acute febrile disease
3. Auxiliary treatment of tuberculosis

Precaution: Though this formula has the heat-clearing and fire-reducing function, it emphasizes the nourishment of yin and does not have a strong heat-clearing action. So for those with excessive fire, this formula is not suitable.

Associated Formulas:

1. Major Yin-Replenishing Pill（大补阴丸, da bu yin wan）*Danxi's Experiential Therapy* 《丹溪心法》

This is comprised of Chinese Corktree Bark（黄柏, Huangbai）, Common Anemarrhena Rhizome（知母, Zhimu）, Prepared Rehmannia Root（熟地黄, Shudihuang）, Tortoise Shell and Plastron（龟版, Guiban）and Pig Spinal Cord（猪脊髓, Zhujisui）. Its actions are nourishing yin of both the liver and kidney to eliminate fire. It is indicated for the syndrome of yin deficiency and hyperactivity of fire due to stirring up of deficient fire resulting from yin deficiency of the kidney and liver.

2. Lung-Clearing Decoction（清肺汤, qing fei tang）*Curative Measures for Diseases* 《万病回春》

The composition of this formula is Baikal Skullcap Root（黄芩, Huangqin）, Balloonflower Root（桔梗, Jiegeng）, Tangerine Peel（橘皮, Jupi）, Tuckahoe（茯苓, Fuling）, Apricot Seed（杏仁, Xingren）, Chinese Angelica Root（当归, Danggui）, Licorice Root（甘草, Gancao）, Tendrilleaf Fritillary Bulb（贝母, Beimu）, White Mulberry Root-Bark（桑白皮, Sangbaipi）, Cochinchinese Asparagus Root（天门冬, Tianmendong）, Cape Jasmine Fruit（山栀子, Shanzhizi）, Dwarf Lilyturf Root（麦门冬, Maimendong）, Chinese Magnoliavine Fruit（五味子, Wuweizi）, Fresh Ginger（生姜, Shengjiang）and Chinese Date（大枣, Dazao）. Its actions are clearing away lung-heat, regulating flow of qi, removing phlegm and relieving cough. It is indicated for lung diseases. Comparatively, Yin-Nourishing and Fire-Eliminating Decoction（滋阴降火汤, zi yin jiang huo tang）stresses nourishing yin and reducing fire and is indicated for kidney diseases.

6. Yin-Nourishing Real Treasure Decoction
（滋阴至宝汤, zi yin zhi bao tang）

Source: *Curative Measures for Diseases* 《万病回春》
Composition: Chinese Angelica Root（当归, Danggui）6g
White Peony Root（白芍药, Baishaoyao）9g
Largehead Atractylodes Rhizome（白术, Baizhu）6g
Tuckahoe（茯苓, Fuling）6g
Tangerine Peel（橘皮, Jupi）6g
Common Aemarrhena Rhizome（知母, Zhimu）6g

Tendrilleaf Fritillary Bulb (贝母, Beimu)9g
Nutgrass Galingale Rhizome (香附, Xiangfu) 3g
Chinese Wolfberry Root-Bark (地骨皮, Digupi)9g
Dwarf Lilyturf Root (麦门冬, Maimendong)9g
Wild Mint Herb (薄荷, Bohe)3g
Licorice Root (甘草, Gancao)3g
Chinese Thorowax Root (柴胡, Chaihu)6g
Roasting Ginger (煨姜, Weijiang)3g

Actions: Nourishing yin and clearing away lung-heat, dispersing stagnated liver-qi and alleviating depression, invigorating the spleen and regulating yingfen.

Applied Syndrome: Consumptive diseases due to attack of the lung by liver fire resulting from stagnation of the liver qi and deficiency of the spleen. It is manifested as low fever for a long period, cough with sputum, asthma, hectic fever, listlessness, tiredness, spontaneous sweating and night sweating, feeling of fullness and stuffiness in the chest, poor appetite, thin, white and dry tongue coating, wiry, thin and rapid pulse.

Yin-Nourishing Real Treasure Decoction
(Liver-Soothing and Lung-Clearing Method)

Ingredients	Effects	Combined Effects	Syndrome	Chief Symptoms
Chinese Angelica Root (当归, Danggui)6g White Peony Root (白芍药, Baishaoyao)9g Largehead Atractylodes Rhizome (白术, Baizhu)6g Tuckahoe (茯苓, Fuling)6g Wild Mint Herb (薄荷, Bohe)3g Licorice Root (甘草, Gancao)3g Chinese Thorowax Root (柴胡, Chaihu)6g Roasting Ginger (煨姜, Weijiang)3g	Regulating the liver and spleen	Regulating the liver and spleen, nourishing yin and reducing fever	Comsuptive diseases (stagnation of the liver qi and deficiency of the spleen, liver fire attacking the lung)	Low fever for a long time, hectic fever, cough with sputum and asthma, listlessness, tiredness, spontaneous sweating and night sweating, feeling of fullness and stuffiness in the chest, poor appetite, thin, white and dry tongue coating, wiry, thin and rapid pulse
Common Anemarrhena Rhizome (知母, Zhimu)6g Tendrilleaf Fritillary Bulb (贝母, Beimu)9g	Clearing away heat and resolving phlegm			
Chinese Wolfberry Root-Bark (地骨皮, Digupi)9g Dwarf Lilyturf Root (麦门冬, Maimendong)9g	Nourishing yin and reduce fever			
Tangerine Peel (橘皮, Jupi)6g Nutgrass Galingale Rhizome (香附, Xiangfu) 3g	Dispersing the stagnated liver-qi			

Points in Constitution: This formula uses the ingredients of Merry Life Powder(逍遥散, xiao yao san) to coordinate the function of the liver and spleen. By adding Dwarf Lilyturf Root(麦门冬, Maimendong), Chinese Wolfberry Root-Bark(地骨皮, Digupi) and also Common Anemarrhena Rhizome(知母, Zhimu) to nourish yin and eliminate heat. The addition of Common Anemarrhena Rhizome(知母, Zhimu) and Tendrilleaf Fritillary Bulb(贝母, Beimu) is to clear away heat and ressolve phlegm. The use of Nutgrass Galingale Rhizome(香附, Xiangfu) and Tangerine Peel(橘皮, Jupi) is to reinforce the actions of liver qi. Although it is named Yin-Nourishing Real Treasure Decoction(滋阴至宝汤, zi yin zhi bao tang), it emphasizes dispersing stagnated liver qi, clearing away lung-heat and invigorating the spleen so that the liver can't reversedly restrict the lung and over restrict the spleen. Therefore, productive cough of consumptive diseases can be healed with this indirect treatment.

Indications:
1. Low fever for a long period
2. Chronic bronchitis

Precution: This formula is good at soothing the liver and regulating the circulation of qi. In addition, it has the actions of nousishing yin and removing heat. It is indicated for those with the syndrome of stagnation of the liver qi and deficiency of the spleen accompanied with little fire.

Associated Formula:

Modified Merry Life Powder(加味逍遥散, jia wei xiao yao san) *Abstracts of Chinese Internal Medicine*《内科摘要》

This is comprised of Chinese Thorowax Root(柴胡, Chaihu), Chinese Angelica Root(当归, Danggui), Largehead Atractylodes Rhizome(白术, Baizhu), White Peony Root(白芍药, Baishaoyao), Tuckahoe(茯苓, Fuling), Licorice Root(甘草, Gancao), Tree Peony Bark(牡丹皮, Mudanpi) and Cape Jasmine Fruit(山栀子, Shanzhizi). This formula is good at dispersing the stagnated liver-qi, clearing away heat, invigorating the spleen, regulating blood and menstruation. It is mainly indicated for heat syndrome due to incoordination between the liver and spleen, stagnation of liver-qi and blood deficiency.

7. Lily Bulb Decoction for Strengthening the Lung (百合固金汤, bai he gu jin tang)

Source: *Collection of Formulae with Notes*《医方集解》
Composition: Lily Bulb(百合, Baihe)12g
Dried Rehmannia Root(生地黄, Shengdihuang)6g
Prepared Rehmannia Root(熟地黄, Shudihuang)9g
Dwarf Lilyturf Root(麦门冬, Maimendong)6g
Figwort Root(玄参, Xuanshen)3g
Chinese Angelica Root(当归, Danggui)3g

White Peony Root (白芍药, Baishaoyao) 3g
Tendrilleaf Fritillary Bulb (贝母, Beimu) 3g
Balloonflower Root (桔梗, Jiegeng) 3g
Licorice Root (甘草, Gancao) 3g

Actions: Nourishing yin and eliminating fire, moistening the lung and resolving phlegm.

Applied Syndrome: Stirring up of deficient fire due to yin deficiency of both lung and kidney manifested by cough and hemoptysis, asthma and chest pain, dry and sore throat, hoarseness, feverish sensation in the five centers, red tongue with little coating, thin and rapid pulse.

Lily Bulb Decoction for Strengthening the Lung
(Yin-Nourishing and Dryness-Removing Method)

Ingredients	Effects	Combined Effects	Syndrome	Chief Symptoms
Lily Bulb (百合, Baihe) 12g Dried Rehmannia Root (生地黄, Shengdihuang) 6g Dwarf Lilyturf Root (麦门冬, Maimendong) 6g Figwort Root (玄参, Xuanshen) 3g	Nourishing yin and eliminating fire	Nourishing yin and eliminating fire, moistening the lung and resolving phlegm	Attacking of the lung by deficient fire resulting from deficient yin of both the lung and kidney	Cough with scanty sputum, hemoptysis, asthma and chest pain, dry and sore throat, hoarseness, feverish sensation in the five centers, red tongue with little coating, thin and rapid pulse
Prepared Rehmannia Root (熟地黄, Shudihuang) 9g Chinese Angelica Root (当归, Danggui) 3g White Peony Root (白芍药, Baishaoyao) 3g	Enriching blood and nourishing yin			
Tendrilleaf Fritillary Bulb (贝母, Beimu) 3g Balloonflower Root (桔梗, Jiegeng) 3g Licorice Root (甘草, Gancao) 3g	Resolving phlegm and stopping cough			

Points in Constitution: Lily Bulb (百合, Baihe), which has the actions of tonifying the kidney, moistening the lung and tranquilizing the mind, is the key drug of this formula. When it is combined with Prepared Rehmannia Root (熟地黄, Shudihuang) which greatly nourishes the kidney yin, it has the interpromoting function, i.e. generation between metal and water. When they are combined with Dwarf Lilyturf Root (麦门冬, Maimendong) and Figwort Root (玄参, Xuanshen), they can nourish yin to reduce pathogenic fire and moistening the lung to relieve cough. The use of ingredients of Four Herbs Decoction (四物汤, si wu tang) without Szechwan Lovage Rhizome (川芎, Chuanxiong) is to enrich blood and nourish yin. Tendrilleaf Fritillary

Bulb (贝母, Beimu), Balloonflower Root (桔梗, Jiegeng) and Licorice Root (甘草, Gancao) are used together to clear away lung heat, resolve phlegm and stop cough. In a word, this formula consists of yin-nourishing and blood-tonifying herbs with a view to nourishing yin, reducing fire, moistening the lung and stopping cough.

Indications:
1. Pulmonary tuberculosis
2. Chronic bronchitis
3. Hemoptysis due to bronchiectasis
4. Chronic laryngopharyngectomy

Precautions:

1. Most of the drugs in the formula are sweet, cold and sticky in nature. Thus, this formula should be used cautiously for those with diarrhea due to deficiency of the spleen.

2. It is contraindicated in cough with bloody expectoration due to attack of the lung by liver fire or excessive heat in the lung meridian.

Associated Formulas:

1. Lung-Nourishing Decoction (养金汤, yang jin tang) *Source and Cause of Miscellaneous Diseases* 《杂病源流犀烛》

This is comprised of Dried Rehmannia Root (生地黄, Shengdihuang), Ass-hide Glue (阿胶, Ejiao), Apricot Seed (杏仁, Xingren), Common Anemarrhena Rhizome (知母, Zhimu), Coastal Glehnia Root and Fourleaf Ladybell Root (沙参, Shashen), Dwarf Lilyturf Root (麦门冬, Maimendong), White Mulberry Root-Bark (桑白皮, Sangbaipi). Its actions are nourishing yin and moistening dryness. It is manily indicated for dryness and pain in the throat due to stirring up of deficient fire.

2. Hundred Flowers Pill (百花丸, bai hua wan) *Selected Prescriptions of Chinese Medicine of Beijin* 《北京市中药处方选集》

This is comprised of Common Coltsfoot Flower (款冬花, Kuandonghua), Chinese Magnoliavine Fruit (五味子, Wuweizi), Tatarian Aster Root (紫菀, Ziyuan), Snakegourd Root (天花粉, Tianhuafen), Tree Peony Bark (牡丹皮, Mudanpi), Balloonflower Root (桔梗, Jiegeng), Tangerine Peel (橘皮, Jupi), Dwarf Lilyturf Root (麦门冬, Maimendong), Whiteflower Hogfennel Root (前胡, Qianhu), Lily Bulb (百合, Baihe), Figwort Root (玄参, Xuanshen), Coastal Glehnia Root and Fourleaf Ladybell Root (沙参, Shashen), Wild Mint Herb (薄荷, Bohe), Carbonized Cattail Pollen (炒蒲黄, Chao Puhuang), Apricot Seed (杏仁, Xingren), Persimmon Frost (柿霜, Shishuang) and Tendrilleaf Fritillary Bulb (川贝母, Chuan Beimu). Its actions are clearing away heat, moistening the lung, relieving cough and stopping asthma. It is indicated for cough with expectoration and asthma, dry mouth, difficulty in sounding (or aphonia) and bloody expectoration due to attack of the lung by deficient fire.

3. Dwarf Lilyturf Decoction (麦门冬汤, mai men dong tang) *Synopsis of Golden Cabinet* 《金匮要略》

This is comprised of Dwarf Lilyturf Root (麦门冬, Maimendong), Pinellia Rhizome (半夏, Banxia), Licorice Root (甘草, Gancao), Ginseng (人参, Renshen), Rice (粳米, Jingmi) and

Chinese Date (大枣, Dazao). Its actions are benefiting the stomach, promoting the production of body fluid and keeping the adverse qi downward. It is indicated for consumptive lung disease due to deficiency of the stomach, insufficiency of body fluid and stirring up of deficient fire.

4. Decoction for Nourishing the Lung and Removing Heat (补肺清金饮, bu fei qing jin yin) *Ma Peizhi's Records on Surgery* 《马培之外科医案》

This is comprised of Common Yam Rhizome (山药, Shanyao), Coastal Glehnia Root and Fourleaf Ladybell Root (沙参, Shashen), Dendrobium Herb (石斛, Shihu), Snakegourd Peel (瓜蒌皮, Gualoupi), Dwarf Lilyturf Root (麦门冬, Maimendong), Apricot Seed (杏仁, Xingren), Tuckahoe (茯苓, Fuling), Thunberg Fritillary Bulb (浙贝母, Zhe Beimu), Tangerine Peel (橘红, Juhong) and Lotus Seed (莲子, Lianzi). Its actions are nourishing the lung and clearing away heat from the lung. It is indicated for pigeon breast and humpback with weak and rapid pulse due to yin deficiency and lung-heat.

5. Lung-Clearing Decoction (清肺汤, qing fei tang) *Source and Cause of Miscellaneous Diseases* 《杂病源流犀烛》

This is comprised of Indian Bread Pink Epidermis (赤茯苓, Chifuling), Tangerine Peel (橘皮, Jupi), Chinese Angelica Root (当归, Danggui), Dried Rehmannia Root (生地黄, Shengdihuang), Red Peony Root (赤芍, Chishao), Cochinchinese Asparagus Root (天门冬, Tianmendong), Dwarf Lilyturf Root (麦门冬, Maimendong), Cape Jasmine Fruit (山栀子, Shanzhizi), Baikal Skullcap Root (黄芩, Huangqin), Tatarian Aster Root (紫菀, Ziyuan), White Mulberry Root-Bark (桑白皮, Sangbaipi), Ass-hide Glue (阿胶, Ejiao), Licorice Root (甘草, Gancao) and Chinese Date (大枣, Dazao). Its actions are moistening the lung and nourishing yin, removing phlegm and arresting bleeding. It is indicated for cough with expectoration of phlegm and hemoptysis.

6. Ass-hide Glue plus Four Herbs Decoction (阿胶四物汤, e jiao si wu tang) *Source and Cause of Miscellaneous Diseases* 《杂病源流犀烛》

This is comprised of Chinese Angelica Root (当归, Danggui), Prepared Rehmannia Root (熟地黄, Shudihuang), White Peony Root (白芍药, Baishaoyao), Szechwan Lovage Rhizome (川芎, Chuanxiong) and Ass-hide Glue (阿胶, Ejiao). Its actions are enriching blood and relieving cough. It is indicated for chronic cough due to blood deficiency.

8. Harmony-Preserving Decoction
(保和汤, bao he tang)

Source: *Miraculous Book of Ten kinds of Dosage Form* 《十药神书》
Composition: Common Anemarrhena Rhizome (知母, Zhimu)9g
Tendrilleaf Fritillary Bulb (贝母, Beimu)9g
Cochinchinese Asparagus Root (天门冬, Tianmendong)9g
Common Coltsfoot Flower (款冬花, Kuandonghua)9g
Snakegourd Root (天花粉, Tianhuafen)6g

Coix Seed (薏苡仁, Yiyiren) 6g
Apricot Seed (杏仁, Xingren) 6g
Chinese Magnoliavine Fruit (五味子, Wuweizi) 6g
Licorice Root (甘草, Gancao) 3g
Dutchmanspipe Fruit (马兜铃, Madouling) 6g
Tatarian Aster Root (紫菀, Ziyuan) 6g
Lily Bulb (百合, Baihe) 9g
Balloonflower Root (桔梗, Jiegeng) 6g
Ass-hide Glue (阿胶, Ejiao) 9g
Chinese Angelica Root (当归, Danggui) 9g
Dried Rehmannia Root (生地黄, Shengdihuang) 9g
Perilla Leaf (紫苏, Zisu) 9g
Wild Mint Herb (薄荷, Bohe) 6g
Sessile Stemona Root (百部, Baibu) 9g

Actions: Nourishing yin and moistening the lung, stopping cough and resolving phlegm.

Applied Syndrome: Consumptive lung disease due to dryness of the lung, yin deficiency and accumulation of turbid phlegm in the interior manifested as cough, asthma, dry throat and hoarseness, expectoration, stuffiness sensation in the chest, red tongue, weak and rapid pulse.

Points in Constitution: The combination of Common Anemarrhena Rhizome (知母, Zhimu) and Tendrilleaf Fritillary Bulb (贝母, Beimu), which is called Ermu Power (二母散, er mu san), is mainly used for tuberculosis with pathogenic heat, for which the warm and tonifying drugs should be forbidden. Tendrilleaf Fritillary Bulb (贝母, Beimu) resolves phlegm and purges lung-fire while Common Anemarrhena Rhizome (知母, Zhimu) nourishes the kidney and clears the lung. The combination of the two, bitter in taste and cold in property, can clear away heat and eliminate dryness by moistening the lung. In this formula, a large dose of yin-nourishing drugs, together with cough-relieving and phlegm-resolving drugs, are used, which means that a large amount of drugs must be applied for severe cases. Since this kind of treatment may cause damage to the stomach, it should be used cautiously, especially for those with a weak body. Furthermore, there are various pathogenesis for consumptive lung diseases, this formula may be used for the later stage of consumptive lung diseases with scorched lung lobes due to remained lung-heat and impairment of lung-yin. It is not suitable for those with powerful lung-heat or deficiency of both qi and yin.

Indications:
1. Pulmonary fibrosis
2. Pulmonary atelectasis
3. Pulmonary cirrhosis, pulmonary emphysema
4. Chronic bronchitis

Precaution: Most drugs in this formula are sweet, cold and sticky in nature. Thus, it should be used cautiously for those with diarrhea and poor appetite due to deficiency of the spleen.

Harmony-Preserving Decoction
(Yin-Nourishing and Lung-Clearing Method)

Ingredients	Effects	Combined Effects	Syndrome	Chief Symptoms
Common Anemarrhena Rhizome (知母, Zhimu)9g Tendrilleaf Fritillary Bulb (贝母, Beimu)9g	Clearing away heat and moistening dryness, stopping cough and resolving phlegm	Nourishing yin and moistening the lung, stopping cough and resolving phlegm	Consumptive lung disease (dryness of the lung and yin deficiency, accumulation of turbid phlegm in the interior)	Cough, asthma, dry throat and hoarseness, expectoration, stuffiness sensation in the chest, red tongue, weak and rapid pulse
Apricot Seed (杏仁, Xingren)6g Coix Seed (薏苡仁, Yiyiren)6g Dutchmanspipe Fruit (马兜铃, Madouling)6g Tatarian Aster Root (紫菀, Ziyuan)6g Balloonflower Root (桔梗, Jiegeng)6g Sessile Stemona Root (百部, Baibu)9g Common Coltsfoot Flower (款冬花, Kuandonghua)9g Chinese Magnoliavine Fruit (五味子, Wuweizi)6g	Stopping cough and resolvinging phlegm			
Ass-hide Glue (阿胶, Ejiao)9g Chinese Angelica Root (当归, Danggui)9g Dried Rehmannia Root (生地黄, Shengdihuang)9g Cochinchinese Asparagus Root (天门冬, Tianmendong)9g Snakegourd Root (天花粉, Tianhuafen)6g Lily Bulb (百合, Baihe)9g	Nourishing yin and moistening dryness			
Perilla Leaf (紫苏, Zisu)9g Wild Mint Herb (薄荷, Bohe)6g	Slightly dispersing and regulating lung qi			
Licorice Root (甘草, Gancao)3g	Coordinating the actions of the above herbs			

Associated Formulas:

1. Prepared Licorice Decoction (炙甘草汤, zhi gan cao tang) *Treatise on Exogenous Febrile Diseases* 《伤寒论》

This is comprised of Prepared Licorice Root (炙甘草, Zhi Gancao), Dried Rehmannia Root (生地黄, Shengdihuang), Ass-hide Glue (阿胶, Ejiao), Ginseng (人参, Renshen), Dwarf Lilyturf Root (麦门冬, Maimendong), Fresh Ginger (生姜, Shengjiang), Chinese Date (大枣, Dazao), Cassia Twig (桂枝, Guizhi) and Hemp Seed (麻仁, Maren). This formula is good at replenishing qi, enriching blood, nourishing yin and moistening dryness. It is mainly indicated for consumptive lung disease manifested as protracted cough with profuse expectoration due to deficiency of both qi and yin which results in dryness of the lung.

2. Dwarf Lilyturf Decoction (麦门冬汤, mai men dong tang) *Synopsis of Golden Cabinet* 《金匮要略》

This is comprised of Dwarf Lilyturf Root (麦门冬, Maimendong), Pinellia Rhizome (半夏, Banxia), Licorice Root (甘草, Gancao), Ginseng (人参, Renshen), Rice (粳米, Jingmi) and Chinese Date (大枣, Dazao). Its actions are moistening the lung, benefiting the stomach and keeping the adverse qi downwards. It is chiefly indicated for consumptive lung disease due to impairment of body fluid and stirring up of deficient fire resulting from yin deficiency of both the lung and stomach.

3. Ginseng and Giant Gecko Powder (人参蛤蚧散, ren shen ge jie san) *The Precious Mirror of Hygiene* 《卫生宝鉴》

This is comprised of Giant Gecko (蛤蚧, Gejie), Ginseng (人参, Renshen), Common Anemarrhena Rhizome (知母, Zhimu), Tendrilleaf Fritillary Bulb (贝母, Beimu), White Mulberry Root-Bark (桑白皮, Sangbaipi), Apricot Seed (杏仁, Xingren), Tuckahoe (茯苓, Fuling) and Licorice Root (甘草, Gancao). This formula is good at benefiting the lung and kidney, moistening the lung, removing phlegm, relieving cough and stopping asthma. It is mainly indicated for consumptive lung disease due to deficiency of both the lung and kidney, insufficiency of qi and yin and accumulation of turbid phlegm in the interior.

4. Lung-Rising Decoction (举肺汤, ju fei tang) *Source and Cause of Miscellaneous Diseases* 《杂病源流犀烛》

This is comprised of Balloonflower Root (桔梗, Jiegeng), Licorice Root (甘草, Gancao), Cochinchinese Asparagus Root (天门冬, Tianmendong), Bamboo Shavings (竹茹, Zhuru), Ass-hide Glue (阿胶, Ejiao), Coastal Glehnia Root and Fourleaf Ladybell Root (沙参, Shashen), Tendrilleaf Fritillary Bulb (贝母, Beimu) and Lily Bulb (百合, Baihe). Its actions are nourishing yin and moistening the lung. It is indicated for consumptive lung disease due to deficiency of lung yin and interior heat resulting from deficiency of yin.

9. Lunar Corona Pill (月华丸, yue hua wan)

Source: *Comprehension of Medicine* 《医学心悟》
Composition: Cochinchinese Asparagus Root (天门冬, Tianmendong)6g

Dwarf Lilyturf Root (麦门冬, Maimendong) 6g
Dried Rehmannia Root (生地黄, Shengdihuang) 6g
Prepared Rehmannia Root (熟地黄, Shudihuang) 6g
Coastal Glehnia Root and Fourleaf Ladybell Root (沙参, Shashen) 6g
Common Yam Rhizome (山药, Shanyao) 6g
Tuckahoe (茯苓, Fuling) 6g
Mulberry Leaf (桑叶, Sangye) 3g
Chrysanthemum Flower (菊花, Juhua) 3g
Tendrilleaf Fritillary Bulb (川贝母, Chuan Beimu) 6g
Ass-hide Glue (阿胶, Ejiao) 6g (melting in decoction)
Sanchi Root (三七, Sanqi) 6g
Essile Stemona Root (百部, Baibu) 6g
Otter Liver (獭肝, Tagan) 15g, it can be replaced by Aweto (冬虫夏草, Dongchongxiacao) 6g

Actions: Nourishing yin and moistening the lung, relieving cough and arresting bleeding, poisoning parasites and treating consumptive diseases.

Applied Syndrome: Consumptive lung disease due to yin deficiency and interior heat manifested by hectic fever and night sweating, cough with bloody expectoration, irritability and dry mouth, thin, red tongue with less coating or thin and yellow coating, thin and rapid pulse.

Points in Constitution: The main function of this formula is nourishing yin, moistening the lung, arresting bleeding and relieving cough. In this formula, Otter Liver (獭肝, Tagan) is for nourishing yin and arresting bleeding, Sanchi Root (三七, Sanqi) for activating blood circulation and arresting bleeding, and Ass-hide Glue (阿胶, Ejiao) for nourishing blood and arresting bleeding. The combination of the three is indicated for hemoptysis by arresting bleeding. Aweto (冬虫夏草, Dongchongxiacao) may be used instead of Otter Liver (獭肝, Tagan), which is difficult to be obtained.

Indications:
1. Infiltrative pulmonary tuberculosis
2. Bronchiectasis

Associated Formulas:

1. Lily Bubus Decoction for Strengthening the Lung (百合固金汤, bai he gu jin tang) *Posthumous Writings in Cautious Room* 《慎斋遗书》

This is comprised of Lily Bulb (百合, Baihe), Prepared Rehmannia Root (熟地黄, Shudihuang), Dried Rehmannia Root (生地黄, Shengdihuang), Chinese Angelica Root (当归, Danggui), White Peony Root (白芍药, Baishaoyao), Licorice Root (甘草, Gancao), Balloonflower Root (桔梗, Jiegeng), Figwort Root (玄参, Xuanshen), Tendrilleaf Fritillary Bulb (贝母, Beimu) and Dwarf Lilyturf Root (麦门冬, Maimendong). Its actions are nourishing the lung and kidney, relieving cough and removing phlegm. It is indicated for consumptive lung diseases due to deficiency of lung-yin and stirring up of deficient fire.

2. Lung-Invigorating Ass-hide Glue Decoction (补肺阿胶汤, bu fei e jiao tang) *Key to Therapeutics of Children's Diseases* 《小儿药证直诀》

Lunar Corona Pills
(Yin-Nourishing and Lung-Moistening Method)

Ingredients	Effects	Combined Effects	Syndrome	Chief Symptoms
Cochinchinese Asparagus Root (天门冬, Tianmendong)6g Dwarf Lilyturf Root (麦门冬, Maimendong)6g Dried Rehmannia Root (生地黄, Shengdihuang)6g Prepared Rehmannia Root (熟地黄, Shudihuang)6g Coastal Glehnia Root and Fourleaf Ladybell Root (沙参, Shashen)6g	Nourishing yin and moistening the lung	Nourishing yin and moistening the lung, stopping cough and arresting bleeding, poisoning parasites and treating consumptive diseases	Consumptive lung disease (yin deficiency and interior heat)	Hectic fever and night sweating, cough with bloody expectoration, irritability and dry mouth, thin, red tongue and less coating or thin and yellow coating, thin and rapid pulse
Common Yam Rhizome (山药, Shanyao)6g Tuckahoe (茯苓, Fuling)6g	Invigorating the spleen and benefiting the lung			
Mulberry Leaf (桑叶, Sangye)3g Chrysanthemum Flower (菊花, Juhua)3g	Clearing away heat in the liver and lung			
Tendrilleaf Fritillary Bulb (川贝母, Chuan Beimu)6g	Moistening the lung and dissipating blockages, stopping cough and resolving phlegm			
Ass-hide Glue (阿胶, Ejiao)6g	Nourishing yin, arresting bleeding and moistening the lung			
Sanchi Root (三七, Sanqi)6g	Activating blood circulation and arresting bleeding			
Otter Liver (獭肝, Tagan)15g Sessile Stemona Root (百部, Baibu)6g	Special drugs for poisoning parasites and treating consumptive diseases			

This is comprised of Ass-hide Glue (阿胶, Ejiao), Great Burdock Achene (牛蒡子, Niubangzi), Licorice Root (甘草, Gancao), Dutchmanspipe Fruit (马兜铃, Madouling), Apricot Seed (杏仁, Xingren) and Sticky Rice (糯米, Nuomi). Its actions are nourishing yin and invigorating the lung, clearing away heat and arresting bleeding. It is indicated for cough and hemoptysis due to deficient heat of the lung.

10. Ten Charred Herbs Powder
(十灰散, shi hui san)

Source: *Miraculous Book of Ten kinds of Dosage Form* 《十药神书》
Composition: Japanese Thistle Herb or Root (大蓟, Daji) 9g
Common Cephalanoploris Herb (小蓟, Xiaoji) 9g
Lotus Leaf (荷叶, Heye) 9g
Chinese Arborvitae Leafytwig (侧柏叶, Cebaiye) 9g
Lalang Grass Rhizome (白茅根, Baimaogen) 9g
Tree Peony Bark (牡丹皮, Mudanpi) 12g
Charred Rhubarb (大黄炭, Dahuangtan) 15g
India Madder Root (茜草根, Qiancaogen) 15g
Charred Fortune Windmillpalm Petiole (棕榈炭, Zonglütan) 15g
Cape Jasmine Fruit (山栀子, Shanzhizi) 15g

Actions: Removing heat from the blood to arrest bleeding.

Applied Syndrome: Hemorrhage syndrome due to attack of blood-heat manifested as acute and severe upper hemorrhages with a large quantity of bright blood, red tongue and rapid pulse, such as hematemesis, hemoptysis, bleeding from the gum and epistaxis.

Points in Constitution: Most of the ingredients of this formula are the drugs for removing heat from the blood and arresting bleeding. Rhubarb (大黄, Dahuang) and Cape Jasmine Fruit (山栀子, Shanzhizi) are added to clear away heat, purge fire and induce the heat downward, while Tree Peony Bark (牡丹皮, Mudanpi) is used for removing blood stasis and arresting bleeding without leaving stasis.

Indications:

1. Hemoptysis due to pulmonary tuberculosis, bronchiectasis and bronchitis
2. Nasal hemorrhage due to pathogenic heat damaging the lung meridian
3. Metrorrhagia and metrostaxis (hemorrhage of hysteromyoma, dysfunctional uterine bleeding etc.)
4. Hemorrhage of wounds
5. Hemorrhage of stomach and duodenal ulcer, esophagitis

Precautions:

1. This formula is designed for hemorrhage due to heat. Thus, it is forbidden for hemorrhage due to deficient cold.

Ten Charred Herbs Powder
(Blood-Cooling and Bleeding-Arresting Method)

Ingredients	Effects	Combined Effects	Syndrome	Chief Symptoms
Japanese Thistle Herb or Root (大蓟, Daji) 9g Common Cephalanoploris Herb (小蓟, Xiaoji) 9g Lotus Leaf (荷叶, Heye) 9g India Madder Root (茜草根, Qiancaogen) 15g Lalang Grass Rhizome (白茅根, Baimaogen) 9g	Cooling blood to arrest bleeding	Removing heat from the blood to arrest bleeding	Hemorrhage due to attack of blood heat	Acute and severe hematemesis, hemoptysis and apostaxis, usually in a large quantity of bright blood, red tongue and rapid pulse
Charred Fortune Windmill-palm Petiole (棕榈炭, Zonglütan) 15g Chinese Arborvitae Leafy Twig (侧柏叶, Cebaiye) 9g	Astringing to arrest bleeding			
Cape Jasmine Fruit (山栀子, Shanzhizi) 15g	Clearing away liver fire			
Charred Rhubarb (大黄炭, Dahuangtan) 15g	Leading heat downwards			
Tree Peony Bark (牡丹皮, Mudanpi) 12g	Removing heat from the blood and dissolving blood stasis			

2. This is a formula for the secondary aspect of a disease and can not be used excessively for a long period of time. For hemorrhage, once the bleeding stops, the cause should be examined and the primary symptom be treated as soon as possible.

Associated Formulas:

1. Four Fresh Herbs Pill (四生丸, si sheng wan) *The Complete Effective Prescriptions for Diseases of Women* 《妇人良方大全》

This is comprised of Chinese Arborvitae Leafy Twig (生侧柏叶, Shengcebaiye), Dried Rehmannia Root (生地黄, Shengdihuang), Lotus Leaf (生荷叶, Shengheye) and Argy Wormwood Leaf (生艾叶, Shengaiye). Its actions are removing heat from the blood to arrest bleeding. It is indicated for hematemesis and apostaxis due to attack of blood heat, manifested as bright red blood, dry throat and mouth, wiry, rapid and powerful pulse.

2. Two Fresh Herbs Decoction (二鲜饮, er xian yin) *Records of Traditional Chinese and Western Medicine in Combination* 《医学衷中参西录》

This is comprised of Fresh Lalang Grass Rhizome (鲜茅根, Xian Maogen) and Fresh Lotus Root (鲜藕, Xian Ou). Its actions are dissolving blood stasis and arresting bleeding. It is indicated for hematemesis, apostaxis, hematochezia and hematuria due to attack of blood heat.

3. Mysterious Red Pellet (秘红丹, mi hong dan) *Records of Traditional Chinese and Western Medicine in Combination* 《医学衷中参西录》

This is comprised of Rhubarb (生大黄, Sheng Dahuang), Cassia Bark (肉桂, Rougui) and Hematite (代赭石, Daizheshi). Its actions are calming the liver and regulating the stomach, keeping the adverse qi downwards and arresting bleeding. It is indicated for hematemesis and apostaxis due to stagnation of liver-qi, irritability and reversed flow of the stomach-qi.

11. Divaricate Saposhnikovia Miraculous Powder (防风通圣散, fang feng tong sheng san)

Source: *Formulae and Expositions* 《宣明论方》
Composition: Chinese Angelica Root (当归, Danggui) 6g
Szechwan Lovage Rhizome (川芎, Chuanxiong) 6g
White Peony Root (白芍药, Baishaoyao) 6g
Rhubarb (大黄, Dahuang) 6g
Wild Mint Herb (薄荷, Bohe) 6g
Ephedra (麻黄, Mahuang) 6g
Weeping Forsythia Capsule (连翘, Lianqiao) 6g
Mirabilite (芒硝, Mangxiao) 6g
Gypsum (石膏, Shigao) 12g
Baikal Skullcap Root (黄芩, Huangqin) 12g
Balloonflower Root (桔梗, Jiegeng) 6g
Talc (滑石, Huashi) 15g
Licorice Root (甘草, Gancao) 6g
Fineleaf Schizonepeta Herb (荆芥, Jingjie) 6g
Largehead Atractylodes Rhizome (白术, Baizhu) 6g
Cape Jasmine Fruit (山栀子, Shanzhizi) 6g
Divaricate Saposhnikovia Root (防风, Fangfeng) 6g

Actions: Expelling wind and relieving the exterior syndrome, clearing away heat and relaxing the bowels.

Applied Syndrome: Syndrome of excess both in the exterior and interior due to attack of the exterior by wind and accumulation of heat in the interior. The manifestations are aversion to cold and high fever, diaphoresis, dizziness, red eyes and painful eyeball, bitter taste in the mouth and dry throat, uncomfortable feeling in the throat, thick tears and saliva, constipation, dysuria with dark urine, yellow and greasy tongue coating, rapid and powerful pulse. This formula is also applied to sores, hematochezia and piles, red nose and urticaria.

Divaricate Saposhnikovia Miraculous Powder
(Exterior-Relieving and Interior-Clearing Method)

Ingredients	Effects	Combined Effects	Syndrome	Chief Symptoms
Ephedra (麻黄, Mahuang)6g Fineleaf Schizonepeta Herb (荆芥, Jingjie)6g Divaricate Saposhnikovia Root (防风, Fangfeng)6g Wild Mint Herb (薄荷, Bohe)6g	Expelling wind and relieving the exterior syndrome	Expelling wind and relieving the exterior syndrome, clearing away heat to loosen the bowels	Excess in both the exterior and interior due to accumulation of excessive wind and heat	Aversion to cold and high fever, diaphoresis, dizziness, red eyes and painful eyeball, bitter taste in the mouth and dry throat, uncomfortable feeling in the throat, constipation and dysuria, yellow and greasy tongue coating, rapid and powerful pulse
Rhubarb (大黄, Dahuang)6g Mirabilite (芒硝, Mangxiao)6g	Expelling heat to loosen the bowels			
Talc (滑石, Huashi)15g	Clearing away heat and promoting diuresis			
Cape Jasmine Fruit (山栀子, Shanzhizi)6g Gypsum(石膏,Shigao)12g Weeping Forsythia Capsule (连翘, Lianqiao)6g Baikal Skullcap Root (黄芩, Huangqin)12g Balloonflower Root (桔梗, Jiegeng)6g	Clearing away heat, purging fire and clearing away toxic material			
Chinese Angelica Root (当归, Danggui)6g White Peony Root (白芍药, Baishaoyao)6g Szechwan Lovage Rhizome (川芎, Chuanxiong)6g	Enriching blood and regulating blood flow			
Largehead Atractylodes Rhizome (白术, Baizhu)6g	Invigorating the spleen and clearing away dampness			
Licorice Root (甘草, Gancao)6g	Coordinating the actions of the above herbs			

Points in Constitution: This formula, in fact, is the combination of Stomach-Regulating Purgative Decoction (调胃承气汤, tiao wei cheng qi tang) and Antiphlogistic Powder (败毒散, bai du san). It includes the four methods of diaphoresis, diuresis, heat-clearing and purgation and the exterior and interior syndromes are treated simultaneously. In addition, the pathogens in the upper and lower jiao are expelled seperatedly. Diaphoresis does not harm the exterior while purgation does not harm the interior. Therefore, it is widely used in the clinic for the syndrome of excessive heat in the interior with pathogenic wind in the exterior.

Indications:
1. Cold, influenza
2. Furuncle on head and face
3. Acute conjunctivitis
4. Obesity
5. Habitual constipation, hemorrhoidal pain
6. Urticaria, eczema, drug eruption, zoster, psoriasis, brandy nose, etc.

Precaution:
This formula is indicated for the syndrome of excess in both the exterior and interior. Thus, it is forbidden for weak persons and pregnant women.

Associated Formula:
Double Expelling Powder (双解散, shuang jie san) *Complete Works for Treating Sores* 《疡医大全》

This is comprised of Divaricate Saposhnikovia Root (防风, Fangfeng), Szechwan Lovage Rhizome (川芎, Chuanxiong), Chinese Angelica Root (当归, Danggui), White Peony Root (白芍, Baishao), Rhubarb (大黄, Dahuang), Wild Mint Herb (薄荷, Bohe), Weeping Forsythia Capsule (连翘, Lianqiao), Gypsum (石膏, Shigao), Balloonflower Root (桔梗, Jiegeng), Baikal Skullcap Root (黄芩, Huangqin), Cassia Twig (桂枝, Guizhi), Spike of Fineleaf Schizonepeta Herb (荆芥穗, Jingjiesui), Talc (滑石, Huashi) and Licorice Root (甘草, Gancao). Its actions are relieving the exterior syndrome, removing toxin, purging heat and relaxing the bowels. It is indicated for early stage of pox due to accumulation of wind and heat, manifested as aversion to cold, fever, constipation, scanty and dark urine, red tongue with slight yellow and greasy coating, rapid and excessive pulse.

12. Five Retentions Powder (五积散, wu ji san)

Source: *Prescriptions of Peaceful Benevolent Dispensary* 《和剂局方》
Composition: Ephedra (麻黄, Mahuang) 6g
Dahurican Angelica Aoot (白芷, Baizhi) 6g
Swordlike Atractylodes Ahizome (苍术, Cangzhu) 6g
Officinal Magnolia Bark (厚朴, Houpo) 6g
Pinellia Rhizome (半夏, Banxia) 6g
Tangerine Peel (橘皮, Jupi) 6g

Fresh Ginger (生姜, Shengjiang)6g
Tuckahoe (茯苓, Fuling)6g
Bitter Orange (枳壳, Zhiqiao)6g
Balloonflower Root (桔梗, Jiegeng)6g
Dried Ginger (干姜, Ganjiang)3g
Cassia Bark (肉桂, Rougui)3g
Chinese Angelica Root (当归, Danggui)6g
Szechwan Lovage Rhizome (川芎, Chuanxiong)6g
White Peony Root (白芍药, Baishaoyao)6g
Prepared Licorice Root (炙甘草, Zhi Gancao)6g

Actions: Relieving the exterior syndrome and warming the interior, regulating flow of qi and resolving phlegm, regulating flow of blood and alleviating pain.

Applied Syndrome:

1. Attack of the exterior by exogenous wind-cold with the damage to the interior due to eating cold food manifested as aversion to cold, fever with diaphoresis, headache and pain all over the body, subjective sensation of contraction in the neck and back, feeling of fullness in the chest, anorexia, vomiting, abdominal pain, white and greasy tongue coating, floating, l wiry or tense pulse.

2. Incoordination of qi and blood in women with attack of exogenous cold manifested by pericardial and abdominal pain, irregular menstruation, wiry, tense or slow pulse.

Points in Constitution: This formula consists of the ingredients of Stomach-Calming Powder (平胃散, ping wei san) plus some cold-dispelling, interior-warming and blood-regulating herbs. It firstly regulates stomach-qi to expel cold, remove dampness, regulate flow of qi, activate circulation of blood and resolve phlegm. Therefore, it is named Powder for Treating Five Retentions (五积散, wu ji san).

Indications:

1. Common cold of wind-cold type with signs of stomach and intestine diseases
2. Chronic bronchitis, acute pulmonary infection
3. Malnutrition and indigestion syndrome in children

Precaution: This formula is designed for the syndrome of wind-cold in the exterior and stagnation of cold in the interior. It is not suitable for those with heat in the interior and cold in the exterior or exterior syndrome due to wind heat.

Associated Formulas:

1. Ephedra, Aconite and Manchurian Wildginger Decoction (麻黄附子细辛汤, ma huang fu zi xi xin tang) *Treatise on Exogenous Febrile Diseases*《伤寒论》

This is comprised of Ephedra (麻黄, Mahuang), Prepared Aconite Root (附子, Fuzi) and Manchurian Wildginger Herb (细辛, Xixin). Its actions are restoring yang and relieving the exterior syndrome. It is indicated for the exterior syndrome due to yang deficiency manifested as high fever, severe aversion to cold which can not be relieved by wearing thick clothes and quilt, lassitude, deep and weak pulse.

Five Retentions Powder
(Exterior-Relieving and Interior-Warming Method)

Ingredients	Effects	Combined Effects	Syndrome	Chief Symptoms
Ephedra (麻黄, Mahuang) 6g Dahurican Angelica Root (白芷, Baizhi) 6g Fresh Ginger (生姜, Shengjiang) 6g	Relieving the exterior syndrome and expelling cold	Relieving the exterior syndrome and warming the interior, regulating flow of qi and resolving phlegm, regulating circulation of blood and alleviating pain	Attack of exterior by exogenous wind-cold with damage to the interior due to eating cold food	Fever with diaphoresis, headache and pain all over the body, vomiting, abdominal pain in woman and irregular menstruation, white and greasy tongue coating, floating, wiry or tense pulse
Dried Ginger (干姜, Ganjiang) 3g Cassia Bark (肉桂, Rougui) 3g	Warming the middle-jiao to expel cold			
Swordlike Atractylodes Rhizome (苍术, Cangzhu) 6g Officinal Magnolia Bark (厚朴, Houpo) 6g Pinellia Rhizome (半夏, Banxia) 6g Tangerine Peel (橘皮, Jupi) 6g Tuckahoe (茯苓, Fuling) 6g	Removing dampness and invigorating the spleen, regulating qi and resolving phlegm			
Chinese Angelica Root (当归, Danggui) 6g Szechwan Lovage Rhizome (川芎, Chuanxiong) 6g White Peony Root (白芍药, Baishaoyao) 6g	Regulating flow of blood and alleviating pain			
Bitter Orange (枳壳, Zhiqiao) 6g Balloonflower Root (桔梗, Jiegeng) 6g	Regulating the upper and downward movement of qi			
Prepared Licorice Root (炙甘草, Zhi Gancao) 6g	Coordinating the actions of the above herbs			

2. Stagnation-Relieving Pill (越鞠丸, yue ju wan) *Danxi's Experiential Therapy* 《丹溪心法》

This is comprised of Swordlike Atractylodes Rhizome (苍术, Cangzhu), Nutgrass Galingale Rhizome (香附, Xiangfu), Szechwan Lovage Rhizome (川芎, Chuanxiong), Medicated Leaven (神曲, Shenqu) and Cape Jasmine Fruit (山栀子, Shanzhizi). Its actions are activating flow of qi and relieving the depressed liver. It is applied for stuffiness sensation in the chest and hypochondrium, distention and pain in the abdomen and epigastrium, acid regurgitation and vomiting and indigestion due to depressed qi, blood stasis, stagnation of phlegm, accumulation of fire and retention of dampness and food.

3. Digestion-Promoting Pill for Five Infantile Malnutrition (五疳消食丸, wu gan xiao shi wan) *Prescriptions of Peaceful Benevolent Dispensary*《和剂局方》

This is comprised of Stir-Baked Malt (炒麦芽, Chaomaiya), Stir-Baked Rangooncreeper Fruit (炒使君子, Chao Shijunzi), Stir-Baked Coptis Rhizome (炒黄连, Chao Huanglian), Tangerine Peel (橘红, Juhong), Chinese Gentian Root (龙胆草, Longdancao) and Bigfruit Elm Fruit (芜荑, Wuyi). Its actions are clearing away heat, promoting digestion and relieving infantile malnutrition. It is indicated for infantile malnutrition manifested as yellowish complexion, thin body, big abdomen with blue veins, ulcerative gingivitis and halitosis; or abdominal pain and dysentery due to parasitic infection.

Additional Formulas

Qi-Dispersing and Lung-Regulating Pill
(通宣理肺丸, tong xuan li fei wan)

Source: Collection of Chinese Patent Medicines of Peking《北京市中成药方选集》
Composition: Perilla Leaf (紫苏叶, Zisuye)9g
Baikal Skullcap Root (黄芩, Huangqin)9g
Bitter Orange (枳壳, Zhiqiao)9g
Apricot Seed (杏仁, Xingren)6g
Tangerine Peel (橘皮, Jupi)6g
Balloonflower Root (桔梗, Jiegeng)6g
Tuckahoe (茯苓, Fuling)9g
Whiteflower Hogfennel Root (前胡, Qianhu)6g
Ephedra (麻黄, Mahuang)6g
Pinellia Rhizome (半夏, Banxia)6g
Licorice Root (甘草, Gancao)6g

Actions: Relieving the exterior and dispersing the lung, stopping cough and resolving phlegm.

Applied Syndrome: Cough due to wind and cold. The lung is attacked by wind-cold, which causes failure of the lung in dispersion and descent manifested as fever and aversion to cold, headache, diaphoresis, cough with white sputum, running nose, tiredness, thin and white tongue coating, floating and tense pulse.

Points in Constitution: This formula is based on Three Drugs Decoction(三拗汤, san ao tang), Two Vintage Herbs Decoction(二陈汤, er chen tang) and Nutgrass Flatsedge and Perilla Leave Powder(香苏散, xiang shu san). It is indicated for cough and asthma caused by exogenous wind-cold. In this formula, Baikal Skullcap Root (黄芩, Huangqin), which is bitter in taste, cold in property and has the heat-removing action to prevent either the pathogenic cold from entering the interior to change into heat or the warm and dry herbs exert their effects excessively to damage yin, is used to clear away heat so that the exterior cold can not attack the interior and change into heat syndrome.

Indications:
1. Cold
2. Acute bronchitis
3. Acute attack of chronic bronchitis

Precaution: This formula is suitable for cough due to attack of exogenous wind-cold. It is forbidden for cough due to wind-heat or phlegm-heat.

Associated Formulas:
1. Compound Tablet of Extract of Tendrilleaf Fritillary Bulb (复方川贝精片, fu fang chuan

Qi-Dispersing and Lung-Regulating Pill
(Exterior-Relieving and Lung-Dispesing Method)

Ingredients	Effects	Combined Effects	Syndrome	Chief Symptoms
Perilla Leaf (紫苏叶, Zisuye)9g Ephedra (麻黄, Mahuang)6g	Inducing diaphoresis to relieve the exterior syndrome, dispersing the lung and relieving asthma	Relieving the exterior syndrome and dispersing the lung, stopping cough and resolving phlegm	Cough and asthma (due to attack of the lung by wind-cold)	Fever and aversion to cold, headache, diaphoresis, cough with white sputum, running nose, tiredness, thin and white tongue coating, floating and tense pulse
Apricot Seed (杏仁, Xingren)6g Whiteflower Hogfennel Root (前胡, Qianhu)6g Balloonflower Root (桔梗, Jiegeng)6g	Promoting the dispersing and descending function of the lung and stopping cough			
Bitter Orange (枳壳, Zhiqiao)9g Tangerine Peel (橘皮, Jupi)6g Tuckahoe (茯苓, Fuling)9g 法 Pinellia Rhizome (半夏, Banxia)6g Licorice Root (甘草, Gancao)6g	Removing dampness and resolving phlegm			
Baikal Skullcap Root (黄芩, Huangqin)9g	Clearing away lung heat			

bei jing pian) *Practical Prescriptions for Respiratory Diseases*《呼吸系病实用方》

This is comprised of Tendrilleaf Fritillary Bulb (川贝母, Chuan Beimu), Chinese Magnoliavine Fruit (五味子, Wuweizi), Ephedra (麻黄, Mahuang), Thinleaf Milkwort Root (远志, Yuanzhi), Tangerine Peel (橘皮, Jupi), Pinellia Rhizome (半夏, Banxia), Balloonflower Root (桔梗, Jiegeng) and Licorice Root (甘草, Gancao). Its actions are moistening the lung and removing phlegm, relieving cough and stopping asthma. It is indicated for cough and asthma with expectoration of phlegm due to attack of the lung by wind and cold.

2. Inula Herb Powder (金沸草散, jin fei cao san) *Prescriptions of Peaceful Benevolent Dispensary*《和剂局方》

This is comprised of Inula Flower (旋覆花, Xuanfuhua), Pinellia Rhizome (半夏, Banxia), Licorice Root (甘草, Gancao), Ephedra (麻黄, Mahuang), Whiteflower Hogfennel Root (前胡, Qianhu), Spike of Fineleaf Schizonepeta Herb (荆芥穗, Jingjiesui), Red Peony Root (赤芍药, Chishaoyao), Fresh Ginger (生姜, Shengjiang) and Chinese Date (大枣, Dazao). Its actions are expelling wind-cold, keeping the adverse qi downward, relieving cough and removing phlegm. It is indicated for cough due to exogenous wind-cold.

Pleurisy Decoction Number One
（胸膜炎汤Ⅰ号，xiong mo yan tang yi hao）

Source: *Medical Records and Prescriptions in Clinic*《临床医案医方》
Composition: Inula Flower（旋覆花，Xuanfuhua）6g
Hematite（代赭石，Daizheshi）12g
Tangerine Peel（橘皮，Jupi）9g
Bitter Orange（枳壳，Zhiqiao）6g
Snakegourd Fruit（全瓜蒌，Quangualou）18g
Longstamen Onion Bulb（薤白，Xiebai）9g
Balloonflower Root（桔梗，Jiegeng）6g
Urmeric Root-tuber（郁金，Yujin）9g
Tangerine Leaf（橘叶，Juye）9g
Reed Rhizome（芦根，Lugen）15g
Weeping Forsythia Capsule（连翘，Lianqiao）15g
Apricot Seed（杏仁，Xingren）9g

Actions: Regulating flow of qi and alleviating pain, lowering the adverse qi downwards and removing phlegm.

Applied Syndrome: Pleurisy. Retention of turbid phlegm in the chest and hypochondrium leads to disorder of the movement of qi in the collaterals manifested as pain in the chest and hypochondrium which may become severe when coughing or breathing deeply, hypopnea, cough with sputum, oppressed feeling in the chest, thin and white tongue coating, wiry pulse.

Points in Constitution: This formula emphasizes regulating flow of qi and removing mass to relieve pain. It is the combination of modified Inulae and Red Ochre Decoction（旋覆代赭汤，xuan fu dai zhe tang）and Frichosanthes, Macrostem Onion and Liquor Decoction（瓜蒌薤白白酒汤，gua lou xie bai bai ju tang）. In this formula, Turmeric Root-Tuber（郁金，Yujin）and Tangerine Leaf（橘叶，Juye）are the habitual drugs for relieving pain in the chest and hypochondria.

Indications:
1. Dry pleurisy
2. Intercosal neuralgia

Precaution: This formula is suitable for dry pleurisy due to qi stagnation and phlegm retention. It is contraindicated in exudative pleurisy due to accumulation of water and heat or when it is acccompanied with deficiency of healthy qi.

Associated Formulas:
1. Modified Cold Limbs Powder（加减四逆散，jia jian si ni san）*Essentials on Diagnosis and Treatment of Chinese Internal Medicine*《中医内科证治备要》

Pleurisy Decoction Number One
(Qi-Regulating and Phlegm-Resolving Method)

Ingredients	Effects	Combined Effects	Syndrome	Chief Symptoms
Inula Flower (旋覆花, Xuanfuhua)6g Hematite (代赭石, Daizheshi)12g	Lowering the adverse flow of qi and removing phlegm	Regulating flow of qi and alleviating pain, keeping the adverse qi downwards and removing phlegm	Pleurisy (retention of turbid phlegm and pain due to qi stagnation)	Pain in the chest and hypochondrium, which becoming severe when cough or deep breathing, cough, oppressed feeling in the chest, thin and white tongue coating, wiry pulse
Snakegourd Fruit (全瓜蒌, Quangualou)18g Longstamen Onion Bulb (薤白, Xiebai)9g	Dispersing the obstruction of qi in the chest and dissipating blockages, warming and promoting flow of qi and alleviating pain			
Balloonflower Root (桔梗, Jiegeng)6g Bitter Orange (枳壳, Zhiqiao)6g Apricot Seed (杏仁, Xingren)9g Tangerine Peel (橘皮, Jupi)9g	Regulating activities of qi, removing phlegm and stopping cough			
Turmeric Root-Tuber (郁金, Yujin)9g Tangerine Leaf (橘叶, Juye)9g	Regulating flow of qi to relieve the depressed liver, alleviating pain in the chest and hypochondrium			
Reed Rhizome (芦根, Lugen)15g Weeping Forsythia Capsule (连翘, Lianqiao)15g	Clearing away heat and toxic material			

This is comprised of Chinese Thorowax Root (柴胡, Chaihu), Immature Bitter Orange (枳实, Zhishi), White Peony Root (白芍药, Baishaoyao), Turmeric Root-Tuber (郁金, Yujin), Green Tangerine Peel (青皮, Qingpi), Tangerine Peel (橘皮, Jupi), Yanhusuo (元胡, Yuanhu), Peach Seed (桃仁, Taoren), White Mustard Seed (白芥子, Baijiezi), Snakegourd Fruit (全瓜蒌, Quangualou), Licorice Root (甘草, Gancao) and Safflower (红花, Honghua). Its actions are regulating flow of qi, activating blood circulation and alleviating pain. It is indicated for pleurisy with pain in the chest and hypochondrium due to qi stagnation and blood stasis.

2. Eagle Wood Qi-Lowering Powder (沉香降气散 chen xiang jiang qi san) *Prescriptions of Peaceful Benevolent Dispensary*《和剂局方》

This is comprised of Chinese Eagle Wood (沉香, Chenxiang), Prepared Licorice Root (炙甘草, Zhi Gancao), Villous Amomum Fruit (砂仁, Sharen) and Nutgrass Galingale Rhizome (香附, Xiangfu). Its actions are removing stagnation of qi and keeping the adverse qi downwards. It is indicated for pain in the hypochondrium due to stagnation of qi and abnormal rising of qi.

3. Qi-Restoration and Blood-Activating Decoction (复元活血汤, fu yuan huo xue tang) *Invention of Medicine*《医学发明》

This is comprised of Chinese Thorowax Root (柴胡, Chaihu), Snakegourd Root (天花粉, Tianhuafen), Chinese Angelica Root (当归, Danggui), Safflower (红花, Honghua), Licorice Root (甘草, Gancao), Pangolin Scales (穿山甲, Chuanshanjia), Rhubarb (大黄, Dahuang) and Peach Seed (桃仁, Taoren). Its actions are activating blood circulation, removing blood stasis, dispersing the stagnated liver-qi and dredging the collaterals. It is indicated for pain in the hypochondrium due to stagnation of qi and stasis of blood resulting from depressed liver-qi.

Pleurisy Decoction Number Two
(胸膜炎汤 II 号, xiong mo yan tang er hao)

Source: *Medical Records and Prescriptions in Clinic*《临床医案医方》
Composition: Chinese Waxgourd Seed (冬瓜子, Dongguazi)30g
Pepperweed Seed (葶苈子, Tinglizi)9g
Coix Seed (薏苡仁, Yiyiren)30g
Tuckahoe (茯苓, Fuling)12g
Tangerine Peel (橘皮, Jupi)9g
Snakegourd Fruit (瓜蒌, Gualou)12g
Longstamen Onion Bulb (薤白, Xiebai)9g
Balloonflower Root (桔梗, Jiegeng)6g
Inula Flower (旋覆花, Xuanfuhua)6g
Hematite (代赭石, Daizheshi)12g
Apricot Seed (杏仁, Xingren)9g
Bitter Orange (枳壳, Zhiqiao)6g
Actions: Purging lung, promoting urination and relieving cough.
Applied Syndrome: Pleural effusion. Water retention in the chest and hypochondrium results in disorder of activities of qi manifested as pain in the hypochondrium which is aggravated by coughing and spitting, pain in the chest aggravated by breathing, distention and fullness in the chest and hypochondrium, shortness of breath, tachypnea, cough, white and greasy tongue coating, wiry or deep wiry pluse.

Pleurisy Decoction Number Two
(Lung-Purging and Urination-Promoting Method)

Ingredients	Effects	Combined Effects	Syndrome	Chief Symptoms
Chinese Waxgourd Seed (冬瓜子, Dongguazi) 30g	Clearing away heat and removing phlegm	Purging the lung, promoting urination and relieving cough	Pleural effusion (Water retention in the chest and hypochondrium, with disorder of activities of qi)	Pain in the hypochondrium which is aggravated by coughing and spitting, distention and fullness in the chest and hypochondrium, shortness of breath, tachypnea, cough, white and greasy tongue coating, wiry or deep wiry pluse
Pepperweed Seed or Flixweed Tansymustard Seed (葶苈子, Tinglizi) 9g	Purging lung and promoting urination			
Coix Seed (薏苡仁, Yiyiren) 30g Tuckahoe (茯苓, Fuling) 12g	Promoting urination and inducing diuresis to cure pleural effusion			
Inula Flower (旋覆花, Xuanfuhua) 6g Hematite (代赭石, Daizheshi) 12g	Keeping the adverse qi downwards and relieving cough			
Snakegourd Fruit (瓜蒌, Gualou) 12g Longstamen Onion Bulb (薤白, Xiebai) 9g	Relieving the obstruction of yang-qi, resolving phlegm and dispersing accumulation of pathogen			
Tangerine Peel (橘皮, Jupi) 9g Balloonflower Root (桔梗, Jiegeng) 6g Apricot Seed (杏仁, Xingren) 9g Bitter Orange (枳壳, Zhiqiao) 6g	Regulating flow of qi and benefiting the lung			

Points in Constitution: This formula is the Pleurisy Decoction Number One (胸膜炎汤Ⅰ号, xiong mo yan tang yi hao) without Turmeric Root-Tuber (郁金, Yujin), Tangerine Leaf (橘叶, Juye), Reed Rhizome (芦根, Lugen) and Weeping Forsythia Capsule (连翘, Lianqiao) but plus Pepperweed Seed (葶苈子, Tinglizi), Chinese Waxgourd Seed (冬瓜子, Dongguazi), Coix Seed (薏苡仁, Yiyiren) and Tuckahoe (茯苓, Fuling) to enhance the functions of purging the lung, inducing diuresis and eliminating phlegm. The main indication of Number One Decoction is pain due to qi stagnation, while that of Number Two Decoction is pleural effusion. From the above-mentioned modification the marvelous effect is shown in the two decoctions.

Indications:
1. Exudative pleurisy
2. Thoracic cavity amass fluid

Precaution: This formula is suitable for pleural effusion due to fluid retention in the chest and hypochondrium and disordered activities of qi. For pleural effusion accompanied with qi deficiency, this formula should be used together with other herbs.

Associated Formulas:

1. Ten Chinese Date Decoction (十枣汤, shi zao tang) *Treatise on Exogenous Febrile Diseases* 《伤寒论》

This is comprised of Lilac Daphne Flower-Bud (芫花, Yuanhua), Kansui Root (甘遂, Gansui), Peking Euphorbia Root (大戟, Daji) and Chinese Date (大枣, Dazao). Its action is removing water retention by purgation. It is indicated for pleural effusion due to fluid retention in the chest and hypochondrium.

2. Saliva-Controlling Pellet (控涎丹, kong xian dan) *Treatise on the Triple-Pathogenic Doctrine of Etiology* 《三因极一病证方论》

This is comprised of Kansui Root (甘遂, Gansui), Peking Euphorbia Root (大戟, Daji) and White Mustard Seed (白芥子, Baijiezi). Its actions are removing phlegm and expelling retention of water. It is indicated for pain in the chest, back, neck, nape, waist and thigh due to retention of phlegm and water in the chest and hypochondrium.

Chapter Two
Formulas for Diseases of the Circulatory System

There is a saying in the theory of traditional Chinese medicine that "the heart controls blood and vessels". Thus, the diseases of the circulatory system are mainly considered as the problem of the heart though some of them are related to the liver, lung, kidney and spleen. The main causes of this disease are mostly the stimulation of seven emotions and the main pathogenesis is deficiency of qi and blood or blockage of phlegm or blood stasis. There are corresponding prescriptions, sometimes combined with western medicine, for various diseases such as palpitation, arrhythmia, angina pectoris, hypertension, hypotension, heart failure and myocarditis.

1. Liver-Subduing and Wind-Stopping Decoction
（镇肝息风汤，zhen gan xi feng tang）

Source: Records of Traditional Chinese and Western Medicine in Combination 《医学衷中参西录》

Composition: Achyranthes Root（怀牛膝，Huainiuxi）30g
Hematite（代赭石，Daizheshi）30g
Dragon's Bone（生龙骨，Sheng Longgu）15g
Oyster Shell（生牡蛎，Sheng Muli）15g
Tortoise Shell and Plastron（龟版，Guiban）15g
Figwort Root（玄参，Xuanshen）15g
Cochinchinese Asparagus Root（天门冬，Tianmendong）15g
White Peony Root（白芍药，Baishaoyao）15g
Capillary Wormwood Herb（茵陈，Yinchen）6g
Szechwan Chinaberry Fruit（川楝子，Chuanlianzi）6g
Malt（麦芽，Maiya）6g
Licorice Root（甘草，Gancao）3g

Actions: Calming the liver to stop the wind, nourishing yin and checking exuberance of yang.

Applied Syndrome: Wind-stroke or aura of wind-stroke. Yin deficiency of both the liver and kidney brings about failure of water in nourishing wood, thus leading to hyperactivity of yang and stirring of wind. The manifestations are vertigo, or deviation of the mouth, fainting, or hemiplegia, or dysphoria with smothery sensation, flushed complexion, eye distention and tinnitus, powerful and long wiry pulse.

Liver-Subduing and Wind-Stopping Decoction
(Liver-Calming and Endogeneous Wind-Stopping Method)

Ingredients	Effects	Combined Effects	Syndrome	Chief Symptoms
Achyranthes Root (怀牛膝, Huainiuxi) 30g White Peony Root (白芍药, Baishaoyao) 15g	Leading blood flowing downwards and nourishing the liver and kidney	Calming the liver and stopping the wind, nourishing yin and checking exuberance of yang	Yin deficiency of liver and kidney, hyperactivity of yang and stirring of wind	Vertigo, or deviation of the mouth, or faint, or hemiplegia, powerful and long wiry pulse
Hematite (代赭石, Daizheshi) 30g Dragon's Bone (生龙骨, Sheng Longgu) 15g Oyster Shell (生牡蛎, Sheng Muli) 15g	Checking hyperactivity of liver yang			
Tortoise Shell and Plastron (龟版, Guiban) 15g Figwort Root (玄参, Xuanshen) 15g Cochinchinese Asparagus Root (天门冬, Tianmendong) 15g	Nourishing yin of liver and kidney			
Capillary Wormwood Herb (茵陈, Yinchen) 6g Szechwan Chinaberry Fruit (川楝子, Chuanlianzi) 6g Malt (麦芽, Maiya) 6g	Clearing away heat and dispersing the stagnated liver-qi			
Licorice Root (甘草, Gancao) 3g	Coordinating the actions of the above drugs			

Points in Constitution: In this formula, a large dosage of Hematite (代赭石, Daizheshi), Dragon's Bone (生龙骨, Sheng Longgu) and Oyster Shell (生牡蛎, Sheng Muli) are used for calming the liver to stop the wind and tranquilizing the mind. The combination of Tortoise Shell and Plastron (龟版, Guiban) and Oyster Shell (牡蛎, Muli) is to calm the liver and check exuberance of yang. The use of Figwort Root (玄参, Xuanshen), Cochinchinese Asparagus Root (天门冬, Tianmendong) and White Peony Root (白芍药, Baishaoyao) is to nourish yin and liver. Capillary Wormwood Herb (茵陈, Yinchen), Malt (麦芽, Maiya) and Szechwan Chinaberry Fruit (川楝子, Chuanlianzi) are used to clear away heat and disperse the stagnated liver-qi so as to correspond with the nature of the liver. The heavy use of Achyranthes Root (怀牛膝, Huainiuxi) is to induce the blood circulating downward. This formula has the functions of calming the liver, nourishing liver-yin and dispersing the stagnated liver-qi, which result in calming the liver and stopping interior wind and hyperactivity of yang.

Indications:
1. Hypertension
2. Hypertensive encephalopathy
3. Cerebrovascular accident (CAV)
4. Cerebral arteriosclerosis
5. Hyperthyroidism
6. Pheochromocytoma
7. Primary hyperaldosteronism

Precaution: This formula is indicated for the syndrome of yin deficiency and hyperactivity of yang accompanied with liver-wind stirring inside the body. It is not suitable for hyperactivity of yang without yin deficiency.

Associated Formulas:

1. Sweeping Down Decoction for Tension Hypertension(建瓴汤, jian ling tang) *Records of Traditional Chinese and Western Medicine in Combination* 《医学衷中参西录》

This is comprised of Common Yam Rhizome (怀山药, Huaishanyao), Hematite (生赭石, Sheng Zheshi), Dragon's Bone (生龙骨, Sheng Longgu), Oyster Shell (生牡蛎, Sheng Muli), Dried Rehmannia Root (生地黄, Shengdihuang), White Peony Root (白芍药, Baishaoyao), Twotooth Achyranthes Root (牛膝, Niuxi) and Chinese Arborvitae Seed (柏子仁, Baiziren). Its actions are calming the liver, stopping the wind, nourishing yin and tranquilizing the mind. It is indicated for dizziness, palpitation, irritability and insomnia due to hyperactivity of liver yang. The actions of the Liver-Calming and Wind-Stopping Decoction(镇肝息风汤, zhen gan xi feng tang) are stronger than those of the Sweeping Down Decoction for Tension Hypertension (建瓴汤, jian ling tang). Thus in the clinic, the former is ususlly applied to the aura of wind-stroke in an emergency, while the latter is aimed to prevent the occurance of wind-stroke by nourishing yin.

2. Wind-Calming Decoction (镇风汤, zhen feng tang) *Records of Traditional Chinese and Western Medicine in Combination* 《医学衷中参西录》

This is comprised of Gambirplant Hooked Stem and Branch (钩藤, Gouteng), Chinese Gentian Root (龙胆草, Longdancao), Natural Indigo (青黛, Qingdai), Pinellia Rhizome (半夏, Banxia), Indian Bread with Hostwood (茯神, Fushen), Silkworm with Batrytis Larva (僵蚕, Jiangcan), Antelope Horn (羚羊角, Lingyangjiao), Leaf of Wild Mint Herb (薄荷叶, Boheye) and Cinnabar (朱砂, Zhusha). Its actions are stopping the wind and clearing away heat, calming the liver and checking exuberance of yang. It is indicated for acute infantile convulsion.

3. Hemiplegia-Treating and Stroke-Healing Decoction (补偏愈风汤, bu pian yu feng tang) *Brief Explanation on Prescriptions* 《医方简义》

It is comprised of Ginseng (人参, Renshen), Tuckahoe (茯苓, Fuling), Toasted Membranous Milkvetch Root (炙黄芪, Zhi Huangqi), Chinese Angelica Root (当归, Danggui), Eucommia Bark (杜仲, Duzhong), Achyranthes Root (怀牛膝, Huainiuxi), Prepared Rehmannia Root (熟

地, Shudi), Membranous Milkvetch Root (生黄芪, Sheng Huangqi), Largehead Atractylodes Rhizome (白术, Baizhu), Red Peony Root (赤芍, Chishao), Incised Notopterygium Rhizome or Root (羌活, Qianghuo), Doubleteeth Pubescent Angelica Root (独活, Duhuo), Cassia Twig (桂枝, Guizhi) and Chinese Taxillus Twig (桑寄生, Sangjisheng). Its actions are replenishing qi, enriching blood and calming the liver to stop the wind. It is indicated for atrophy of hands and feet due to increased activity of the liver resulting from deficiency of qi and blood.

2. Sweeping Down Decoction for Tension Hypertension (建瓴汤, jian ling tang)

Source: *Records of Traditional Chinese and Western Medicine in Combination* 《医学衷中参西录》
Composition: Dried Rehmannia Root (生地黄, Shengdihuang) 18g
Dragon's Bone (生龙骨, Sheng Longgu) 18g
Oyster Shell (生牡蛎, Sheng Muli) 18g
Achyranthes Root (怀牛膝, Huainiuxi) 30g
Common Yam Rhizome (生山药, Sheng Shanyao) 30g
Hematite (代赭石, Daizheshi) 24g
White Peony Root (白芍药, Baishaoyao) 12g
Chinese Arborvitae Seed (柏子仁, Baiziren) 12g
Actions: Calming the liver to stop the wind, nourishing yin and checking exuberance of yang.
Applied Syndrome: Cerebral hemorrhage due to hyperactivity of liver yang resulting from yin deficiency of the liver and kidney which leads to failure of water in nourishing wood. This is manifested as dizziness, feeling of heaviness, distention and pain in the head, aphasis, tinnitus and eye distention, palpitation and amnesia, insomnia and dreaminess, red tongue, wiry, hard and long pulse.
Points in Constitution: In this formula, Common Yam Rhizome (山药, Shanyao), Dried Rehmannia Root (生地黄, Shengdihuang) and White Peony Root (白芍药, Baishaoyao) are used to nourish the organs in lower jiao, which treats the primary cause of wind-stroke. The application of heavy materials is to suppress hyperactivity of yang and the use of Twotooth Achyranthes Root (牛膝, Niuxi) is to induce blood circulating downward so as to attain the purpose of treating the primary, the secondary, the upper and the lower together. Zhang Xichun, a famous ancient physician, said:"After taking this formula, encephalic blood stasis goes downwards as water pours down from a high place. Thus, cerebral hemorrhage will be healed of itself."
Indications:
1. Hypertension
2. Neurasthenia
3. Angioneurotic headache
4. Cerebrovascular accident (CAV)
5. Climacteric syndrome

Sweeping Down Decoction for Tension Hypertension
(Yin-Nourishing and Exuberant Yang-Checking Method)

Ingredients	Effects	Combined Effects	Syndrome	Chief Symptoms
Dried Rehmannia Root (生地黄, Shengdihuang) 18g White Peony Root (白芍药, Baishaoyao) 12g Common Yam Rhizome (生山药, Sheng Shanyao) 30g	Nourishing the liver and kidney	Calming the liver to stop the wind, nourishing yin and checking exuberance of yang	Cerebral hemorrhage (Hyperactivity of liver yang caused by yin deficiency of liver and kidney)	Dizziness, tinnitus and eye distention, palpitation and amnesia, insomnia and dreaminess, red tongue, wiry, hard and long pulse
Dragon's Bone (生龙骨, Sheng Longgu) 18g Oyster Shell (生牡蛎, Sheng Muli) 18g Hematite (代赭石, Daizheshi) 24g	Checking exuberance of yang and keeping the adverse qi downwards			
Achyranthes Root (怀牛膝, Huainiuxi) 30g	Nourishing the liver and kidney, causing blood to flow downwards			
Chinese Arborvitae Seed (柏子仁, Baiziren) 12g	Nourishing heart and tranquilizing the mind			

Precaution: It is contraindicated in vertigo and headache due to excessive fire of liver and gallbladder, or occurrence of wind resulting from extreme heat.

Associated Formulas:

1. Barbary Wolfberry, Chrysanthemum and Rehmannia Pill (杞菊地黄丸, qi ju di huang wan) *Medical Rank* 《医级》

This is comprised of the ingredients of Bolus of Six Drugs Containing Rhizome Rehmanniae Peaeparatae (六味地黄丸, liu wei di huang wan) plus Barbary Wolfberry Fruit (枸杞子, Gouqizi) and Chrysanthemum Flower (菊花, Juhua). Its actions are nourishing the liver and kidney and improving acuity of sight. It is indicated for blurred vision, failure in eyesight, dry eyes, epiphora induced by wind, dizziness, red tongue with little coating, thin and rapid pulse due to yin deficiency of the liver and kidney.

2. Yin-Nourishing and Wind-Calming Decoction (滋阴息风汤, zi yin xi feng tang) *Supplement to Essence of Medicine* 《医醇賸义》

This is comprised of Prepared Rehmannia Root（熟地黄，Shudihuang）, Chinese Angelica Root（当归，Danggui）, Barbary Wolfberry Fruit（枸杞子，Gouqizi）, Chinese Dodder Seed（菟丝子，Tusizi）, Chrysanthemum Flower（菊花，Juhua）, Medicinal Indian Mulberry Root（巴戟天，Bajitian）, Common St. Paulswort Herb（豨莶草，Xixiancao）, Tall Gastrodia Rhizome（天麻，Tianma）, Doubleteeth Pubescent Angelica Root（独活，Duhuo）, Chinese Date（大枣，Dazao）and Fresh Ginger（生姜，Shengjiang）. Its actions are replenishing the liver and kidney, nourishing yin and checking exuberance of yang. It is indicated for dizziness, convulsion and numbness of the limbs due to yin deficiency of the liver and kidney.

3. Gambirplant Hooked Stem and Branch Powder
（钩藤散，gou teng san）

Source: *Effective Prescriptions for Universal Relief*《普济本事方》
Composition: Gambirplant Hooked Stem and Branch（钩藤，Gouteng）9g
Chrysanthemum Flower（菊花，Juhua）9g
Gypsum（生石膏，Shengshigao）15g
Divaricate Saposhnikovia Root（防风，Fangfeng）6g
Dwarf Lilyturf Root（麦门冬，Maimendong）9g
Pinellia Rhizome（半夏，Banxia）6g
Tangerine Peel（橘皮，Jupi）6g
Indian Bread with Hostwood（茯神，Fushen）6g
Fresh Ginger（生姜，Shengjiang）3g
Licorice Root（甘草，Gancao）3g
Ginseng（人参，Renshen）3g
Actions: Clearing away liver heat, stopping wind and removing phlegm.
Applied Syndrome: Upper attacks of wind-phlegm due to stirring of the wind inside the body resulting from liver heat, manifested by dizziness, headache and irritability, epigastric fullness, vomiting and bitter taste in the mouth, red tongue with greasy coating, wiry pulse.
Points in Constitution: When Gambirplant Hooked Stem and Branch（钩藤，Gouteng）and Gypsum（生石膏，Shengshigao）are combined, they have the same actions of Antelope Horn（羚羊角，Lingyangjiao）, which are good at clearing away liver heat and calming the liver wind. If they are combined again with Two Vintage Herbs Decoction（二陈汤，er chen tang）, they can expel wind-phlegm. This formula can clear away liver heat, stop the wind and remove phlegm. Thus, it is very suitable for occurrence of wind syndrome in case of extreme heat. For those whose promordial qi is not impaired, Ginseng（人参，Renshen）should not be used.
Indications:
1. Neurosis
2. Hypertension
3. Climacteric syndrome

Gambirplant Hooked Stem and Branch Powder
(Heat-Removing and Wind-Stopping Method)

Ingredients	Effects	Combined Effects	Syndrome	Chief Symptoms
Gambirplant Hooked Stem and Branch (钩藤, Gouteng)9g Chrysanthemum Flower (菊花, Juhua)9g	Clearing away liver heat to relieve dizziness	Clearing away liver heat to stop the wind, resolving phlegm	Stirring of the wind inside the body due to liver heat, upper attacks of wind-phlegm	Dizziness, headache and irritability, epigastric fullness, vomiting and bitter taste in the mouth, red tongue with greasy coating, wiry pulse
Gypsum (生石膏, Shengshigao)15g Divaricate Saposhnikovia Root (防风, Fangfeng)6g	Clearing away heat to stop the wind			
Dwarf Lilyturf Root (麦门冬, Maimendong)9g	Nourishing yin and tranquilizing the mind			
Pinellia Rhizome (半夏, Banxia)6g Indian Bread with Hostwood (茯神, Fushen)6g Tangerine Peel (橘皮, Jupi)6g Fresh Ginger (生姜, Shengjiang)3g Licorice Root (甘草, Gancao)3g	Resolving phlegm and regulating stomach qi			
Ginseng (人参, Renshen)3g	Replenishing qi and promoting the production of body fluid			

Associated Formulas:

1. Gambirplant Hooked Stem and Branch Decoction (钩藤饮, gou teng yin) *The Golden Mirror of Medicine* 《医宗金鉴》

This is comprised of Ginseng (人参, Renshen), Scorpion (全蝎, Quanxie), Antelope Horn (羚羊角, Lingyangjiao), Tall Gastrodia Rhizome (天麻, Tianma), Prepared Licorice Root (炙甘草, Zhigancao) and Gambirplant Hooked Stem and Branch (钩藤, Gouteng). Both this decoction and the Gambirplant Hooked Stem and Branch Powder(钩藤散, gou teng yin) have the action of clearing away heat to stop the wind. But the decoction, compared with the powder, has a strong spasm-relieving action and is good at treating infantile convulsion due to up-stirring of the liver resulting from excessive heat.

2. Antelope Horn and Gambirplant Hooked Stem and Branch Decoction (羚角钩藤汤, ling jiao gou teng tang) *Popular Version of Treatise on Exogenous Febrile Diseases* 《通俗伤寒论》

This is comprised of Antelope Horn (羚羊角, Lingyangjiao), Mulberry Leaf (桑叶, Sangye), Tendrilleaf Fritillary Bulb (川贝母, Chuan Beimu), Dried Rehmannia Root (生地黄, Shengdihuang), Gambirplant Hooked Stem and Branch (钩藤, Gouteng), Chrysanthemum Flower (菊

花, Juhua), Indian Bread With Hostwood (茯神木, Fushenmu), White Peony Root (杭芍药, Hangshaoyao), Licorice Root (生甘草, Shenggancao) and Bamboo Shavings (淡竹茹, Danzhuru). Both this Antelope Horn and Gambirplant Hooked Stem and Branch Decoction(羚角钩藤汤, ling jiao gou teng tang) and the Gambirplant Hooked Stem and Branch Powder(钩藤散, gou teng san) have the action of clearing away heat to stop the wind. But the Antelope Horn and Gambirplant Hooked Stem and Branch Decoction(羚角钩藤汤, ling jiao gou teng tang) also has the actions of nourishing yin and promoting the production of body fluid, and is good for treating the syndrome of up-stirring of the liver accompanied by impairment of yin resulting from extreme heat.

4. Chinese Angelica, Gentian and Aloes Pill (当归龙荟丸, dang gui long hui wan)

Source: *Danxi's Experiential Therapy*《丹溪心法》
Composition: Chinese Angelica Root (当归, Danggui)9g
Chinese Gentian Root (龙胆草, Longdancao)6g
Cape Jasmine Fruit (山栀子, Shanzhizi)9g
Aloes (芦荟, Luhui)3g
Coptis Rhizome (黄连, Huanglian)6g
Chinese Corktree Bark (黄柏, Huangbai)6g
Baikal Skullcap Root (黄芩, Huangqin)6g
Rhubarb (大黄, Dahuang)3g
Common Aucklandia Root (木香, Muxiang)3g
Musk (麝香, Shexiang)0.15g taking it separately with water.
Actions: Clearing the liver and purging fire.
Applied Syndrome: Syndrome of excessive fire of the liver and gallbladder, manifested as dizziness, irritability, zealotry and delirium, constipation, dysuria with dark urine, red tongue with yellow coating, wiry, rapid and strong pulse.
Points in Constitution: Aloes (芦荟, Luhui) functions best at clearing the liver and removing heat; meanwhile it also can relax the bowels. When it is combined with Chinese Angelica Root (当归, Danggui), it enriches blood, moistens the intestines, purges fire without impairing yin and clear away heat without causing stagnation of blood. The characteristic of this formula lies in the good use of Common Aucklandia Root (木香, Muxiang) which can, by regulating functional activities of qi, prevent the cool-natured drugs from damaging the stomach. The use of Musk (麝香, Shexiang) is to induce resuscitation to treat mental disorder due to heat.
Indications:
1. Hypertension
2. Angioneurotic headache
3. Acute hepatitis, acute cholecystitis

Chinese Angelica, Gentian and Aloes Pill
(Liver-Clearing and Fire-Purging Method)

Ingredients	Effects	Combined Effects	Syndrome	Chief Symptoms
Chinese Angelica Root (当归, Danggui) 9g	Enriching blood, moistening the intestines to relax the bowels	Clearing and purging excessive fire of the liver and gallbladder	Syndrome of excessive fire of the liver and gallbladder	Dizziness, irritability, zealotry and delirium, constipation, dysuria with dark urine, red tongue with yellow coating, wiry, rapid and strong pulse
Aloes (芦荟, Luhui) 3g Rhubarb (大黄, Dahuang) 3g	Purging heat and relaxing the bowels			
Chinese Gentian Root (龙胆草, Longdancao) 6g	Clearing and purging heat-dampness of the liver and gallbladder			
Cape Jasmine Fruit (山栀子, Shanzhizi) 9g Coptis Rhizome (黄连, Huanglian) 6g Baikal Skullcap Root (黄芩, Huangqin) 6g Chinese Corktree Bark (黄柏, Huangbai) 6g	Clearing away heat and purging fire			
Common Aucklandia Root (木香, Muxiang) 3g	Activating flow of qi and alleviating pain			
Musk (麝香, Shexiang) 0.15g	Inducing resuscitation with the fragrant herbs			

4. Acute conjunctivitis
5. Mania

Precaution: This formula is especially designed for the syndrome of excessive heat of the liver and gallbladder. It is not suitable for the syndrome of hyperactivity of yang due to deficiency of yin.

Associated Formulas:

1. Gentian Liver-Purging Decoction (龙胆泻肝汤, long dan xie gan tang) *Collection of Formulae with Notes* 《医方集解》

This is comprised of Chinese Gentian Root (龙胆草, Longdancao), Baikal Skullcap Root (黄芩, Huangqin), Cape Jasmine Fruit (山栀子, Shanzhizi), Oriental Waterplantain Rhizome (泽泻, Zexie), Plantain Seed (车前子, Cheqianzi), Akebia Stem (木通, Mutong), Chinese Angelica Root (当归, Danggui), Dried Rehmannia Root (生地黄, Shengdihuang), Chinese Thorowax Root (柴胡, Chaihu) and Licorice Root (生甘草, Shenggancao). Both this decoction and the Chinese Angelica, Gentian and Aloes Pill (当归龙荟丸, dang gui long hui wan) have the functions of clearing away heat and promoting diuresis. Comparatively, the Chinese Angelica, Gentian and Aloes Pill (当归龙荟丸, dang gui long hui wan) has a strong heat-clearing action while the Gentianae Liver-Purging Decoction (龙胆泻肝汤, long dan xie gan tang) has a strong diuresis-inducing action and is good at treating the syndrome of flaming-up of excessive fire of the liver and gallbladder and attack of lower-jiao by damp-heat in the liver meridian.

2. Blue-Purging Pill (泻青丸, xie qing wan) *Key to Therapeutics of Children's Diseases* 《小儿药证直诀》

This is comprised of Chinese Angelica Root (当归, Danggui), Chinese Gentian Root (龙胆草, Longdancao), Szechwan Lovage Rhizome (川芎, Chuanxiong), Cape Jasmine Fruit (山栀子, Shanzhizi), Rhubarb (大黄, Dahuang), Incised Notopterygium Rhizome or Root (羌活, Qianghuo) and Divaricate Saposhnikovia Root (防风, Fangfeng). Both this formula and Chinese Angelica, Gentian and Aloes Pill(当归龙荟丸, dang gui long hui wan) can clear the liver and purging fire, but the Blue-Purging Pill(泻青丸, xie qing wan) is good at treating bitter taste in the mouth, red eyes, irritability, red tongue with yellow coating, taut and rapid pulse due to stagnation of liver-fire.

3. Left Golden Pill (左金丸, zuo jin wan) *Danxi's Experiential Therapy* 《丹溪心法》

This is comprised of Coptis Rhizome (黄连, Huanglian) and Medicinal Evodia Fruit (吴茱萸, Wuzhuyu). Its actions are clearing away heat and purging fire, keeping the adverse qi downwards to stop vomiting. It is indicated for distention and pain in the hypochondrium, feeling of a fullness and depression in the gastric cavity, belching, gastric upset with acid regurgitation, bitter taste in the mouth, vomiting, yellow and the Chinese Angelica, Gentian and Aloes Pill(当归龙荟丸, dang gui long hui wan) and coating and taut pulse due to attack of the stomach by liver-fire.

Additional Formulas

Yang Hyperactivity-Checking Decoction with Seven Drugs
（七物降下汤，qi wu jiang xia tang）

Source: *Hall for Repairing Musical Instrument* 《修琴堂》
Composition: Chinese Angelica Root（当归，Danggui）6g
Szechwan Lovage Rhizome（川芎，Chuanxiong）6g
White Peony Root（白芍药，Baishaoyao）9g
Prepared Rehmannia Root（熟地黄，Shudihuang）9g
Membranous Milkvetch Root（黄芪，Huangqi）6g
Gambirplant Hooked Stem and Branch（钩藤，Gouteng）15g
Chinese Corktree Bark（黄柏，Huangbai）9g
Actions: Nourishing yin, enriching blood and stopping the wind.
Applied Syndrome: Hyperactivity of liver yang with yin deficiency due to protracted or chronic diseases, manifested as dizziness, tinnitus, or edema in the lower limbs, pale tongue with less coating, deep, wiry and thin pulse.

Yang Hyperactivity-Checking Decoction with Seven Drugs
(Blood-Enriching and Wind-Stopping Method)

Ingredients	Effects	Combined Effects	Syndrome	Chief Symptoms
Chinese Angelica Root（当归，Danggui）6g Prepared Rehmannia Root（熟地黄，Shudihuang）9g Szechwan Lovage Rhizome（川芎，Chuanxiong）6g White Peony Root（白芍药，Baishaoyao）9g	Enriching blood and regulating the flow of blood	Enriching blood and dispersing the stagnated liver-qi	Hyperactivity of liver yang	Dizziness, tinnitus, headache, or edema in the lower limbs, pale tongue with little coating, deep, wiry and thin pulse
Gambirplant Hooked Stem and Branch（钩藤，Gouteng）15g Chinese Corktree Bark（黄柏，Huangbai）9g	Removing heat from the liver to stop the wind			
Membranous Milkvetch Root（黄芪，Huangqi）6g	Replenishing the primary qi			

Points in Constitution: The ingredients of Four Herbs Decoction (四物汤, si wu tang) are combined with Gambirplant Hooked Stem and Branch (钩藤, Gouteng) and Chinese Corktree Bark (黄柏, Huangbai) to clear the liver and remove heat from the blood. Membranous Milkvetch Root (黄芪, Huangqi) not only replenishes qi but also reduces blood pressure and promotes urination. The combination of Membranous Milkvetch Root (黄芪, Huangqi), which ascends qi, and Gambirplant Hooked Stem and Branch (钩藤, Gouteng), which descends qi, can mediate circulation of qi, thus water and blood circulation will be normalized and wind is stopped.

Indications:
1. Nephridial hypertension
2. Nephrotic syndrome
3. Terminal toxemia of pregnancy

Associated Formula:

Ass-hide Glue and Yolk Decoction (阿胶鸡子黄汤, e jiao ji zi huang tang) *Popular Version of Treatise on Exogenous Febrile Diseases*《通俗伤寒论》

This is comprised of Ass-Hide Glue (阿胶, Ejiao), White Peony Root (白芍药, Baishaoyao), Abalone Shell (石决明, Shijueming), Gambirplant Hooked Stem and Branch (钩藤, Gouteng), Dried Rehmannia Root (生地黄, Shengdihuang), Prepared Licorice Root (炙甘草, Zhi Gancao), Oyster Shell (生牡蛎, Sheng Muli), Chinese Starjasmine Stem (络石藤, Luoshiteng), Indian Bread With Hostwood (茯神木, Fushenmu) and Yolk (鸡子黄, Jizihuang). Its actions are nourishing yin, clearing away heat and calming the liver. It is indicated for dizziness, tinnitus, headache, red tongue with little coating, deep, wiry and thready pulse due to stirring-up of endopathogenic wind and deficiency of both yin and blood resulting from pathogenic heat impairing yin.

Blood Pressure-Reducing Decoction
(降压汤, jiang ya tang)

Source: *Jiangxi Journal of Traditional Chinese Medicine*《江西中医药》
Composition: Abalone Shell (石决明, Shijueming) 30g
Dan-shen Root (丹参, Danshen) 30g
Puncturevine Caltrop Fruit (刺蒺藜, Cijili) 30g
Common Selfheal Fruit-spike (夏枯草, Xiakucao) 30g
Plantain Seed (车前子, Cheqianzi) 45g
Actions: Stopping wind, clearing away heat and reducing blood pressure.
Applied Syndrome: Hypertension caused by attack of the head due to excessive fire and stirring-up of wind resulting from protracted stagnation of liver-qi and mental disorder, manifested as dizziness, headache, oppressing feeling in the chest, high blood pressure, irritability, insomnia and dreaminess, tender and red tongue with little coating, wiry, thin and rapid pulse.

Blood Pressure-Reducing Decoction
(Liver-Calming and Exuberant Yang-Checking Method)

Ingredients	Effects	Combined Effects	Syndrome	Chief Symptoms
Abalone Shell (石决明, Shijueming) 30g	Calming the liver and checking exuberance of yang, clearing away liver heat and improving acuity of sight	Checking exuberance of yang and clearing away heat, stopping the wind and reducing blood pressure	Hypertension (hyperactivity of liver-yang and excessive heat in the liver meridian)	High blood pressure, dizziness and headache, oppressed feeling in the chest and irritability, insomnia and dreaminess, tender and red tongue with little coating, wiry, thin and rapid pulse
Puncturevine Caltrop Fruit (刺蒺藜, Cijili) 30g Common Selfheal Fruit-Spike (夏枯草, Xiakucao) 30g	Dispersing the stagnated liver-qi and clearing away heat			
Plantain Seed (车前子, Cheqianzi) 45g	Clearing away heat and promoting urination			
Dan-Shen Root (丹参, Danshen) 30g	Activating blood circulation and removing blood stasis			

Points in Constitution: The characteristic of this formula is to combine several drugs which have been proved to have an obvious pressure-reducing action by modern research into a formula. But originally, it does not turn aside from the method of clearing away liver-heat.

Indications:
1. Hypertension
2. Climacteric syndrome
3. Vegetative nerve functional disturbance
4. Angioneurotic headache

Precaution: One of the main symptoms of the syndrome is wiry, thready and rapid pulse, which is the manifestation of deficiency of yin and excess of heat. However, there are not the drugs for nourishing yin and promoting the production of body fluid. So in the clinic, this formula should be modified when it is used for vertigo due to yin deficiency and hyperactivity of fire.

Associated Formulas:

1. Antelope Horn and Gambirplant Hooked Stem and Branch Decoction (羚角钩藤汤, ling jiao gou teng tang) *Popular Version of Treatise on Exogenous Febrile Diseases* 《通俗伤寒论》

This is comprised of Antelope Horn (羚角, Lingjiao), Mulberry Leaf (桑叶, Sangye), Tendrilleaf Fritillary Bulb (川贝母, Chuan Beimu), Dried Rehmannia Root (生地黄, Shengdihuang), Gambirplant Hooked Stem and Branch (钩藤, Gouteng), Chrysanthemum Flower (菊花, Juhua), Indian Bread with Hostwood (茯神, Fushen), White Peony Root (白芍药,

Baishaoyao), Bamboo Shavings (竹茹, Zhuru) and Licorice Root (甘草, Gancao). Both this formula and the Blood Pressure-Reducing Decoction(降压汤, jiang ya tang) have the actions of clearing away heat, stopping the wind and reducing blood pressure, but Antelope Horn and Gambirplant Hooked Stem and Branch Decoction(羚角钩藤汤, ling jiao gou teng tang) is good at treating high fever, restlessness, convulsion, dry and crimson tongue, wiry, rapid and forceful pulse due to excessive heat in the liver meridian which results in up-stirring of the liver. Blood Pressure-Reducing Decoction (降压汤, jiang ya tang) is good at treating high blood pressure, dizziness, oppressed feeling in the chest, irritability, dreaminess, wiry, thin and rapid pulse due to hyperactivity of liver yang which leads to stirring-up of the liver by calming the liver and checking exuberance of yang.

2. Liver-Calming and Wind-Stopping Decoction (镇肝息风汤, zhen gan xi feng tang) *Records of Traditional Chinese and Western Medicine in Combination*《医学衷中参西录》

This is comprised of Twotooth Achyranthes Root (牛膝, Niuxi), Hematite (代赭石, Daizheshi), Dragon's Bone (生龙骨, Sheng Longgu), Oyster Shell (牡蛎, Muli), Tortoise Shell and Plastron (龟版, Guiban), White Peony Root (杭芍药, Hangshaoyao), Figwort Root (玄参, Xuanshen), Cochinchinese Asparagus Root (天门冬, Tianmendong), Szechwan Chinaberry Fruit (川楝子, Chuanlianzi), Malt (麦芽, Maiya), Capillary Wormwood Herb (茵陈, Yinchen) and Licorice Root (甘草, Gancao). Both Blood Pressure-Reducing Decoction(降压汤, jiang ya tang) and this Liver-Calming and Wind-Stopping Decoction(镇肝息风汤, zhen gan xi feng tang) have the actions of stopping the wind, checking exuberance of yang and reducing blood pressure. The latter also has yin-nourishing action and is good at treating vertigo, tinnitus, dysphoria with smothery sensation, or gradual atrophy of the limbs, deviation of the eye and mouth or faint and flaccidity, wiry, long and forceful pulse due to yin deficiency of both the liver and kidney and stirring-up of the liver resulting from hyperactivity of yang.

3. Tall Gastrodia and Gambirplant Hooked Stem and Branch Decoction (天麻钩藤饮, tian ma gou teng yin) *New Explanation of Diagnosis and Treatment of Miscellaneous Disease*《杂病证治新义》

This is comprised of Tall Gastrodia Rhizome (天麻, Tianma), Gambirplant Hooked Stem and Branch (钩藤, Gouteng), Abalone Shell (石决明, Shijueming), Cape Jasmine Fruit (山栀子, Shanzhizi), Baikal Skullcap Root (黄芩, Huangqin), Twotooth Achyranthes Root (牛膝, Niuxi), Eucommia Bark (杜仲, Duzhong), Motherwort Herb (益母草, Yimucao), Chinese Taxillus Twig (桑寄生, Sangjisheng), Indian Bread with Hostwood (茯神, Fushen) and Fleece-Flower Stem (夜交藤, Yejiaoteng). Its actions are calming the liver to stop dizziness, benefiting the kidney and tranquilizing the mind. This formula is good at treating vertigo and insomnia due to upward attack of the head and inward disturbance of the mind by hyperactivity of yang.

Qi-Replenishing and Yin-Nourishing Decoction
(益气养阴汤, yi qi yang yin tang)

Source: *Hubei Journal of Traditional Chinese Medicine*《湖北中医杂志》

Composition: Pilose Asiabell Root (党参, Dangshen)15g
Dwarf Lilyturf Root (麦门冬, Maimendong)9g
Chinese Magnoliavine Fruit (五味子, Wuweizi)6g
Toasted Membranous Milkvetch Root (炙黄芪, Zhi Huangqi)15g
Cassia Bark (肉桂, Rougui)3g
Prepared Licorice Root (炙甘草, Zhi Gancao)9g
Shriveled Wheat (浮小麦, Fuxiaomai)30g
Chinese Date (大枣, Dazao)9g

Actions: Replenishing qi, nourishing yin and raising blood pressure.

Applied Syndrome: Hypotension due to habitual weakness or deficiency of both qi and blood after severe or chronic diseases. Deficiency of qi causes failure of yang to ascend and insufficiency of blood leads to failure of the brain in nourishment, thus bringing about the manifestations of vertigo, headache, listlessness, tiredness, restlessness of deficiency type and spontaneous sweating, pale tongue with white coating, feeble and weak pulse.

Qi-Replenishing and Yin-Nourishing Decoction
(Method of Replenishing both Qi and Yin)

Ingredients	Effects	Combined Effects	Syndrome	Chief Symptoms
Pilose Asiabell Root (党参, Dangshen)15g Toasted Membranous Milkvetch Root (炙黄芪, Zhi Huangqi)15g	Replenishing qi and lifting yang	Replenishing qi, nourishing yin and raising blood pressure	Hypotension (deficiency of both qi and yin)	Low blood pressure, vertigo, headache, listlessness and tiredness, restlessness, spontaneous sweating, pale tongue with white coating, feeble and weak pulse
Dwarf Lilyturf Root (麦门冬, Maimendong)9g Chinese Magnoliavine Fruit (五味子, Wuweizi)6g	Nourishing yin and promoting the production of body fluid			
Cassia Bark (肉桂, Rougui)3g	Warming qi and blood			
Shriveled Wheat (浮小麦, Fuxiaomai)30g	Replenishing qi and arresting perspiration			
Chinese Date (大枣, Dazao)9g Prepared Licorice Root (炙甘草, Zhi Gancao)9g	Replenishing qi and regulating the middle-jiao			

Points in Constitution: This formula is the combination of Pulse-Activating Decoction (生脉饮, sheng mai yin) and Licorice, Wheat and Chinese Date Decoction (甘麦大枣汤, gan mai da zao tang) plus Membranous Milkvetch Root (黄芪, Huangqi), and Cassia Bark (肉桂, Rougui).

It replenishes qi and nourishes yin to enrich blood, which benefits the recovery of blood pressure.

Indications:

1. Hypotension
2. Low blood sugar
3. Neurosis, vegetative nerve functional disturbance
4. Qi and Yin deficiency due to nutritional anemia, severe disease, chronic disease or operation

Precaution: This formula is especially designed for vertigo due to failure to ascend clear yang resulting from deficiency of qi and yin. It is not suitable for vertigo caused by hyperactivity of liver yang, or excessive phlegm-dampness or hyperactivity of yang due to deficiency of yin.

Associated Formulas:

1. Eight Treasures Decoction（八珍汤，ba zhen tang）*Classification and Treatment of Traumatic Diseases*《正体类要》

This is comprised of Chinese Angelica Root（当归，Danggui）, Szechwan Lovage Rhizome（川芎，Chuanxiong）, White Peony Root（白芍药，Baishaoyao）, Prepared Rehmannia Root（熟地黄，Shudihuang）, Ginseng（人参，Renshen）, Largehead Atractylodes Rhizome（白术，Baizhu）, Tuckahoe（茯苓，Fuling）, Fresh Ginger（生姜，Shengjiang）, Chinese Date（大枣，Dazao）and Prepared Licorice Root（炙甘草，Zhi Gancao）. This formula and the Qi-Replenishing and Yin-Nourishing Decoction（益气养阴汤，yi qi yang yin tang）can both replenish qi, tonify blood and treat dizziness, listlessness and tiredness due to deficiency of qi and yin. However, Qi-Replenishing and Yin-Nourishing Decoction（益气养阴汤，yi qi yang yin tang）particularly emphasizes tonifying the heart and benefiting the kidney while Eight Treasures Decoction（八珍汤，ba zhen tang）stresses tonifying the heart and Spleen.

2. Ten Strong Tonic Herbs Pill（十全大补汤，shi quan da bu tang）*Prescriptions of Peaceful Benevolent Dispensary*《和剂局方》

This consists of the ingredients of Four Gentlemen Decoction（四君子汤，si jun zi tang）, Four Herbs Decoction（四物汤，si wu tang）and Membranous Milkvetch Root（黄芪，Huangqi）and Cassia Bark（肉桂，Rougui）. On the basis of replenishing qi, which is the action of Four Gentlemen Decoction（四君子汤，si jun zi tang）and enriching the blood, which is the action of Four Herbs Decoction（四物汤，si wu tang）, this formula enhances the action of replenishing kidney-qi. It is usually applied for consumptive diseases with cough, emission, soreness of loin, unhealing of skin and external desease, metrorrhagia and metrostaxis in woman due to severe deficiency of the kidney and unconsolidation of the kidney-qi.

Lipide-Lowering and Vessels-Dredging Decoction
（降脂通脉饮，jiang zhi tong mai yin）

Source: *Journal of Traditional Chinese Medicine*《中医杂志》
Composition: Prepared Tuber Fleeceflower Root（制何首乌，Zhi Heshouwu）30g
Cherokee Rose Fruit（金樱子，Jinyingzi）30g

Cassia Seed (决明子, Juemingzi)30g
Coix Seed (薏苡仁, Yiyiren)30g
Capillary Wormwood Herb (茵陈, Yinchen)24g
Oriental Waterplantain Rhizome (泽泻, Zexie)24g
Hawthorn Fruit (山楂, Shanzha)18g
Chinese Thorowax Root (柴胡, Chaihu)12g
Turmeric Root-Tuber (郁金, Yujin)12g
Rhubarb (大黄, Dahuang) (fried with wine)6g

Actions: Tonifying the liver and kidney, clearing the liver and removing phlegm, regulating flow of qi and activating blood circulation.

Applied Syndrome: Hyperlipemia, caused by accumulation of turbid phlegm which results from disturbance in qi transformation and yin deficiency of both the liver and kidney. It is manifested as vertigo, corpulence, tiredness, palpitation and oppressing feeling in the chest, anorexia, red tongue with white coating, wiry and thin pulse.

Lipide-Lowering and Vessels-Dredging Decoction
(Blood-Enriching, Dampness-Removing and Blood Flow-Activating Method)

Ingredients	Effects	Combined Effects	Syndrome	Chief Symptoms
Prepared Fleeceflower Root (制何首乌, Zhi Heshouwu)30g Cherokee Rose Fruit (金樱子, Jinyingzi)30g	Tonifying the liver and kidney, supplementing essence and enriching blood	Tonifying the liver and kidney, clearing the liver and removing phlegm, regulating flow of qi and activating circulation of blood	Hyperlipemia (stagnation of qi and blood due to accumulation of turbid phlegm and deficiency of the liver and kidney)	Hyperlipemia, vertigo, fatness, or tiredness, palpitation and oppressing feeling in the chest, anorexia, red tongue with white coating, wiry and thin pulse
Cassia Seed (决明子, Juemingzi)30g Coix Seed (薏苡仁, Yiyiren)30g Capillary Wormwood Herb (茵陈, Yinchen)24g Oriental Waterplantain Rhizome (泽泻, Zexie)24g	Calming the liver, checking exuberance of yang and clearing away phlegm heat			
Chinese Thorowax Root (柴胡, Chaihu)12g Turmeric Root-Tuber (郁金, Yujin)12g Hawthorn Fruit (生山楂, Sheng Shanzha)18g	Dispersing the liver and regulating the flow of qi, activating blood circulation and removing blood stasis			
Prepared Rhubarb with Wine (酒大黄, Jiu Dahuang) (fired with wine)6g	Slowly purging pathogen retention, activating blood circulation and removing blood stasis			

Points in Constitution: This formula is applied for hyperlipemia by tonifying the kidney, removing phlegm and activating blood circulation. It is a method for strengthening body resistance and eliminating pathogenic factors at the same time. Among this formula the Hawthorn Fruit (山楂, Shanzha), Prepared Rhubarb with Wine (酒大黄, Jiu Dahuang), Oriental Waterplantain Rhizome (泽泻, Zexie) and Capillary Wormwood Herb (茵陈, Yinchen) are the common drugs for lowering blood-fat.

Indications:
1. Hyperlipemia
2. Coronary heart disease

Precaution: It is not suitable to hyperlipemia and vertigo due to hyperactivity of liver yang.

Associated Formulas:

1. Tall Gastrodia and Gambirplant Hooked Stem and Branch Decoction (天麻钩藤饮, tian ma gou teng yin) *New Explanation of Diagnosis and Treatment of Miscellaneous Disease*《杂病证治新义》

This is comprised of Tall Gastrodia Rhizome (天麻, Tianma), Gambirplant Hooked Stem and Branch (钩藤, Gouteng), Abalone Shell (石决明, Shijueming), Cape Jasmine Fruit (山栀子, Shanzhizi), Baikal Skullcap Root (黄芩, Huangqin), Twotooth Achyranthes Root (牛膝, Niuxi), Eucommia Bark (杜仲, Duzhong), Motherwort Herb (益母草, Yimucao), Chinese Taxillus Twig (桑寄生, Sangjisheng), Fleece-Flower Stem (夜交藤, Yejiaoteng) and Indian Bread with Hostwood (茯神, Fushen). Both this Tall Gastrodia and Gambirplant Hooked Stem and Branch Decoction (天麻钩藤饮, tian ma gou teng yin) and the Lipide-Lowering and Vessels-Dredging Decoction (降脂通脉饮, jiang zhi tong mai yin) can be applied to calm the liver and check exuberance of yang to treat vertigo, but comparatively, the former [Tall Gastrodia and Gambirplant Hooked Stem and Branch Decoction (天麻钩藤饮, tian ma gou teng yin)] is stronger than the latter [Lipide-Lowering and Vessels-Dredging Decoction (降脂通脉饮, jiang zhi tong mai yin)] in the action of nourishing the liver and kidney. The latter is better than the former in tha actions of clearing away heat and tranquilizing the mind.

2. Back to the Left Pill (左归丸, zuo gui wan) *Jingyue's Complete Works*《景岳全书》

This is comprised of Prepared Rehmannia Root (熟地黄, Shudihuang), Common Yam Rhizome (山药, Shanyao), Barbary Wolfberry Fruit (枸杞子, Gouqizi), Asiatic Cornelian Cherry Fruit (山茱萸, Shanzhuyu), Twotooth Achyranthes Root (牛膝, Niuxi), Chinese Dodder Seed (菟丝子, Tusizi), Antler Glue (鹿角胶, Lujiaojiao) and Glue of Tortoise Shell and Plastron (龟版胶, Guibanjiao). Both this formula and the Lipide-Lowering and Vessels-Dredging Decoction (降脂通脉饮, jiang zhi tong mai yin) can treat vertigo due to kidney deficiency, but the Back to the Left Pill (左归丸, zuo gui wan) is stronger than Lipide-Lowering and Vessels-Dredging Decoction (降脂通脉饮, jiang zhi tong mai yin) in nourishing yin and invigorating kidney and is used for vertigo, soreness and weakness of the loins and knees, night sweating, dryness of the mouth and throat, emission and spermatorrhea due to extreme deficiency of kidney yin.

3. Pinellia, Largehead Atractylodes and Tall Gastrodia Decoction (半夏白术天麻汤, ban xia bai zhu tian ma tang) *Medicine Comprehended*《医学心悟》

This is comprised of Pinellia Rhizome (半夏, Banxia), Largehead Atractylodes Rhizome (白

术，Baizhu)，Tall Gastrodia Rhizome（天麻，Tianma)，Tuckahoe（茯苓，Fuling)，Tangerine Peel（橘红，Juhong)，Licorice Root（甘草，Gancao)，Fresh Ginger（生姜，Shengjiang) and Chinese Date（大枣，Dazao). Both this Pinellia, Largehead Atractylodes and Tall Gastrodia Decoction（半夏白术天麻汤，ban xia bai zhu tian ma tang) and Lipide-Lowering and Vessels-Dredging Decoction（降脂通脉饮，jiang zhi tong mai yin) can be used to treat vertigo. However, since the Pinellia, Largehead Atractylodes and Tall Gastrodia Decoction（半夏白术天麻汤，ban xia bai zhu tian ma tang) has strong phlegm-resolving and wind-Stopping actions, but not the action of nourishing the liver and kidney, it is only good at treating vertigo due to upward attack of the head by wind-phlegm.

Coronary Heart Disease Tablet Number Two
冠心Ⅱ号（guan xin er hao）
Coronary Heart Disease Tablet（冠心片，guan xin pian）

Source: *Reference of Study on Traditional Chinese Medicine*《中医药研究参考》
Composition: Dan-Shen Root（丹参，Danshen)30g
Szechwan Lovage Rhizome（川芎，Chuanxiong)15g
Safflower（红花，Honghua)15g
Red Peony Root（赤芍药，Chishaoyao)15g
Rosewood（降香，Jiangxiang)15g

Actions: Promoting blood circulation and removing blood stasis, activating flow of qi and alleviating pain. Applied Syndrome: Obstruction of qi or pain in the chest, caused by blockage of coronary arteries resulting from stagnation of qi and blood and manifested as stabbing pain in the chest which may radiate to the back, shortness of breath and oppressing feeling in the chest, dark purple tongue, deep and unsmooth pulse.

Points in Constitution: In this formula, Dan-Shen Root（丹参，Danshen), Szechwan Lovage Rhizome（川芎，Chuanxiong), Safflower（红花，Honghua) and Red Peony Root（赤芍，Chishao) are all the drugs for activating blood circulation and removing blood stasis. The herb of Rosewood（降香，Jiangxiang) has the action of promoting flow of qi and alleviating pain. Modern research has shown that this formula has a good effect on coronary heart disease and angina pectoris.

Indications:
1. Coronary heart disease, angina pectoris
2. Myocardial infarction (MI)
3. Gastroduodenal ulcer
4. Menalgia

Associated Formulas:
1. Palpitation-Relieving Decoction（宁心汤，ning xin tang) *Liaoning Journal of Traditonal Chinese Medicine*《辽宁中医杂志》Number 6, 1983

Coronary Heart Disease Tablet Number Two
(Method of Activating Blood Circulation and Removing Blood Stasis)

Ingredients	Effects	Combined Effects	Syndrome	Chief Symptoms
Dan-Shen Root (丹参, Danshen) 30g	Enriching blood and activating blood circulation	Activating blood circulation and removing blood stasis, promoting flow of qi and alleviating pain	Coronary heart disease (obstruction of coronary artery due to stagnation of qi and blood)	Stabbing pain in the chest which radiates to the back, shortness of breath and oppressing feeling in the chest, dark purple tongue, deep and unsmooth pulse
Szechwan Lovage Rhizome (川芎, Chuanxiong) 15g	Activating blood circulation, promoting flow of qi and alleviating pain			
Safflower (红花, Honghua) 15g Red Peony Root (赤芍, Chishao) 15g	Activating blood circulation and removing blood stasis			
Rosewood (降香, Jiangxiang) 15g	Activating blood circulation, promoting flow of qi and alleviating pain			

This is comprised of the ingredients of Peech Seed and Safflower Decoction Containing Four Drugs (桃红四物汤, tao hong si wu tang) plus Heterophylly Falsestarwort Root (太子参, Taizishen), Dan-Shen Root (丹参, Danshen), Tuckahoe (茯苓, Fuling), Common Aucklandia Root (木香, Muxiang) and Licorice Root (甘草, Gancao). Its actions are activating blood circulation and removing blood stasis, replenishing qi and nourishing yin. It is indicated for obstruction of qi in the chest due to obstruction of yang in the chest and stagnation of qi and blood.

2. Dan-Shen Decoction (丹参饮, dan shen yin) *Current Formulae in Verse* 《时方歌括》

This is comprised of Dan-Shen Root (丹参, Danshen), Sandalwood (檀香, Tanxiang) and Villous Amomum Fruit (砂仁, Sharen). Its actions are activating blood circulation and dissolving blood stasis, activating flow of qi and alleviating pain. It is indicated for various pericardial and gastric pain due to stagnation of qi and blood.

3. Blood-House Blood Stasis-Dispelling Decoction (血府逐瘀汤, xue fu zhu yu tang) *Correction of Medical Classics* 《医林改错》

This is comprised of the ingredients of Peech Seed and Safflower Decoction Containing Four Drugs (桃红四物汤, tao hong si wu tang) plus Twotooth Achyranthes Root (牛膝, Niuxi), Balloonflower Root (桔梗, Jiegeng), Chinese Thorowax Root (柴胡, Chaihu), Bitter Orange (枳壳, Zhiqiao) and Licorice Root (甘草, Gancao). Its actions are activating blood circulation and dissolving blood stasis, activating flow of qi and alleviating pain. It is indicated for chronic localized stabbing pain in the chest and head due to blood stasis and also due to qi stagnation.

4. Snakegourd, Longstamen Onion and Liquor Decoction (瓜蒌薤白白酒汤, gua lou xie bai bai jiu tang) *Synopsis of Golden Cabinet*《金匮要略》

This is comprised of Snakegourd Fruit (瓜蒌, Gualou), Longstamen Onion Bulb (薤白, Xiebai) and Distilled Spirit (白酒, Baijiu). Its actions are relieving the obstruction of yang-qi and dissipating blockages, activating flow of qi and removing phlegm. It is indicated for obstruction of qi in the chest with slight turbid phlegm.

5. Snakegourd, Longstamen Onion and Pinellia Decoction (瓜蒌薤白半夏汤, gua lou xie bai ban xia tang) *Synopsis of Cabinet*《金匮要略》

This is comprised of the ingredients of Snakegourd, Longstamen Onion and Liquor Decoction (瓜蒌薤白半夏汤, gua lou xie bai ban xia tang) plus Pinellia Rhizome (半夏, Banxia). It is good at warming and relieving the obstruction of yang in the chest, eliminating phlegm and dissipating blockages. It is indicated for obstruction of qi in the chest with excessive turbid phlegm manifested as severe asthma which causes the inability to lie flat.

6. Immature Bitter Orange, Longstamen Onion and Cassia Twig Decoction (枳实薤白桂枝汤, zhu shi xie bai gui zhi tang) *Synopsis of Golden Cabinet*《金匮要略》

This is comprised of Immature Bitter Orange (枳实, Zhishi), Longstamen Onion Bulb (薤白, Xiebai), Officinal Magnolia Bark (厚朴, Houpo), Cassia Twig (桂枝, Guizhi) and Snakegourd Fruit (瓜蒌, Gualou). Its actions are relieving the obstruction of yang-qi and dissipating stasis, activating flow of qi and alleviating pain. It is indicated for obstruction of qi in the chest with severe accumulation of phlegm and stagnation of qi manifested as fullness and oppression in the chest and feeling of gas rushing up from the hypochondrium to the thorax.

7. Storesin Pill for Coronary Heart Disease (冠心苏合丸, guan xin su he wan) *Pharmacopoeia of the People's Republic of China*《中华人民共和国药典》

This is comprised of Storesin (苏合香, Suhexiang), Borneol (冰片, Bingpian), Olibanum (乳香, Ruxiang), Sandalwood (檀香, Tanxiang) and Dutchmanspipe Root (青木香, Qingmuxiang). Its actions are regulating flow of qi, dispersing the obstructed qi in the chest and alleviating pain. It is indicated for an oppressing feeling and pain in the chest due to obstruction of qi resulting from failure of yang-qi in transportation.

8. Storesin Pill (苏合香丸, su he xiang wan) *Prescriptions of Peaceful Benevolent Dispensary*《和剂局方》

This is comprised of Largehead Atractylodes Rhizome (白术, Baizhu), Dutchmanspipe Root (青木香, Qingmuxiang), Nutgrass Galingale Rhizome (香附, Xiangfu), Cinnabar (朱砂, Zhusha), Medicine Terminalia Fruit (诃子, Hezi), Sandalwood (檀香, Tanxiang), Benzoin (安息香, Anxixiang), Chinese Eaglewood Wood (沉香, Chenxiang), Musk (麝香, Shexiang), Clove Flower-Bud (丁香, Dingxiang), Long Pepper Fruit (荜茇, Biba), Borneol (冰片, Bingpian), Prepared Frankincense (薰陆香, Xunluxiang), Storesin Oil (苏合香油, Suhexiangyou) and Asiatic Rhinoceros Horn (犀角, Xijiao). Its actions are warming and activating yang, inducing resuscitation, relieving the depressed qi and eliminating turbid evils. It is indicated for pain in the chest due to accumulation of cold in the blood vessels resulting from stagnation of qi and stasis of blood.

Heart-Stimulating Decoction
(强心饮, qiang xin yin)

Source: *Liaoning Journal of Traditonal Chinese Medicine*《辽宁中医杂志》
Composition: Pilose Asiabell Root (党参, Dangshen)15g
Membranous Milkvetch Root (黄芪, Huangqi)15g
Prepared Aconite Root (附子, Fuzi)9~15g
Shorthorned Epimedium Herb (淫羊藿, Yinyanghuo)12g
Dan-Shen Root (丹参, Danshen)15g
Motherwort Herb (益母草, Yimucao)30g
Siberian Solomonseal Rhizome (黄精, Huangjing)12g
Dwarf Lilyturf Root (麦门冬, Maimendong)15g
Licorice Root (甘草, Gancao)6g
Actions: Warming yang and replenishing qi, activating blood circulation and invigorating pulse-beating.
Applied Syndrome: Obstruction of qi in the chest, palpitation and severe palpitation due to obstruction of yang-qi and deficiency of both qi and yin, manifested as an oppressing feeling in the chest and shortness of breath, palpitation and severe palpitation, intolerance of cold, pale and corpulent tongue, thin or knotted and intermittent pulse.

Heart-Stimulating Decoction
(Yang-Warming and Qi-Replenishing Method)

Ingredients	Effects	Combined Effects	Syndrome	Chief Symptoms
Pilose Asiabell Root (党参, Dangshen)15g Membranous Milkvetch Root (黄芪, Huangqi)15g Licorice Root (甘草, Gancao)6g	Replenishing qi and supporting the healthy qi	Warming yang and replenishing qi, activating blood circulation and invigorating pulse-beating	Obstruction of coronary artery due to deficiency of yang-qi	Oppressing feeling in the chest and shortness of breath, palpitation and sever palpitation, intolerance of cold, pale and corpulent tongue, thin or knotted and intermittent pulse
Prepared Aconite Root (附子, Fuzi)9~15g Shorthorned Epimedium Herb (淫羊藿, Yinyanghuo)12g	Warming and restoring yang-qi			
Dan-Shen Root (丹参, Danshen)15g Motherwort Herb (益母草, Yimucao)30g	Activating blood circulation and enriching blood			
Siberian Solomonseal Rhizome (黄精, Huangjing)12g Dwarf Lilyturf Root (麦门冬, Maimendong)15g	Replenishing qi and nourishing yin			

Points in Constitution: Combination of prepared Aconite Root（附子，Fuzi）, Membranous Milkvetch Root（黄芪，Huangqi）and Pilose Asiabell Root（党参，Dangshen）can warm yang and replenish qi. Coordination of Dan-Shen Root（丹参，Danshen）and Motherwort Herb（益母草，Yimucao）can activate blood circulation and invigorate the pulse. The combination of these two groups of drugs results in sufficiency of yang-qi of the heart and regular blood circulation.

Indications:
1. Sick sinus syndrome
2. Auriculo-ventricular block (AVB)
3. Coronary heart disease
4. Sinus bradycardia
5. Chronic cardiac insufficiency

Associated Formulas:

1. Cassia Twig, Licorice, Dragon's Bone and Oyster Shell Decoction（桂枝甘草龙骨牡蛎汤, gui zhi gan cao long gu mu li tang）*Treatise on Exogenous Febrile Diseases*《伤寒论》

This is comprised of Cassia Twig（桂枝，Guizhi）, Licorice Root（甘草，Gancao）, Dragon's Bone（龙骨，Longgu）and Oyster Shell（牡蛎，Muli）. Its actions are warming and replenishing heart-yang, tranquilizing the mind and relieving palpitation. It is indicated for palpitation due to deficiency of heart yang.

2. Cassia Twig and Licorice Decoction（桂枝甘草汤, gui zhi gan cao tang）*Treatise on Exogenous Febrile Diseases*《伤寒论》

This is comprised of Cassia Twig（桂枝，Guizhi）and Licorice Root（甘草，Gancao）. Its actions are benefiting the heart and restoring yang. It is indicated for palpitation which can be relieved if pressed by hands, mostly due to deficiency of heart-yang resulting from extreme diaphoresis.

3. Devine Black Bird Decoction（真武汤, zhen wu tang）*Treatise on Exogenous Febrile Diseases*《伤寒论》

This is comprised of Tuckahoe（茯苓，Fuling）, White Peony Root（白芍药，Baishaoyao）, Largehead Atractylodes Rhizome（白术，Baizhu）, Fresh Ginger（生姜，Shengjiang）and Prepared Aconite Root（附子，Fuzi）. Its actions are warming yang and excreting water. It is indicated for palpitation and twitching of different parts of the body and eyes due to yang deficiency and retention of water evils.

Heart Failure Mixture
（心衰合剂，xin shuai he ji）

Source: *Journal of Traditional Chinese Medicine*《中医杂志》
Composition: Pepperweed Seed（葶苈子，Tinglizi）30g
White Mulberry Root-Bark（桑白皮，Sangbaipi）30g
Plantain Seed（车前子，Cheqianzi）(wrapped with cloth for boiling)30g

Oriental Waterplantain Rhizome (泽泻, Zexie)15g
Membranous Milkvetch Root (生黄芪, Sheng Huangqi)30g
Heterophylly Falsestarwort Root (太子参, Taizishen)30g
Chinese Magnoliavine Fruit (五味子, Wuweizi)12g
Dwarf Lilyturf Root (麦门冬, Maimendong)15g
Dan-shen Root (丹参, Danshen)30g
Chinese Angelica Root (当归, Danggui)12g

Actions: Purging lung and promoting urination, replenishing qi and nourishing yin, activating blood circulation and invigorating pulse-beating.

Applied Syndrome: Congestive heart failure. Insufficiency of the heart qi leads to blockage of blood vessels, retention of body fluid and obstruction of lung qi and is manifested as palpitation, shortness of breath, cough, asthma with scanty foamy sputum or sputum with bloody streaks, feeling of distention and fullness in the chest, hypochondrium and abdomen, oliguria, edema, pale tongue or with petechia, deep, slow and unsmooth pulse, or deep and unsmooth pulse.

Heart Failure Mixture
(Qi-Replenishing and Urination-Inducing Method)

Ingredients	Effects	Combined Effects	Syndrome	Chief Symptoms
Membranous Milkvetch Root (生黄芪, Sheng Huangqi)30g Heterophylly Falsestarwort Root(太子参,Taizishen)30g	Replenishing the heart and lung	Purging the lung and inducing urination, replenishing qi and nourishing yin, activating blood circulation and invigorating pulse-beating	Heart failure. (Obstruction of the lung due to deficiency of qi, blood stasis and retention of body fluid)	Palpitation, shortness of breath, cough and asthma with scanty foamy sputum, feeling of distention and fullness in the chest and hypochondrium and abdomen, oliguria and edema, pale tongue or with petechia, deep, slow and unsmooth pulse or deep and unsmooth pulse
Pepperweed Seed or Flixweed Tansymustard Seed(葶苈子,Tinglizi)30g White Mulberry Root-Bark (桑白皮, Sangbaipi)30g	Purging the lung and relieving asthma, inducing urination to relieve edema			
Plantain Seed (车前子, Cheqianzi)30g Oriental Waterplantain Rhizome(泽泻,Zexie)15g	Inducing urination to eliminate dampness			
Dan-Shen Root (丹参, Danshen)30g Chinese Angelica Root (当归, Danggui)12g	Enriching blood and activating blood circulation			
Dwarf Lilyturf Root (麦门冬, Maimendong)15g	Nourishing yin and tranquilizing the mind			
Chinese Magnoliavine Fruit (五味子, Wuweizi)12g	Astringing the lung qi			

Points in Constitution: The main action of this formula is inducing diuresis though it can also replenish qi, exert the tonic effect of the heart, enrich blood and activate blood circulation. This formula can also be viewed as the modified Pulse-Activating Decoction(生脉饮, sheng mai yin). With different dosages, this formula has a reinforcing action, or purging action, or both reinforcing and purging actions.

Indications:
1. Chronic cardiac insufficiency
2. Rheumatic heart disease, cor pulmonale with chronic cardiac insufficiency
3. Cor pulmonale

Precaution: This formula is indicated for heart failure due to qi deficiency, blood stasis and water retention in the interior. For severe cases two prescriptions should be taken in four times a day; for mild cases one prescription a day for several days to consolidate the effect.

Associated Formulas:

1. Himalayan Teasel Decoction (续断饮, xu duan yin) *Guiding Prescriptions of Ren Zhai* 《仁斋直指方》

This is comprised of Corydalis Tuber (延胡索, Yanhusuo), Chinese Angelica Root (当归, Danggui), Szechwan Lovage Rhizome (川芎, Chuanxiong), Twotooth Achyranthes Root (牛膝, Niuxi), Himalayan Teasel Root (续断, Xuduan), Red Peony Root (赤芍药, Chishaoyao), Cassia Bark (肉桂, Rougui), Dahurican Angelica Root (白芷, Baizhi), Trogopterus Dung (五灵脂, Wulingzhi), Incised Notopterygium Rhizome or Root (羌活, Qianghuo), Tuckahoe (茯苓, Fuling), Pharbitis Seed (牵牛子, Qianniuzi), Pinellia Rhizome (半夏, Banxia) and Prepared Licorice Root (炙甘草, Zhi Gancao). Its actions are activating blood and excreting water. It is indicated for chronic heart failure manifested as edema of the limbs due to blood stasis, or even mass, distension and pain in the hypochondrium due to blood stasis of the liver.

2. Bitter Apricot and Pepperweed Pill (苦葶苈丸, ku ting li wan) *Imperial Medical Encyclopaedia* 《圣济总录》

This is comprised of Pepperweed Seed (葶苈子, Tinglizi), Apricot Seed (杏仁, Xingren), Tangerine Peel (橘皮, Jupi), Fourstamen Stephania Root (防己, Fangji), Indian Bread Pink Epidermis (赤茯苓, Chifuling) and Perilla Leaf (紫苏, Zisu). Its actions are purging lung and promoting urination. It is indicated for chronic heart failure due to water accumulation in the lung manifested as asthma, dysuria with dark urine, edema in the loins and legs which causes difficulty in sleeping

3. Devine Black Bird Decoction (真武汤, zhen wu tang) *Treatise on Exogenous Febrile Diseases* 《伤寒论》

This is comprised of Tuckahoe (茯苓, Fuling), White Peony Root (白芍药, Baishaoyao), Largehead Atractylodes Rhizome (白术, Baizhu), Fresh Ginger (生姜, Shengjiang) and Prepared Aconite Root (炮附子, Pao Fuzi). Its actions are warming yang and inducing diuresis. It is indicated for chronic heart failure due to yang deficiency of the heart and kidney and water retention. The manifestations are dysuria, heaviness sensation and pain in the limbs, or edema in the limbs, pale tongue with white coating, deep and slow pulse.

Heart Rhythm-Adjusting Mixture
(整律合剂, zheng lu he ji)

Source: *Fujian Journal of Traditional Chinese Medicine*《福建中医药》
Composition: Pilose Asiabell Root (党参, Dangshen) 30g
Dan-shen Root (丹参, Danshen) 30g
Lightyellow Sophora Root (苦参, Kushen) 30g
Prepared Licorice Root (炙甘草, Zhi Gancao) 15g
Chinese Arborvitae Seed (柏子仁, Baiziren) 9g
Antifebrile Dichroa Root (常山, Changshan) 9g
Actions: Replenishing qi, resolving phlegm, activating blood circulation and enriching blood.
Applied Syndrome:
Arrhythmia. Insufficincy of the heart-yang or qi deficiency of the heart and spleen may bring about stagnation of blood which leads to retention of phlegm-dampness. The manifestations are palpitation, listlessness and tiredness, vertigo, dark red tongue with white and greasy coating, knotted and intermittent pulse.

Heart Rhythm-Adjusting Mixture
(Heart-Nourishing and Mind-Tranquilizing Method)

Ingredients	Effects	Combined Effects	Syndrome	Chief Symptoms
Pilose Asiabell Root (党参, Dangshen) 30g Prepared Licorice Root (炙甘草, Zhi Gancao) 15g	Benefiting and invigorating heart qi	Invigorating heart qi, resolving phlegm-dampness, activating blood circulation and enriching blood	Arrhythmia (Internal blockage of phlegm, dampness and blood stasis resulting from deficiency of the heart qi)	Palpitation, listlessness and tiredness, vertigo, dark red tongue with white and greasy coating, knotted and intermittent pulse
Dan-Shen Root (丹参, Danshen) 30g	Activating blood circulation and removing blood stasis			
Chinese Arborvitae Seed (柏子仁, Baiziren) 9g	Nourishing the heart and tranquilizing the mind			
Lightyellow Sophora Root (苦参, Kushen) 30g	Removing dampness and resolving phlegm, adjusting rhythm of the heart			
Antifebrile Dichroa Root (常山, Changshan) 9g	Expelling dampness and resolving phlegm			

Points in Constitution: Antifebrile Dichroa Root (常山, Changshan) is a drastic herb with a strong action for eliminating phlegm, while Lightyellow Sophora Root (苦参, Kushen) can dry dampness and resolve phlegm. The combination of them two can eliminate turbid phlegm. When they are combined again with Dan-Shen Root (丹参, Danshen), they are applied for palpitation due to blockage of the blood vessels by damp-phlegm.

Indications:
1. Frequent attack or abiogenesis supraventricular premature beat
2. Atrial fibrillation
3. Sinus tachycardia
4. Sinus bradycardia
5. Coronary heart disease
6. Cardiac insufficiency

Precaution: This formula is designed for palpitation due to deficiency of yang-qi, which is the principal cause, and retention of phelgm with blood stasis, which is the secondary cause. Thus, it is not suitable for palpitation due to simple excessive phlegm-dampness or pure weakness of body resistance.

Associated Formulas:

1. Prepared Licorice Decoction (炙甘草汤, zhi gan cao tang) *Treatise on Exogenous Febrile Diseases*《伤寒论》

This is comprised of Prepared Licorice Root (炙甘草, Zhi Gancao), Fresh Ginger (生姜, Shengjiang), Cassia Twig (桂枝, Guizhi), Ginseng (人参, Renshen), Dried Rehmannia Root (生地黄, Shengdihuang), Ass-hide Glue (阿胶, Ejiao), Dwarf Lilyturf Root (麦门冬, Maimendong), Hemp Seed (火麻仁, Huomaren) and Chinese Date (大枣, Dazao). Both this formula and Mixture for Adjusting Rhythm of the Heart (整律合剂, zheng lu he ji) can treat arrhythmia, but the latter has the actions of warming and replenishing yang-qi, drying dampness, resolving phlegm, activating blood circulation and removing blood stasis. It is mainly indicated for palpitation due to deficiency of qi and weakness of yang, obstruction of blood vessels and blockage of collaterals by phlegm and dampness. While Prepared Licorice Decoction (炙甘草汤, zhi gan cao tang) emphasizes replenishing qi and invigorating the spleen, it is good at treating palpitation and knotted and intermittent pulse due to failure of the heart in nourishment resulting from insufficient production of qi and blood.

2. Modified Pulse-Restoring Decoction (加减复脉汤, jia jian fu mai tang) *Detailed Analysis of Epidemic Febrile Diseases*《温病条辨》

This is comprised of Prepared Licorice Root (炙甘草, Zhi Gancao), Dried Rehmannia Root, Prepared Rehmannia Root (干地黄, Gandihuang), White Peony Root (白芍药, Baishaoyao), Dwarf Lilyturf Root (麦门冬, Maimendong), Ass-hide Glue (阿胶, Ejiao) and Hemp Seed (火麻仁, Huomaren). Its actions are nourishing yin, promoting the production of body fluid and moistening dryness. It is indicated for dysphoria with smothery sensation, thirst and dry mouth, feeble and large pulse due to impairment of yin fluid resulting from long-time accumulation of pathogenic heat.

Palpitation-Relieving Decoction
(宁心汤, ning xin tang)

Source: *Jiangsu Journal of Traditional Chinese Medicine*《江苏中医杂志》
Composition: Ginseng (人参, Renshen) 9g
Dwarf Lilyturf Root (麦门冬, Maimendong) 9g
Dried Rehmannia Root (生地黄, Shengdihuang) 15g
Spine Date Seed (酸枣仁, Suanzaoren) 9g
Cassia Twig (桂枝, Guizhi) 6g
Snakegourd Peel (瓜蒌皮, Gualoupi) 9g
Fleece-flower Stem (夜交藤, Yejiaoteng) 20g
Dan-shen Root (丹参, Danshen) 15g
Prepared Licorice Root (炙甘草, Zhi Gancao) 9g

Actions: Replenishing qi and nourishing yin, calming the heart and tranquilizing the mind.

Applied Syndrome: Palpitation. Insufficiency of the heart qi and deficiency of yin and blood may result in inability of blood to circulate, leading to stagnation of blood or blood stasis in the vessles. The manifestations are palpitation and oppressing feeling in the chest, shortness of breath, precordial discomfort which becomes severe after over-labouring, pale tongue with white coating and thin pulse.

Palpitation-Relieving Decoction
(Method of Replenishing both Qi and Blood)

Ingredients	Effects	Combined Effects	Syndrome	Chief Symptoms
Ginseng (人参, Renshen) 9g Dwarf Lilyturf Root (麦门冬, Maimendong) 9g Dried Rehmannia Root (生地黄, Shengdihuang) 15g	Replenishing qi, nourishing yin and promoting the production of body fluid	Replenishing qi and nourishing yin, calming the heart and tranquilizing the mind	Palpitation (blood stasis in the vessles due to deficiency of qi and yin)	Palpitation and oppressing feeling in the chest, shortness of breath, precordial discomfort, which become severe after over labour, pale tongue with white coating, thin pulse
Cassia Twig (桂枝, Guizhi) 6g Dan-Shen Root (丹参, Danshen) 15g Snakegourd Peel (瓜蒌皮, Gualoupi) 9g	Warming the channels, activating blood circulation, activating colleterals			
Fleece-Flower Stem (夜交藤, Yejiaoteng) 20g Spine Date Seed (酸枣仁, Suanzaoren) 9g	Nourishing the heart and tranquilizing the mind			
Prepared Licorice Root (炙甘草, Zhi Gancao) 9g	Replenishing qi and regulating the middle-jiao			

Points in Constitution: Based on the drugs for replenishing qi and yin, this formula consists of the blood-activating and mind-tranquilizing drugs so as to attain the purpose of replenishing both qi and yin, activating bood circulation and calming the heart.

Indications:
1. Arrhythmia
2. Coronary heart disease
3. Chronic cardiac insufficiency
4. Vegetative nerve functional disturbance

Precaution: This formula is especially designed for palpitation due to deficiency of both qi and yin which leads to insufficiency of heart blood. It is not suitable to palpitation due to excessive heart fire which causes attack of the heart by excessive heat.

Associated Formula:

Heart Rhythm-Regulating Decoction(调律汤, tiao lu tang) *Huang Yanshou's prescriptions of Guangzhou College of Traditional Chinese Medicine*《广州中医学院黄衍寿方》

This is comprised of Dried Rehmannia Root (生地黄, Shengdihuang), Pilose Asiabell Root (党参, Dangshen), Dwarf Lilyturf Root (麦门冬, Maimendong), Chinese Magnoliavine Fruit (五味子, Wuweizi), Chinese Angelica Root (当归, Danggui), Green Tangerine Peel (青皮, Qingpi) and Antifebrile Dichroa Root (常山, Changshan). Both this Palpitation-Relieving Decoction (宁心汤, ning xin tang) and Heart Rhythm-Regulating Decoction(调律汤, tiao lu tang) can replenish qi and yin of the heart. But the latter contains the drugs which are fragrant in flavor and have the actions of activating flow of qi and inducing resuscitation. So it is mainly used to treat arrhythmia. The former mainly consists of drugs for activating blood circulation and dredging the collaterals and is mainly used to treat palpitation or severe palpitation.

Chapter Three
Formulas for Diseases of the Digestive

Chinese drugs and prescriptions have good effects on diseases of the dig... diseases are, according to differentiation of symptom-complex, usually cons... of the spleen and stomach although they have close relations with the liver... causes are mostly attributable to impairment of the spleen due to excessive... moderate diet or irregular food intake. The principal pathogenesis is stagnation... sufficiency of the spleen and retention of food. For many diseases such as acute... and acute enteritis, chronic enteritis, peptic ulcer, gastroneurosis, gastrospasm and... there are corresponding prescriptions which are widely used in clinic.

1. Middle-Soothing Powder
(安中散, an zhong san)

Source: *Prescriptions of Peaceful Benevolent Dispensary*《和剂局方》
Composition: Corydalis Tuber (延胡索, Yanhusuo) 6g
Lesser Galangal Rhizome (高良姜, Gaoliangjiang) 6g
Fennel Fruit (小茴香, Xiaohuixiang) 6g
Cassia Bark (肉桂, Rougui) 3g
Calcined Oyster Shell (煅牡蛎, Duan Muli) 9g
Villous Amomum Fruit (砂仁, Sharen) 6g
Licorice Root (甘草, Gancao) 6g
Actions: Warming the middle-jiao and alleviating pain.
Applied Syndrome:
1. Abdominal pain due to attack of the stomach by pathogenic cold or deficiency of middle-jiao yang, manifested as acute or chronic epigastric and abdominal pain, acid regurgitation, feeling of distention and fullness in the chest which usually radiates to the hypochondrium, nausea, vomiting, tiredness, pale tongue with white coating, deep, slow and weak pulse.
2. Abdominal stabbing pain in women due to stagnation of qi and blood or accumulation of cold, marked by spasm and pain in the lower abdomen, feeling of cold and pain in the lumbaosacral region.

Middle-Shoothing Powder
(Middle-Warming and Pain-Alleviating Method)

Ingredients	Effects	Combined Effects	Syndrome	Chief Symptoms
...rk (肉桂, Rougui) ...alangal Rhizome (高良姜, Gaoliangjiang)6g ...l Fruit (小茴香, Xiaohuixiang)6g	Warming the middle-jiao and expelling cold, drying dampness and alleviating pain	Warming the middle-jiao and expelling cold, regulating the stomach qi and alleviating pain	Abdominal pain due to cold in the middle-jiao	Epigastric and abdominal pain, acid regurgitation, poor appetite with splatering sound in the gastric region, nausea, vomiting, tiredness, soft stool or diarrhea, pale tongue with white coating, deep, slow and weak pulse
Villous Amomum Fruit (砂仁, Sharen)6g	Regulating flow of qi and alleviating pain, regulating the stomach qi to stop vomiting			
Corydalis Tuber (延胡索, Yanhusuo)6g Lesser Galangal Rhizome (高良姜, Gaoliangjiang)6g	Activating blood circulation, promoting flow of qi and alleviating pain			
Calcined Oyster Shell (煅牡蛎, Duan Muli)9g	Inducing astringency and relieving gastric hyperacidity			
Prepared Licorice Root (炙甘草, Zhi Gancao)6g	Replenishing qi and regulating the middle-jiao			

Points in Constitution: Blood and qi will flow freely if they are in a warm condition. In this formula, the drugs of Cassia Bark (肉桂, Rougui), Fennel Fruit (小茴香, Xiaohuixiang) and Lesser Galangal Rhizome (高良姜, Gaoliangjiang), which are warm and hot in nature, are used to warm and activate flow of qi and blood. Then, Villous Amomum Fruit (砂仁, Sharen) and Yanhusuo (元胡索, Yuanhusuo) which have the actions of activating flow of both qi and blood and alleviating pain are added to relieve effectively various pains due to accumulation of cold, stagnation of qi and blood stasis. The use of Oyster Shell (牡蛎, Muli) which should be calcined can not only stop diarrhea by inducing astringency but also protect the stomach by relieving gastric hyperacidity.

Indications:

1. Nervous gastritis

2. Chronic gastritis
3. Gastroatonia
4. Gastroneurosis

Precaution: This formula is mainly indicated for epigastric or abdominal pain due to cold retention and qi stagnation. It is not suitable for gastric pain due to heat.

Associated Formulas:

1. Galangal and Cyperus Pill (良附丸, liang fu wan) *Collection of Effective Formulaes* 《良方集腋》

This is comprised of Lesser Galangal Rhizome (高良姜, Gaoliangjiang) and Cyperus tuber (香附, Xiangfu). Its actions are warming the middle-jiao and expelling cold, regulating qi and relieving the depressed liver-qi. It is indicated for pain in the hypochondrium, abdominal or epigastric pain and oppressed feeling in the chest due to stagnation of liver qi and retention of cold in the stomach.

2. Middle-Regulating Pill (理中丸, li zhong wan) *Treatise on Exogenous Febrile Diseases* 《伤寒论》

This is comprised of Ginseng (人参, Renshen), Dried Ginger (干姜, Ganjiang), Largehead Atractylodes Rhizome (白术, Baizhu) and Prepared Licorice Root (炙甘草, Zhi Gancao). Its actions are warming the middle-jiao to expel cold, replenishing qi and invigorating the spleen. It is indicated for abdominal pain which can be relieved when warmed and pressed, feeling of fullness in the abdomen, poor appetite and loose stool due to deficiency and cold of the spleen and stomach. It is also indicated for blood loss due to yang deficiency or chronic infantile convulsion due to deficiency and cold of the middle-jiao.

3. Major Middle-Strengthening Decoction (大建中汤, da jian zhong tang) *Synopsis of Golden Cabinet* 《金匮要略》

This is comprised of Princklyash Peel (蜀椒, Shujiao), Dried Ginger (干姜, Ganjiang) and Ginseng (人参, Renshen). Its actions are warming and replenishing the middle-jiao, keeping the adverse qi downwards and alleviating pain. It is indicated for severe epigastric or abdominal pain, feeling of fullness in the abdomen and vomiting due to deficiency of the middle-jiao yang and excessive cold in the interior. Besides, it also treats severe abdominal megalgia due to deficiency cold of the spleen and stomach or due to ascarid.

4. Evodia, Fresh Ginger plus Chinese Angelica Cold Limbs Decoction (当归四逆加吴茱萸生姜汤, dang gui si ni jia wu zhu yu sheng jiang tang) *Treatise on Exogenous Febrile Diseases* 《伤寒论》

This is comprised of Chinese Angelica Root (当归, Danggui), Cassia Twig (桂枝, Guizhi), White Peony Root (白芍药, Baishaoyao), Manchurian Wildginger Herb (细辛, Xixin), Medicinal Evodia Fruit (吴茱萸, Wuzhuyu), Fresh Ginger (生姜, Shengjiang), Chinese Date (大枣, Dazao) and Licorice Root (甘草, Gancao). Its actions are warming the meridian and expelling cold, enriching blood and invigorating pulse-beating. It is indicated for cold limbs, extremely thin pulse, or dysmenorrhea, or flaccid constriction of penis.

2. Chinese Angelica Decoction
(当归汤, dang gui tang)

Source: *Prescriptions of Peaceful Benevolent Dispensary*《和剂局方》
Composition: Chinese Angelica Root (当归, Danggui) 9g
White Peony Root (白芍药, Baishaoyao) 6g
Membranous Milkvetch Root (黄芪, Huangqi) 6g
Ginseng (人参, Renshen) 3g
Dried Ginger (干姜, Ganjiang) 3g
Princklyash Peel (蜀椒, Shujiao) 3g
Pinellia Rhizome (半夏, Banxia) 6g
Prepared Licorice Root (炙甘草, Zhi Gancao) 3g
Officinal Magnolia Bark (厚朴, Houpo) 6g

Actions: Warming the middle-jiao and expelling cold, replenishing qi and enriching the blood, regulating flow of qi and keeping the adverse qi downward.

Applied Syndrome: Pericardial and abdominal pain due to deficiency of qi and blood or cold of deficiency type and stagnation of qi. This is manifested as colicky pain in the chest and abdomen, cold feeling in the back, oppression and fullness in the chest and abdomen, tiredness and listlessness, cold limbs, pale tongue with littlle coating, or white and moist coating, deep, thin and weak pulse.

Points in Constitution: In this formula, the ingredients of Princklyash Peel (蜀椒, Shujiao), Dried Ginger (干姜, Ganjiang) and Ginseng (人参, Renshen) in Major Middle-Strengthening Decoction (大建中汤, da jian zhong tang) are used to warm and replenish the middle-jiao, keep the adverse qi downward and alleviate pain. The ingredients of Peony and Licorice Decoction (芍药甘草汤, shao yao gan cao tang) are used to relieve muscular spasm and alleviate pain. The ingredients of Membranous Milkvetch Root (黄芪, Huangqi) and Chinese Angelica Root (当归, Danggui) in Chinese Angelica Blood-Enriching Decoction (当归补血汤, dang gui bu xue tang) are used to replenish qi and enrich blood. Pinellia Rhizome (半夏, Banxia) and Officinal Magnolia Bark (厚朴, Houpo) are added to regulate flow of qi and harmonize the function of the stomach. This formula has both the replenishing and warming characteristics, thus it is suitable for gastric and abdominal pain due to a weak body with excess cold.

Indications:
1. Gastrospasm
2. Chronic gastritis
3. Gastroneurosis
4. Menalgia

Precaution: This formula is not suitable for epigastric or abdominal pain due to accumulation of cold in the interior while qi is not impaired.

Chinese Angelica Decoction
(Middle-Warming and Adverse Qi-Lowering Method)

Ingredients	Effects	Combined Effects	Syndrome	Chief Symptoms
Princklyash Peel(蜀椒, Shujiao)3g Dried Ginger (干姜, Ganjiang)3g	Warming the middle-jiao and expelling cold	Warming the middle-jiao and expelling cold, replenishing qi and enriching the blood, regulating flow of qi and keeping the adverse qi downwards	Cold pain in the chest (stomach) and abdomen	Clicky pain in the chest and abdomen, cold feeling in the back, oppression and fullness in the chest and abdomen, tiredness and listlessness, cold limbs, or dysmenorrhea, pale tongue with little coating or white and moist coating, deep, thin and weak pulse
White Peony Root (白芍药, Baishaoyao)6g Chinese Angelica Root (当归, Danggui)9g Membranous Milkvetch Root (黄芪, Huangqi)6g Ginseng (人参, Renshen)3g Prepared Licorice Root (炙甘草, Zhi Gancao)3g	Warming and replenishing the middle-jiao, relieving muscular spasm and alleviating pain			
Officinal Magnolia Bark (厚朴, Houpo)6g Pinellia Rhizome (半夏, Banxia)6g	Warming the middle-jiao and regulating flow of qi, regulating the stomach qi and keeping the adverse qi downwards			

Associated Formulas:

1. Middle-Soothing Powder (安中散, an zhong san) *Prescriptions of Peaceful Benevolent Dispensary* 《和剂局方》

This is comprised of Corydalis Tuber (延胡索, Yanhusuo), Lesser Galangal Rhizome (高良姜, Gaoliangjiang), Fennel Fruit (小茴香, Xiaohuixiang), Cassia Bark (肉桂, Rougui), Oyster Shell (牡蛎, Muli), Villous Amomum Fruit (砂仁, Sharen) and Licorice Root (甘草, Gancao). Its actions are warming the middle-jiao and alleviating pain. It is indicated for severe abdominal pain due to cold retention and qi stagnation.

2. Chinese Angelica Decoction (当归汤, dang gui tang) *Key to Therapeutics of Children's Diseases* 《小儿药证直诀》

This is comprised of Chinese Angelica Root (当归, Danggui), White Peony Root (白芍药, Baishaoyao), Ginseng (人参, Renshen), Balloonflower Root (桔梗, Jiegeng), Tangerine Peel

(橘皮, Jupi) and Prepared Licorice Root (炙甘草, Zhi Gancao). Its actions are warming the middle-jiao to expel cold, replenishing qi and invigorating the spleen. It is indicated for a child's abdominal pain with cold limbs due to catching of cold during sleep.

3. Major Middle-Strengthening Decoction (大建中汤, da jian zhong tang) *Synopsis of Golden Cabinet*《金匮要略》

This is comprised of Princklyash Peel (蜀椒, Shujiao), Dried Ginger (干姜, Ganjiang) and Ginseng (人参, Renshen). Its actions are warming and replenishing the middle-jiao, keeping the adverse qi downwards and alleviating pain. It is indicated for severe epigastric or abdominal pain, feeling of fullness in the abdomen and vomiting due to yang deficiency of the middle-jiao and excessive cold in the interior or for abdominal megalgia due to deficiency cold of the spleen and stomach or due to ascarid.

3. Dan-Shen Decoction
(丹参饮, dan shen yin)

Source: *Current Formulae in Verse*《时方歌括》
Composition: Dan-shen Root (丹参, Danshen) 30g
Sandalwood (檀香, Tanxiang) 4.5g
Villous Amomum Fruit (砂仁, Sharen) 4.5g
Actions: Activating blood circulation and dissolving blood stasis, promoting flow of qi and alleviating pain.

Dan-Shen Decoction
(Method of Activating Blood Circulation and Regulating Flow of Qi)

Ingredients	Effects	Combined Effects	Syndrome	Chief Symptoms
Dan-Shen Root (丹参, Danshen) 30g	Activating blood circulation and dissolving blood stasis	Promoting blood circulation and dissolving blood stasis, activating flow of qi and alleviating pain	Various pericardial and gastric pain (due to qi stagnation and blood stasis)	Pain in the pericardium, chest or the gastric region, localized stabbing pain, red tongue with yellow coating, wiry and rapid pulse
Sandalwood (檀香, Tanxiang) 4.5g	Promoting flow of qi and alleviating pain			
Villous Amomum Fruit (砂仁, Sharen) 4.5g	Warming the middle-jiao and activating flow of qi			

Applied Syndrome: Variety of pericardial and gastric pains due to stagnation of qi and blood stasis which accumulate in the middle-jiao and transform into heat after a long time. The manifestations are pain in the pericardium, chest or gastric region; localized stabbing or dull pain, red tongue with yellow coating, wiry and rapid pulse.

Points in Constitution: There are only three drugs which are mild in nature in this formula. Among them Dan-Shen Root (丹参, Danshen) is the main drug used for activating blood circulation and removing blood stasis. The other drugs Sandalwood (檀香, Tanxiang) and Villous Amomum Fruit (砂仁, Sharen) are the adjuvant drugs used for activating flow of qi, regulating the middle-jiao and alleviating pain. The combination of the three results in regular circulation of qi and blood. Hence, the relief of pain.

Indications:
1. Gastroduodenal ulcer
2. Gastroneurosis
3. Menalgia
4. Coronary heart disease, angina pectoris
5. Hepatosplenomegaly

Precaution: This formula is suitable for stagnancy or heat syndrome which is manifested as localized stabbing pain, red tongue with yellow coating, wiry and rapid pulse.

Associated Formulas:

1. Laughing Powder (失笑散, shi xiao san) *Prescriptions of Peaceful Benevolent Dispensary* 《和剂局方》

This is comprised of Trogopterus Dung (五灵脂, Wulingzhi) and Carbonized Cattail Pollen (炒蒲黄, Chao Puhuang). Its actions are activating blood circulation and dissolving blood stasis, dissipating blockages and alleviating pain. It is indicated for various localized stabbing pain due to blood stasis in the liver meridian.

2. Four Herbs Stasis-Dissolving Decoction (四物化郁汤, si wu hua yu tang) *Differential Diagnosis and Treatment of Diseases* 《类证治裁》

This is comprised of Chinese Angelica Root (当归, Danggui), White Peony Root (白芍药, Baishaoyao), Prepared Rehmannia Root (熟地黄, Shudihuang), Szechwan Lovage Rhizome (川芎, Chuanxiong), Peach Seed (桃仁, Taoren), Safflower (红花, Honghua), Natural Indigo (青黛, Qingdai) and Nutgrass Galingale Rhizome (香附, Xiangfu). Its actions are regulating flow of qi, activating blood circulation and removing blood stasis. It is indicated for blood stasis with unsmooth and hollow pulse.

3. Four Herbs with Corydalis Tuber Decoction (四物延胡汤, si wu yan hu tang) *Source and Cause of Miscellaneous Diseases* 《杂病源流犀烛》

This is comprised of Chinese Angelica Root (当归, Danggui), Corydalis Tuber (延胡索, Yanhusuo), White Peony Root (白芍药, Baishaoyao), Dried Rehmannia Root (生地黄, Shengdihuang), Szechwan Lovage Rhizome (川芎, Chuanxiong), Peach Seed (桃仁, Taoren), Safflower (红花, Honghua) and Twotooth Achyranthes Root (牛膝, Niuxi). Its actions are activating blood circulation and dissolving blood stasis, activating flow of qi and alleviating pain. It is indicated for periappendicular abscess with rigidity and pain in the lower abdomen due to blood stasis.

4. Blood-House Blood Stasis-Dispelling Decoction （血府逐瘀汤, xue fu zhu yu tang） *Correction of Medical Classics*《医林改错》

This is comprised of Chinese Angelica Root （当归, Danggui）, Balloonflower Root （桔梗, Jiegeng）, Red Peony Root （赤芍, Chishao）, Dried Rehmannia Root （生地黄, Shengdihuang）, Szechwan Lovage Rhizome （川芎, Chuanxiong）, Peach Seed （桃仁, Taoren）, Safflower （红花, Honghua）, Twotooth Achyranthes Root （牛膝, Niuxi）, Licorice Root （甘草, Gancao）, Bitter Orange （枳壳, Zhiqiao） and Chinese Thorowax Root （柴胡, Chaihu）. Its actions are activating blood circulation and dissolving blood stasis, activating flow of qi and alleviating pain. It is indicated for localized stabbing pain in the chest due to qi stagnation and blood stasis in the chest.

5. Four Herbs with Rubia Root and Inula Flower Decoction （四物绛覆汤, si wu jiang fu tang） *Revised Popular Treatise on Exogenous Febrile Diseases*《重订通俗伤寒论》

This is comprised of Chinese Angelica Root （当归, Danggui）, Rubia Root（新绛, xinjiang）, White Peony Root （白芍药, Baishaoyao）, Dried Rehmannia Root （生地黄, Shengdihuang）, Szechwan Lovage Rhizome （川芎, Chuanxiong）, Tangerine Pith （橘络, Juluo）, Inula Flower （旋覆花, Xuanfuhua） and Scallion （青葱管, Qingcongguan）. Its actions are activating blood circulation and removing blood stasis, regulating flow of qi and alleviating pain. It is indicated for pain in the epigastrium and hypochondrum due to stagnation of qi and blood.

6. Powder of Ending Part of Chinese Angelica Root （当归须散, dang gui xu san） *An Introduction to Medicine*《医学入门》

This is comprised of Ending Part of Chinese Angelica Root （当归尾, Dangguiwei）, Licorice Root （甘草, Gancao）, Red Peony Root （赤芍, Chishao）, Commbined Spicebush Root （乌药, Wuyao）, Nutgrass Galingale Rhizome （香附, Xiangfu）, Peach Seed （桃仁, Taoren）, Safflower （红花, Honghua）, Sappan Wood （苏木, Sumu） and Cassia Bark （官桂, Guangui）. Its actions are dissipating blood stasis, activating blood circulation and alleviating pain. It is indicated for pain in the chest and hypochondrium or chills and fever due to stagnation of qi and blood.

4. Immortal Viscera-Nourishing Decoction
（真人养脏汤, zhen ren yang zang tang）

Source: *Prescriptions of Peaceful Benevolent Dispensary*《和剂局方》
Composition: Ginseng （人参, Renshen）6g
Chinese Angelica Root （当归, Danggui）9g
Largehead Atractylodes Rhizome （白术, Baizhu）12g
Nutmeg Seed （肉豆蔻, Roudoukou）12g
Cassia Bark （肉桂, Rougui）3g
White Peony Root （白芍药, Baishaoyao）15g
Common Aucklandia Root （木香, Muxiang）9g
Medicine Terminalia Fruit （诃子, Hezi）12g

Poppy Capsule（罂粟壳，Yingsuqiao）9g

Actions: Warming and tonifying the spleen and kidney, astringing the intestines to stop diarrhea.

Applied Syndrome: Chronic diarrhea and dysentery due to deficiency-cold of the spleen and kidney, manifested as incontinence of the feces due to loose bowel, abdominal pain which may be relieved by warmth and pressure, fartigue or tiredness, poor appetite, pale tongue, deep and slow pulse; or dysentery or passing stool with blood and pus day and night, tenesmus, pain around the umbilicus.

Immortal Viscera-Nourishing Decoction
(Intestines-Astringing and Diarrhea-Stopping Method)

Ingredients	Effects	Combined Effects	Syndrome	Chief Symptoms
Poppy Capsule（罂粟壳，Yingsuqiao）9g Medicine Terminalia Fruit（诃子，Hezi）12g	Astringing the intestines to stop diarrhea	Warming and tonifying the spleen and kidney, astringing the intestines to stop diarrhea	Protracted diarrhea and dysentery due to deficiency-cold of the spleen and kidney	Incontinence of the feces due to loose bowels, abdominal pain or pain around umbilicus which may be relieved by warmth and pressure, fartigue or tiredness, poor appetite, pale tongue, deep and slow pulse; or dysentery or passing stool with blood and pus day and night, tenesmus, pale tongue, deep and slow pulse
Cassia Bark（肉桂，Rougui）3g Nutmeg Seed（肉豆蔻，Roudoukou）12g	Warming and tonifying the spleen and kidney			
Ginseng（人参，Renshen）6g Largehead Atractylodes Rhizome（白术，Baizhu）12g	Replenishing qi and invigorating the spleen			
Chinese Angelica Root（当归，Danggui）9g White Peony Root（白芍药，Baishaoyao）15g	Tonifying blood and nourishing yin			
Common Aucklandia Root（木香，Muxiang）9g	Regulating flow of qi and activating the spleen qi			

Points in Constitution: The characteristic of this formula is that the drugs for astringing the intestines to stop diarrhea and the drugs for warming and replenishing qi and blood are used simultaneously and that the primary and secondary aspects of the disease are treated at the same time. The combination of Cassia Bark（肉桂，Rougui）with Chinese Angelica Root（当归，Danggui）can warm and nourish blood while Common Aucklandia Root（木香，Muxiang）can regulate flow of qi. It should be pointed out that astringent drugs must be used very cautiously when the evil has not been expelled entirely. They can only be used to treat the secondary aspect of the disease in an emergency or acute case.

Indications:
1. Chronic colitis
2. Chronic bacillary dysentery
3. Intestinal tuberculosis
4. Colon cancer
5. Colon's disease

Precautions:
1. Alcohol, meat, cold, sea or oil food should be avoided when this formula is used.
2. It should be cautiously used for diarrhea withou complete relief of pathogens.

Associated Formulas:

1. Peach Blossom Decoction (桃花汤, tao hua tang) *Treatise on Exogenous Febrile Diseases* 《伤寒论》

This is comprised of Red Halloysite (赤石脂, Chishizhi), Dried Ginger (干姜, Ganjiang) and Rice (粳米, Jingmi). Its actions are warming the middle-jiao, astringing the intestines and arresting bleeding. It is indicated for prolonged dysentery and purulent and bloody stool due to yang deficiency in the middle-jiao.

2. Red Halloysite and Limonite Decoction (赤石脂禹余粮汤, chi shi zhi yu yu liang tang) *Treatise on Exogenous Febrile Diseases* 《伤寒论》

This is comprised of Red Halloysite (赤石脂, Chishizhi) and Limonite (禹余粮, Yuyuliang). It is good at treating the secondary aspect of the disease and its action is astringing the intestines to stop diarrhea. It is indicated for stubbon cronic diarrhea.

3. Four Miraculous Herbs Pill (四神丸, si shen wan) *Standard for Diagnosis and Treatment* 《证治准绳》

This is comprised of Nutmeg Seed (肉豆蔻, Roudoukou), Malaytea Scurfpea Fruit (补骨脂, Buguzhi), Chinese Magnoliavine Fruit (五味子, Wuweizi) and Medicinal Evodia Fruit (吴茱萸, Wuzhuyu). Its actions are replenishing the kidney and inducing astringency. It is indicated for diarrhea before dawn, poor appetite or anorexia, soreness and weakness of both the loins and knees due to deficiency-cold of the spleen and kidney.

5. Common Aucklandia and Areca Seed Pill
(木香槟榔丸, mu xiang bing lang wan)

Source: *Confucian's Duties to Their Parents* 《儒门事亲》
Composition: Areca Seed (槟榔, Binglang) 6g
Nutgrass Galingale Rhizome (香附, Xiangfu) 9g
Green Tangerine Peel (青皮, Qingpi) 6g
Tangerine Peel (橘皮, Jupi) 6g

Pharbitis Seed (牵牛, Qianniu) 6g

Rhubarb (大黄, Dahuang) 9g

Common Aucklandia Root (木香, Muxiang) 6g

Kwangsi Turmeric Rhizome (莪术, Ezhu) 6g

Coptis Rhizome (黄连, Huanglian) 6g

Chinese Corktree Bark (黄柏, Huangbai) 9g

Actions: Promoting flow of qi to remove stagnation, eliminating food retention and purging heat.

Common Aucklandia and Areca Seed Pill
(Food Retention-Eliminating and Qi Stagnation-Removing Method)

Ingredients	Effects	Combined Effects	Syndrome	Chief Symptoms
Common Aucklandia Root (木香, Muxiang) 6g Areca Seed (槟榔, Binglang) 6g	Activating flow of qi to remove the stagnation, eliminating distention and alleviating pain	Promoting flow of qi to remove the stagnation, eliminating food retention and purging heat	Indigestion and dysentery (due to irregular diet and accumulation of heat and dampness)	Feeling of distention, fullness and pain in the gastric and abdominal region, constipation, or dysentery with purulent and bloody discharge, yellow and greasy coating, deep and forceful pulse
Green Tangerine Peel (青皮, Qingpi) 6g Tangerine Peel (橘皮, Jupi) 6g Nutgrass Galingale Rhizome (香附, Xiangfu) 9g	Activating flow of qi and eliminating food retention			
Pharbitis Seed (牵牛, Qianniu) 6g Rhubarb (大黄, Dahuang) 9g	Eliminating food retention, purging heat and relaxing the bowels			
Kwangsi Turmeric Rhizome (莪术, Ezhu) 6g	Promoting blood circulation and activating flow of qi, alleviating pain by eliminating food retention			
Coptis Rhizome (黄连, Huanglian) 6g Chinese Corktree Bark (黄柏, Huangbai) 9g	Clearing away heat, drying dampness and stopping dysentery			

Applied Syndrome: Indigestion and dysentery. An irregular diet may cause food retention and stagnation of qi in the interior, which results in accumulation of dampness and transformation of heat. The manifestations are feeling of distention, fullness and pain in the gastric or abdominal region, constipation, or dysentery with pus and blood, yellow and greasy tongue coating, deep and forceful pulse.

Points in Constitution: This formula uses Common Aucklandia Root (木香, Muxiang) and Areca Seed (槟榔, Binglang) as the main drugs to activate flow of qi and remove stagnation. Besides, some other heat-clearing, blood-activating and purging drugs are added especially to induce purgation and elimination. Therefore, it is only suitable for the case of exuberance of the genuine qi with excessive evils. If it is erroneously applied to the defficiency case, it may injure the stomach-qi.

Indications:
1. Acute colitis
2. Acute bacillary dysentery
3. Indigestion
4. Gastrolithiasis
5. Intestinal obstruction

Precautions:
1. Since this formula has drastic actions of removing retention and relieving the stagnation of qi, it is only applied to those who have both strong bodies and excessiveness of qi. For those who are very weak or accompanied with exterior syndrome, this formula should be forbidden.

2. It should be cautiously used for indigestion due to deficiency of the spleen and stomach.

Associated Formulas:
1. Common Aucklandia and Areca Seed Pill (木香槟榔丸, mu xiang bing lang wan) *The Precious Mirror of Hygiene*《卫生宝鉴》

This is the formula of Common Aucklandia and Areca Seed Pill(木香槟榔丸, mu xiang bing lang wan) recorded in *Confucian's Duties to Their Parents*《儒门事亲》plus Bitter Orange (枳壳, Zhiqiao). Of the two formulas, the one recorded in *The Precious Mirror of Hygiene*《卫生宝鉴》is mainly to further strengthen the qi-activating and stagnation-removing actions. It is indicated for obvious stagnation of qi resulting from retention of damp-heat.

2. Common Aucklandia and Areca Seed Pill (木香槟榔丸, mu xiang bing lang wan) *Collections of Formulae with Notes*《医方集解》

This is the formula of Common Aucklandia and Areca Seed Pill(木香槟榔丸, mu xiang bing lang wan) recorded in *The Precious Mirror of Hygiene*《卫生宝鉴》plus Common Burreed Rhizome (三棱, Sanleng) and Mirabilite (芒硝, Mangxiao). The characteristic of this formula is to strenghthen the retention-eliminating and stagnation-removing actions. It is mainly used for constipation due to retention of food or indigestion.

3. Common Aucklandia and Areca Seed Pill (木香槟榔丸, mu xiang bing lang wan) *Prescriptions of Peaceful Benevolent Dispensary*《和剂局方》

This is comprised of Chinese Bushcherry Seed (郁李仁, Yuliren), Chinese Honeylocusy Fruit

(皂角, Zaojiao), Pinellia Rhizome (半夏, Banxia), Areca Seed (槟榔, Binglang), Bitter Orange (枳壳, Zhiqiao), Common Aucklandia Root (木香, Muxiang), Apricot Seed (杏仁, Xingren) and Green Tangerine Peel (青皮, Qingpi). Its action is activating flow of qi to remove stagnation. It is indicated for fullness and expression in the epigastric and abdominal region due to retention of phlegm and food and stagnation of qi in the three-jiao.

4. Common Aucklandia Stagnation-Removing Pill (木香导滞丸, mu xiang dao zhi wan) *Expounding of Pediatrics* 《幼科发挥》

This is comprised of Fried Immature Bitter Orange (炒枳实, Chao Zhishi), Officinal Magnolia Bark (厚朴, Houpo), Areca Seed (槟榔, Binglang), Baikal Skullcap Root (黄芩, Huangqin), Coptis Rhizome (黄连, Huanglian), Chinese Corktree Bark (黄柏, Huangbai), Rhubarb (大黄, Dahuang), Pharbitis Seed (牵牛子, Qianniuzi) and Common Aucklandia Root (木香, Muxiang). Its actions are removing stagnation and eliminating retention. It is indicated for dysentery in the early stage.

5. Common Aucklandia Stagnation-Removing Pill (木香导滞丸, mu xiang dao zhi wan) *Songyan's Medical Shortcut* 《松崖医径》

This is comprised of Immature Bitter Orange (枳实, Zhishi), Medicated Leaven (神曲, Shenqu), Tuckahoe (茯苓, Fuling), Baikal Skullcap Root (黄芩, Huangqin), Coptis Rhizome (黄连, Huanglian), Largehead Atractylodes Rhizome (白术, Baizhu), Rhubarb (大黄, Dahuang), Areca Seed (槟榔, Binglang), Common Aucklandia Root (木香, Muxiang) and Oriental Waterplantain Rhizome (泽泻, Zexie). Its actions are clearing away heat, eliminating dampness and removing stagnation. It is indicated for dyspepsia, fullness and stuffiness sensation and restlessness due to accumulation of damp-heat in the intestines.

6. Common Aucklandia Qi-Soothing Powder (木香顺气散, mu xiang shun qi san) *Standard for Diagnosis and Treatment* 《证治准绳》

This is comprised of Bitter Orange (枳壳, Zhiqiao), Nutgrass Galingale Rhizome (香附, Xiangfu), Green Tangerine Peel (青皮, Qingpi), Tangerine Peel (橘皮, Jupi), Officinal Magnolia Bark (厚朴, Houpo), Swordlike Atractylodes Rhizome (苍术, Cangzhu), Villous Amomum Fruit (砂仁, Sharen), Areca Seed (槟榔, Binglang), Common Aucklandia Root (木香, Muxiang), Prepared Licorice Root (炙甘草, Zhi Gancao) and Fresh Ginger (生姜, Shengjiang). Its actions are activating flow of qi, dissipating depressed qi and alleviating pain. It is mainly indicated for abdominal pain due to stagnation of qi.

6. Immature Bitter Orange Stagnation-Dispelling Pill
(枳实导滞丸, zhi shi dao zhi wan)

Source: *Differentiation on Endogenous and Exogenous Diseases* 《内外伤辨惑论》
Composition: Immature Bitter Orange (枳实, Zhishi) 15g
Tuckahoe (茯苓, Fuling) 9g
Oriental Waterplantain Rhizome (泽泻, Zexie) 6g

Largehead Atractylodes Rhizome（白术，Baizhu）9g
Medicated Leaven（神曲，Shenqu）15g
Rhubarb（大黄，Dahuang）9g
Coptis Rhizome（黄连，Huanglian）9g
Baikal Skullcap Root（黄芩，Huangqin）9g

Actions: Eliminating food retention and qi stagnation, clearing away heat and expelling dampness.

Applied Syndrome: Indigestion due to heat-dampness. Excessive eating and drinking results in heat and dampness, which accumulates in the stomach and intestines. The manifestations are distention and pain in the abdomen and epigastrium, eructation with fetid odour and acid regurgitation, anorexia and vomiting, or diarrhea, or dysentery, or constipation, scanty and dark urine, yellow and greasy tongue coating, deep and forceful pulse.

Immature Bitter Orange Stagnation-Dispelling Pill
(Food Retention-Eliminating and Qi Stagnation-Removing Method)

Ingredients	Effects	Combined Effects	Syndrome	Chief Symptoms
Rhubarb（大黄，Dahuang）9g	Eliminating food retention and purging heat	Eliminating food retention and removing stagnation, clearing away heat and expelling dampness	Indigestion due to heat-dampness	Distention and pain in the abdomen and epigastrium, eructation with fetid odour and acid regurgitation, anorexia and vomiting, or diarrhea, or dysentery, or constipation, scanty and dark urine, yellow and greasy tongue coating, deep and forceful pulse
Immature Bitter Orange（枳实，Zhishi）15g	Promoting flow of qi to relieve distention			
Coptis Rhizome（黄连，Huanglian）9g Baikal Skullcap Root（黄芩，Huangqin）9g	Clearing away heat and drying dampness, benefiting the intestines to stop dysentery			
Tuckahoe（茯苓，Fuling）9g Oriental Waterplantain Rhizome（泽泻，Zexie）6g	Removing dampness and and inducing diuresis			
Largehead Atractylodes Rhizome（白术，Baizhu）9g	Invigorating the spleen and removing dampness			
Medicated Leaven（神曲，Shenqu）15g	Promoting digestion and invigorating the spleen			

Points in Constitution: The characteristic of this formula is that the heat-removing and purgative drugs are used together with the drugs for activating flow of qi and eliminating retention of food to treat various diseases due to damp-heat and food retention. Since the treatment of dirrhea and dysentery belongs to "treating diarrhea with purgatives instead of astringents", it is only indicated for the case caused by stagnation of heat due to food retention.

Indications:
1. Acute or chrolic gastroenteritis
2. Begin of acute bacillary dysentery
3. Indigestion
4. Enteroparalysis
5. Cirrhosis ascites
6. Incomplete intestinal obstruction

Precautions:
1. This formula should be cautiously used to prolonged dysentery with weak body or diarrhea without indigestion.
2. It is also cautiously used to indigestion with deficiency of the spleen and stomach.

Associated Formulas:

1. Harmony-Preserving Pill (保和丸, bao he wan) *Danxi's Experiential Therapy* 《丹溪心法》

This is comprised of Hawthorn Fruit (山楂, Shanzha), Medicated Leaven (神曲, Shenqu), Pinellia Rhizome (半夏, Banxia), Tuckahoe (茯苓, Fuling), Tangerine Peel (橘皮, Jupi), Weeping Forsythia Capsule (连翘, Lianqiao) and Radish Seed (莱菔子, Laifuzi). Its actions are promoting digestion and regulating the stomach qi. It is indicated for mild cases of variety of indigestion.

2. Eaglewood Wood Indigestion-Relieving Pill (沉香化滞丸, chen xiang hua zhi wan) *Supplement to Curative Measures for Diseases* 《增补万病回春》

This is comprised of Chinese Eaglewood Wood (沉香, Chenxiang), Kwangsi Turmeric Rhizome (莪术, Ezhu), Nutgrass Galingale Rhizome (香附, Xiangfu), Tangerine Peel (橘皮, Jupi), Common Aucklandia Root (木香, Muxiang), Villous Amomum Fruit (砂仁, Sharen), Wrinkled Gianthyssop Herb (藿香, Huoxiang), Fried Malt (炒麦芽, Chao Maiya), Fried Medicated Leaven (炒神曲, Chao Shenqu) and Prepared Licorice Root (炙甘草, Zhi Gancao). Its actions are eliminating food retention, removing phlegm, expelling evils and relieving retention due to drinking wine. It is indicated for fullness in the middle-jiao, manifested by vomiting of the fetid and nausea.

3. Eaglewood Qi Stagnation-Dissipating Pill (沉香化气丸, chen xiang hua qi wan) *Standard for Diagnosis and Treatment* 《证治准绳》

This is comprised of Rhubarb (大黄, Dahuang), Baikal Skullcap Root (黄芩, Huangqin), Ginseng (人参, Renshen), Largehead Atractylodes Rhizome (白术, Baizhu), Chinese Eaglewood Wood (沉香, Chenxiang) and Bamboo Juice (竹沥, Zhuli). Its actions are activating flow of qi and removing food retention. It is indicated for various syndromes of dysentery.

4. Immatures Bitter Orange Stuffiness-Removing Pill (枳实消痞丸, zhi shi xiao pi wan) *Secret Record of the Chamber of Orchids* 《兰室秘藏》

This is comprised of Dried Ginger (干姜, Ganjiang), Prepared Licorice Root (炙甘草, Zhi Gancao), Malt (麦芽, Maiya), Tuckahoe (茯苓, Fuling), Largehead Atractylodes Rhizome (白术, Baizhu), Pinellia Rhizome (半夏, Banxia), Ginseng (人参, Renshen), Immature Bitter Orange (枳实, Zhishi), Officinal Magnolia Bark (厚朴, Houpo) and Coptis Rhizome (黄连, Huanglian). Its actions are removing stuffiness and fullness, invigorating the spleen and regulating the stomach-qi. It is indicated for feeling of fullness and stuffiness due to deficiency of the spleen accompanied with obvious stagnation of qi and heat.

5. Aucklandia, Amomum Fruit, Immature Bitter Orange and Largehead Atractylodes Pill (香砂枳术丸, xiang sha zhi zhu wan) *Jingyue's Complete Works* 《景岳全书》

This is comprised of Immature Bitter Orange (枳实, Zhishi), Villous Amomum Fruit (砂仁, Sharen), Largehead Atractylodes Rhizome (白术, Baizhu) and Common Aucklandia Root (木香, Muxiang). Its actions are activating flow of qi and removing food retention. It is indicated for indigestion due to stagnation of qi.

6. Aucklandia, Amomum Fruit, Immature Bitter Orange and Largehead Atractylodes Pill (香砂枳术丸, xiang sha zhi zhu wan) *Manual of Preparation of Traditional Chinese Medicine* 《中药制剂手册》

This is comprised of Immature Bitter Orange (枳实, Zhishi), Villous Amomum Fruit (砂仁, Sharen), Largehead Atractylodes Rhizome (白术, Baizhu), Common Aucklandia Root (木香, Muxiang), Medicated Leaven (神曲, Shenqu), Fried Malt (炒麦芽, Chao Maiya), Tangerine Peel (橘皮, Jupi), Nutgrass Galingale Rhizome (香附, Xiangfu) and Hawthorn Fruit (山楂, Shanzha). Its actions are soothing flow of qi and dispersing the obstruction of qi in the chest, regulating the stomach qi and activating flow of the spleen qi. It is indicated for epigastric and abdominal pain and dyspepsia due to incoordination of the spleen and stomach, stagnation of qi and indigestion.

7. Immature Bitter Orange Stagnation-Removing Decoction (枳实化滞汤, zhi shi hua zhi tang) *Syndrome-Cause-Pulse-Treatment* 《症因脉治》

This is comprised of Immature Bitter Orange (枳实, Zhishi), Tangerine Peel (橘皮, Jupi), Officinal Magnolia Bark (厚朴, Houpo), Medicated Leaven (神曲, Shenqu), Malt (麦芽, Maiya), Radish Seed (莱菔子, Laifuzi) and Villous Amomum Fruit (砂仁, Sharen). Its actions are activating flow of qi, eliminating food retention and removing stagnation. It is indicated for abdominal pain or feeling of distention and fullness in the chest and abdomen due to indigestion.

7. Spleen-Warming Decoction
(温脾汤, wen pi tang)

Source: *Prescriptions Worth a Thousand Gold for Emergencies* 《备急千金要方》
Composition: Rhubarb (大黄, Dahuang) 12g

Prepared Aconite Root (附子, Fuzi)9g
Dried Ginger (干姜, Ganjiang)6g
Ginseng (人参, Renshen)9g
Licorice Root (甘草, Gancao)3g

Actions: Warming and replenishing the spleen yang, purging the accumulation of cold.

Applied Syndrome: Constipation due to deficiency of the spleen-yang and accumulation of cold, manifested as cold feeling and pain around the umbilicus which is relieved with warmth and pressure, constipation or protracted dysentery with pus and blood, cold extremities, white tongue coating, deep and wiry pulse.

Spleen-Warming Decoction
(Yang-Warming and Bowels-Relaxing Method)

Ingredients	Effects	Combined Effects	Syndrome	Chief Symptoms
Rhubarb (大黄, Dahuang)12g	Removing food retention	Warming and replenishing the spleen yang, purging the accumulated cold.	Constipation due to deficiency of the spleen yang and the accumulation of cold	Cold feeling and pain around the umbilicus which may be relieved by warming and pressing, constipation, or prolonged dysentery with purulent and bloody discharge, cold extremities, white tongue coating, deep and wiry pulse
Prepared Aconite Root (附子, Fuzi)9g Dried Ginger (干姜, Ganjiang)6g	Warming and replenishing the spleen yang			
Ginseng (人参, Renshen)9g Licorice Root (甘草, Gancao)3g	Replenishing qi and invigorating the spleen			

Points in Constitution: The excess-syndrome should be treated by purgation while the deficiency-syndrome should be treated with tonic therapy. In this formula, the warming and replenishing drugs are used simultaneously with purgatives. Rhubarb (大黄, Dahuang) is cold in nature and has a purging action. When combined with the hot-natured Prepared Aconite Root (附子, Fuzi) and Dried Ginger (干姜, Ganjiang), Rhubarb (大黄, Dahuang) can purge the accumulation of cold without impairing the spleen-yang because its cold nature is eliminated and its actions remain.

Indications:
1. Peptic ulcer
2. Uremia, urinaemia
3. Intestinal obstruction
4. Chronic dysentery

Precaution: This formula is not suitable for constipation due to accumulation of heat in the stomach and intestines.

Associated Formulas:

1. Rhubarb and Prepared Aconite Decoction (大黄附子汤, da huang fu zi tang) *Synopsis of Golden Cabinet*《金匮要略》

This is comprised of Rhubarb (大黄, Dahuang), Prepared Aconite Root (附子, Fuzi) and Manchurian Wildginger Herb (细辛, Xixin). Its actions are dissipating the accumulation of cold in the stomach and intestines. It is indicated for a cold feeling and pain in the abdomen, constipation and cold limbs due to accumulation of cold in the stomach and intestines.

2. Three Herbs Emergency Pill (三物备急丸, san wu bei ji wan) *Synopsis of Golden Cabinet*《金匮要略》

This is comprised of Rhubarb (大黄, Dahuang), Dried Ginger (干姜, Ganjiang) and Croton Fruit (巴豆, Badou). Its action is purging the accumulation of cold. It is indicated for distention and stabbing pain in the pericardial and abdominal regions, constipation, blue complexion and dyspnea due to rapid accumulation of yin-cold in the stomach and intestines.

3. Pinellia and Sulfur Pill (半硫丸, ban liu wan) *Prescriptions of Peaceful Benevolent Dispensary*《和剂局方》

This is comprised of Pinellia Rhizome (半夏, Banxia), Sulfur (硫黄, Liuhuang) and Fresh Ginger (生姜, Shengjiang). Its actions are warming the kidney to expel cold, relieving the obstruction of yang-qi and purging turbid evils. It is indicated for constipation of deficiency-cold type, intolerance of cold, anorexia, vomiting and slow pulse due to insufficiency of fire from the gate of life.

8. Intestines-Moistening Pill
(润肠丸, run chang wan)

Source: *Shen's Work on the Importance of Life Preservation*《沈氏尊生书》

Composition: Chinese Angelica Root (当归, Danggui) 9g

Prepared Rehmannia Root (熟地黄, Shudihuang) 30g

Peach Seed (桃仁, Taoren) 9g

Hemp Seed (麻子仁, Maziren) 15g

Bitter Orange (枳壳, Zhiqiao) 9g

Actions: Moistening the intestines and relaxing the bowels, nourishing yin and tonifying the blood.

Applied Syndrome: Constipation due to deficiency of yin and blood, manifested as discomfort around the umbilicus, constipation, pale or red tongue, thin and rapid pulse.

Points in Constitution: This formula combines the yin-nourishing drugs with the intestines-moistening drugs to relax the bowels. It is the regular method for constipation due to yin deficiency, which means that more water in the river gives higher speed to a boat. Bitter Orange (枳壳, Zhiqiao) is used to benefit the lung, improve appetite, descend qi and relax the bowels.

Intestines-Moistening Pill
(Intestines-Moistening and Bowels-Relaxing Method)

Ingredients	Effects	Combined Effects	Syndrome	Chief Symptoms
Chinese Angelica Root (当归, Danggui) 9g Prepared Rehmannia Root (熟地黄, Shudihuang) 30g	Enriching blood and moistening the intestines	Moistening the intestines to relax the bowels, nourishing yin and tonifying the blood	Constipation due to yin deficiency	Discomfort around the umbilicus, constipation, pale tongue or red tongue, thin and rapid pulse
Peach Seed (桃仁, Taoren) 9g Hemp Seed (麻子仁, Maziren) 15g	Moistening the intestines to relax the bowels			
Bitter Orange (枳壳, Zhiqiao) 9g	Activating flow of qi and relieving distention			

Indications:
1. Habitual constipation
2. Women constipation post partum

Precautions:
1. This formula is not suitable for constipation due to accumulation of heat in the stomach and intestines.
2. It is also not suitable for sudden constipation due to rapid accomunication of yin-cold in the stomach and intestines, or constipation of deficiency-cold type due to decline of fire from the gate of life.

Associated Formulas:

1. Hemp Seed Pill (麻子仁丸, ma zi ren wan) *Treatise on Exogenous Febrile Diseases* 《伤寒论》

This is comprised of Hemp Seed (麻子仁, Maziren), White Peony Root (白芍药, Baishaoyao), Immature Bitter Orange (枳实, Zhishi), Rhubarb (大黄, Dahuang), Officinal Magnolia Bark (厚朴, Houpo), Apricot Seed (杏仁, Xingren) and Honey (蜂蜜, Fengmi). Its actions are purging heat and moistening the intestines to relax the bowels. It is indicated for constipation due to spleen deficiency resulting from insufficient fluid and heat-dryness in the stomach and intestines.

2. Five Kinds of Kernels Pills (五仁丸, wu ren wan) *Effective Prescriptions from Physicians of Successive Generation* 《世医得效方》

This is comprised of Peach Seed (桃仁, Taoren), Apricot Seed (杏仁, Xingren), Chinese Arborvitae Seed (柏子仁, Baiziren), Pine Seed (松子仁, Songziren), Chinese Bushcherry Seed

(郁李仁, Yuliren) and Tangerine Peel (橘皮, Jupi). Its actions are moistening dryness and relaxing the bowels. It is indicated for constipation due to deficiency of body fluid and dryness of the intestines.

9. Coptis Decoction
(黄连汤, huang lian tang)

Source: *Treatise on Exogenous Febrile Diseases*《伤寒论》
Composition: Coptis Rhizome (黄连, Huanglian) 9g
Prepared Licorice Root (炙甘草, Zhi Gancao) 9g
Pinellia Rhizome (半夏, Banxia) 9g
Dried Ginger (干姜, Ganjiang) 6g
Cassia Twig (桂枝, Guizhi) 6g
Ginseng (人参, Renshen) 6g
Chinese Date (大枣, Dazao) 3g

Actions: Equally harmonizing the heat in the upper and cold in the lower to regulate the stomach-qi and keep the adverse qi downwards.

Applied Syndrome: Syndrome of heat in the upper-jiao and cold in the lower-jiao. Heat in the upper-jiao leads to failure of the stomach qi in harmony and descent and cold in the lower-jiao brings about inability of the spleen to be warmed. The manifestations are feeling of fullness in the gastric region, vomiting, abdominal pain, irritability and stuffiness in the chest, borborygmus and diarrhea, yellow and white tongue coating, wiry and slow pulse.

Points in Constitution: In this formula, Coptis Rhizome (黄连, Huanglian) which is bitter in taste and cold in nature is used to clear away heat in the upper; Dried Ginger (干姜, Ganjiang) which is pungent in taste and warm in nature is used to expel cold in the middle; Cassia Twig (桂枝, Guizhi) is used to relieve the obstruction of yang-qi; Ginseng (人参, Renshen), Licorice Root (甘草, Gancao) and Chinese Date (大枣, Dazao) are used to regulate the stomach qi and replenish the middle-jiao; and Pinellia Rhizome (半夏, Banxia) is used to keep the adverse qi downwards to stop vomiting. In one word, this is a formula for dispersion with pungent drugs, descent with bitter drugs, clearing the upper, warming the lower, regulating the stomach qi and keeping the adverse qi downward.

Indications:
1. Acute gastritis
2. Gastroenteritis

Precaution: This formula is suitable for the syndrome of heat in the upper-jiao and cold in the lower-jiao. It is contraindicated in gastrointestinal tract diseases due to simple cold or heat.

Associated Formulas:
1. Pinellia Heart-Purging Decoction (半夏泻心汤, ban xia xie xin tang) *Treatise on Exogenous Febrile Diseases*《伤寒论》

Coptis Decoction
(The Upper-Clearing and Lower-Warming Method)

Ingredients	Effects	Combined Effects	Syndrome	Chief Symptoms
Coptis Rhizome (黄连, Huanglian) 9g	Clearing away heat (from the heart and stomach)	Equally harmonizing the heat in the upper and cold in the lower to regulate the stomach-qi	The syndrome of heat in the stomach and cold in the intestines	Feeling of fullness and oppression in the gastric region, vomiting, irritability, abdominal pain and stuffiness in the chest, borborygmus and diarrhea, yellow and white tongue coating, wiry and slow pulse
Dried Ginger (干姜, Ganjiang) 6g	Dispelling cold (from the abdomen and intestines)			
Cassia Twig (桂枝, Guizhi) 6g	Relieving the obstruction of yang-qi			
Pinellia Rhizome (半夏, Banxia) 9g	Lowering the adverse qi downwards to stop vomiting			
Prepared Licorice Root (炙甘草, Zhi Gancao) 9g Ginseng (人参, Renshen) 6g Chinese Date (大枣, Dazao) 3g	Replenishing qi and regulating qi in the middle-jiao			

This is comprised of Pinellia Rhizome (半夏, Banxia), Dried Ginger (干姜, Ganjiang), Baikal Skullcap Root (黄芩, Huangqin), Coptis Rhizome (黄连, Huanglian), Ginseng (人参, Renshen), Licorice Root (甘草, Gancao) and Chinese Date (大枣, Dazao). Its actions are regulating the stomach-qi, keeping the adverse qi downwards, eliminating mass and relieving fullness. It is indicated for epigastric fullness due to penetration of pathogenic factors into the interior and accumulation of both heat and cold.

2. Fresh Ginger Heart-Purging Decoction (生姜泻心汤, sheng jiang xie xin tang) *Treatise on Exogenous Febrile Diseases*《伤寒论》

This is comprised of the ingredients of Pinellia Heart-Purging Decoction (半夏泻心汤) plus Fresh Ginger (生姜, Shengjiang). In this formula a large dose of Fresh Ginger (生姜, Shengjiang) is used, which stresses the actions of regulating the stomach qi, keeping the adverse qi downwards, dissipating water retention and relieving fullness. It is indicated for epigastric fullness due to penetration of pathogenic factors into the interior and accumulation of both water and heat.

3. Licorice Heart-Purging Decoction (甘草泻心汤, gan cao xie xin tang) *Treatise on Exogenous Febrile Diseases* 《伤寒论》

The composition of this formula is similar to that of Pinellia Heart-Purging Decoction (半夏泻心汤). However, it emphasizes the heavy application of Licorice Root (甘草, Gancao). This formula has the actions of replenishing qi and regulating the stomach, relieving fullness and stopping dysentery. It is indicated for epigastric fullness due to penetration of pathogenic factors into the interior, deficiency of the stomach and stagnation of qi.

10. Dysentery-Stopping Pill
(驻车丸, zhu che wan)

Source: *Prescriptions Worth a Thousand Gold for Emergencies* 《备急千金要方》
Composition: Coptis Rhizome (黄连, Huanglian) 9g
Ass-hide Glue (阿胶, Ejiao) 12g
Chinese Angelica Root (当归, Danggui) 12g
Dried Ginger (干姜, Ganjiang) 9g
Actions: Nourishing yin and tonifying blood, clearing away heat and removing dampness.
Applied Syndrome: Dysentery due to damp-heat. Accumulation of damp-heat leads to obstruction of qi and blood, bringing about impairment of yin fluid, manifested as dysentery with pus and blood, continuous abdominal pain, dysphoria with smothery sensation, dry mouth and throat, red tongue with little coating, thin and rapid pulse.

Dysentery-Stopping Pill
(Blood-Tonifying and Dysentery-Stopping Method)

Ingredients	Effects	Combined Effects	Syndrome	Chief Symptoms
Coptis Rhizome (黄连, Huanglian) 9g	Clearing away heat, removing dampness and stopping dysentery	Nourishing yin and enriching blood, clearing away heat and removing dampness	Impairment of yin fluid due to interior accumulation of damp-heat	Dysentery with pus and blood, continuous, abdominal pain, dysphoria with smothery sensation, dry mouth and throat, red tongue with less coating, thin and rapid pulse
Dried Ginger (干姜, Ganjiang) 9g	Drying dampness and relieving diarrhea			
Ass-hide Glue (阿胶, Ejiao) 12g	Nourishing yin and tonifying blood			
Chinese Angelica Root (当归, Danggui) 12g	Enriching blood, promoting flow of blood and alleviating pain			

Points in Constitution: In this formula, Coptis Rhizome (黄连, Huanglian) which is bitter in taste and cold in nature the descending and purging actions while Dried Ginger (干姜, Ganjiang) which is pungent in taste and warm in nature has the dispersing and dredging actions. The combination of these two drugs has both the dispersing and descending actions to remove the accumulated damp-heat. Ass-hide Glue (阿胶, Ejiao) can tonify kidney-water, nourish liver-yin and moisten dryness of the lung. When the Ass-hide Glue (阿胶, Ejiao) is combined with Dried Ginger (干姜, Ganjiang), they can not only replenish the damaged yin but also prevent the pathogens from remaining.

Indications:
1. Bacillary dysentery
2. Amebic dysentery
3. Chronic colitis
4. Chronic gastroenteritis

Precaution: This formula is applied for chronic dysentery due to mixture of deficiency and excess. It is not suitable for dysentery simply due to heat-dampness.

Associated Formulas:

1. White Peony Decoction (芍药汤, shao yao tang) *Collection of Pathogenesis for Protecting Healthy Qi from Plain Question* 《素问病机气宜保命集》

This is comprised of White Peony Root (白芍药, Baishaoyao), Chinese Angelica Root (当归, Danggui), Coptis Rhizome (黄连, Huanglian), Areca Seed (槟榔, Binglang), Common Aucklandia Root (木香, Muxiang), Licorice Root (甘草, Gancao), Rhubarb (大黄, Dahuang), Baikal Skullcap Root (黄芩, Huangqin) and Cassia Bark (肉桂, Rougui). Its actions are clearing and purging heat-dampness and regulating flow of both qi and blood. It is indicated for dysentery due to heat-dampness manifested as abdominal pain, tenesmus with purulent and bloody discharge, burning sensation in the anus, yellow and greasy tongue coating.

2. Baikai Skullcap Decoction (黄芩汤, huang qin tang) *Treatise on Exogenous Febrile Diseases* 《伤寒论》

This is comprised of White Peony Root (白芍药, Baishaoyao), Baikal Skullcap Root (黄芩, Huangqin), Licorice Root (甘草, Gancao) and Chinese Date (大枣, Dazao). Its actions are clearing away heat to stop dysentery, regulating the middle-jiao to alleviate pain. It is indicated for dysentery of heat type manifested by abdominal pain, red tongue with yellow coating and rapid pulse.

3. Lobed Kudzuvine, Baikal Skullcap and Coptis Decoction (葛根黄芩黄连汤, ge gen huang qin huang lian tang) *Treatise on Exogenous Febrile Diseases* 《伤寒论》

This is comprised of Lobed Kudzuvine Root (葛根, Gegen), Licorice Root (甘草, Gancao), Baikai Skullcap Root (黄芩, Huangqin) and Coptis Rhizome (黄连, Huanglian). Its actions are relieving the exterior syndrome and clearing away heat in the interior. It is indicated for dysentery of heat type accompanied with exterior syndrome.

4. Chinese Pulsatilla Decoction (白头翁汤, bai tou weng tang) *Treatise on Exogenous Febrile Diseases* 《伤寒论》

This is comprised of Chinese Pulsatilla Root (白头翁, Baitouweng), Chinese Corktree Bark (黄柏, Huangbai), Coptis Rhizome (黄连, Huanglian) and Largeleaf Chinese Ash Bark (秦皮, Qinpi). Its actions are clearing away heat and toxic material, removing heat from the blood to stop dysentery. It is indicated for dysentery of heat type which affects the blood system and is manifested as dysentery with less purulent and more blood discharge, thirst with desire for drinking.

5. Chinese Pulsatilla Decoction plus Ass-hide Glue (白头翁加阿胶汤, bai tou weng jia e jiao tang) *Synopsis of Golden Cabinet* 《金匮要略》

This is comprised of Chinese Pulsatilla Root (白头翁, Baitouweng), Ass-hide Glue (阿胶, E-jiao), Licorice Root (甘草, Gancao), Chinese Corktree Bark (黄柏, Huangbai), Coptis Rhizome (黄连, Huanglian) and Largeleaf Chinese Ash Bark (秦皮, Qinpi). Its actions are removing heat from the blood and nourishing yin to stop dysentery. It is indicated for dysentery with purulent and blood discharge, abdominal pain and tenesmus, thirst and restlessness, red tongue with yellow coating, weak and rapid pulse due to deficiency of yin and blood.

6. White Peony and Coptis Decoction (芍药黄连汤, shao yao huang lian tang) *Essentials of Diagnosis and Treatment* 《治法机要》

This is comprised of White Peony Root (白芍药, Baishaoyao), Chinese Angelica Root (当归, Danggui), Rhubarb (大黄, Dahuang), Cassia Bark (肉桂, Rougui), Coptis Rhizome (黄连, Huanglian) and Prepared Licorice Root (炙甘草, Zhi Gancao). Its actions are clearing away heat, inducing diuresis and regulating yingfen. It is indicated for abdominal pain with bloody discharge after defecation.

7. Common Aucklandia and Areca Seed Pill (木香槟榔丸, mu xiang bing lang wan) *Confucian's Duties to Their Parents* 《儒门事亲》

This is comprised of Areca Seed (槟榔, Binglang), Nutgrass Galingale Rhizome (香附, Xiangfu), Green Tangerine Peel (青皮, Qingpi), Tangerine Peel (橘皮, Jupi), Pharbitis Seed (牵牛, Qianniu), Rhubarb (大黄, Dahuang), Common Aucklandia Root (木香, Muxiang), Kwangsi Turmeric Rhizome (莪术, Ezhu), Coptis Rhizome (黄连, Huanglian) and Chinese Corktree Bark (黄柏, Huangbai). Its actions are activating flow of qi to remove stagnation, eliminating food retention to purge heat. It is indicated for feeling of distention, fullness and pain in the gastric and abdominal region, constipation, or dysentery with purulent and bloody discharge, tenesmus and abdominal pain due to transformation of heat resulting from indigestion and stagnation of qi.

8. Common Aucklandia and Coptis Decoction (木香黄连汤, mu xiang huang lian tang) *Effective Prescriptions* 《奇效良方》

It is comprised of Akebia Stem (木通, Mutong), Bitter Orange (枳壳, Zhiqiao), Tangerine Peel (橘皮, Jupi), Rhubarb (大黄, Dahuang), Common Aucklandia Root (木香, Muxiang), Coptis Rhizome (黄连, Huanglian) and Chinese Corktree Bark (黄柏, Huangbai). Its actions are activating flow of qi, expelling dampness, purging heat and stopping dysentery. It is indicated for dysentery with purulent and bloody discharge or tenesmus.

11. "B" Character Decoction
(乙字汤, yi zi tang)

Source: *Essay on Ye Guiting's Medical Work*《叶桂亭医事小言》
Composition: Chinese Thorowax Root（柴胡, Chaihu）9g
Baikal Skullcap Root（黄芩, Huangqin）9g
Shunk Bugbane Rhizome（升麻, Shengma）6g
Rhubarb（大黄, Dahuang）3g
Licorice Root（甘草, Gancao）6g
Chinese Angelica Root（当归, Danggui）9g
Actions: Eliminating damp-heat from the blood.
Applied Syndrome: Hemorrhoid with hemorrhage, swelling and pain in the anus or prolapse of rectum with symptoms of damp-heat such as red tongue with yellow and greasy coating, wiry and smooth pulse.

"B" Character Decoction
(Heat-Clearing and Pain-Relieving Method)

Ingredients	Effects	Combined Effects	Syndrome	Chief Symptoms
Chinese Thorowax Root（柴胡, Chaihu）9g Shunk Bugbane Rhizome（升麻, Shengma）6g	Clearing away heat and dispelling wind	Clearing away heat and purging fire, regulating flow of blood and alleviating pain	Hemorrhoid	Hemorrhoid with hemorrhage, prolapse of rectum, swelling and pain in the anus, constipation, red tongue with yellow and greasy coating, wiry and smooth pulse
Baikal Skullcap Root（黄芩, Huangqin）9g Rhubarb（大黄, Dahuang）3g	Removing heat and toxic material			
Chinese Angelica Root（当归, Danggui）9g 〔Rhubarb（大黄, Dahuang）〕	Regulating flow of blood and alleviating pain			
Licorice Root（甘草, Gancao）6g	Clearing away toxic material			

Points in Constitution: Most of diseases of the anus are due to damp-heat, blood stasis and toxic material. Rhubarb（大黄, Dahuang）, the drug for treating disorder of qi in the blood, not only relaxes the bowels and clears away toxic material but also has the actions of activating blood circulation, removing blood stasis and arresting bleeding. In this formula, the application of Rhubarb (大黄, Dahuang) is creative and original. Chinese Thorowax Root (柴胡, Chaihu) and Shunk Bugbane Rhizome (升麻, Shengma) can keep the turbid yin downward by lifting clear yang, which purges stagnated heat, thus ensuring the relief of stagnations.

Indications:
1. Hemorrhoid hemorrhage
2. Proctoptosis
3. Anus pain and tumefaction

Precaution: This formula should not be used singly for bleeding or hemorrhage due to hemorrhoid accompanied with deficiency of qi and blood.

Associated Formulas:

Sophora Flower Powder (槐花散, huai hua san) *Proven Effective Formulae*《本事方》

This is comprised of Sophora Flower (槐花, Huaihua), Chinese Arborvitae Leafy Twig (侧柏叶, Cebaiye), Spike of Fineleaf Schizonepeta Herb (荆芥穗, Jingjiesui) and Bitter Orange (枳壳, Zhiqiao). Its actions are clearing away heat from the intestines to cool the blood, expelling wind and descending qi. It is indicated for hematochezia and hemorrhoid with bleeding.

12. Yang-Lifting and Stomach-Benefiting Decoction (升阳益胃汤, sheng yang yi wei tang)

Source: *Differentiation on Endogenous and Exogenous Diseases*《内外伤辨惑论》
Composition: Membranous Milkvetch Root (黄芪, Huangqi)30g
Pinellia Rhizome (半夏, Banxia)9g
Ginseng (人参, Renshen)9g
Licorice Root (甘草, Gancao)9g
Doubleteeth Pubescent Angelica Root (独活, Duhuo)9g
Divaricate Saposhnikovia Root (防风, Fangfeng)9g
White Peony Root (白芍药, Baishaoyao)9g
Notopterygium Rhizome or Root (羌活, Qianghuo)9g
Tangerine Peel (橘皮, Jupi)6g
Tuckahoe (茯苓, Fuling)6g
Chinese Thorowax Root (柴胡, Chaihu)6g
Oriental Waterplantain Rhizome (泽泻, Zexie)6g
Largehead Atractylodes Rhizome (白术, Baizhu)6g
Coptis Rhizome (黄连, Huanglian)30g
Fresh Ginger (生姜, Shengjiang)3g
Chinese Date (大枣, Dazao)3g

Actions: Replenishing qi and lifting yang, removing dampness and strengthening the stomach.

Applied Syndrome: Accumulation of dampness in the middle-jiao due to deficiency of the spleen and stomach, manifested as laziness, somnolence, inability of the limbs to flex, heaviness sensation of the body and joint, edema, bitter taste and dry tongue, poor appetite or anorexia, tastelessness, indigestion, irregular stool, frequency of micturition, pale tongue with thin coating, weak and feeble pulse.

Yang-Lifting and Stomach-Benefiting Decoction
(Qi-Replenishing and Yang-Lifting Method)

Ingredients	Effects	Combined Effects	Syndrome	Chief Symptoms
Membranous Milkvetch Root (黄芪, Huangqi)30g Ginseng (人参, Renshen)9g Largehead Atractylodes Rhizome (白术, Baizhu)6g	Replenishing qi and invigorating the stomach	Replenishing qi and lifting yang, removing dampness and strengthening the stomach	Transformation of heat due to accumulation of dampness resulting from deficiency of the spleen and stomach	Laziness, somnolence, inability of the limbs to flex, heaviness sensation of the body and joint edema, bitter taste in the mouth and dry tongue, anorexia and tastelessness, indigestion, irregular stool, frequency of micturition, pale tongue with thin coating, weak and feeble pulse
Chinese Thorowax Root (柴胡, Chaihu)6g Divaricate Saposhnikovia Root (防风, Fangfeng)9g Incised Notopterygium Rhizome or Root (羌活, Qianghuo)9g Doubleteeth Pubescent Angelica Root (独活, Duhuo)9g	Lifting clear yang, expelling wind and removing dampness			
Pinellia Rhizome (半夏, Banxia)9g Tangerine Peel (橘皮, Jupi)6g	Removing dampness with the pungent and bitter drugs			
Tuckahoe (茯苓, Fuling)6g Oriental Waterplantain Rhizome (泽泻, Zexie)6g	Removing dampness and inducing diuresis			
Coptis Rhizome (黄连, Huanglian)30g	Clearing away heat and drying dampness			
White Peony Root (白芍药, Baishaoyao)9g	Inducing astringency and regulating yinfen			
Fresh Ginger (生姜, Shengjiang)3g Chinese Date (大枣, Dazao)3g Licorice Root (甘草, Gancao)9g	Regulating yingfen and weifen			

Points in Constitution: Based on Middle-Reinforcing and Qi-Benefiting Decoction (补中益气汤), this formula strengthens the dampness-removing action, which is very suitable for the syndrome of retention of dampness in three-jiao accompanied with failure of clearing yang to rise.

Indications:
1. Gastritis
2. Prolapse of gastric mucosa
3. Urticaria
4. Other idiopathic fever

Precautions:
1. The wind-expelling herbs in the formula should be used in a small dose. Otherwise, this formula will reverse the order of primary and secondary, which means it is far from lifting yang but makes the spleen and stomach more deficient.

2. After administration, it is necessary to take some nutritive and digestible food. The fat and greasy food should be avoided.

3. After taking the medicine, it is advisable for the patients to take up some slight activities to promote the digestion of food and absorption of the medicine, but strain or extreme fatigue should be avoided.

Associated Formula:

Yang-Lifting Decoction (升阳汤, sheng yang tang) *Treatise on the Spleen and Stomach* 《脾胃论》

This is comprised of Chinese Thorowax Root (柴胡, Chaihu), Sharpleaf Galangal Fruit (益智仁, Yizhiren), Main Part of Chinese Angelica Root (当归身, Dangguishen), Tangerine Peel (橘皮, Jupi), Shunk Bugbane Rhizome (升麻, Shengma), Licorice Root (甘草, Gancao) and Safflower (红花, Honghua). Its actions are replenishing qi, lifting yang, warming the spleen and stopping diarrhea. It is indicated for loose stool characterized by 3-4 times a day with small amount, or occasional diarrhea, borborygmus and yellow urine.

13. Common Burreed and Kwangsi Turmeric Decoction (荆蓬煎丸, ji peng jian wan)

Source: *The Precious Mirror of Hygiene* 《卫生宝鉴》
Composition: Common Aucklandia Root (木香, Muxiang) 9g
Green Tangerine Peel (青皮, Qingpi) 9g
Fennel Fruit (茴香, Huixiang) 6g
Bitter Orange (枳壳, Zhiqiao) 9g
Areca Seed (槟榔, Binglang) 9g
Common Burreed Rhizome (三棱, Sanleng) 9g
Kwangsi Turmeric Rhizome (莪术, Ezhu) 9g
Actions: Regulating flow of qi and removing retention of food, eliminating mass and relieving

fullness sensation.

Applied Syndrome: Abdominal mass or hypochondriac lump due to accumulation of phlegm, characterized by being soft and localized and manifested as fullness, stuffiness, distention and pain in the abdomen, thin and white tongue coating, wiry pulse.

Common Burreed and Kwangsi Turmeric Decoction
(Qi-Regulating and Blood-Activating Method)

Ingredients	Effects	Combined Effects	Syndrome	Chief Symptoms
Common Aucklandia Root (木香, Muxiang) 9g Green Tangerine Peel (青皮, Qingpi) 9g Fennel Fruit (茴香, Huixiang) 6g Bitter Orange (枳壳, Zhiqiao) 9g Areca Seed (槟榔, Binglang) 9g	Regulating flow of qi and dissipating blockages	Regulating flow of qi and activating blood circulation, dredging the collaterals and eliminating mass	Accumulation or mass in the abdomen due to stagnation of qi and blood	The early stage of abdominal mass syndrome characterized by being soft and localized, distention and pain in the abdomen, thin and white coating, wiry pulse.
Common Burreed Rhizome (三棱, Sanleng) 9g Kwangsi Turmeric Rhizome (莪术, Ezhu) 9g	Activating blood circulation and eliminating abdominal mass			

Points in Constitution: This formula concludes various qi-regulating drugs and has the actions of regulating qi, activating blood circulation, promoting digestion, dissipating blockages and expelling phlegm. In the original formula, Bitter Orange (枳壳, Zhiqiao) is fried with Croton Fruit (巴豆, Badou) to strengthen the actions of dissipating blockages, expelling phlegm and eliminating mass.

Indications:

1. Gastrointestinal functional disturbance
2. Incomplete intestinal obstruction
3. Cirrhosis, splenomegaly
4. Chronic pelvic inflammation in women

Precautions:

1. It is contraindicated in pregnant woman.
2. It is forbidden for those without abdominal mass.
3. Raw and cold food should be avoided.

Associated Formulas:

Abdominal Mass-Removing Pill（化积丸，hua ji wan）*Source and Cause of Miscellaneous Diseases*《杂病源流犀烛》

This is comprised of Common Burreed Rhizome（三棱，Sanleng）, Kwangsi Turmeric Rhizome（莪术，Ezhu）, Chinese Asafetida（阿魏，Awei）, Pumice（海浮石，Haifushi）, Nutgrass Galingale Rhizome（香附，Xiangfu）, Red Orpiment（雄黄，Xionghuang）, Areca Seed（槟榔，Binglang）, Sappan Wood（苏木，Sumu）, Ark Shell（瓦楞子，Walengzi）and Trogopterus Dung（五灵脂，Wulingzhi）. Its actions are removing blood stasis and abdominal mass. It is indicated for hard abdominal mass due to prolonged retention of foodwhich gives severe pains and brings about poor appetite.

Additional Formulas:

Heat-Removing Decoction for Acute Pancreatitis
（胰腺清化汤, yi xian qing hua tang）

Source: *Common Acute Abdomen*《常见急腹症》
Composition: Chinese Thorowax Root（柴胡, Chaihu）15g
White Peony Root（白芍药, Baishaoyao）15g
Baikal Skullcap Root（黄芩, Huangqin）15g
Officinal Magnolia Bark（厚朴, Houpo）12g
Immature Bitter Orange（枳实, Zhishi）9g
Fortune Eupatorium Herb（佩兰, Peilan）9g
Rhubarb（大黄, Dahuang）9g
Honeysuckle Flower（金银花, Jinyinhua）30g
Indigowoad Leaf（大青叶, Daqingye）30g
Mirabilite（芒硝, Mangxiao）6g

Actions: Clearing away heat and purging fire, regulating flow of qi and alleviating pain.

Applied Syndrome: Acute pancreatitis. Engorgement or eating too much fat leads to heat accumulating in the epigastrical region, manifested as sudden onset of epigastralgia which is severe as if stabbed by a knife, nausea and vomiting, low fever or high fever, scanty and dark urine, or jaundice, red tongue with yellow and greasy coating, wiry or bounding and rapid pulse.

Points in Constitution: This formula is the combination of Major Bupleurum Decoction（大柴胡汤, da chai hu tang）without Pinellia Rhizome（半夏, Banxia）and Major Purgative Decoction（大承气汤, da cheng qi tang）plus other ingredients. Major Purgative Decoction（大承气汤）has the actions of clearing away heat, relaxing the bowels and purging the accumulation of heat, while Major Bupleurum Decoction（大柴胡汤, da chai hu tang）has the actions of expelling evils exteriorly, purging heat interiorly and alleviating pain. Honeysuckle Flower（金银花, Jinyinhua）and Indigowoad Leaf（大青叶, Daqingye）, which have the actions of clearing away heat and removing toxic material and Fortune Eupatorium Herb（佩兰, Peilan）, which has the actions of promoting diuresis and eliminating turbid evils, are used to clear the accumulated damp-heat. Thus, this formula is able to exert all the actions of clearing away heat, purging fire, regulating flow of qi and alleviating pain.

Indications:
1. Acute pancreatitis
2. Acucte holecystitis

Precaution: It should be cautiously used for pregnant woman because there are some purgative drugs in this formula.

Heat-Removing Decoction for Acute Pancreatitis
(Heat-Removing, Fire-Purging, Qi-Regulating and Dampness-Eliminating Method)

Ingredients	Effects	Combined Effects	Syndrome	Chief Symptoms
Chinese Thorowax Root (柴胡, Chaihu) 15g Baikal Skullcap Root (黄芩, Huangqin) 15g	Harmonizing the functions of Shaoyang system and reducing fever	Clearing away heat and purging fire, regulating flow of qi and alleviating pain	Acute pancreatitis (due to accumulation of heat in the epigastric region)	Sudden onset of epigastralgia which is severe as if cut by a knife, nausea and vomiting, low fever or high fever, scanty and dark urine, or jaundice, red tongue with yellow and greasy coating, wiry or bounding and rapid pulse.
Honeysuckle Flower (金银花, Jinyinhua) 30g Indigowoad Leaf (大青叶, Daqingye) 30g	Clearing away heat and toxic material			
Fortune Eupatorium Herb (佩兰, Peilan) 9g	Regulating the stomach qi to stop vomiting			
Officinal Magnolia Bark (厚朴, Houpo) 12g Immature Bitter Orange (枳实, Zhishi) 9g White Peony Root (白芍药, Baishaoyao) 15g	Regulating flow of qi and alleviating pain			
Rhubarb (大黄, Dahuang) 9g Mirabilite (芒硝, Mangxiao) 6g	Purging heat and removing stagnation			

Associated Formulas:

1. Minor Chinese Thorowax Decoction (小柴胡汤, xiao chai hu tang) *Treatise on Exogenous Febrile Diseases* 《伤寒论》

This is comprised of Chinese Thorowax Root (柴胡, Chaihu), Ginseng (人参, Renshen), Baikal Skullcap Root (黄芩, Huangqin), Pinellia Rhizome (半夏, Banxia), Licorice Root (甘草, Gancao), Fresh Ginger (生姜, Shengjiang) and Chinese Date (大枣, Dazao). Its actions are treating shaoyang disease by mediation and dispersing the stagnated liver-qi. It is indicated for the syndrome of shaoyang.

2. Modified Chinese Thorowax Decoction (加味柴胡汤, jia wei chai hu tang) *Source and*

Cause of Miscellaneous Diseases《杂病源流犀烛》

This is comprised of Capillary Wormwood Herb（茵陈，Yinchen）, Chinese Thorowax Root（柴胡，Chaihu）, Baikal Skullcap Root（黄芩，Huangqin）, Pinellia Rhizome（半夏，Banxia）, Coptis Rhizome（黄连，Huanglian）, Fermented Soybean（淡豆豉，Dandouchi）, Lobed Kudzu-vine Root（葛根，Gegen） and Rhubarb（大黄，Dahuang）. Its actions are clearing away heat and drying dampness, mediating shaoyang and alleviating pain. It is indicated for pain in the hypochondrium and jaundice due to accumulation of heat and dampness in the liver and gallbladder. Points in Constitution: Six fu-organs must be unobstructed in order to function well. This formula is the modified Rhubarb and Tree Peony Bark Decoction（大黄牡丹皮汤, da huang mu dan pi tang）. In the formula, Rhubarb（大黄，Dahuang） is used to relax the bowels, purge heat and remove blood stasis. Peach Seed（桃仁，Taoren） and Tree Peony Bark（牡丹皮，Mudanpi） are used to activate blood circulation and remove blood stasis. Szechwan Chinaberry Fruit Powder（金铃子散，Jinglingzisan）, which includes Corydalis Tuber（延胡索，Yanhusuo） and has the actions of removing blood stasis and alleviating pain, is the key prescription for treating periappendicular abscess due to excessive heat when it is combined with Honeysuckle Flower（金银花，Jinyinhua）, which can clear away heat and toxic material, and Common Aucklandia Root（木香，Muxiang）, which can activate flow of qi.

Blood Stasis-Removing Decoction for Acute Appendicitis
（阑尾化瘀汤，lan wei hua yu tang）

Source: *Manual for Acute Abdomen*《急腹症手册》
Composition: Tree Peony Bark（牡丹皮，Mudanpi）9g
Peach Seed（桃仁，Taoren）9g
Corydalis Tuber（延胡索，Yanhusuo）9g
Common Aucklandia Root（木香，Muxiang）9g
Szechwan Chinaberry Fruit（川楝子，Chuanlianzi）15g
Rhubarb（大黄，Dahuang）9g
Honeysuckle Flower（金银花，Jinyinhua）15g

Actions: Clearing away heat and toxic material, removing blood stasis and dissipating blockages.

Applied Syndrome: Periappendicular abscess due to accumulation of damp-heat and stagnation of qi and blood, manifested as fever, epigastric distention and stuffiness, belching and anorexia, nausea, pain in right lower abdomen, localized pain with tenderness or a lump, constipation, scanty and dark urine, yellow and greasy tongue coating, wiry tense or wiry, smooth pulse.

Indications:
1. Acute appendicitis
2. Acute pelvic inflammation
3. Inflammation after tubal ligation operation

Blood Stasis-Removing Decoction for Acute Appendicitis
(Heat-Clearing and Stasis-Removing Method)

Ingredients	Effects	Combined Effects	Syndrome	Chief Symptoms
Rhubarb (大黄, Dahuang)9g	Purging heat and removing blood stasis	Clearing away heat and toxic material, removing blood stasis and dissipating blockages	Periappendicular abscess (due to accumulation of damp-heat and stagnation of qi and blood)	Fever, gastric and abdominal distention and stuffiness, belching and anorexia, nausea, pain in right lower abdomen, localized pain, tenderness or with lump, constipation, scanty and dark urine, yellow and greasy coating, wiry tense or wiry smooth pulse
Peach Seed (桃仁, Taoren)9g Tree Peony Bark (牡丹皮, Mudanpi)9g	Breaking and dispelling blood stasis			
Honeysuckle Flower (金银花, Jinyinhua) 15g	Clearing away heat and toxic material, reducing swelling and dissipating blockages			
Szechwan Chinaberry Fruit (川楝子, Chuanlianzi)15g Corydalis Tuber (延胡索, Yanhusuo)9g Common Aucklandia Root (木香, Muxiang)9g	Activating flow of qi and alleviating pain			

Precaution: This formula is applied for periappendicular abscess due to accumulation of heat-dampness and stagnation of qi and blood. It is not suitable for periappendicular abscess due to accumulation of cold, dampness and blood stasis.

Associated Formulas:

1. Heat-Clearing and Stasis-Removing Decoction for Acute Appendicitis(阑尾清化汤, Lan wei qing hua tang) *Manual for Acute Abdomen*《急腹症手册》

This is comprised of Rhubarb (大黄, Dahuang), Peach Seed (桃仁, Taoren), Tree Peony Bark (牡丹皮, Mudanpi), Szechwan Chinaberry Fruit (川楝子, Chuanlianzi), Licorice Root (甘草, Gancao), Red Peony Root (赤芍, Chishao), Honeysuckle Flower (金银花, Jinyinhua) and Dandelion (蒲公英, Pugongying). Its actions are clearing away heat and toxic material, activating flow of qi and blood circulation. It is indicated for acute appendicitis in the heat-accumulating stage.

2. Coix Seed, Prepared Aconite and Whiteflower Patrinia Powder (薏苡附子败酱散, yi yi fu zi bai jiang san) *Synopsis of Golden Cabinet*《金匮要略》

This is comprised of Coix Seed (薏苡仁, Yiyiren), Prepared Aconite Root (附子, Fuzi) and Whiteflower Patrinia Herb (败酱草, Baijiangcao). Its actions are evacuating pus and reducing swelling. It is indicated for periappendicular abscess due to mixture of cold-dampness and blood stasis.

Gallstones-Removing Decoction
(胆道排石汤, dan dao pai shi tang)

Source: *Common Acute Abdomen in Surgery Treated by the Combination of Traditonal Chinese Medicine and Western Medicine*《中西医结合治疗常见外科急腹症》

Composition: Christina Loosestrife Herb（金钱草, Jinqiancao）30g

Capillary Wormwood Herb（茵陈蒿, Yinchenhao）30g

Turmeric Root-tuber（郁金, Yujin）30g

Common Aucklandia Root（木香, Muxiang）9g

Immature Bitter Orange（枳实, Zhishi）9g

Rhubarb（大黄, Dahuang）6~9g

Actions: Clearing away heat and inducing diuresis, promoting flow of qi and alleviating pain, normalizing function of the gallbladder to discharge the stone.

Applied Syndrome:

Cholelithiasis due to qi stagnation of both the liver and gallbladder and accumulation of damp-heat in the interior. The manifestations are severe megalgia in the right upper abdomen, fever or alternating attacks of chills and fever, bitter taste in the mouth and dry throat, red tongue with yellow and greasy coating, wiry or wiry and rapid pulse.

Points in Constitution: This formula is the modified Oriental Wormwood Decoction(茵陈蒿汤, yin chen hao tang), which has the actions of clearing away heat, inducing diuresis and relieving jaundice. When it is combined with Christina Loosestrife Herb（金钱草, Jinqiancao）and Turmeric Root-Tuber（郁金, Yujin）, it can clear away heat from the gallbladder, promote diuresis and drain the stone away. It is a main prescription for cholelithiasis.

Indications:

1. Acute cholecystitis

2. Cholelithiasis

3. Toxic hepatitis

4. Acute infectious icterus hepatitis

5. Biliary ascariasis

6. Icterus due to leptospirosis

Precaution: It should be used cautiously for those who are weak and accompanied with loose stool.

Associated Formulas:

1. Liver-Dispersing and Gallbladder-Benefiting Decoction（疏肝利胆汤, shu gan li dan tang）*New Traditional Chinese Medicine*《新中医》1986.11

This is comprised of Chinese Thorowax Root（柴胡, Chaihu）, Immature Bitter Orange（枳实, Zhishi）, White Peony Root（白芍, Baishao）, Common Aucklandia Root（木香, Muxiang）, Turmeric Root-Tuber（郁金, Yujin）, Baikal Skullcap Root（黄芩, Huangqin）, Mirabilite（芒

硝，Mangxiao), Chicken Gizzard Membrane (鸡内金，Jineijin), Officinal Magnolia Bark (厚朴，Houpo), Rhubarb (大黄，Dahuang), Coptis Rhizome (黄连，Huanglian) and Licorice Root (甘草，Gancao). Its actions are dispersing the stagnated liver-qi, normalizing functioning of the gall-bladder, clearing away heat and draining the stone away. It is indicated for cholelithiasis due to stagnation of liver-qi and accumulation of heat-dampness in the liver and gallbladder.

Gallstones-Removing Decoction
(Heat-Clearing, Dampness-Removing, Qi-Regulating and Pain-alleviating Method)

Ingredients	Effects	Combined Effects	Syndrome	Chief Symptoms
Rhubarb (大黄，Dahuang)6~9g	Purging heat and relaxing the bowels	Clearing away heat and inducing diuresis, activating flow of qi and alleviating pain, normalizing the secretory function of the gallbladder to discharge the stone	Cholelithiasis (due to qi stagnation of both the liver and gallbladder and the accumulation of damp-heat in the interior)	Severe megalgia in the right upper abdomen, fever or alternating episodes of chills and fever, bitter taste in the mouth and dry throat, red tongue with yellow and greasy coating, wiry or wiry and rapid pulse
Christina Loosestrife Herb (金钱草，Jinqiancao)30g	Clearing away heat of the gallbladder, inducing diuresis and eliminating the stone			
Turmeric Root-Tuber (郁金，Yujin) 30g Immature Bitter Orange (枳实，Zhishi)9g Common Aucklandia Root (木香，Muxiang)9g	Regulating the activities of qi in the liver, gallbladder, spleen and stomach			
Capillary Wormwood Herb (茵陈蒿，Yinchenhao) 30g	Clearing away heat of the gallbladder, inducing diuresis and relieving jaundice			

2. Gallbladder-Calming Decoction (安胆汤，an dan tang) *Zhejiang Journal of Traditional Chinese Medicine*《浙江中医杂志》1982. 11-12

This is comprised of Christina Loosestrife Herb (金钱草，Jinqiancao), White Peony Root (白芍药，Baishaoyao), Rhubarb (大黄，Dahuang), Chinese Thorowax Root (柴胡，Chaihu) and Capillary Wormwood Herb (茵陈蒿，Yinchenhao). Its actions are clearing away heat, inducing diuresis, relieving the depressed qi and removing stagnation. It is indicated for cholecystitis and Cholelithiasis.

3. Capillary Wormwood Decoction (茵陈蒿汤，yin chen hao tang) *Treatise on Exogenous*

Febrile Diseases《伤寒论》

This is comprised of Cape Jasmine Fruit（栀子，Zhizi）, Rhubarb（大黄，Dahuang）and Capillary Wormwood Herb（茵陈蒿，Yinchenhao）. Its actions are clearing away heat, inducing diuresis and relieving jaundice. It is indicated for jaundice due to heat-dampness.

4. Ascaris-Expelling Decoction Number One（驱蛔汤一号，qu hui tang yi hao）*Acute Abdomen Treated by the Combination of Traditonal Chinese Medicine and Western Medicine*《中西医结合治疗急腹症》

This is comprised of Areca Seed（槟榔，Binglang）, Rangooncreeper Fruit（使君子，Shijunzi）, Szechwan Chinaberry Bark（苦楝皮，Kulianpi）, Smoked Plum（乌梅，Wumei）, Common Aucklandia Root（木香，Muxiang）, Bitter Orange（枳壳，Zhiqiao）, Pricklyash Peel（川椒，Chuanjiao）, Manchurian Wildginger Herb（细辛，Xixin）, Dried Ginger（干姜，Ganjiang）and Weathered Sodium Sulfate（元明粉，Yuanmingfen）. Its actions are expelling ascaris and alleviating pain. It is indicated for the early stage of ascariasis of the biliary tract with severe pain.

5. Ascaris-Expelling Decoction Number Two（驱蛔汤二号，qu hui tang er hao）*Acute Abdomen Treated by the Combination of Traditonal Chinese Medicine and Western Medicine*《中西医结合治疗急腹症》

This is comprised of Chinese Thorowax Root（柴胡，Chaihu）, Turmeric Root-Tuber（郁金，Yujin）, Cape Jasmine Fruit（山栀子，Shanzhizi）, Common Aucklandia Root（木香，Muxiang）, Bitter Orange（枳壳，Zhiqiao）, Capillary Wormwood Herb（茵陈蒿，Yinchenhao）, Oyster Shell（牡蛎，Muli）and Baked Alumon（枯矾，Kufan）. Its actions are normalizing functioning of the gallbladder and expelling ascaris. It is indicated for ascariasis of the biliary tract with died ascarid.

6. Ascaris-Expelling Decoction Number Three（驱蛔汤三号，qu hui tang san hao）*Acute Abdomen Treated by the Combination of Traditonal Chinese Medicine and Western Medicine*《中西医结合治疗急腹症》

This is comprised of Areca Seed（槟榔，Binglang）, Rangooncreeper Fruit（使君子，Shijunzi）, Szechwan Chinaberry Bark（苦楝皮，Kulianpi）, Stone-Like Omphalia（雷丸，Leiwan）, Rhubarb（大黄，Dahuang）, Officinal Magnolia Bark（厚朴，Houpo）and Bitter Orange（枳壳，Zhiqiao）. Its actions are expelling ascaris and relaxing the bowels. It is indicated for ascariasis of the biliary tract and used to expelling the ascaris from the intestines.

7. Gentian Liver-Purging Decoction（龙胆泻肝汤，long dan xie gan tang）*Secret Record of the Chamber of Orchids*《兰室秘藏》

This is comprised of Chinese Gentian Root（龙胆草，Longdancao）, Dried Rehmannia Root（生地黄，Shengdihuang）, Chinese Angelica Root（当归，Danggui）, Chinese Thorowax Root（柴胡，Chaihu）, Oriental Waterplantain Rhizome（泽泻，Zexie）, Plantain Seed（车前子，Cheqianzi）, Cape Jasmine Fruit（栀子，Zhizi）, Baikal Skullcap Root（黄芩，Huangqin）, Licorice Root（甘草，Gancao）and Akebia Stem（木通，Mutong）. Its actions are purging excessive fire of the liver and gallbladder and clearing away heat-dampness of the three-jiao. It is indicated for the syndrome of downward attack of heat-dampness in the liver meridian and flaming-up of excessive fire of the liver and gallbladder.

8. Capillary Wormwood, Chinese Thorowax Gallbladder-Clearing Decoction（茵柴清胆汤，yin

chai qing dan tang) *Ran's Experienced Prescriptions*《冉氏经验方》

It is comprised of Chinese Thorowax Root (柴胡, Chaihu), Rhubarb (大黄, Dahuang), Coptis Rhizome (黄连, Huanglian), Tree Peony Bark (牡丹皮, Mudanpi), Honeysuckle Flower (金银花, Jinyinhua), Indigowoad Leaf (大青叶, Daqingye), Cape Jasmine Fruit (山栀子, Shanzhizi), Commbined Spicebush Root (乌药, Wuyao), Immature Bitter Orange (枳实, Zhishi), Capillary Wormwood Herb (茵陈蒿, Yinchenhao), Umbellate Pore Fungus (猪苓, Zhuling) and Licorice Root (甘草, Gancao). Its actions are clearing away heat, inducing diuresis, normalizing functioning of the gallbladder and curing jaundice. It is indicated for acute cholecystitis due to heat-dampness in the liver and gallbladder.

Liver-Soothing Decoction
(舒肝饮, shu gan yin)

Source: *Curative Li Congfu's Medical Records*《李聪甫医案》
Composition: Pilose Asiabell Root (党参, Dangshen) 9g
Largehead Atractylodes Rhizome (白术, Baizhu) 9g
Turmeric Root-tuber (郁金, Yujin) 9g
Common Aucklandia Root (木香, Muxiang) 6g
Bitter Orange (枳壳, Zhiqiao) 6g
Tuckahoe (茯苓, Fuling) 12g
Licorice Root (甘草, Gancao) 3g
Tangerine Peel (橘皮, Jupi) 6g
Dan-shen Root (丹参, Danshen) 12g
Chinese Angelica Root (当归, Danggui) 9g
White Peony Root (白芍药, Baishaoyao) 9g
Green Tangerine Peel (青皮, Qingpi) 6g
Turtle Carapace (鳖甲, Biejia) 15g

Actions: Dispersing the stagnated liver-qi and regulating the spleen, promoting flow of qi and activating blood circulation.

Applied Syndrome: Stagnation of qi and stasis of blood due to depression of the liver and deficiency of the spleen. The manifestations are mass in the hypochondrium with feelings of distention and pain, vascular spider in the head, neck, chest and arm, poor appetite, tiredness, pale tongue, ecchymosis on margin of tongue, wiry and thin pulse.

Points in Constitution: The action of this formula is dispersing the stagnated liver-qi and invigorating the spleen. It is similar to Merry Life Powder(逍遥散, xiao yao san) in action. But, the ingredients and dosage of this formula are heavier than those of Merry Life Powder(逍遥散, xiao yao san). Instead of Chinese Thorowax Root (柴胡, Chaihu) and Wild Mint Herb (薄荷, Bohe), the use of Turmeric Root-Tuber (郁金, Yujin), Green Tangerine Peel (青皮, Qingpi), Dan-Shen Root (丹参, Danshen) and Bitter Orange (枳壳, Zhiqiao) in this formula lies in the reason that the syndrome belongs to xuefen. In this formula, the five ingredients of Miraculous Effect Powder(异功散, yi gong san) can replenish qi, invigorate the spleen, activate flow of qi and remove stagnation. According to Zhang Zhongjing, who was a famous ancient physician and designed the formula of Decocted Turtle Shell Pill(鳖甲煎丸, bie jia jian wan), Carapace (鳖甲, Biejia), which has the actions of activating flow of qi, promoting blood circulation, softening hardness and eliminating mass, is used for hepatosplenomegaly.

Liver-Soothing Decoction
(Qi-Replenishing and Blood-Activating Method)

Ingredients	Effects	Combined Effects	Syndrome	Chief Symptoms
Pilose Asiabell Root (党参, Dangshen)9g Largehead Atractylodes Rhizome (白术, Baizhu)9g Tuckahoe (茯苓, Fuling)12g Licorice Root (甘草, Gancao)3g Tangerine Peel (橘皮, Jupi)6g	Replenishing qi and invigorating the spleen, regulating flow of qi and removing stagnation	Dispersing the stagnated liver-qi and invigorating the spleen, activating flow of qi and activating blood circulation, dissipating blockages and eliminating mass	Mass in the hypochondrium (due to qi stagnation and blood stasis resulting from stagnation of the liver qi and deficiency of the spleen)	Mass in the hypochondrium with feelings of distention and pain, vascular spider in the head, neck, chest and arm, poor appetite, tiredness, pale tongue, ecchymosis on margin of tongue, wiry and thin pulse
Common Aucklandia Root (木香, Muxiang)6g Bitter Orange (枳壳, Zhiqiao)6g	Regulating flow of qi, activating the spleen and benefiting the activities of qi			
Dan-Shen Root (丹参, Danshen)12g Chinese Angelica Root (当归, Danggui)9g White Peony Root (白芍药, Baishaoyao)9g	Activating blood circulation and enriching blood, nourishing liver yin and alleviating pain			
Turmeric Root-Tuber (郁金, Yujin)9g Green Tangerine Peel (青皮, Qingpi)6g Turtle Carapace (鳖甲, Biejia)15g	Soothing the liver and removing blood stasis, soften hardness and dissipating blockages			

Indications:

1. Begin of cirrhosis

2. Hepatitis B

Precaution: This formula has a better effect on chronic liver diseases. It is not suitable for jaundice, cholelithiasis and cholecystitis due to accumulation of heat-dampness and stagnation of qi and blood.

Associated Formulas:

1. Merry Life Powder（逍遥散，xiao yao san）*Prescriptions of Peaceful Benevolent Dispensary*《和剂局方》

This is comprised of Chinese Thorowax Root（柴胡，Chaihu）, Chinese Angelica Root（当归，Danggui）, White Peony Root（白芍药，Baishaoyao）, Largehead Atractylodes Rhizome（白术，Baizhu）, Tuckahoe（茯苓，Fuling）, Licorice Root（甘草，Gancao）, Wild Mint Herb（薄荷，Bohe）and Roasting Ginger（煨姜，Weijiang）. Its actions are soothing the liver and regulating the circulation of qi, invigorating the spleen and regulating yingfen. It is indicated for pain in the hypochondrium, alternate attacks of chills and fever, weak and wiry pulse due to depressed liver-qi and blood deficiency.

2. Qi-Replenishing, Retention-Removing and Poison-Clearing Decoction（益气化积解毒汤，yi qi hua ji jie du tang）*Jilin Journal of Traditional Chinese Medicine*《吉林中医药》

This is comprised of Membranous Milkvetch Root（黄芪，Huangqi）, Dan-Shen Root（丹参，Danshen）, Largehead Atractylodes Rhizome（白术，Baizhu）, Tuckahoe（茯苓，Fuling）, Turmeric Root-Tuber（郁金，Yujin）, Chinese Angelica Root（当归，Danggui）, Dried Rehmannia Root（生地黄，Shengdihuang）, Hirsute Shiny Bugleweed Herb（泽兰叶，Zelanye）, Indigowood Root（板蓝根，Banlangen）, Whiteflower Patrinia Herb（败酱草，Baijiangcao）, Chicken Gizzard Membrane（鸡内金，Jineijin）, Siberian Solomonseal Rhizome（黄精，Huangjing）and Dried Human Placenta（紫河车，Ziheche）. Its actions are replenishing qi, removing food retention, clearing away toxic material and inducing diuresis. It is indicated for tympanites, abdominal mass and jaundice due to deficiency of the spleen and kidney which brings about stagnation of liver blood and accumulation of heat-dampness.

3. Chinese Thorowax Liver-Clearing Decoction（柴胡清肝饮，chai hu qing gan yin）*Syndrome-Cause-Pulse-Treatment*《症因脉治》

This is comprised of Chinese Thorowax Root（柴胡，Chaihu）, Green Tangerine Peel（青皮，Qingpi）, Bitter Orange（枳壳，Zhiqiao）, Cape Jasmine Fruit（山栀子，Shanzhizi）, Akebia Stem（木通，Mutong）, Gambirplant Hooked Stem and Branch（钩藤，Gouteng）, Perilla Stem（苏梗，Sugeng）, Baikal Skullcap Root（黄芩，Huangqin）, Common Anemarrhena Rhizome（知母，Zhimu）and Licorice Root（甘草，Gancao）. Its actions are dispersing the stagnated liver-qi and clearing away heat. It is indicated for stabbing pain in the chest, hypochondrium and epigastrium due to heat in the liver and gallbladder.

4. Chinese Thorowax Liver-Soothing Powder（柴胡疏肝散，chai hu shu gan san）*Jingyue's Complete Works*《景岳全书》

It is comprised of Tangerine Peel（橘皮，Jupi）, Chinese Thorowax Root（柴胡，Chaihu）, Szechwan Lovage Rhizome（川芎，Chuanxiong）, Bitter Orange（枳壳，Zhiqiao）, White Peony Root（白芍药，Baishaoyao）, Nutgrass Galingale Rhizome（香附，Xiangfu）and Prepared Licorice

Root (炙甘草, Zhi Gancao). Its actions are dispersing the stagnated liver-qi, activating flow of qi, promoting blood circulation and alleviating pain. It is indicated for pain in the chest and hypochondrium, alternate spells of chills and fever due to stagnation of liver-qi.

5. Minor Chinese Thorowax Decoction (小柴胡汤, xiao chai hu tang) *Treatise on Exogenous Febrile Diseases* 《伤寒论》

This is comprised of Chinese Thorowax Root (柴胡, Chaihu), Ginseng (人参, Renshen), Baikal Skullcap Root (黄芩, Huangqin), Pinellia Rhizome (半夏, Banxia), Licorice Root (甘草, Gancao), Fresh Ginger (生姜, Shengjiang) and Chinese Date (大枣, Dazao). Its actions are treating shaoyang disease by mediation, soothing the liver and regulating the circulation of qi. It is indicated for shaoyang diseases manifested as a feeling of fullness in the chest and hypochondrium, alternate attacks of chills and fever, bitter taste in the mouth and dry throat.

6. Liver-Soothing and Spleen-Regulating Pill (舒肝理脾丸, shu gan li pi wan) *The Foundation of Clinical Traditional Chinese Medicine* 《中医临床学基础》

This is comprised of Turtle Carapace (鳖甲, Biejia), Lalang Grass Rhizome (白茅根, Baimaogen), Chinese Angelica Root (当归, Danggui), Red Peony Root (赤芍, Chishao), Trogopterus Dung (五灵脂, Wulingzhi), Cattail Pollen (蒲黄, Puhuang), Madder Root (茜草, Qiancao), Chinese Thorowax Root (柴胡, Chaihu), Turmeric Root-Tuber (郁金, Yujin), Earth Worm (地龙, Dilong), Chicken Gizzard Membrane (鸡内金, Jineijin), Green Tangerine Peel (青皮, Qingpi) and Bitter Orange (枳壳, Zhiqiao). Its actions are dispersing the stagnated liver-qi and regulating the spleen, activating blood circulation and removing blood stasis. It is indicated for distending pain in the hypochondrium, oppressed feeling in the chest, poor appetite and abdominal mass.

Liver-Recuperating Pill
(复肝丸, fu gan wan)

Source: *Shanghai Journal of Traditional Chinese Medicine* 《上海中医药杂志》
Composition: Dried Human Placenta (紫河车, Ziheche)6g
Red Ginseng Stigma (红参须, Hongshenxu)6g
Stir-backed Ground Bettle (炙地鳖虫, Zhi Dibiechong)6g
Sanchi Root (三七, Sanqi)6g
Turmeric Rhizome (姜黄, Jianghuang)6g
Turmeric Root-tuber (郁金, Yujin)6g
Chicken Gizzard Membrane (鸡内金, Jineijin)6g
Stir-backed Pangolin Scales (炙穿山甲, Zhi Chuanshanjia)6g
Actions: Replenishing qi and activating blood circulation, removing blood stasis and eliminating mass.
Applied Syndrome: Mass and tympanites due to stagnation of liver-blood, manifested as a lump in the hypochondrium which is characterized by localized distention and pain, emaciated body,

dark complexion, dark, reddish tongue or with ecchymosis, wiry and unsmooth or wiry and thin pulse.

Liver-Recuperating Pill
(Fullness-Relieving and Mass-Removing Method)

Ingredients	Effects	Combined Effects	Syndrome	Chief Symptoms
Dried Human Placenta (紫河车, Ziheche)6g Red Ginseng Stigma (红参须, Hongshenxu)6g	Potently replenishing qi and blood, restoring the healthy qi and reinforcing the origin	Replenishing qi and activating blood circulation, removing blood stasis and eliminating mass	Mass and tympanites (due to impairment of healthy qi resulting from depressed liver-qi and stagnation of blood	Lump in the hypochondrium characterized by localized distention and pain, emaciated body, dark complexion, dark reddish tongue or with ecchymosis, wiry and unsmooth or wiry and thin pulse.
Stir-Backed Ground Bettle (炙地鳖虫, Zhi Dibiechong)6g Sanchi Root (三七, Sanqi)6g Stir-Backed Pangolin Scales (炙穿山甲, Zhi Chuanshanjia)6g	Activating blood circulation and removing blood stasis, dredging the collaterals and eliminating mass			
Turmeric Rhizome (姜黄, Jianghuang)6g Turmeric Root-Tuber (郁金, Yujin)6g	Regulating flow of qi, activating blood circulation and alleviating pain			
Chicken Gizzard Membrane (生鸡内金, Sheng Jineijin)6g	Strengthening the stomach, promoting digestion and eliminating mass			

Points in Constitution: This formula is comprised of Ginseng (人参, Renshen), which is mainly for reinforcing the body resistance, Sanchi Root (三七, Sanqi), which is mainly for dissipating the stagnation, Dried Human Placenta (紫河车, Ziheche), which is strongly for replenishing qi and blood, and the other drugs of Ground Bettle (地鳖虫, Dibiechong), Pangolin Scales (穿山甲, Chuanshanjia), Turmeric Root-Tuber (郁金, Yujin) and Turmeric Rhizome (姜黄, Jianghuang) which are for activating blood circulation, eliminating mass and alleviating pain. The use of Chicken Gizzard Membrane (鸡内金, Jineijin) is for strengthening the stomach and eliminating mass. The combination of these drugs exert the effects of replenishing qi, activating blood circulation, removing blood stasis and eliminating mass.

Indications:

1. Initial of cirrhosis

2. Infectious hepatitis
3. Hypersplenism
4. Cholecystitis

Precaution: Since this formula has the qi-replenishing and blood-activating actions and its nature is comparatively warm, it should be cautiously used to those who are accompanied with heat due to yin deficiency.

Associated Formulas:

1. Liver-Strengthening and Hardness-Softening Decoction (强肝软坚汤, qiang gan ruan jian tang) *Research Data on the Combination of Traditional Chinese Medicine with Western Medicine in Shanxi Province*, *Volume Eight* 《山西省中西医结合研究资料第八集》1977.11

This is comprised of Chinese Angelica Root (当归, Danggui), White Peony Root (白芍药, Baishaoyao), Dan-Shen Root (丹参, Danshen), Turmeric Root-Tuber (郁金, Yujin), Whiteflower Patrinia Herb (败酱草, Baijiangcao), Cape Jasmine Fruit (山栀子, Shanzhizi), Tree Peony Bark (牡丹皮, Mudanpi), Dried Rehmannia Root (生地黄, Shengdihuang), Largehead Atractylodes Rhizome (白术, Baizhu), Tuckahoe (茯苓, Fuling), Turtle Carapace (鳖甲, Biejia), Membranous Milkvetch Root (黄芪, Huangqi), Dried Human Placenta (紫河车, Ziheche), Hawthorn Fruit (山楂, Shanzha) and Capillary Wormwood Herb (茵陈, Yinchen). Its actions are restoring the body resistance, resolving blood stasis, eliminating hardness, clearing away heat, inducing diuresis and dissipating blockages. It is indicated for abdominal mass and tympanites due to stagnation of liver blood and accumulation of heat.

2. Liver-Strengthening and Hardness-Softening Decoction Number Two (强肝软坚汤二号, qiang gan ruan jian tang er hao) *Research Data on the Combination of Traditional Chinese Medicine with Western Medicine in Shanxi Province*, *Volume Eight* 《山西省中西医结合研究资料第八集》1977.11

This is the formula of Liver-Strengthening and Hardness-Softening Decoction (强肝软坚汤, qiang gan ruan jian tang) by removing Whiteflower Patrinia Herb (败酱草, Baijiangcao), Tree Peony Bark (牡丹皮, Mudanpi), Dried Rehmannia Root (生地黄, Shengdihuang), Hawthorn Fruit (山楂, Shanzha), Dried Human Placenta (紫河车, Ziheche) and Largehead Atractylodes Rhizome (白术, Baizhu) but adding Swordlike Atractylodes Rhizome (苍术, Cangzhu), Pilose Asiabell Root (党参, Dangshen), Common Yam Rhizome (山药, Shanyao), Nutmeg Seed (肉豆蔻, Roudoukou), Common Aucklandia Root (木香, Muxiang) and Siberian Solomonseal Rhizome (黄精, Huangjing). Its actions are invigorating the spleen and removing blood stasis. It is indicated for cirrhosis mainly due to spleen deficiency.

3. Liver-Strengthening and Hardness-Softening Decoction Number Three (强肝软坚汤三号, qiang gan ruan jian tang san hao) *Research Data on the Combination of Traditional Chinese Medicine with Western Medicine in Shanxi Province*, *Volume Eight* 《山西省中西医结合研究资料第八集》1977.11

This is the formula of Liver-Strengthening and Hardness-Softening Decoction Number Two (强肝软坚汤二号, qiang gan ruan jian tang er hao) without Membranous Milkvetch Root (黄芪, Huangqi), Siberian Solomonseal Rhizome (黄精, Huangjing), Swordlike Atractylodes Rhizome

(苍术, Cangzhu), Tuckahoe (茯苓, Fuling) and Common Yam Rhizome (山药, Shanyao) but with Suberect Spatholobus Stem (鸡血藤, Jixueteng), Peach Seed (桃仁, Taoren), Stir-Backed Pangolin Scales (炮山甲, Pao shanjia) and Common Cephalanoploris Herb (小蓟, Xiaoji). Its actions are dissolving blood stasis, activating blood circulation and dreging collaterals. It is indicated for cirrhosis mainly due to blood stasis in the collaterals.

4. Liver-Strengthening and Hardness-Softening Decoction Number Four (强肝软坚汤四号, qiang gan ruan jian tang si hao) *Research Data on the Combination of Traditional Chinese Medicine with Western Medicine in Shanxi Province Volume Eight* 《山西省中西医结合研究资料第八集》1977.11

This is the formula of Liver-Strengthening and Hardness-Softening Decoction Number Three (强肝软坚汤三号, qiang gan ruan jian tang san hao) without Suberect Spatholobus Stem (鸡血藤, Jixueteng), Peach Seed (桃仁, Taoren), Stir-Backed Pangolin Scales (炮山甲, Pao shanjia) and Common Cephalanoploris Herb (小蓟, Xiaoji) but with Coastal Glehnia Root and Fourleaf Ladybell Root (沙参, Shashen), Dwarf Lilyturf Root (麦门冬, Maimendong) and Barbary Wolfberry Fruit (枸杞子, Gouqizi). Its action is tonifying the liver and kidney. It is indicated for cirrhosis mainly due to deficiency of liver yin and kidney yin.

5. Liver-Strengthening and Hardness-Softening Decoction Number Five (强肝软坚汤五号, qiang gan ruan jian tang wu hao) *Research Data on the Combination of Traditional Chinese Medicine with western Medicine in Shanxi Province*, *Volume Eight* 《山西省中西医结合研究资料第八集》1977.11

This is the formula of Liver-Strengthening and Hardness-Softening Decoction Number Four(强肝软坚汤四号, qiang gan ruan jian tang si hao) by removing such yin-nourishing herbs as Coastal Glehnia Root and Fourleaf Ladybell Root (沙参, Shashen), Dwarf Lilyturf Root (麦门冬, Maimendong), Barbary Wolfberry Fruit (枸杞子, Gouqizi) but adding Poria Peel (茯苓皮, Fulingpi), Plantain Seed (车前子, Cheqianzi), Rhubarb (大黄, Dahuang) and Chinese Lobelia Herb (半边莲, Banbianlian). Its actions are removing blood stasis and promoting urination. It is indicated for cirrhosis mainly due to accumulation of qi and water.

6. Liver-Strengthening and Hardness-Softening Decoction Number Six (强肝软坚汤六号, qiang gan ruan jian tang liu hao) *Research Data on the Combination of Traditional Chinese Medicine with Western Medicine in Shanxi Province*, *Volume Eight* 《山西省中西医结合研究资料第八集》1977.11

This is the formula of Liver-Strengthening and Hardness-Softening Decoction Number Five(强肝软坚汤五号, qiang gan ruan jian tang wu hao) plus Dried Human Placenta (紫河车, Ziheche) and Ass-hide Glue (阿胶, Ejiao). Its actions are nourishing yin and enriching the blood. It is indicated for cirrhosis with ascites due to yin deficiency.

7. Liver-Soothing Pill (舒肝丸, shu gan wan) *Selected Prescriptions of National Chinese Patent Medicine in Tianjin* 《全国中成药处方集》天津方

This is comprised of White Peony Root (白芍药, Baishaoyao), Turmeric Rhizome (姜黄, Jianghuang), Round Cardamon Seed (白豆蔻, Baidoukou), Officinal Magnolia Bark (厚朴, Houpo), Bitter Orange (枳壳, Zhiqiao), Corydalis Tuber (延胡索, Yanhusuo), Chinese Eaglewood Wood (沉香, Chenxiang), Villous Amomum Fruit (砂仁, Sharen), Common Aucklandia Root (木香, Muxiang), Tangerine Peel (橘皮, Jupi), Szechwan Chinaberry Fruit (川楝子, Chuanlianzi) and Tuckahoe (茯苓, Fuling). Its actions are soothing the liver and regulating circulation of qi. It is indicated for stabbing pain in the bilateral hypochondrium due to stagnation of liver qi.

8. Hardness-Removing Decoction (化坚汤, hua jian tang) *Longevity and Life Prescription* 《寿世保元》

This is comprised of Largehead Atractylodes Rhizome (白术, Baizhu), Nutgrass Galingale Rhizome (香附, Xiangfu), Hawthorn Fruit (山楂, Shanzha), Tangerine Peel (橘皮, Jupi), Pinellia Rhizome (半夏, Banxia), Tuckahoe (茯苓, Fuling), Chinese Angelica Root (当归, Danggui), Szechwan Lovage Rhizome (川芎, Chuanxiong), Immature Bitter Orange (枳实, Zhishi), Kwangsi Turmeric Rhizome (莪术, Ezhu), Peach Seed (桃仁, Taoren), Safflower (红花, Honghua), Licorice Root (甘草, Gancao) and Fresh Ginger (生姜, Shengjiang). Its actions are removing blood stasis and eliminating abdominal mass. It is indicated for food retention, abdominal mass, water retention and indigestion.

9. Decoction for Dispersing the Stagnated Qi and Recuperating the Middle-jiao (达郁宽中汤, da yu kuan zhong tang) *Elite of Characteristic Experience of Famous Doctors* 《名医特色经验精华》

This is comprised of Chinese Eaglewood Wood (沉香, Chenxiang), Chinese Angelica Root (当归, Danggui), White Peony Root (白芍药, Baishaoyao), Chinese Thorowax Root (柴胡, Chaihu), Peel of Citron Fruit (香橼皮, Xiangyuanpi), Silkworm Feculae (晚蚕沙, Wancansha), Chicken Gizzard Membrane (鸡内金, Jineijin), Lalang Grass Rhizome (白茅根, Baimaogen) and Fresh Shallot (鲜葱, Xiancong). Its actions are dispersing the stagnated liver-qi, regulating the spleen, activating flow of qi and promoting urination. It is indicated for tympanites due to stagnated liver-qi and abnormal activities of qi in the three-jiao.

Esophagitis Pill
(食道炎丸, shi dao yan wan)

Source: *Fujian Journal of Traditional Chinese Medicine* 《福建中医药》
Composition: Coastal Gehnia Root and Fourleaf Ladybell Root (沙参, Shashen)9g
Dwarf Lilyturf Root (麦门冬, Maimendong)9g
Balloonflower Root (桔梗, Jiegeng)9g
Honeysuckle Flower (金银花, Jinyinhua)9g
Weeping Forsythia Capsule (连翘, Lianqiao)9g
Boat-fruited Sterculia Seed (胖大海, Pangdahai)6g
Licorice Root (甘草, Gancao)9g
Actions: Clearing away heat and toxic material, dispersing the lung and benefiting the stomach, promoting the production of body fluid and nourishing yin.

Applied Syndrome: Esophagitis due to impairment of yin and body fluid resulting from attack on the lung and stomach by noxious heat. The manifestations are burning and stabbing pain behind the sternum, vomiting and acid regurgitation, anorexia, red tongue with yellow coating, wiry and rapid pulse.

Esophagitis Pill
(Yin-Nourishing and Phlegm-Resolving Method)

Ingredients	Effects	Combined Effects	Syndrome	Chief Symptoms
Coastal Glehnia Root and Fourleaf Ladybell Root (沙参, Shashen)9g Dwarf Lilyturf Root (麦门冬, Maimendong)9g	Clearing away heat, promoting the production of body fluid, nourishing the lung and stomach	Clearing away heat and toxic material, nourishing yin and relieving sore throat	Esophagitis (due to impairment of yin and body fluid resulting from exogenous toxic heat attacking the lung and stomach)	Burning and stabbing pain behind the sternum, vomiting and acid regurgitation, anorexia, red tongue with yellow coating, wiry and rapid pulse
Balloonflower Root (桔梗, Jiegeng)9g	Promoting the dispersing function of the lung			
Honeysuckle Flower (金银花, Jinyinhua)9g Weeping Forsythia Capsule (连翘, Lianqiao)9g	Clearing away heat and toxic material			
Boat-Fruited Sterculia Seed (胖大海, Pangdahai)6g	Clearing away heat and relieving sore throat, moistening the intestine and relaxing the bowels			
Licorice Root (甘草, Gancao)9g	Being sweety and slowly clearing away toxic material			

Points in Constitution: This formula combines the drugs which have the actions of nourishing yin and promoting the production of body fluid with the drugs which have the actions of clearing away heat and toxic material to exert a collective effect. In Traditional Chinese Medicine, the stomach belongs to dry earth and the lung is a tender viscera. Thus, most of the drugs in this formula are mild, moist and have the dispersing and descending function to correspond to the pathogenesis.

Indications:
1. Esophagitis
2. Begining of carcinoma of esophagus

3. Acute laryngopharyngitis
4. Acute tonsillitis

Precaution: This formula should be modified when it is used for esophagitis due to accumulation of excessive phlegm-heat and disturbance of flow of qi.

Associated Formulas:

1. Left Golden Pill (左金丸, zuo jin wan) *Danxi's Experiential Therapy*《丹溪心法》

This is comprised of Coptis Rhizome (黄连, Huanglian) and Medicinal Evodia Fruit (吴茱萸, Wuzhuyu). Its actions are clearing away heat, purging fire and keeping the adverse qi downwards to stop vomiting. It is indicated for distention and pain in the chest and hypochondrium, gastric upset, acid regurgitation and vomiting of bitter liquid due to attack of the stomach by liver-fire which is transformed from depressed liver-qi.

2. Diaphragm-Cooling Powder (凉膈散, liang ge san) *Prescriptions of Peaceful Benevolent Dispensary*《和剂局方》

This is comprised of Rhubarb (大黄, Dahuang), Mirabilite (芒硝, Mangxiao), Licorice Root (甘草, Gancao), Cape Jasmine Fruit (山栀子, Shanzhizi), Wild Mint Herb (薄荷, Bohe), Baikal Skullcap Root (黄芩, Huangqin), Weeping Forsythia Capsule (连翘, Lianqiao) and Tophatherum Leaf (竹叶, Zhuye). Its action is clearing away heat and toxic material. It is indicated for dysphoria with smothery sensation in the chest, thirst, sore throat, constipation and yellowish urine due to accumulation of heat in the chest, diaphragm or hyponchondrium which impairs body fluid.

3. Inflammation-Diminishing and Membrane-Protecting Formula (消炎护膜方, xiao yan hu mo fang) *Shanghai Journal of Traditional Chinese Medicine*《上海中医药杂志》

This is comprised of Coptis Rhizome (黄连, Huanglian), Talc (滑石, Huashi), Bitter Orange (枳壳, Zhiqiao), Tangerine Peel (橘皮, Jupi) and Licorice Root (甘草, Gancao). Its actions are clearing away heat, activating flow of qi and relieving sore throat. It is indicated for regurgitated esophagitis and gastritis.

Dryness-Moistening and Stomach-Nourishing Decoction
(润燥养胃汤, run zao yang wei tang)

Source: *Zhejiang Journal of Traditional Chinese Medicine*《浙江中医杂志》
Composition: Coastal Glehnia Root (北沙参, Beishashen) 15g
Dendrobium Herb (石斛, Shihu) 15g
Dwarf Lilyturf Root (麦门冬, Maimendong) 12g
Dried Rehmannia Root (生地黄, Shengdihuang) 12g
White Peony Root (白芍药, Baishaoyao) 12g
Chinese Angelica Root (当归, Danggui) 9g
Smoked Plum (炙乌梅, Zhi Wumei) 9g
Szechwan Chinaberry Fruit (川楝子, Chuanlianzi) 9g

Fragrant Solomonseal Rhizome (玉竹, Yuzhu)12g

Actions: Nourishing yin, moistening dryness and benefiting the stomach.

Applied Syndrome: Gastritis due to impairment of the stomach by heat of deficiency type which results from yin deficiency of the lung and stomach. The manifestations are unbearable dull and burning pain in the gastric region, dry mouth and throat, thirst with desire to drink, dry stool, yellowish urine, thin, small and light red tongue with little coating, thin and rapid pulse.

Dryness-Moistening and Stomach-Nourishing Decoction
(Yin-Nourishing and Dryness-Moistening Method)

Ingredients	Effects	Combined Effects	Syndrome	Chief Symptoms
Coastal Glehnia Root (北沙参, Beishashen) 15g Dendrobium Herb (石斛, Shihu)15g Dwarf Lilyturf Root (麦门冬, Maimendong)12g Dried Rehmannia Root (生地黄, Shengdihuang)12g Fragrant Solomonseal Rhizome (玉竹, Yuzhu)12g White Peony Root (白芍药, Baishaoyao)12g	Nourishing yin and promoting the production of body fluid to moist dryness	Nourishing yin, moistening dryness and benefiting the stomach	Gastritis (due to impairment of the stomach by deficiency heat which results from yin deficiency of the lung and stomach)	Unbearable dull and burning pain in the gastric region, dry mouth and throat, thirst with desire to drink, dry stool, yellowish urine, thin, small and light red tongue with little coating, thin and rapid pulse
Chinese Angelica Root (当归, Danggui)9g	Regulating blood and alleviating pain			
Smoked Plum (炙乌梅, Zhi Wumei)9g	Promoting the production of body fluid and regulating the stomach qi			
Szechwan Chinaberry Fruit (川楝子, Chuanlianzi)9g	Activating flow of qi and alleviating pain			

Points in Constitution: This formula is a modification of Coastal Glehnia and Dwarf Lilyturf Decoction (沙参麦冬汤) and the principle of its design is similar to that of Decoction Worth A Thousand Copper Coins(一贯煎). The main drugs of this formula are sweet and sour in favour, which can nourish yin.

Indications:

1. Chronic gastritis
2. Gastroduodenal ulcer

Precaution: This formula is not suitable for syndrome of deficiency and cold of the stomach-qi.

Associated Formulas:

1. Coastal Glehnia and Ophiopogon Decoction (沙参麦门冬汤, sha shen mai men dong tang) *Detailed Analysis of Epidemic Febrile Diseases*《温病条辨》

This is comprised of Coastal Glehnia Root and Fourleaf Ladybell Root (沙参, Shashen), Dwarf Lilyturf or Ophiopogon Root (麦门冬, Maimendong), Fragrant Solomonseal Rhizome (玉竹, Yuzhu), Licorice Root (生甘草, Shenggancao), Winter Mulberry Leaf (冬桑叶, Dong Sangye), White Hyacinth Bean (生扁豆, Sheng Biandou), Snakegourd Root (天花粉, Tianhuafen). Its actions are clearing and nourishing the lung and stomach, promoting the production of body fluid and moistening dryness. It is indicated for dry throat and thirst, or fever, or dry cough with scanty sputum due to impairment of yin of the lung and stomach by dryness.

2. Ophiopogon Decoction (麦门冬汤, mai men dong tang) *Synopsis of Golden Cabinet*《金匮要略》

This is comprised of Ophiopogon Root (麦门冬, Maimendong), Pinellia Rhizome (半夏, Banxia), Ginseng (人参, Renshen), Rice (粳米, Jingmi), Chinese Date (大枣, Dazao) and Licorice Root (甘草, Gancao). Its actions are nourishing yin of both the lung and stomach. It is indicated for cough with dyspnea, vomiting, difficult expectoration due to flaring up of fire of deficient type and adverse rising of lung-qi resulting from yin deficiency of both the lung and stomach,.

3. Decoction Worth A Thousand Copper Coins (一贯煎, yi guan jian) *Medical Words in Liuzhou*《柳州医话》

This is comprised of Coastal Glehnia Root and Fourleaf Ladybell Root (沙参, Shashen), Dwarf Lilyturf Root (麦门冬, Maimendong), Chinese Angelica Root (当归, Danggui), Dried Rehmannia Root (生地黄, Shengdihuang), Barbary Wolfberry Fruit (枸杞子, Gouqizi) and Szechwan Chinaberry Fruit (川楝子, Chuanlianzi). Its actions are nourishing the liver and kidney and dispersing the stagnated liver-qi. It is indicated for pain in the hypochondrium and epigastric region due to yin deficiency and qi stagnation.

Chapter Four
Formulas for Diseases of the Urogenital System

The diseases of the urogenital system are considered to be problems of the kidney according to the theory of traditional Chinese medicine. They are usually caused by an attack of damp-heat, congenital defect or impairment of the kidney due to sexual indulgence. The main pathogenesis is kidney deficiency and accumulation of damp-heat in the lower-jiao. In TCM, there have been many effective prescriptions for acute or chronic nephritis, nephritic syndrome, acute or chronic urinary tract infection, prostatitis, prostatomegaly, lithangiuria and sexual neurosis, which are widely used in clinic.

1. Field Thistle Decoction
(小蓟饮子, xiao ji yin zi)

Source: *Prescriptions for Rescuring the Sick* 《济生方》
Composition: Lotus Node (藕节, Oujie) 9g
Cattail Pollen (蒲黄, Puhuang) 9g
Talc (滑石, Huashi) 9g (wrapped when decocted)
Akebia Stem (木通, Mutong) 9g
Tophatherum Leaf (竹叶, Zhuye) 9g
Cape Jasmine Fruit (山栀子, Shanzhizi) 9g
Dried Rehmannia Root (生地黄, Shengdihuang) 15g
Chinese Angelica Root (当归, Danggui) 9g
Prepared Licorice Root (炙甘草, Zhi Gancao) 9g

Actions: Removing heat from the blood, arresting bleeding, reducing diuresis and relieving stranguria.

Applied Syndrome: Stranguria of heat type complicated by hematuria, caused by excessive pathogenic heat in the lower-jiao which brings about impairment of blood vessels. The manifestations are hematuria, frequent micturition with dark yellowish color and dripping, hot and painful sensation, red tongue with yellow coating, rapid pulse.

Points in Constitution: This formula combines Common Cephalanoploris Herb (小蓟, Xiaoji), which has the action of removing heat from the blood and arresting bleeding with the ingredients of Fire-Inducing Powder (导赤散, dao chi san) and those of Six to One Powder (六一散, liu yi san) to strengthen the actions of clearing away heat and relieving stranguria. In this formula, all the drugs except Chinese Angelica Root (当归, Danggui) are cold or cool in nature. The use of Chinese Angelica Root (当归, Danggui) which is warm in nature, can not only activate blood circulation and alleviate pain but also prevent the other drugs from being overcold to lead to blood stasis.

Field Thistle Decoction
(Method of Removing Heat from the Blood and Arresting Bleeding)

Ingredients	Effects	Combined Effects	Syndrome	Chief Symptoms
Common Cephanoploris Herb (小蓟, Xiaoji) 9g Dried Rehmannia Root (生地黄, Shengdihuang) 15g	Removing heat from the blood and arresting bleeding	Removing heat from the blood and arresting bleeding, reducing diuresis and treating stranguria	Impairment of blood vessels due to excessive damp-heat	Hematuria, frequent micturition with dark, yellowish colour and dripping, hot and painful sensation, red tongue with yellow coating, rapid pulse
Cattail Pollen (蒲黄, Puhuang) 9g Lotus Node (藕节, Oujie) 9g	Removing heat from the blood and arresting bleeding, removing blood stasis			
Cape Jasmine Fruit (山栀子, Shanzhizi) 9g Akebia Stem (木通, Mutong) 9g Tophatherum Leaf (竹叶, Zhuye) 9g Prepared Licorice Root (炙甘草, Zhi Gancao) 9g	Clearing away heat, reducing diuresis and treating stranguria			
Talc (滑石, Huashi) 9g Licorice Root (甘草, Gancao)	Clearing away heat and promoting urination			
Chinese Angelica Root (当归, Danggui) 9g	Activating blood circulation and alleviating pain			

Indications:
1. Acute urinary tract infection
2. Acute nephritis
3. Urinary tract calculus

Precaution: This formula is contraindicated in prolonged stranguria complicated by hematuria and deficiency of body resistance.

Associated Formulas:

1. Four Fresh Herbs pill（四生丸, si sheng wan）*The Complete Effective Prescriptions for Diseases of Women*《妇人良方大全》

This is comprised of Lotus Leaf（生荷叶, Sheng Heye）, Argy Wormwood Leaf（生艾叶, Sheng Aiye）, Chinese Arborvitae Leafy Twig（生柏叶, Shengbaiye）and Dried Rehmannia Root（生地黄, Shengdihuang）. Its action is removing heat from the blood to arrest bleeding. It is indicated for bleeding in the upper body such as hematemesis and apostaxis with bright red blood due to excessive heat.

2. Ten Charred Herbs Powder（十灰散, shi hui san）*Miraculous Book of Ten kinds of Dosage Form*《十药神书》

This is comprised of Japanese Thistle Herb or Root（大蓟, Daji）, Common Cephanoploris Herb（小蓟, Xiaoji）, Lotus Leaf（荷叶, Heye）, Chinese Arborvitae Leafy Twig（侧柏叶, Cebaiye）, Lalang Grass Rhizome（白茅根, Baimaogen）, India Madder Root（茜根, Qiangen）, Cape Jasmine Fruit（山栀子, Shanzhizi）, Rhubarb（大黄, Dahuang）, tree Peony Bark（牡丹皮, Mudanpi）and Peel of Fortune Windmillpalm Petiole（棕榈皮, Zonglüpi）. Its actions are removing heat from the blood and arresting bleeding. It is indicated for various bleeding due to excessive blood-heat.

2. Powder for Five Kinds of Stranguria
（五淋散, wu lin san）

Source: *Prescriptions of Peaceful Benevolent Dispensary*《和剂局方》
Composition: Indian Bread Pink Epidermis（赤茯苓, Chifuling）6g
Chinese Angelica Root（当归, Danggui）6g
Licorice Root（生甘草, Shenggancao）6g
Red Peony Root（赤芍, Chishao）6g
Cape Jasmine Fruit（山栀子, Shanzhizi）6g
Baikal Skullcap Root（黄芩, Huangqin）6g
Dried Rehmannia Root（生地黄, Shengdihuang）6g
Talc（滑石, Huashi）9g
Akebia Stem（木通, Mutong）6g
Plantain Seed（车前子, Cheqianzi）9g
Oriental Waterplantain Rhizome（泽泻, Zexie）6g
Actions: Removing heat from the blood, reducing diuresis and treating stranguria.
Applied Syndrome: Hematuria, uropsammus and strangury of heat type, caused by deficiency of kidney qi and heat in the urinary bladder which results in disturbance of activities of qi and blockage of the water passages. The manifestations are frequency and urgency of micturition, dripping and painful urination, pain in the lower abdomen, blood or stone in the urine, distention and pain in the lower abdomen which radiates to the loins, red tongue with yellow and greasy

coating, smooth and rapid pulse.

Powder for Five Kinds of Stranguria
(Heat-Clearing and Stranguria-Treating Method)

Ingredients	Effects	Combined Effects	Syndrome	Chief Symptoms
Dried Rehmannia Root (生地黄, Shengdihuang)6g	Removing heat from the blood and arresting bleeding			
Baikal Skullcap Root (黄芩, Huangqin)6g Cape Jasmine Fruit (山栀子, Shanzhizi)6g	Clearing away heat and toxic material			
Talc (滑石, Huashi)9g Akebia Stem (木通, Mutong)6g Indian Bread Pink Epidermis (赤茯苓, Chifuling)6g Plantain Seed (车前子, Cheqianzi)9g Oriental Waterplantain Rhizome (泽泻, Zexie)6g	Reducing diuresis and treating stranguria	Removing heat from the blood, reducing diuresis and treating stranguria	Stranguria (due to impairment of blood vessels by accumulated damp-heat)	Frequency and urgency of micturition, turbid urine, dripping and painful urination with blood or stone in the urine, distention and pain in the lower abdomen radiating to the loin, red tongue with yellow and greasy coating, smooth and rapid pulse
Red Peony Root (赤芍, Chishao)6g Chinese Angelica Root (当归, Danggui)6g	Activating blood circulation and alleviating pain			
Licorice Root (生甘草, Shenggancao)6g	Clearing away heat and toxic material and co-ordinating the actions of the above drugs			

Points in Constitution: The characteristic of this formula is that in a number of heat-clearing and stranguria-treating drugs, Chinese Angelica Root (当归, Danggui) and Red Peony Root (赤芍, Chishao) are used to activate blood circulation, alleviate pain and relieve spasm in the urinary tract.

Indications:
1. Hematuria

2. Urinary tract calculus

3. Urinary tract infection

Precaution: This formula is applied for stranguria due to pathogenic heat or stranguria complicated by hematuria due to excessive heat. It is contraindicated in stranguria due to qi deficiency or yin deficiency.

Associated Formulas:

1. Eight Corrections Powder (八正散, ba zheng san) *Prescriptions of Peaceful Benevolent Dispensary*《和剂局方》

This is comprised of Plantain Seed (车前子, Cheqianzi), Lilac Pink Herb (瞿麦, Qumai), Common Knotgrass Herb (萹蓄, Bianxu), Talc (滑石, Huashi), Seed of Cape Jasmine Fruit (山栀子仁, Shanzhiziren), Prepared Licorice Root (炙甘草, Zhi Gancao), Akebia Stem (木通, Mutong) and Rhubarb (大黄, Dahuang). Its actions are clearing away heat, purging fire, promoting urination and relieving stranguria. It is indicated for stranguria due to heat-dampness.

2. Japanese Felt Fern Powder (石韦散, shi wei san) *The Complete Effective Prescriptions for Diseases of Women*《妇人大全良方》

This is comprised of Japanese Felt Fern Leaf (石韦, Shiwei), Baikal Skullcap Root (黄芩, Huangqin), Akebia Stem (木通, Mutong), Elm Bark (榆白皮, Yubaipi), Cluster Mallow Fruit (冬葵子, Dongkuizi), Spike of Lilac Pink Herb (瞿麦穗, Qumaisui) and Licorice Root (甘草, Gancao). Its actions are clearing away heat, inducing diuresis and relieving stranguria. It is indicated for stranguria due to pathogenic heat and stranguria resulting from urolithiasis.

3. Sevenlobed Yam Decoction for Clearing Turbid Urine (萆薢分清饮, bi xie fen qing yin)

Source: *Danxi's Experiential Therapy*《丹溪心法》

Composition: Sevenlobed Yam Rhizome (萆薢, Bixie) 9g

Sharpleaf Galangal Fruit (益智仁, Yizhiren) 9g

Commbined Spicebush Root (乌药, Wuyao) 9g

Grassleaf Sweetflag Rhizome (石菖蒲, Shichangpu) 9g

Actions: Warming the kidney, reducing diuresis and clearing the turbid urine.

Applied Syndrome: Cloudy urine or stranguria with chyluria, caused by downward flow of damp-turbidity due to deficiency-cold of the lower-jiao and manifested by cloudy urine or urine just like chyme, frequency of micturition, pale tongue with white coating and a deep pulse.

Points in Constitution: This formula is mainly used for warming the kidney to help qi transformation. However, it also has the action of inducing astringency. Thus, it is applied for deficient but not excessive syndrome.

Indications:

1. Galacturia / chyluria

2. Chronic prostatitis

Sevenlobed Yam Decoction for Clearing Turbid Urine
(Kidney-Warming and Dampness-Removing Method)

Ingredients	Effects	Combined Effects	Syndrome	Chief Symptoms
Sevenlobed Yam Rhizome (萆薢, Bixie) 9g	Reducing diuresis and eliminating the turbid	Warming the kidney, reducing diuresis and clearing the turbid urine	Stranguria with chyluria (due to downward flow of damp-turbidity resulting from deficiency-cold of the lower-jiao)	Turbid urine or urine just like chyme, frequency of micturition, pale tongue with white coating and deep pulse
Sharpleaf Galangal Fruit (益智仁, Yizhiren) 9g Commbined Spicebush Root (乌药, Wuyao) 9g	Warming the kidney, controlling nocturnal emission and decreasing urination			
Grassleaf Sweetflag Rhizome (石菖蒲, Shichangpu) 9g	Being fragrant in smell and eliminating turbid evils, clearing away obstruction in seven orifices and removing dampness			

Precaution: It is contraindicated in stranguria with chyluria due to accumulation of damp-heat in the lower-jiao.

Associated Formulas:

1. Sevenlobed Yam Decoction for Clearing Turbid Urine (萆薢分清饮, bi xie fen qing yin) *Comprehension of Medicine* 《医学心悟》

This is comprised of Sevenlobed Yam Rhizome (萆薢, Bixie), Chinese Corktree Bark (黄柏, Huangbai), Grassleaf Sweetflag Rhizome (石菖蒲, Shichangpu), Tuckahoe (茯苓, Fuling), Largehead Atractylodes Rhizome (白术, Baizhu), Lotus Plumule (莲子心, Lianzixin), Dan-Shen Root (丹参, Danshen) and Plantain Seed (车前子, Cheqianzi). Its actions are clearing away heat, inducing diuresis, clearing turbid urine and eliminating turbid evils. It is indicated for nebulous urine and stranguria with chyluria due to damp-heat in the lower-jiao.

2. Sevenlobed Yam Decoction (萆薢饮, bi xie yin) *Comprehension of Medicine* 《医学心悟》

This is comprised of Sevenlobed Yam Rhizome (萆薢, Bixie), Powder of Giant Gecko (文蛤粉, Wengefen), Japanese Felt Fern Leaf (石韦, Shiwei), Plantain Seed (车前子, Cheqianzi), Tuckahoe (茯苓, Fuling), Common Rush Pith (灯心草, Dengxincao), Lotus Plumule (莲子心, Lianzixin), Grassleaf Sweetflag Rhizome (石菖蒲, Shichangpu) and Chinese Corktree Bark (黄柏, Huangbai). Its actions are clearing away heat and expelling dampness, clearing turbid urine and eliminating turbid evils. It is indicated for stranguria with chyluria.

3. Turbid Urine-Clearing Decoction (分清饮, fen qing yin) *One Hundred Questions in Pedi-*

atrics《婴童百问》

This is comprised of Sharpleaf Galangal Fruit (益智仁, Yizhiren), Sevenlobed Yam Rhizome (萆薢, Bixie), Grassleaf Sweetflag Rhizome (石菖蒲, Shichangpu) and Commbined Spicebush Root (乌药, Wuyao). Its actions are clearing the turbid and eliminating evils. It is indicated for dripping urination and with reddish or whitish turbid urine.

4. Heart-Clearing Lotus Seed Decoction
(清心莲子饮, qing xin lian zi yin)

Source: *Prescriptions of Peaceful Benevolent Dispensary*《和剂局方》
Composition: Baikal Skullcap Root (黄芩, Huangqin) 9g
Dwarf Lilyturf Root (麦门冬, Maimendong) 9g
Chinese Wolfberry Root-bark (地骨皮, Digupi) 9g
Plantain Seed (车前子, Cheqianzi) 9g
Prepared Licorice Root (炙甘草, Zhi Gancao) 6g
Lotus Seed (莲子, Lianzi) 15g
Tuckahoe (茯苓, Fuling) 9g
Membranous Milkvetch Root (黄芪, Huangqi) 9g
Ginseng (人参, Renshen) 6g

Actions: Replenishing qi and yin, clearing away heart-fire and treating stranguria.

Applied Syndrome: Stranguria caused by deficiency of the lung and spleen-qi which results in incoordination between the heart and the kidney with excess in the upper and deficiency in the lower. Or stranguria caused by flaming-up of the heart-fire which brings about yin-deficiency of the lung and kidney and occurence of deficiency-heat in the interior. The manifestations are dry mouth and tongue, emission, leucorrhea with reddish discharge, enuresis, painful urination, restlessness, diabetes, feverish sensation in the five centers, red and dry tongue with little coating. Or stranguria caused by overthinking which impairs the spleen and lung. The manifestations are frequent urination, cloudy urine, tiredness, poor appetite, red and dry tongue with little coating, deep, thin and feeble pulse.

Points in Constitution: The characteristic of this formula lies in clearing away heat from the heart, inducing urination, replenishing qi and nourishing yin simultaneously. It can induce diuresis without impairing yin and replenishing qi without invigorating fire. It is applied for the combined syndrome of both deficiency and excess due to long-time illness or a weak body.

Indications:
1. Urodynia
2. Dysuria
3. Seminal emission

Precaution: This formula is designed for the syndrome of impairment of both qi and yin due to attack of heart-heat to the small intestine. It is not suitable for aphthous stonatitis or sores in the mouth and tongue, irritability and painful urination due to excessive heat in the heart meridian.

Heart-Clearing Lotus Seed Decoction
(Yin-Nourishing and Heat-Clearing Method)

Ingredients	Effects	Combined Effects	Syndrome	Chief Symptoms
Lotus Seed (莲子, Lianzi)15g	Clearing away heart-fire and tranquilizing the mind	Replenishing qi and nourishing yin, clearing away heart-fire and treating stranguria	Stranguria (due to deficiency of qi and impairment of yin resulting from heat in the heart transferring into the small intestine)	Five kinds of Stranguria, painful urination, emission, dry mouth and tongue, feverish sensation in the five centers, spontaneous sweating and night sweating, tiredness, red and dry tongue with little coating, deep, thin and feeble pulse
Baikal Skullcap Root (黄芩, Huangqin)9g Chinese Wolfberry Root-Bark (地骨皮, Digupi)9g	Removing heat from the blood			
Tuckahoe (茯苓, Fuling)9g Plantain Seed (车前子, Cheqianzi)9g	Reducing diuresis and treating stranguria			
Dwarf Lilyturf Root (麦门冬, Maimendong)9g	Nourishing yin and tranquilizing the mind			
Ginseng (人参, Renshen)6g Membranous Milkvetch Root (黄芪, Huangqi)9g Prepared Licorice Root (炙甘草, Zhi Gancao)6g	Replenishing qi and strengthening the body resistance			

5. Lung-Clearing Drink
(清肺饮, qing fei yin)

Source: *Assembled Supplement to Diagnosis and Treatment* 《证治汇补》
Composition: Tuckahoe (茯苓, Fuling)9g
Baikal Skullcap Root (黄芩, Huangqin)9g
White Mulberry Root-Bark (桑白皮, Sangbaipi)12g

Dwarf Lilyturf Root (麦门冬, Maimendong) 15g
Cape Jasmine Fruit (山栀子, Shanzhizi) 12g
Oriental Waterplantain Rhizome (泽泻, Zexie) 9g
Akebia Stem (木通, Mutong) 9g
Plantain Seed (车前子, Cheqianzi) 9g

Actions: Removing lung-heat and clearing water passage.

Applied Syndrome: Uroschesis or retention of urine due to excessive lung-heat, manifested by difficult urination or anuresis, dry throat, irritability and thirst with a desire to drink, tachypnea or cough, thin and yellow tongue coating, rapid pulse.

Lung-Clearing Decoction
(Lung-Clearing and Diuresis-Reducing Method)

Ingredients	Effects	Combined Effects	Syndrome	Chief Symptoms
Baikal Skullcap Root (黄芩, Huangqin) 9g White Mulberry Root-Bark (桑白皮, Sangbaipi) 12g	Clearing away and purging lung heat	Clearing away heat and reducing diuresis	Retention of urine (due to excessive lung-heat)	Difficult urination or anuresis, dry throat, irritability and thirst with desire to drink, tachypnea or cough, thin and yellow tongue coating, rapid pulse
Dwarf Lilyturf Root (麦门冬, Maimendong) 15g	Nourishing yin and moistening the lung			
Plantain Seed (车前子, Cheqianzi) 9g Akebia Stem (木通, Mutong) 9g Cape Jasmine Fruit (山栀子, Shanzhizi) 12g Tuckahoe (茯苓, Fuling) 9g Oriental Waterplantain Rhizome (泽泻, Zexie) 9g	Clearing away heat and promoting urination			

Points in Constitution:

The lung is the upper source of water circulation. This formula combines the method of removing lung-heat with the one of clearing water passage to treat retention of urine.

Indications:

1. Nervous urodialysis
2. Spasm of bladder sphincter
3. Urinary tract calculus, urethrostenosis, urinary injury

4. Hyperplasia of prostate of old man

Precaution: This formula is not suitable for retention of urine due to deficiency of the spleen or kidney.

Associated Formulas:

1. Eight Corrections Powder (八正散, ba zheng san) *Prescriptions of Peaceful Benevolent Dispensary*《和剂局方》

This is comprised of Plantain Seed (车前子, Cheqianzi), Lilac Pink Herb (瞿麦, Qumai), Common Knotgrass Herb (萹蓄, Bianxu), Talc (滑石, Huashi), Cape Jasmine Fruit (山栀子, Shanzhizi), Licorice Root (甘草, Gancao), Akebia Stem (木通, Mutong), Rhubarb (大黄, Dahuang) and Common Rush Pith (灯心草, Dengxincao). Its actions are clearing away heat, purging fire, promoting urination and relieving stranguria. It is indicated for retention of urine or stranguria due to downward attack of damp-heat upon the urinary bladder.

2. Chinese Eaglewood Powder (沉香散, chen xiang san) *Supplement to the Synopsis of Golden Cabinet*《金匮翼》

This is comprised of Chinese Eaglewood Wood (沉香, Chenxiang), Japanese Felt Fern Leaf (石韦, Shiwei), Talc (滑石, Huashi), Chinese Angelica Root (当归, Danggui), Tangerine Peel (橘皮, Jupi), White Peony Root (白芍药, Baishaoyao), Cluster Mallow Fruit (冬葵子, Dongkuizi), Licorice Root (甘草, Gancao) and Cowherb Seed (王不留行, Wangbuliuxing). Its actions are regulating flow of qi and promoting urination. It is indicated for retention of urine or stranguria due to stagnation of liver qi.

6. Chinese Eaglewood Powder
(沉香散, chen xiang san)

Source: *Treatise on the Triple-Pathogenic Doctrine of Etiology*《三因极一病证方论》

Composition: Chinese Eaglewood Wood (沉香, Chenxiang) 6g

Japanese Felt Fern Leaf (石韦, Shiwei) 9g

Talc (滑石, Huashi) 9g

Chinese Angelica Root (当归, Danggui) 9g

Tangerine Peel (橘皮, Jupi) 9g

White Peony Root (白芍药, Baishaoyao) 12g

Cluster Mallow Fruit (冬葵子, Dongkuizi) 9g

Licorice Root (甘草, Gancao) 6g

Cowherb Seed (王不留行, Wangbuliuxing) 9g

Actions: Activating flow of qi, promoting urination and treating stranguria.

Applied Syndrome: Stranguria due to stagnation of qi which results from five depressed emotions, manifested by distention and fullness in the lower abdomen, dripping urination, thin and white tongue coating, deep and wiry pulse.

Chinese Eaglewood Powder
(Urination-Promoting and Stranguria-Treating Method)

Ingredients	Effects	Combined Effects	Syndrome	Chief Symptoms
Chinese Eaglewood Wood (沉香, Chenxiang)6g Tangerine Peel (橘皮, Jupi)9g	Promoting the flow of qi and eliminating water	Promoting the flow of qi, reducing diuresis and treating stranguria	Stranguria (due to stagnation of qi)	Distention and fullness in the lower abdomen, dripping urination, thin and white tongue coating, deep and wiry pulse
Chinese Angelica Root (当归, Danggui)9g	Regulating blood circulation and promoting flow of qi			
White Peony Root (白芍药, Baishaoyao)12g	Relieving spasm and inducing diuresis			
Japanese Felt Fern Leaf (石韦, Shiwei)9g Talc (滑石, Huashi)9g Cluster Mallow Fruit (冬葵子, Dongkuizi)9g Cowherb Seed (王不留行, Wangbuliuxing)9g	Promoting urination and treating stranguria			
Licorice Root (甘草, Gancao)6g	Coordinating the actions of the ingredients			

Points in Constitution: Chinese Eaglewood Wood (沉香, Chenxiang) has the action of improving inspiration by invigorating the kidney-qi which not only keeps the adverse qi downward, but also warms the kidney to improve qi transformation. Therefore, it is the monarch drug. There is a close relationship among qi, blood and water, thus, this formula can treat the problem in flow of qi, inducement of diuresis and circulation of blood.

Indications:
1. Urinary tract infection
2. Prostatitis

Associated Formula:

Substitutive Resistant Pill (代抵当丸, dai di dang wan) *Standard for Diagnosis and Treatment*《证治准绳》

This is comprised of Rhubarb (大黄, Dahuang), Mirabilite (芒硝, Mangxiao), Peach Seed (桃仁, Taoren), Ending Part of Chinese Angelica Root (当归尾, Dangguiwei), Dried Rehmannia Root（生地黄，Shengdihuang）, Pangolin Scales（穿山甲，Chuanshanjia）and Cassia Bark（肉桂，Rougui）. Its actions are activating blood circulation and removing blood stasis. It is indicated for dripping urination or anuresis, distention and pain in the lower abdomen, dark purplish tongue or with petechia, thin and unsmooth pulse.

7. Decoction for Diuresis
（疏凿饮子, shu zaoyin zi）

Source: *Prescriptions for Rescuring the Sick*《济生方》
Composition: Incised Notopterygium Rhizome or Root（羌活，Qianghuo）9g
Largeleaf Gentian Root（秦艽，Qinjiao）9g
Pokeberry Root（商陆，Shanglu）6g
Areca Seed（槟榔，Binglang）9g
Areca Peel（大腹皮，Dafupi）15g
Poria Peel（茯苓皮，Fulingpi）30g
Fresh Ginger Peel（生姜皮，Shengjiangpi）6g
Bunge Tricklyash Seed（椒目，Jiaomu）9g
Akebia Stem（木通，Mutong）12g
Oriental Waterplantain Rhizome（泽泻，Zexie）12g
Rice Bean（赤小豆，Chixiaodou）15g

Actions: Expelling wind and relieving the exterior syndrome, promoting urination and relaxing the bowels.

Applied Syndrome: Severe edema with excess in both the interior and exterior but without deficiency. The manifestations are edema all over the body, asthma and thirst, difficulty in urination and defecation, fullness and stuffiness in the chest and gastric region, irritability, greasy and yellowish tongue coating, soft and rapid pulse.

Points in Constitution: This formula expels excessive fluid or water by inducing diaphoresis, promoting urination and relaxing the bowels. The combined use of these methods of inducing diaphoresis, promoting urination and expelling excessive fluid with potent purgative lies in quickly clearing the water passagee, thus, leading to elimination of edema.

Indications:
1. Edema of chronic nephritis
2. Cirrhosis hydroperitoneum

Precautions:
1. This formula is designed for edema due to excess both in the interior and exterior with severe dampness. Thus, for severe weakness of body resistance or deficiency of yin and blood, or retention of phlegm and dampness without heat, this formula should be used cautiously or used after it is modified.
2. If the condition of the disease is relieved, the formula should be stopped right away. It can

not be taken for long.

Decoction for Diuresis
(Diaphoresis-Inducing, Urination-Promoting and Water-Dispelling Method)

Ingredients	Effects	Combined Effects	Syndrome	Chief Symptoms
Incised Notopterygium Rhizome or Root (羌活, Qianghuo) 9g Largeleaf Gentian Root (秦艽, Qinjiao) 9g	Expelling wind and removing dampness	Expelling wind and relieving the exterior, promoting urination and loosing the bowels	Abundance of dampness with excess in both the interior and exterior	Edema all over the body, asthma and thirst, difficulty in urination and defecation, fullness and stuffiness in the chest and gastric region, irritability, greasy and yellowish tongue coating, soft and rapid pulse
Pokeberry Root (商陆, Shanglu) 6g	Purging and inducing diuresis			
Areca Seed (槟榔, Binglang) 9g	Activating flow of qi and inducing diuresis			
Areca Peel (大腹皮, Dafupi) 15g Poria Peel (茯苓皮, Fulingpi) 30g Fresh Ginger Peel (生姜皮, Shengjiangpi) 6g Rice Bean (赤小豆, Chixiaodou) 15g Oriental Waterplantain Rhizome (泽泻, Zexie) 12g Akebia Stem (木通, Mutong) 12g	Inducing diuresis and promoting urination			
Bunge Tricklyash Seed (椒目, Jiaomu) 9g	Warming the middle-jiao and inducing diuresis			

Associated Formulas:

1. Ten Chinese Dates Decoction (十枣汤, shi zao tang) *Treatise on Exogenous Febrile Diseases* 《伤寒论》

This is comprised of Lilac Daphne Flower-Bud (芫花, Yuanhua), Kansui Root (甘遂, Gansui), Peking Euphorbia Root (大戟, Daji) and Chinese Date (大枣, Dazao). Its actions are expelling extra fluids and eliminating water retention by purgation. It is indicated for pleural effusion manifested as a dragging pain in the chest and hypochondrium, shortness of breath and asthma or ascites, feeling of distention and fullness in the abdomen, difficult urination and defecation.

2. Saliva-Controlling Pill (控涎丹, kong xian dan) *Treatise on the Triple-Pathogenic Doctrine*

of Etiology《三因极一病证方论》

This is comprised of Kansui Root（甘遂, Gansui）, Peking Euphorbia Root（大戟, Daji）and White Mustard Seed（白芥子, Baijiezi）. Its actions are removing phlegm and expelling water-retention. It is indicated for retention of phlegm in the chest manifested as sudden intolerable dull pain in the chest, back, nape, loin and crotch which radiates to bones and muscles, or cold limbs and headache, or faint and somnolence, anorexia, thick and sticky sputum and wheeziness.

3. Boat and Cart Pill（舟车丸, zhou che wan）*Jingyue's Complete Works*《景岳全书》

This is comprised of Pharbitis Seed（牵牛子, Qianniuzi）, Kansui Root（甘遂, Gansui）, Lilac Daphne Flower-Bud（芫花, Yuanhua）, Peking Euphorbia Root（大戟, Daji）, Rhubarb（大黄, Dahuang）, Green Tangerine Peel（青皮, Qingpi）, Tangerine Peel（橘皮, Jupi）, Common Aucklandia Root（木香, Muxiang）, Areca Seed（槟榔, Binglang）and Mercuros Chloride（轻粉, Qingfen）. Its actions are activating flow of qi and expelling excessive fluid. It is indicated for edema, thirst, sounding breath, hardness of abdomen, constipation, white tongue coating, deep and rapid pulse due to accumulation of water and heat in the interior and stagnation of qi.

8. Spleen-Reinforcing Decoction
（实脾饮, shi pi yin）

Source: *Source: Revised Yan's Formulae for Life-Preserving*《重订严氏济生方》
Composition: Dried Ginger（干姜, Ganjiang）6g
Prepared Aconite Root（附子, Fuzi）6g
Largehead Atractylodes Rhizome（白术, Baizhu）6g
Tuckahoe（茯苓, Fuling）6g
Common Floweringquince Fruit（木瓜, Mugua）6g
Officinal Magnolia Bark（厚朴, Houpo）6g
Common Aucklandia Root（木香, Muxiang）6g
Areca Peel（大腹皮, Dafupi）6g
Caoguo（草果, Caoguo）6g
Licorice Root（甘草, Gancao）3g
Fresh Ginger（生姜, Shengjiang）6g
Chinese Date（大枣, Dazao）3g

Actions: Warming yang and reinforcing the spleen, activating flow of qi and inducing diuresis

Applied Syndrome: Edema due to insufficiency of yang resulting from deficiency-cold of the spleen and kidney. The manifestations are edema all over the body, especially below the waist, oliguria, distention and fullness in the chest and abdomen, poor appetite, fatigue or tiredness, white and smooth tongue coating, deep and slow pulse.

Points in Constitution: This formula uses the ingredients of Cold Limbs Decoction（四逆汤, si ni tang）to warm the kidney and restore yang. When they are combined with large quantity of spleen-invigorating and dampness-removing drugs, the cold and damp pathogens can not be accumulated. Thus, the primary cause of water retention will be eliminated.

Spleen-Reinforcing Decoction
(Method of Warming and Removing Water Dampness)

Ingredients	Effects	Combined Effects	Syndrome	Chief Symptoms
Dried Ginger (干姜, Ganjiang)6g Prepared Aconite Root (附子, Fuzi)6g	Warming the kidney and strengthening the spleen	Warming yang and reinforcing the spleen, activating flow of qi and inducing diuresis	Retention of water and dampness in the interior due to yang deficiency of the spleen and kidney	Edema all over the body, especially below the waist, distention and fullness in the chest and abdomen, oliguria, anorexia and tiredness, white and smooth tongue coating, deep and slow pulse
Largehead Atractylodes Rhizome (白术, Baizhu)6g Tuckahoe (茯苓, Fuling)6g Common Floweringquince Fruit (木瓜, Mugua)6g	Reinforcing the spleen and clearing away dampness			
Officinal Magnolia Bark (厚朴, Houpo)6g Common Aucklandia Root (木香, Muxiang)6g Areca Peel (大腹皮, Dafupi)6g Caoguo (草果, Caoguo)6g	Activating flow of qi, invigorating the spleen and drying dampness			
Fresh Ginger (生姜, Shengjiang)6g Chinese Date (大枣, Dazao)3g Licorice Root (甘草, Gancao)3g	Benefiting the stomach and regulating the middle-jiao			

Indications:

1. Chronic nephritis
2. Edema of heart failure
3. Cirrhosis hydroperitoneum
4. Hypothyroidism
5. Chronic renal failure

Precautions:

1. This formula puts emphasis on warming yang and invigorating the spleen and its diuresis-inducing action is not strong. Thus, for severe edema, some urination-promoting drugs should be

added.

2. It is forbidden for those who suffer from accumulation of water and heat.

Associated Formulas:

1. Divine Black Bird Decoction (真武汤, zhen wu tang) *Treatise on Exogenous Febrile Diseases*《伤寒论》

This is comprised of Tuckahoe (茯苓, Fuling), Largehead Atractylodes Rhizome (白术, Baizhu), White Peony Root (白芍药, Baishaoyao), Fresh Ginger (生姜, Shengjiang) and Prepared Aconite Root (炮附子, Pao Fuzi). Its actions are warming yang and promoting urination. It is indicated for the syndrome of retention of water-dampness in the interior due to deficiency of the spleen yang, or edema due to yang deficiency after erroneous administration for diaphoresis in taiyang disease.

2. Prepared Aconite Decoction (附子汤, fu zi tang) *Treatise on Exogenous Febrile Diseases*《伤寒论》

This is comprised of Prepared Aconite Root (炮附子, Pao Fuzi), Tuckahoe (茯苓, Fuling), Ginseng (人参, Renshen), Largehead Atractylodes Rhizome (白术, Baizhu), White Peony Root (白芍药, Baishaoyao). Its actions are warming the kidney and restoring yang, eliminating cold and clearing away dampness. It is indicated for pain in the body and arthralgia due to internal attack by cold-dampness resulting from yang deficiency.

3. Tuckahoe, Cassia Twig, Largehead Atractylodes and Licorice Decoction (苓桂术甘汤, ling gui zhu gan tang) *Synopsis of Golden Cabinet*《金匮要略》

This is comprised of Tuckahoe (茯苓, Fuling), Cassia Twig (桂枝, Guizhi), Largehead Atractylodes Rhizome (白术, Baizhu) and Prepared Licorice Root (炙甘草, Zhi Gancao). Its actions are warming yang and resolving water retention, invigorating the spleen and inducing diuresis. It is indicated for phlegm-retention, feeling of fullness in the chest and hypochondrium, palpitation and shortness of breath, white and slippery tongue coating, wiry and smooth pulse due to deficiency of middle-jiao yang.

4. Five kinds of Peels Decoction (五皮饮, wu pi yin) *Treasured Classics*《中藏经》

This is comprised of Poria Peel (茯苓皮, Fulingpi), Fresh Ginger Peel (生姜皮, Shengjiangpi), White Mulberry Root-Bark (桑白皮, Sangbaipi), Areca Peel (大腹皮, Dafupi) and Tangerine Peel (橘皮, Jupi). Its actions are inducing diuresis and reducing swelling, regulating flow of qi and invigorating the spleen. It is indicated for severe edema, general edema, dysuria, feeling of distention and fullness in the pericardial and abdominal region, white tongue coating, deep and slow pulse due to deficiency of the spleen and excessive phlegm.

5. Licorice, Dried Ginger, Tuckahoe and Largehead Atractylodes Decoction (甘草干姜茯苓白术汤, gan cao gan jiang fu ling bai zhu tang) *Synopsis of Golden Cabinet*《金匮要略》

This is comprised of Tuckahoe (茯苓, Fuling), Dried Ginger (干姜, Ganjiang), Largehead Atractylodes Rhizome (白术, Baizhu) and Licorice Root (甘草, Gancao). Its actions are warming the middle-jiao and eliminating dampness. It is indicated for a heaviness sensation in the body, or cold feeling and pain below the loins due to retention of cold-dampness in the kidney.

6. Tuckahoe Water-Removing Decoction (茯苓导水汤, fu ling dao shui tang) *The Golden Mir-*

ror of Medicine《医宗金鉴》

This is comprised of Tuckahoe (茯苓, Fuling), Areca Seed (槟榔, Binglang), Umbellate Pore Fungus (猪苓, Zhuling), Villous Amomum Fruit (砂仁, Sharen), Common Aucklandia Root (木香, Muxiang), Tangerine Peel (橘皮, Jupi), Oriental Waterplantain Rhizome (泽泻, Zexie), Common Floweringquince Fruit (木瓜, Mugua), Areca Peel (大腹皮, Dafupi), White Mulberry Root-Bark (桑白皮, Sangbaipi), Perilla Stem (苏梗, Sugeng), Fresh Ginger (生姜, Shengjiang) and Largehead Atractylodes Rhizome (白术, Baizhu). Its actions are inducing diuresis, reducing swelling and relieving fullness. It is indicated for edema during pregnancy and asthma which causes inability to lie flat.

9. Water Retention-Removing Decoction
(分消汤, fen xiao tang)

Source: *Curative Measures for Diseases*《万病回春》
Composition: Swordlike Atractylodes Rhizome (苍术, Cangzhu) 6g
Tuckahoe (茯苓, Fuling) 6g
Umbellate Pore Fungus (猪苓, Zhuling) 6g
Oriental Waterplantain Rhizome (泽泻, Zexie) 6g
Officinal Magnolia Bark (厚朴, Houpo) 6g
Tangerine Peel (橘皮, Jupi) 6g
Immature Bitter Orange (枳实, Zhishi) 3g
Nutgrass Galingale Rhizome (香附, Xiangfu) 6g
Common Aucklandia Root (木香, Muxiang) 3g
Areca Peel (大腹皮, Dafupi) 6g
Villous Amomum Fruit (缩砂仁, Suosharen) 3g
Fresh Ginger (生姜, Shengjiang) 3g
Common Rush Pith (灯心草, Dengxincao) 3g

Actions: Promoting flow of qi and relieving distention, inducing diuresis and relieving swelling.

Applied Syndrome: Edema due to qi stagnation and water retention, manifested by edema in the limbs which is sunken when pressed but turns normal when the finger is raised, stuffiness, distention and fullness feeling in the chest and abdomen which becomes severe after meals, belching or acid regurgitation, scanty urine and constipation, deep and forceful pulse.

Points in Constitution: This formula uses the ingredients of Stomach-Calming Powder (平胃散, ping wei san) to restore the transportation and transformation actions of the spleen and those of Poria Decoction with Four Herbs (四苓汤, si ling tang) to promote urination. Common Aucklandia Root (木香, Muxiang), Villous Amomum Fruit (缩砂仁, Suosharen), Immature Bitter Orange (枳实, Zhishi) and Nutgrass Galingale Rhizome (香附, Xiangfu) are applied to activate flow of qi. Thus, qi stagnation and water retention are respectively eliminated and both qi and fluid flows normally.

Water Retention-Removing Decoction
(Qi-Activating and Diuresis-Inducing Method)

Ingredients	Effects	Combined Effects	Syndrome	Chief Symptoms
Tuckahoe (茯苓, Fuling)6g Umbellate Pore Fungus (猪苓, Zhuling)6g Oriental Waterplantain Rhizome (泽泻, Zexie)6g Common Rush Pith (灯心草, Dengxincao)3g	Reinforcing the spleen, inducing diuresis and eliminating dampness	Activating flow of qi to relieve distention, inducing diuresis to relieve swelling	Qi stagnation and water retention	Edema in the limbs which is sunken when pressed but turns normal when the finger is raised, stuffiness and distention and a fullness feeling of the chest and abdomen which becomes severe after meals, belching and acid regurgitation, scanty urine and constipation, deep and forceful pulse
Swordlike Atractylodes Rhizome (苍术, Cangzhu)6g Officinal Magnolia Bark (厚朴, Houpo)6g Tangerine Peel (橘皮, Jupi)6g	Removing dampness and invigorating the spleen, activating flow of qi and regulating the stomach			
Immature Bitter Orange (枳实, Zhishi)3g Common Aucklandia Root (木香, Muxiang)3g Villous Amomum Fruit (缩砂仁, Suosharen)3g Nutgrass Galingale Rhizome (香附, Xiangfu)6g	Regulating the stomach qi			
Areca Peel (大腹皮, Dafupi)6g	Descending qi and promoting urination			
Fresh Ginger (生姜, Shengjiang)3g	Warming the middle-jiao to stop vomiting			

Indications:
1. Initial hydroperitoneum
2. Excess-syndrome edema

Associated Formulas:
1. Spleen-Reinforcing Decoction (实脾饮, shi pi yin) *Revised Yan's Formulae for Life-Preserving* 《重订严氏济生方》

This is comprised of Officinal Magnolia Bark (厚朴, Houpo), Largehead Atractylodes Rhizome (白术, Baizhu), Common Floweringquince Fruit (木瓜, Mugua), Common Aucklandia Root (木香, Muxiang), Caoguo (草果, Caoguo), Areca Peel (大腹皮, Dafupi), Prepared Aconite Root (附子, Fuzi), Tuckahoe (茯苓, Fuling), Dried Ginger (干姜, Ganjiang) and Licorice Root (甘草, Gancao). Its actions are warming yang and invigorating the spleen, activating flow of qi and inducing diuresis. It is indicated for edema, especially in the lower body, feeling of distention and fullness in the chest and abdomen, heaviness sensation in the body, poor appetite or anorexia, cold extremities, loose stool and oliguria due to yang deficiency.

2. Tuckahoe and Oriental Waterplantain Decoction (茯苓泽泻汤, fu ling ze xie tang) *Synopsis of Golden Cabinet*《金匮要略》

This is comprised of Tuckahoe (茯苓, Fuling), Oriental Waterplantain Rhizome (泽泻, Zexie), Largehead Atractylodes Rhizome (白术, Baizhu), Cassia Twig (桂枝, Guizhi), Fresh Ginger (生姜, Shengjiang) and Licorice Root (甘草, Gancao). Its actions are invigorating the spleen, inducing diuresis and stopping vomiting. It is indicated for frequent vomiting with a desire to drink due to water retention in the stomach.

10. Golden Lock Pill for Solidating Essence (金锁固精丸, jin suo gu jing wan)

Source: *Collection of Formulae with Notes*《医方集解》
Composition: Flatstem Milkvetch Seed (沙苑蒺藜, Shayuanjili) 30g
Lotus Stamen (莲须, Lianxu) 30g
Gordon Euryale Seed (芡实, Qianshi) 30g
Dragon's Bone (龙骨, Longgu) 15g
Oyster Shell (牡蛎, Muli) 15g
Lotus Seed (莲子, Lianzi) 30g
Actions: Tonifying the kidney to arrest spontaneous emission.
Applied Syndrome: Spontaneous emission due to inability of the kidney to store the essence, manifested by emission and spermatorrhea, lumbago and tinnitus, listlessness and tiredness, pale tongue with white coating, thin and feeble pulse.
Points in Constitution: This formula invigorates the kidney and astringes essence simultaneously, but emphasizes the astringing action. Thus, this formula mainly treats the secondary aspect of the diseases.
Indications:
1. Nocturnal emission, spermatorrhea
2. Enuresis
Precaution: Most of the drugs in this formula are the ones for inducing astringency and the main action of them is invigorating the kidney to arrest spontaneous emission. Therefore, this formula is contraindicated in seminal emission due to damp-heat in the lower-jiao.

Golden Lock Pill for Solidating Essence
(Kidney-Tonifying and Emission-Arresting Method)

Ingredients	Effects	Combined Effects	Syndrome	Chief Symptoms
Flatstem Milkvetch Seed (沙苑蒺藜, Shayuanjili)30g	Tonifying the liver and kidney, keeping essence and stopping emission	Invigorating the kidney to arrest spontaneous emission	Spontaneous emission due to inability of the kidney to store the essence	Emission and spermatorrhea, lumbago and tinnitus, listlessness and tiredness, pale tongue with white coating, thin and feeble pulse
Lotus Seed (莲子, Lianzi)30g Gordon Euryale Seed (芡实, Qianshi)30g	Strengthening the kidney to arrest spontaneous emission, invigorating the spleen and nourishing the heart			
Dragon's Bone (龙骨, Longgu)15g Oyster Shell (牡蛎, Muli)15g	Checking exuberance of yang to arrest spontaneous emission, calming the heart and tranquilizing the mind			
Lotus Stamen (莲须, Lianxu)30g	Astringing essence and arresting apontaneous emission			

Associated Formulas:

1. Land and Water Two Fairies Pellet (水陆二仙丹, shui lu er xian dan) *The Effective Prescriptions for Longevity* 《扶寿精方》

This is comprised of Gordon Euryale Seed (芡实, Qianshi) and Cherokee Rose Fruit (金樱子, Jinyingzi). Its actions are invigorating the kidney to arrest spontaneous emission. It is indicated for male emission and nebulous urine or female leucorrhea simply due to deficiency of the kidney.

2. Origin-Reinforcing and Essence-Locking Pill (固本锁精丸, gu ben suo jing wan) *Standard for Diagnosis and Treatment* 《证治准绳》

This is comprised of Common Yam Rhizome (山药, Shanyao), Barbary Wolfberry Fruit (枸杞子, Gouqizi), Chinese Magnoliavine Fruit (五味子, Wuweizi), Asiatic Cornelian Cherry Fruit (山茱萸, Shanzhuyu), Songaria Cynomorium Herb (锁阳, Suoyang), Chinese Corktree Bark (黄柏, Huangbai), Common Anemarrhena Rhizome (知母, Zhimu), Ginseng (人参, Renshen), Membranous Milkvetch Root (黄芪, Huangqi), Lotus Seed(石莲肉, Sshilianrou) and Powder of Clam Shell (海蛤粉, Haigefen). Its actions are invigorating the kidney and controlling nocturnal emission. It is indicated for nocturnal emission, profuse night sweating and spermatorrhea due to deficiency of kidney-yang and unconsolidation of essence and qi.

3. Emission-Condolidating Pill(固精丸, gu jing wan) *Prescriptions for Rescuring the Sick*《济生方》

This is comprised of Desertliving Cistanche Herb (肉苁蓉, Roucongrong), Actinolite (阳起石, Yangqishi), Hairy Antler (鹿茸, Lurong), Red Halloysite (赤石脂, Chishizhi), Medicinal Indian Mulberry Root (巴戟天, Bajitian), Fried Tuber Onion Seed (炒韭子, Chao Jiuzi), Tuckahoe (茯苓, Fuling), Deglued Antler Powder (鹿角霜, Lujiaoshuang), Dragon's Bone (生龙骨, Sheng Longgu) and Prepared Aconite Root (附子, Fuzi). Its actions are invigorating the kidney and controlling nocturnal emission. It is indicated for emission and nebulous urine due to deficiency of the kidney essence and inability to keep essence resulting from excessive sexual indulgence.

4. Essence-Astringing Pill (约精丸, yue jing wan) *Source and Cause of Miscellaneous Diseases*《杂病源流犀烛》

This is comprised of Tuber Onion Seed (韭子, Jiuzi) and Dragon's Bone (龙骨, Longgu). Its actions are astringing essence and arresting spontaneous emission. It is indicated for idiopathic continuous emission both in the night and day.

5. Mantis Egg-Case Powder(桑螵蛸散, sang piao xiao san) *Amplified Herbology*《本草衍义》

This is comprised of Mantis Egg-Case (桑螵蛸, Sangpiaoxiao), Thinleaf Milkwort Root (远志, Yuanzhi), Grassleaf Sweetflag Rhizome (石菖蒲, Shichangpu), Dragon's Bone (龙骨, Longgu), Ginseng (人参, Renshen), Indian Bread with Hostwood (茯神, Fushen), Chinese Angelica Root (当归, Danggui) and Tortoise Shell and Plastron (龟版, Guiban). Its actions are regulating and tonifying the heart and kidney, astringing essence and arresting spontaneous emission. It is indicated for frequency of micturition, or enuresis and spermatorrhea due to deficiency of the heart and kidney.

11. Kidney Yang-Strengthening Pill
(壮阳丹, zhuang yang dan)

Source: *Ancestral Summary on Expanding Heirs of Wang's Family*《万氏家传广嗣纪要》
Composition: Prepared Rehmannia Root (熟地黄, Shudihuang)15g
Medicinal Indian Mulberry Root (巴戟天, Bajitian)9g
Malaytea Scurfpea Fruit (破故纸, Poguzhi)9g
Shorthorned Epimedium Herb (仙灵脾, Xianlingpi)9g
Mantis Egg-Case (桑螵蛸, Sangpiaoxiao)6g
Actinolite (阳起石, Yangqishi)6g
Actions: Reinforcing the kidney and supporting yang.

Applied Syndrome: Sexual impotence due to insufficiency of kidney yang and deficiency-cold of essence and qi. The manifestations are sexual impotence, pallor, dizziness, listlessness, soreness and weakness of the loins and knees, pale tongue with white coating, deep and thin pulse.

Kidney Yang-Strengthening Pill
(Kidney-Reinforcing and Yang-Supoorting Method)

Ingredients	Effects	Combined Effects	Syndrome	Chief Symptoms
Medicinal Indian Mulberry Root (巴戟天, Bajitian)9g Shorthorned Epimedium Herb (仙灵脾, Xianlingpi)9g Malaytea Scurfpea Fruit (破故纸, Poguzhi)9g	Tonifying the kidney and strengthening yang	Tonifying the kidney and supporting yang	Sexual impotence (due to deficiency of the kidney yang and deficiency-cold of essence and qi)	Sexual impotence, pallor, dizziness, listlessness, soreness and weakness of the loin and knees, pale tongue with white coating, deep and thin pulse
Actinolite (阳起石, Yangqishi)6g	Warming the kidney and strengthening yang			
Mantis Egg-Case (桑螵蛸, Sangpiaoxiao)6g	Tonifying the kidney and restoring yang, astringing essence and arresting spontaneous emission			
Prepared Rehmannia Root (熟地黄, Shudihuang)15g	Nourishing yin and blood			

Points in Constitution: edicinal Indian Mulberry Root (巴戟天, Bajitian) and Actinolite (阳起石, Yangqishi) have the actions of warming the kidney and strengthening yang to cure impotence. When combined with Prepared Rehmannia Root (熟地黄, Shudihuang), they can invigorate kidney-qi and nourishing essence and blood. Thus, sexual impotence will be cured. Among the ingredients of the formula, Mantis Egg-Case (桑螵蛸, Sangpiaoxiao) is used to exert both the nourishing and astringing effects and is most suitable for emission and enuresis due to deficiency of the kidney.

Indications:
1. Sexual neurasthenia
2. Chronic weakness disease

Precaution: This formula is designed for sexual impotence due to deficiency of the kidney yang. Thus, it is not suitable for sexual impotence due to depressed liver qi or accumulation of damp-heat in the interior.

Associated Formulas:

1. Procreation-Helping Pellet (赞育丹, zan yu dan) *Jingyue's Complete Works*《景岳全书》

This is comprised of Prepared Rehmannia Root (熟地黄, Shudihuang), Largehead Atractylodes Rhizome (白术, Baizhu), Chinese Angelica Root (当归, Danggui), Barbary Wolfberry Fruit (枸杞子, Gouqizi), Eucommia Bark (杜仲, Duzhong), Common Curculigo Rhizome (仙茅, Xianmao), Medicinal Indian Mulberry Root (巴戟天, Bajitian), Asiatic Cornelian Cherry Fruit (山茱萸, Shanzhuyu), Shorthorned Epimedium Herb (淫羊藿, Yinyanghuo), Desertliving Cistanche Herb (肉苁蓉, Roucongrong), Tuber Onion Seed (韭子, Jiuzi), Common Cnidium Fruit (蛇床子, Shechuangzi), Prepared Aconite Root (附子, Fuzi) and Cassia Bark (肉桂, Rougui). Its actions are invigorating the kidney, restoring yang and supplementing essence. It is indicated for infertility due to sexual impotence, insufficiency of essence and cold of deficiency type resulting from deficiency of the kidney yang.

2. Liver-Soothing Four Drugs Powder (疏肝四味散, shu gan si wei san) *Practical Internal Medicine of Traditional Chinese Medicine*《实用中医内科学》

This is comprised of Centipede (蜈蚣, Wugong), Chinese Angelica Root (当归, Danggui), White Peony Root (白芍药, Baishaoyao) and Licorice Root (甘草, Gancao). Its actions are dispersing the stagnated liver-qi, nourishing blood and dredging meridians and collaterals. It is indicated for sexual impotence due to stagnated liver-qi and blood stasis in the meridians.

3. Chinese Gentian, Earth Worm, Impotence-Treating Decoction (龙胆地龙起痿汤, long dan di long qi wei tang) *Journal of Traditional Chinese Medicine*《中医杂志》

This is comprised of Chinese Gentian Root (龙胆草, Longdancao), Prepared Rhubarb (制大黄, Zhi Dahuang), Centipede (蜈蚣, Wugong), Earth Worm (地龙, Dilong), Chinese Angelica Root (当归, Danggui), Dried Rehmannia Root (生地黄, Shengdihuang), Chinese Thorowax Root (柴胡, Chaihu), Plantain Seed (车前子, Cheqianzi), Akebia Stem (木通, Mutong), Oriental Waterplantain Rhizome (泽泻, Zexie), Common Cnidium Fruit (蛇床子, Shechuangzi) and Tuckahoe (茯苓, Fuling). Its actions are clearing away heat, inducing diuresis, dredging the collaterals and curing impotence. It is indicated for sexual impotence due to downward attack by damp-heat on the lower-jiao, which causes the damp-heat to accumulate in the liver meridian and penis.

12. Liver-Warming Decoction
(暖肝煎, nuan gan jian)

Source: *Jingyue's Complete Works*《景岳全书》
Composition: Chinese Angelica Root (当归, Danggui) 9g
Barbary Wolfberry Fruit (枸杞子, Gouqizi) 9g
Tuckahoe (茯苓, Fuling) 6g

Fennel Fruit (小茴香, Xiaohuixiang)6g
Cassia Bark (肉桂, Rougui)6
Commbined Spicebush Root (乌药, Wuyao)6g
Chinese Eaglewood Wood (沉香, Chenxiang)6g
Fresh Ginger (生姜, Shengjiang)6g

Actions: Warming and replenishing the liver and kidney, activating flow of qi and alleviating pain.

Applied Syndrome: Hernia due to deficiency-cold of the liver and kidney, manifested by pain in the lower abdomen, or swelling, hard, cold and pain in the scrotum which may even radiate to the lower abdomen, intolerance of cold and desire for warming, cold body and limbs, pale tongue with white coating, deep and slow pulse.

Liver-Warming Decoction
(Liver-Warming and Cold-Expelling Method)

Ingredients	Effects	Combined Effects	Syndrome	Chief Symptoms
Cassia Bark (肉桂, Rougui)6 Fennel Fruit (小茴香, Xiaohuixiang)6g	Expelling cold and alleviating pain	Replenishing the liver and kidney, warming yang, expelling cold, activating flow of qi and alleviating pain	Hernia (due to cold retention and qi stagnation resulting from deficiency-cold of the liver and kidney)	Pain in the lower abdomen, cold and pain in the scrotum which is relieved when warmed, pale tongue with white coating, deep and taut pulse.
Commbined Spicebush Root (乌药, Wuyao)6g Chinese Eaglewood Wood (沉香, Chenxiang)6g	Activating flow of qi and alleviating pain			
Chinese Angelica Root (当归, Danggui)9g Barbary Wolfberry Fruit (枸杞子, Gouqizi)9g	Enriching blood to easy tendons			
Tuckahoe (茯苓, Fuling)6g	Invigorating the spleen and inducing diuresis			
Fresh Ginger (生姜, Shengjiang)6g	Warming and expelling cold retention			

Points in Constitution: Testicle is the confluence of urogenital region and its diseases are treated by dealing with the liver. This formula has all the warming, activating and replenishing actions and the drugs used in the formula are related to the liver meridian.

Indications:

1. Cold pain of testicle or lower abdomen

2. Varicocele
3. Inguinoproperitoneal hernia
4. Hydrocele testis

Precaution:

This formula is suitable for pain in the lower abdomen and hernia caused by deficiency-cold of the liver and kidney which leads to qi stagnation. It is contraindicated in redness, swelling and hot pain of the scrotum due to excessive heat syndrome.

Associated Formula:

Tiantai Combined Spicebush Powder（天台乌药散, tian tai wu yao san）*Invention of Medicine*《医学发明》

This is comprised of Commbined Spicebush Root（乌药, Wuyao）, Common Aucklandia Root（木香, Muxiang）, Fennel Fruit（茴香, Huixiang）, Green Tangerine Peel（青皮, Qingpi）, Lesser Galangal Rhizome（高良姜, Gaoliangjiang）, Areca Seed（槟榔, Binglang）, Szechwan Chinaberry Fruit（川楝子, Chuanlianzi）and Croton Fruit（巴豆, Badou）. Its actions are activating flow of qi, dispersing the stagnated liver-qi, expelling cold and alleviating pain. It is indicated for hernia of the small intestine, pain in the lower abdomen which may radiate to the testicle, pale tongue with white coating, deep and slow pulse or wiry pulse, caused by cold accumulation and qi stagnation. The herb Combined Spicebush Powdert(天台乌药, tian tai wu yao san) has strong warming and dispersing actions and is indicated for hernia and abdominal pain due to accumulation of cold and stagnation of qi while Liver-Warming Decoction(暖肝煎, nuan gan jian) not only has the the warming and dispersing actions but also has the nourishing or replenishing effect. It is often used for hernia and abdominal pain due to accumulation of cold and stagnation of qi resulting from deficiency of both the liver and kidney.

13. Tangerine Seed Pill
（橘核丸, ju he wan）

Source: *Prescriptions for Rescuring the Sick*《济生方》
Composition: Tangerine Seed（橘核, Juhe）9g
Seaweed（海藻, Haizao）9g
Kelp（昆布, Kunbu）18g
Szechwan Chinaberry Fruit（川楝子, Chuanlianzi）9g
Peach Seed（桃仁, Taoren）9g
Officinal Magnolia Bark（厚朴, Houpo）9g
Akebia Sem（木通, Mutong）9g
Immature Bitter Orange（枳实, Zhishi）9g
Corydalis Tuber（延胡索, Yanhusuo）9g
Cassia Bark（桂心, Guixin）9g
Common Aucklandia Root（木香, Muxiang）9g

Actions: Activating flow of qi and alleviating pain, softening hardness and dissipating blockage.

Applied Syndrome: Swelling of the scrotum due to cold-dampness, manifested by swelling and deflected drop of testicle, or hard as stone, or pain radiating to umbilicus and abdomen, pale tongue with white coating, deep and slow pulse or deep and wiry pulse.

Tangerine Seed Pill
(Qi-Activating and Blockage-Dissipating Method)

Ingredients	Effects	Combined Effects	Syndrome	Chief Symptoms
Tangerine Seed (橘核, Juhe)9g Szechwan Chinaberry Fruit (川楝子, Chuanlianzi)9g	Activating flow of qi, dissipating blockage and alleviating pain, (the special drugs for hernia)	Activating flow of qi and alleviating pain, expelling cold and removing dampness, softening hardness and dissipating blockage	Swelling of the scrotum (due to stagnation of qi and blood resulting from attack of cold upon the liver meridian)	Swelling and deflected drop of testicle, pain radiating to lower abdomen, white and greasy tongue coating, wiry pulse
Seaweed (海藻, Haizao)9g Kelp (昆布, Kunbu) 18g	Softening hardness and dissipating blockage			
Corydalis Tuber (延胡索, Yanhusuo)9g Peach Seed (桃仁, Taoren)9g	Activating blood circulation and alleviating pain			
Common Aucklandia Root (木香, Muxiang) 9g Officinal Magnolia Bark (厚朴, Houpo)9g Immature Bitter Orange (枳实, Zhishi)9g	Activating flow of qi and alleviating pain, removing dampness and breaking hardness			
Cassia Bark (桂心, Guixin) 9g	Warming and expelling cold retention			
Akebia Stem (木通, Mutong)9g	Dredging blood vessels			

Points in Constitution: The main action of this formula is promoting flow of qi, which can immediately alleviate pain and dissipate blockages. Under warm conditions, blood and qi can flow regularly, thus Cassia Bark (肉桂, Rougui) is used to warm the kidney.

Indications:
1. Hydrocele testis
2. Acute and chronic testitis, epididymitis
3. Tuberculocele

Precaution: This formula is indicated for hernia due to cold-dampness. For redness, swelling, itching and pain of scrotum due to transformation of heat by cold-dampness, this formula may be modified by removing Cassia Bark (肉桂, Rougui) but adding Chinese Corktree Bark (黄柏, Huangbai), Glabrous Greenbrier Rhizome (土茯苓, Tufuling) and Plantain Seed (车前子, Cheqianzi) to clear away damp-heat.

Associated Formula:

Combined Spicebush Root Powder (天台乌药散, tian tai wu yao san) *Invention of Medicine* 《医学发明》

This is comprised of Combined Spicebush Root (乌药, Wuyao), Common Aucklandia Root (木香, Muxiang), Fennel Fruit (茴香, Huixiang), Green Tangerine Peel (青皮, Qingpi), Lesser Galangal Rhizome (高良姜, Gaoliangjiang), Areca Seed (槟榔, Binglang), Szechwan Chinaberry Fruit (川楝子, Chuanlianzi) and Croton Fruit (巴豆, Badou). Its actions are activating flow of qi and dispersing the stagnated liver-qi, expelling cold and alleviating pain. It is indicated for hernia of the small intestine, pain in the lower abdomen which radiates to the testicles, pale tongue with white coating, deep and slow or wiry pulse due to accumulation of cold and stagnation of qi.

14. Bank-Consolidating Pill
(巩堤丸, gong di wan)

Source: *Jingyue's Complete Works* 《景岳全书》
Composition: Prepared Rehmannia Root (熟地黄, Shudihuang) 9g
Chinese Dodder Seed (菟丝子, Tusizi) 9g
Largehead Atractylodes Rhizome (白术, Baizhu) 9g
Chinese Magnoliavine Fruit (五味子, Wuweizi) 6g
Sharpleaf Galangal Fruit (益智仁, Yizhiren) 6g
Malaytea Scurfpea Fruit (破故纸, Poguzhi) 9g
Prepared Aconite Root (附子, Fuzi) 3g
Tuckahoe (茯苓, Fuling) 9g
Tuber Onion Seed (韭子, Jiuzi) 3g

Actions: Warming and tonifying kidney-yang and astringing urination.

Applied Syndrome: Enuresis due to kidney deficiency, manifested by enuresis during sleeping, clear and prolonged urination, or even many times in the night, listlessness and tiredness, pallor, cold limbs, lassitude of the loins and legs, poor memory or dull intelligence, pale tongue with little coating, thin pulse.

Bank-Consolidating Pill
(Kidney-Tonifying and Astringcy-Inducing Method)

Ingredients	Effects	Combined Effects	Syndrome	Chief Symptoms
Prepared Aconite Root (附子, Fuzi)3g Sharpleaf Galangal Fruit (益智仁, Yizhiren)6g Malaytea Scurfpea Fruit (破故纸, Poguzhi)9g Tuber Onion Seed (韭子, Jiuzi)3g	Warming yang and invigorating the kidney	Warming and tonifying kidney-yang and astringing urination	Unconsolidation of the kidney qi	Enuresis during sleeping, listlessness and tiredness, pallor, cold limbs, pale tongue with little coating, thin pulse
Prepared Rehmannia Root (熟地黄, Shudihuang)9g	Nourishing the kidney yin			
Largehead Atractylodes Rhizome (白术, Baizhu)9g Tuckahoe (茯苓, Fuling)9g	Invigorating the spleen and replenishing qi			
Chinese Dodder Seed (菟丝子, Tusizi)9g Chinese Magnoliavine Fruit (五味子, Wuweizi)6g	Astringing the lower-jiao			

Points in Constitution: The characteristics of this formula are 1). to invigorate yang and nourish yin simultaneously but emphasize nourishment of yang; 2). to reinforce the kidney and induce astringency at the same time but stress the inducement of astringency, which can not be ignored when this formula is used.

Indications: Enuresis

Precaution: It is contraindicated in enuresis due to deficiency of yin which results from excessive fire of the heart and liver.

Associated Formula:

Hairy Antler Pill (鹿茸丸, lu rong wan) *Treatise on the Triple-Pathogenic Doctrine of Etiology* 《三因极一病证方论》

This is comprised of Hairy Antler (鹿茸, Lurong), Dwarf Lilyturf Root (麦门冬, Maimendong), Prepared Rehmannia Root (熟地黄, Shudihuang), Membranous Milkvetch Root (黄芪, Huangqi), Ginseng (人参, Renshen), Chinese Magnoliavine Fruit (五味子, Wuweizi), Desertliving Cistanche Herb (肉苁蓉, Roucongrong), Chicken Gizzard Membrane (鸡内金, Jineijin), Malaytea Scurfpea Fruit (补骨脂, Buguzhi), Twotooth Achyranthes Root (牛膝, Niuxi), Figwort Root (玄参, Xuanshen), Tuckahoe (茯苓, Fuling), Chinese Wolfberry Root-Bark (地骨皮, Digupi) and Asiatic Cornelian Cherry Fruit (山茱萸, Shanzhuyu). Its actions are warming yang and consolidating the kidney. It is indicated for frequent urination and diabetes involving the lower-jiao due to kidney deficiency.

15. Sancai Marrow-Preserving Pill Containing Cochinchinese Asparagus, Rehmannia and Ginseng (三才封髓丹, san cai feng sui dan)

Source: *The Precious Mirror of Hygiene* 《卫生宝鉴》
Composition: Cochinchinese Asparagus Root (天门冬, Tianmendong) 15g
Prepared Rehmannia Root (熟地黄, Shudihuang) 15g
Ginseng (人参, Renshen) 6g
Chinese Corktree Bark (黄柏, Huangbai) 6g
Villous Amomum Fruit (砂仁, Sharen) 6g
Prepared Licorice Root (炙甘草, Zhi Gancao) 6g
Desertliving Cistanche Herb (肉苁蓉, Roucongrong) 15g

Actions: Nourishing yin and eliminating fire, tonifying blood and controlling nocturnal emission.

Applied Syndrome: Emaciated body due to deficiency of yin and hyperactivity of fire, manifested as dry sensation in pharynx and throat, cough with bloody sputum, dizziness, nocturnal emission, lassitude of the loin and knees, constipation with weak body, red tongue with little coating, thin and rapid pulse.

Points in Constitution: The ancient physician called the three drugs of Cochinchinese Asparagus Root (天门冬, Tianmendong), Prepared Rehmannia Root (熟地黄, Shudihuang) and Ginseng (人参, Renshen) Sancai (i.e. heaven, earth and human) which means that the human body may be regarded as a small uinverse, of which the above is the heaven and the below is the earth. This formula replenishes all the three organs of the lung, spleen and kidney simultaneously without bringing about heat. Thus, it is an effective prescription for deficiency of yin.

Indications:
1. Sexual neurasthenia
2. Resce oral cavity ulcer
3. Chronic pharyngitis

Precaution: This formula should be used cautiously for the case of loose stool.

Associated Formula:
Procreation-Helping Pellet (赞育丹, zan yu dan) *Jingyue's Complete Works* 《景岳全书》

Sancai Marrow-Preserving Pill Containing Cochinchinese Asparagus, Rehmannia and Ginseng
(Yin-Nourishing and Fire-Eliminating Method)

Ingredients	Effects	Combined Effects	Syndrome	Chief Symptoms
Cochinchinese Asparagus Root (天门冬, Tianmendong) 15g	Nourishing yin and moistening the lung	Nourishing yin and eliminating fire, enriching blood and controlling nocturnal emission	Deficiency of yin and hyperactivity of fire	Emaciated body, lassitude of the loin and knees, dizziness, dry sensation in pharynx and throat, cough with blood in sputum, nocturnal emission, constipation with weak body, red tongue with little coating, thin and rapid pulse
Prepared Rehmannia Root (熟地黄, Shudihuang) 15g	Nourishing yin and tonifying blood			
Ginseng (人参, Renshen) 6g	Invigorating the spleen and replenishing qi			
Desertliving Cistanche Herb (肉苁蓉, Roucongrong) 15g	Promoting the production of essence and tonifying marrow			
Chinese Corktree Bark (黄柏, Huangbai) 6g	Clearing away heat and eliminating fire			
Villous Amomum Fruit (砂仁, Sharen) 6g	Activating spleen-qi and eliminating stagnation			
Prepared Licorice Root (炙甘草, Zhi Gancao) 6g	Coordinating the actions of the above drugs			

This is comprised of Prepared Rehmannia Root (熟地黄, Shudihuang), Eucommia Bark (杜仲, Duzhong), Chinese Angelica Root (当归, Danggui), Medicinal Indian Mulberry Root (巴戟肉, Bajirou), Desertliving Cistanche Herb (肉苁蓉, Roucongrong), Shorthorned Epimedium Herb (淫羊藿, Yinyanghuo), Common Cnidium Fruit (蛇床子, Shechuangzi), Cassia Bark (肉桂, Rougui), Largehead Atractylodes Rhizome (白术, Baizhu), Barbary Wolfberry Fruit (枸杞子, Gouqizi), Common Curculigo Rhizome (仙茅, Xianmao), Asiatic Cornelian Cherry Fruit (山茱萸, Shanzhuyu), Tuber Onion Seed (韭子, Jiuzi), Prepared Aconite Root (附子, Fuzi), [or addingGinseng (人参, Renshen) and Hairy Antler (鹿茸, Lurong)]. Its actions are warming and recuperating the gate of life. It is indicated for sexual impotence due to declination of fire from the gate of life which are manifested by sexual impotence, scanty and cold sperm, dizziness, tinnitus, listlessness, soreness and weakness of the loin and knees, cold body and extremities, pale tongue with white coating, deep and thin pulse.

Additional Formulas

Pilose Asiabell, Membranous Milkvetch Decoction for Stranguria due to Overstrain
(参芪劳淋汤, shen qi lao lin tang)

Source: *Journal of Traditional Chinese Medicine*《中医杂志》
Composition: Membranous Milkvetch Root（黄芪, Huangqi）15g
Pilose Asiabell Root（党参, Dangshen）15g
Tuckahoe（茯苓, Fuling）15g
Dwarf Lilyturf Root（麦门冬, Maimendong）9g
Chinese Wolfberry Root-bark（地骨皮, Digupi）9g
Plantain Seed（车前子, Cheqianzi）9g
Lotus Seed（莲子, Lianzi）15g
Motherwort Herb（益母草, Yimucao）15g
Lalang Grass Rhizome（白茅根, Baimaogen）30g
Spreading Hedyotis Herb（白花蛇舌草, Baihuasheshecao）15g
Licorice Root（甘草, Gancao）6g
Actions: Replenishing qi and yin, clearing away heat and promoting diuresis.
Applied Syndrome: Stranguria due to overstrain or protracted stranguria due to deficiency of qi and yin which results in accumulation of damp-heat in the urinarybladder of lower-jiao. The manifestations are frequency of micturition, feeling of distention and fullness in the lower abdomen, heaviness, soreness and pain in the loins, dry throat and thirst which may relapse when overstrained, listlessness and exhaustion, pale tongue with greasy coating, feeble and weak pulse or thin and smooth pulse.
Points in Constitution: Repeated relapse of stranguria due to overstrain is usually caused by weakened body resistance and remains of pathogenic factors, which is very difficult to eradicate. Thus, this formula combines qi-replenishing and diuresis-inducing drugs. The use of Spreading Hedyotis Herb（白花蛇舌草, Baihuasheshecao）is to strengthen the heat-removing and toxin-clearing actions. This is a formula that treats both the primary and secondary causes of a disease.
  Indications:
  1. Chronic pyelonephritis
  2. Chronic cystitis
Precaution: This formula is designed for prolonged stranguria due to accumulation of damp-heat in the lower abdomen resulting from insufficiency of both qi and yin. It is not suitable for stranguria due to an overstrain with deficiency and cold of kidney-qi.

Pilose Asiabell, Membranous Milkvetch Decoction for Stranguria due to Overstrain

(Qi-Nourishing and Diuresis-Inducing Method)

Ingredients	Effects	Combined Effects	Syndrome	Chief Symptoms
Membranous Milkvetch Root (黄芪, Huangqi) 15g Pilose Asiabell Root (党参, Dangshen) 15g	Replenishing qi and strengthening body resistance	Replenishing qi and yin, clearing away damp-heat	Stranguria due to overstrain (deficiency of qi and yin which results in accumulation of damp-heat in the urinary bladder of lower-jiao)	Frequency of micturition, relapse while overstrain, feeling of distention and fullness in the lower abdomen, heaviness, soreness and pain in the loin, dry throat and thirsty, listlessness and exhausted, pale tongue with greasy coating, feeble and weak pulse or thin and smooth pulse
Dwarf Lilyturf Root (麦门冬, Maimendong) 9g	Nourishing yin fluid			
Plantain Seed (车前子, Cheqianzi) 9g Tuckahoe (茯苓, Fuling) 15g	Inducing diuresis and removing dampness			
Lalang Grass Rhizome (白茅根, Baimaogen) 30g Lotus Seed (莲子, Lianzi) 15g Motherwort Herb (益母草, Yimucao) 15g	Clearing away heat and promoting urination			
Spreading Hedyotis Herb (白花蛇舌草, Baihuasheshecao) 15g	Clearing away damp-heat and toxic material			
Chinese Wolfberry Root-Bark (地骨皮, Digupi) 9g	Removing heat from the blood and reducing the hectic fever due to yin deficiency			
Licorice Root (甘草, Gancao) 6g	Coordinating the actions of the above drugs			

Associated Formulas:

1. Decoction for Stranguria due to Overstrain (劳淋汤, lao lin tang) *Records of Traditional Chinese and Western Medicine in Combination*《医学衷中参西录》

This is comprised of Gordon Euryale Seed (生芡实, Sheng Qianshi), Common Yam Rhizome (生山药, Sheng Shanyao), Common Anemarrhena Rhizome (知母, Zhimu), Ass-hide Glue (阿胶, Ejiao) and White Peony Root (生白芍药, Sheng Baishaoyao). Its actions are reducing fever, decreasing urination and inducing astringency. It is indicated for stranguria due to an overstrain and accumulation of damp-heat in the lower-jiao which results from deficiency of kidney-yin.

2. Membranous Milkvetch Decoction (黄芪汤, huang qi tang) *Imperial Medical Encyclopaedia*《圣济总录》

This is comprised of Membranous Milkvetch Root (黄芪, Huangqi), Ginseng (人参, Renshen), Talc (滑石, Huashi), Chinese Magnoliavine Fruit (五味子, Wuweizi), Tuckahoe (茯苓, Fuling), Magnetite (磁石, Cishi), Yerbadetajo Herb (旱莲草, Hanliancao), White Mulberry Root-Bark (桑白皮, Sangbaipi), Baikal Skullcap Root (黄芩, Huangqin) and Bitter Orange (枳壳, Zhiqiao). Its actions are replenishing qi and benefiting the kidney, inducing diuresis and relieving stranguria. It is indicated for stranguria due to overstrain and accumulation of damp-heat in the urinarybladder which results from insufficiency of kidney-qi.

3. Honeysuckle, Weeping Forsythia and Dendrobium Decoction (银翘石斛汤, yin qiao shi hu tang) *Peking Traditional Chinese Medicine*《北京中医》

This is comprised of Honeysuckle Flower (金银花, Jinyinhua), Weeping Forsythia Capsule (连翘, Lianqiao), Dendrobium Herb (石斛, Shihu), Dried Rehmannia Root (生地黄, Shengdihuang), Prepared Rehmannia Root (熟地黄, Shudihuang), Common Yam Rhizome (山药, Shanyao), Tree Peony Bark (牡丹皮, Mudanpi), tuckahoe (茯苓, Fuling) and Oriental Waterplantain Rhizome (泽泻, Zexie). Its actions are clearing away heat, removing toxic material and nourishing kidney-yin. It is indicated for chronic nephropyelitis or chronic urocystitis due to lingering damp-heat and toxic material remaining in the lower-jiao and deficiency of kidney yin.

Effective Formula for Kidney Recuperation (肾康灵, shen kang ling)

Source: *Sichuan Journal of Traditional Chinese Medicine*《四川中医》
Composition: Christina Loosestrife Herb (金钱草, Jinqiancao) 45g
Chicken Gizzard Membrane (鸡内金, Jineijin) 15g
Japanese Climbing Fern Spores (海金沙, Haijinsha) 30g
Plantain Seed (车前子, Cheqianzi) 15g
Lilac Pink Herb (瞿麦, Qumai) 15g
Common Knotgrass Herb (萹蓄, Bianxu) 15g
Tophatherum Leaf (竹叶, Zhuye) 15g
Akebia Stem (木通, Mutong) 9g
Ricepaperplant Pith (通草, Tongcao) 9g
Common Rush Pith (灯心草, Dengxincao) 9g

Actions: Clearing away heat and inducing diuresis, relieving stranguria and eliminating the stone.

Applied Syndrome: Stranguria due to urinary stone. Heat-dampness attacks the lower-jiao and the urinarybladder fails to conduct its function to transform qi, thus, leading to urine becoming the stone. The manifestations are urine with stone, difficult urination or a sudden break during micturition, stabbing pain in the urethra and dysuria, subjective sensation of contraction in the lower abdomen or angina in the loins and abdomen, even hematuria, red tongue with thin coating, slightly rapid pulse.

Effective Formula for Kidney Recuperation
(Stranguria-Treating and Stone-Eliminating Method)

Ingredients	Effects	Combined Effects	Syndrome	Chief Symptoms
Christina Loosestrife Herb (金钱草, Jinqiancao) 45g Japanese Climbing Fern Spores (海金沙, Haijinsha) 30g	Inducing diuresis, treating stranguria and removing stones	Clearing away heat and promoting diuresis, treating stranguria and eliminating the stone	Blockage of stone in the urinary-bladder (due to attack of the lower-jiao by damp-heat and disturbance in qi transformation of urinary bladder)	Urine with stone, difficult urination or sudden break during micturition, stabbing pain in the urethra and dysuria, subjective sensation of contraction in the lower abdomea or angina in the loin and abdomen, even hematuria, red tongue with thin coating, slightly rapid pulse
Chicken Gizzard Membrane (鸡内金, Jineijin) 15g	Resolving mass and eliminating the stone			
Plantain Seed (车前子, Cheqianzi) 15g Lilac Pink Herb (瞿麦, Qumai) 15g Common Knotgrass Herb (萹蓄, Bianxu) 15g Tophatherum Leaf (竹叶, Zhuye) 15g Akebia Stem (木通, Mutong) 9g Ricepaperplant Pith (通草, Tongcao) 9g Common Rush Pith (灯心草, Dengxincao) 9g	Clearing away heat and dampness, inducing diuresis and treating stranguria			

Points in Constitution: The combination of Christina Loosestrife Herb (金钱草, Jinqiancao), Japanese Climbing Fern Spores (海金沙, Haijinsha) and Chicken Gizzard Membrane (鸡内金, Jineijin) can promote urination, remove stones and treat stranguria. They are the key drugs for urinary tract calculus.

Indication: Urinary tract calculus

Precaution: This formula is designed for stranguria with stones caused by downward attacks of damp-heat upon the lower-jiao. For prolonged stranguria due to urinary calculus accompanied with kidney deficiency, or with insufficiency of both qi and blood, this formula should be used together with other herbs.

Associated Formulas:

1. Pill for Stranguria from Urolithiasis (沙淋丸, sha lin wan) *Records of Traditional Chinese and Western Medicine in Combination* 《医学衷中参西录》

This is comprised of Chicken Gizzard Membrane (生鸡内金, Sheng Jineijin), Membranous Milkvetch Root (生黄芪, Sheng Huangqi), Common Anemarrhena Rhizome (知母, Zhimu), White Peony Root (生杭芍, Shenghangshao), Borax (硼砂, Pengsha), Mirabilite (朴硝, Puxiao) and Niter (硝石, Xiaoshi). Its actions are replenishing qi, regulating blood and eliminating the stone. It is indicated for lingering stranguria due to urinary stone accompanied with deficiency of both qi and blood.

2. Cowherb Seed Powder (王不留行散, wang bu liu xing san) *Imperial Benevolent Prescriptionss of Taiping Period* 《圣惠方》

This is comprised of Cowherb Seed (王不留行, Wangbuliuxing), Kansui Root (甘遂, Gansui), Japanese Felt Fern Leaf (石韦, Shiwei), Cluster Mallow Fruit (冬葵子, Dongkuizi), Akebia Stem (木通, Mutong), Talc (滑石, Huashi), Cattail Pollen (蒲黄, Puhuang), Red Peony Root (赤芍, Chishao), Chinese Angelica Root (当归, Danggui) and Cassia Bark (桂心, Guixin). Its actions are activating blood circulation and removing blood stasis, promoting urination and relieving stranguria. It is indicated for stranguria due to urinary caculus, stranguria complicated by hematuria and urination with bloody streaks and gores.

3. Kidney-Invigorating and Stone-Removing Decoction (补肾通石汤, bu shen tong shi tang) *Jiangsu Traditional Chinese Medicine* 《江苏中医》

This is comprised of Christina Loosestrife Herb (金钱草, Jinqiancao), Yerbadetajo Herb (墨旱莲, Mohanlian), Fleeceflower Root (何首乌, Heshouwu), Barbary Wolfberry Fruit (枸杞子, Gouqizi), Membranous Milkvetch Root (黄芪, Huangqi), Common Anemarrhena Rhizome (知母, Zhimu), Chinese Clematis Root (威灵仙, Weilingxian), Japanese Climbing Fern Spores (海金沙, Haijinsha), Plantain Seed (车前子, Cheqianzi), Cluster Mallow Fruit (冬葵子, Dongkuizi), Japanese Felt Fern Leaf (石韦, Shiwei) and Akebia Stem (木通, Mutong). Its actions are invigorating the kidney, replenishing qi, promoting urination and relieving stranguria. It is indicated for stranguria due to urinary stone accompanied with insufficiency of kidney qi and deficiency of both qi and blood.

4. Decoction for Renal Colic (肾绞痛汤, shen jiao tong tang) *New Traditional Chinese Medicine* 《新中医》

This is comprised of Chinese Thorowax Root (柴胡, Chaihu), Green Tangerine Peel (青皮, Qingpi), Licorice Root (甘草, Gancao), Bitter Orange (枳壳, Zhiqiao), Corydalis Tuber (延胡索, Yanhusuo), Szechwan Chinaberry Fruit (川楝子, Chuanlianzi), Sandalwood (檀香, Tanxiang, to be decocted later), Commbined Spicebush Root (乌药, Wuyao), Red Peony Root (赤芍, Chishao), Common Aucklandia Root (广木香, Guang Muxiang), Twotooth Achyranthes Root (牛膝, Niuxi) and Ovateleaf Holly Bark (救必应, Jiubiying), or Ovateleaf Holly Bark (熊胆木, Xiongdanmu). Its actions are regulating flow of qi, alleviating pain, relieving muscular spasm and convulsion. It is indicated for renal colic due to urinary tract calculus.

Nephritis Decoction
(肾炎汤, shen yang tang)

Source: *Transaction of Hubei College of Traditional Chinese Medicine*《湖南中医学院学报》
Composition: Membranous Milkvetch Root (黄芪, Huangqi) 30g
Tribulus Fruit (白蒺藜, Baijili) 30g
Plantain Herb (车前草, Cheqiancao) 30g
Cicada Slough (蝉蜕, Chantui) 9g
Largehead Atractylodes Rhizome (白术, Baizhu) 9g
Tuckahoe (茯苓, Fuling) 9g
Hirsute Shiny Bugleweed Herb (泽兰, Zelan) 9g
Chinese Dodder Seed (菟丝子, Tusizi) 9g
Licorice Root (甘草, Gancao) 3g

Actions: Replenishing qi and invigorating the spleen, expelling wind and inducing diuresis.

Applied Syndrome: Edema, caused by retention of water-dampness in the exterior which results from deficiency of the spleen with excessive dampness, mostly complicated with weakness of exterior qi and attacks of pathogenic wind. The manifestations are edema, dysuria, aversion to cold and fever, thirst, white tongue, floating pulse.

Points in Constitution: This formula is the modification of Fourstamen Stephania and Membranous Milkvetch Decoction (黄芪防己汤). The use of Tribulus Fruit (白蒺藜) and Cicada Slough (蝉蜕, Chantui), which disperses pathogenic wind to prevent the wind from causing the up-stirring of the liver, shows the insight of clinical doctors.

Indications:
1. Acute and chronic nephritis
2. Rheumatic arthritis

Precaution: This formula is designed for edema caused by insufficiency of both the spleen and kidney yang which results in retention of water and dampness in the interior, mostly complicated with attack of pathogenic wind. Thus, it should be forbidden or used cautiously for edema and dysuria of excess type caused by attack of the exterior of the body by pathogenic wind, cold and dampness.

Associated Formulas:

1. Fourstamen Stephania and Membranous Milkvetch Decoction (防己黄芪汤, fang ji huang qi tang) *Synopsis of Golden Cabinet*《金匮要略》

This is comprised of Fourstamen Stephania Root (防己, Fangji), Membranous Milkvetch Root (黄芪, Huangqi), Largehead Atractylodes Rhizome (白术, Baizhu) and Licorice Root (甘草, Gancao). This formula is good at treating edema which is accompanied with such heat symptoms as scanty and dark urine and thirst. Besides, it is also good at consolidating the superficial qi to remove dampness and is indicated for edema or accomulation of dampness in the exterior due to failure of superficial qi to protect the body manifested as sweating and aversion to wind, heaviness feeling of the body and dysuria.

Nephritis Decoction
(Qi-Replenishing, Kidney-Nourishing and Diuresis-Inducing Method)

Ingredients	Effects	Combined Effects	Syndrome	Chief Symptoms
Membranous Milkvetch Root (黄芪, Huangqi) 30g	Replenishing qi, invigorating the spleen, also promoting urination	Replenishing qi and invigorating the spleen, expelling wind and removing dampness	Retention of water-dampness in the exterior due to deficiency of the spleen with excessive dampness, complicated with attacks of pathogenic wind.	Edema, dysuria, aversion to cold and fever, thirst, white tongue coating, floating pulse
Largehead Atractylodes Rhizome (白术, Baizhu) 9g Tuckahoe (茯苓, Fuling) 9g	Invigorating the spleen and inducing diuresis			
Plantain Herb (车前草, Cheqiancao) 30g	Removing heat and promoting urination			
Hirsute Shiny Bugleweed Herb (泽兰, Zelan) 9g	Activating blood circulation and inducing diuresis			
Tribulus Fruit (白蒺藜) 30g Cicada Slough (蝉蜕, Chantui) 9g	Expelling wind and dredging the collaterals			
Chinese Dodder Seed (菟丝子, Tusizi) 9g	Warming and tonifying the spleen and kidney			
Licorice Root (甘草, Gancao) 3g	Coordinating the actions of the above drugs			

2. Fourstamen Stephania and Tuckahoe Decoction (防己茯苓汤, fang ji fu ling tang) *Synopsis of Golden Cabinet* 《金匮要略》

This is comprised of Fourstamen Stephania Root (防己, Fangji), Membranous Milkvetch Root (黄芪, Huangqi), Cassia Twig (桂枝, Guizhi), Tuckahoe (茯苓, Fuling) and Licorice Root (甘草, Gancao). This formula has the actions of replenishing qi and consolidating the superfical qi besides its wind-dispelling, dampness-removing and yang-qi-activating actions. It is good at treating retention of water due to yang deficiency manifested by edema and involuntary movement of four limbs, cold sensation of limbs and body.

Aconite and Rhubarb Decoction
(附子大黄汤, fu zi da huang tang)

Source: *Shaanxi Journal of Traditional Chinese Medicine* 《陕西中医》
Composition: Prepared Aconite Root (制附子, Zhi Fuzi) 15~30g
Membranous Milkvetch Root (黄芪, Huangqi) 30~60g
Rhubarb (大黄, Dahuang) 15~30g
Mirabilite (芒硝, Mangxiao) 9~15g
Motherwort Herb (益母草, Yimucao) 15~30g
Actions: Warming and tonifying the spleen and kidney, replenishing qi and eliminating turbid evils.
Applied Syndrome: Edema, comsuptive diseases, uroschesis, dysuria and constipation with incessant vomiting due to yang deficiency of the spleen and kidney and excessive dampness and turbidity in the interior. The manifestations are tarnished complexion, intolerance of cold, cold limbs, nausea and vomiting, oliguria, edema all over the body, pale tongue, deep and thin pulse or soft and thin pulse.

Aconite and Rhubarb Decoction
(Interior-Warming and Turbility-Eliminating Method)

Ingredients	Effects	Combined Effects	Syndrome	Chief Symptoms
Prepared Aconite Root (制附子, Zhi Fuzi) 15~30g	Warming and tonifying the spleen and kidney	Warming and replenishing the spleen and kidney, replenishing qi and eliminating turbid evils	Uraemia (due to yang deficiency of the spleen and kidney and excessive dampness in the interior)	Tarnished complexion, intolerance of cold and cold limbs, tiredness, nausea and vomiting, anorexia, oliguria, edema, pale tongue, deep and thin pulse or soft and thin pulse
Membranous Milkvetch Root (黄芪, Huangqi) 30~60g	Replenishing qi and invigorating the spleen, inducing diuresis and relieving swelling			
Rhubarb (大黄, Dahuang) 15~30g Mirabilite (芒硝, Mangxiao) 9~15g	Purging dirty and turbid materials			
Motherwort Herb (益母草, Yimucao) 15~30g	Inducing diuresis and relieving swelling			

Points in Constitution: This formula is the modification of Rhubarb and Prepared Aconite Decoction (大黄附子汤, da huang fu zi tang) recorded in the book of *Synopsis of Golden Cabinet* 《金匮要略》. The original formula is for constipation due to cold retention and pain in the hypochondrium. Thus, Rhubarb (大黄, Dahuang) and Prepared Aconite Root (附子, Fuzi) are combined with Manchurian Wildginger Herb (细辛, Xixin). This formula is for edema due to yang deficiency, thus Rhubarb (大黄, Dahuang) and Prepared Aconite Root (附子, Fuzi) are combined with Membranous Milkvetch Root (黄芪, Huangqi) and Motherwort Herb (益母草, Yimucao).

Indications:
1. Nephropathy syndrome in the last term of chronic nephropathy
2. Uraemia due to various cause
3. Cirrhosis ascites

Precaution: This formula is designed for uraemia due to deficiency of both the spleen and kidney and excessive dampness in the interior. It is not suitable for those who are with excessive damp-heat in the interior.

Associated Formulas:

1. Kidney-Benefiting Decoction (益肾汤, yi shen tang) *Journal of New Medicine* 《新医药杂志》

This is comprised of Chinese Angelica Root (当归, Danggui), Red Peony Root (赤芍, Chishao), Szechwan Lovage Rhizome (川芎, Chuanxiong), Safflower (红花, Honghua), Dan-Shen Root (丹参, Danshen), Peach Seed (桃仁, Taoren), Motherwort Herb (益母草, Yimucao), Honeysuckle Flower (金银花, Jinyinhua), Lalang Grass Rhizome (白茅根, Baimaogen), Indigowoad Root (板蓝根, Banlangen) and Tokyo Violet Herb (紫花地丁, Zihuadiding). Its actions are dissolving blood stasis, reducing swelling, clearing away heat and toxic material. It is indicated for edema and dysuria due to impairment of yang which involves yin and accumulation of blood stasis and heat.

2. Nature Pill (天真丹, tian zhen dan) *Great Treasure of Health Care* 《卫生鸿宝》

This is comprised of Medicinal Indian Mulberry Root (巴戟天, Bajitian), Malaytea Scurfpea Fruit (补骨脂, Buguzhi), Common Fenugreek Seed (葫芦巴, Huluba), Eucommia Bark (杜仲, Duzhong), Cassia Bark (桂心, Guixin), Chinese Eaglewood Wood (沉香, Chenxiang), Fennel Fruit (小茴香, Xiaohuixiang), Amber (琥珀, Hupo), Sevenlobed Yam Rhizome (草薢, Bixie) and Black Pharbitis Seed (黑牵牛, Hei Qianniu). Its actions are warming yang, inducing diuresis, reducing swelling and relieving distention. It is indicated for edema due to yang deficiency in the lower-jiao.

3. Membranous Milkvetch Kidney-Benefiting Decoction (黄芪益肾汤, huang qi yi shen tang) *Zhejiang Journal of Traditional Chinese Medicine* 《浙江中医杂志》

This is comprised of Membranous Milkvetch Root (黄芪, Huangqi), Heartleaf Houttuynia Herb (鱼腥草, Yuxingcao), Spreading Hedyotis Herb (白花蛇舌草, Baihuasheshecao), Earth Worm (地龙, Dilong), Motherwort Herb (益母草, Yimucao), Dan-Shen Root (丹参, Danshen), Cicada Slough (蝉衣, Chanyi), honeysuckle Flower (金银花, Jinyinhua) and Pig Kidney. Its actions are replenishing qi, building up body resistance, clearing away heat and toxic material, activating blood circulation and removing blood stasis. It is indicated for edema, listlessness and asthma due to deficiency of the lung, spleen and kidney which causes remaining of noxious heat and blood stasis.

4. Spleen-Reinforcing Decoction (实脾饮, shi pi yin) *Revised Yan's Formulae for Life-Preserving* 《重订严氏济生方》

This is comprised of Officinal Magnolia Bark (厚朴, Houpo), Largehead Atractylodes Rhizome (白术, Baizhu), Common Floweringquince Fruit (木瓜, Mugua), Common Aucklandia Root (木香, Muxiang), Caoguo Seed (草果仁, Caoguoren), Areca Peel (大腹皮, Dafupi), Prepared Aconite Root (附子, Fuzi), Tuckahoe (茯苓, Fuling), Dried Ginger (干姜, Ganjiang) and Licorice Root (甘草, Gancao). Its actions are warming yang, invigorating the spleen, activating flow of qi and promoting urination. It is indicated for edema, oliguria and loose stool due to yang deficiency.

5. Divine Black Bird Decoction (真武汤, zhen wu tang) *Treatise on Exogenous Febrile Diseases* 《伤寒论》

This is comprised of Tuckahoe (茯苓, Fuling), White Peony Root (白芍药, Baishaoyao), Largehead Atractylodes Rhizome (白术, Baizhu), Fresh Ginger (生姜, Shengjiang) and Prepared Aconite Root (炮附子, Pao Fuzi). Its actions are warming yang and inducing diuresis. It is indicated for accumulation of water dampness in the interior due to deficiency of the spleen and kidney-yang.

6. Kidney-Warming and Toxin-Clearing Decoction (温肾排毒汤, wen shen pai du tang) *New Traditional Chinese Medicine* 《新中医》

This is comprised of Prepared Aconite Root (熟附子, Shu Fuzi), Prepared Pinellia Rhizome with Fresh Ginger (姜半夏, Jiangbanxia), Rhubarb (大黄, Dahuang), Coptis Rhizome (黄连, Huanglian), Pilose Asiabell Root (党参, Dangshen), Largehead Atractylodes Rhizome (白术, Baizhu), Perilla Leaf (紫苏, Zisu), Serissa (六月雪, Liuyuexue), Green Gram Seed (绿豆, Lüdou) and Licorice Root (甘草, Gancao). Its actions are warming and tonifying the spleen and kidney, clearing away toxic material and purging the turbid. It is applied for chronic renal insufficiency and uraemia.

Powder for Urine Retention
(癃闭散, long bi san)

Source: *Journal of Traditional Chinese Medicine* 《中医杂志》
Composition: Cassia Bark (肉桂, Rougui) 3g
Pangolin Scales (穿山甲, Chuanshanjia) 6g
Actions: Warming yang and promoting qi transformation, activating blood circulation and dissolving blood stasis.
Applied Syndrome: Uroschesis or retention of urine due to deficiency of kidney-yang, distur-

bance in qi transformation and blood stasis, manifested as anuria or dysuria, feeling of distention, fullness and pain in the lower abdomen, dark purplish tongue or with petechia, unsmooth or thin and rapid pulse.

Powder for Urine Retention
(Yang-Warming and Orifices-Opening Method)

Ingredients	Effects	Combined Effects	Syndrome	Chief Symptoms
Cassia Bark (肉桂, Rougui) 3g	Warming yang and promoting qi transformation, dispelling cold and removing blood stasis	Warming yang and promoting qi transformation, activating blood circulation and dissolving blood stasis	Retention of urine (due to deficiency of kidney-yang, disturbance in qi transformation and blood stasis)	Anuria or dysuria, distention, fullness and pain in the lower abdomen, dark purplish tongue or with petechia, unsmooth or thin and rapid pulse
Pangolin Scales (穿山甲, Chuanshanjia) 6g	Activating blood circulation and dredging the collaterals			

Points in Constitution: The action of Cassia Bark (肉桂, Rougui) is warming kidney-yang and improving qi transformation to promote urination. And the action of Pangolin Scales (穿山甲, Chuanshanjia) is activating blood circulation and dredging the collaterals. The combination of them can treat retention of urine due to deficiency of the kidney-yang and blood stasis.

Indication: Prostate hypertrophy

Precaution: This formula is designed for retention of urine due to deficiency of the kidney-yang and disturbance in qi transformation. Thus, it is not suitable for those with heat syndrome.

Associated Formulas:

1. Life-Preserving Kidney-Qi Pill (济生肾气丸, ji sheng shen qi wan) *Prescriptions for Rescuring the Sick*《济生方》

This is comprised of Prepared Rehmannia Root (熟地黄, Shudihuang), Fried Common Yam Rhizome (炒山药, Chao Shanyao), Asiatic Cornelian Cherry Fruit (山茱萸, Shanzhuyu), Oriental Waterplantain Rhizome (泽泻, Zexie), Tuckahoe (茯苓, Fuling), Tree Peony Bark (牡丹皮, Mudanpi), Cassia Bark (肉桂, Rougui), Prepared Aconite Root (炮附子, Pao Fuzi), Medicinal Achyranthes Root (川牛膝, Chuan Niuxi) and Plantain Seed (车前子, Cheqianzi). Its actions are warming yang and replenishing qi, improving qi transformation and promoting urination. It is indicated for a heaviness feeling in the loins, edema of the feet and dysuria due to kidney deficiency.

2. Powder for Five Kinds of Stranguria (五淋散, wu lin san) *Prescriptions of Peaceful Benevolent Dispensary*《和剂局方》

This is comprised of Indian Bread Pink Epidermis (赤茯苓, Chifuling), Chinese Angelica Root

(当归, Danggui), Red Peony Root (赤芍, Chishao), Licorice Root (甘草, Gancao) and Cape Jasmine Fruit (山栀子, Shanzhizi). Its actions are clearing away heat and relieving stranguria. It is indicated for dripping urination due to deficiency of kidney-qi and accumulation of heat in the urinary bladder.

3. Eight Corrections Powder (八正散, ba zheng san) *Prescriptions of Peaceful Benevolent Dispensary* 《和剂局方》

This is comprised of Plantain Seed (车前子, Cheqianzi), Lilac Pink Herb (瞿麦, Qumai), Common Knotgrass Herb (萹蓄, Bianxu), Talc (滑石, Huashi), Cape Jasmine Fruit (山栀子, Shanzhizi), Licorice Root (甘草, Gancao), Akebia Stem (木通, Mutong) and Rhubarb (大黄, Dahuang). Its actions are clearing away heat and purging fire, promoting urination and relieving stranguria. It is indicated for stranguria due to pathogenic heat, or stranguria complicated by hematuria manifested as frequency of urination, dysuria and painful urination due to accumulation of damp-heat in the urinary bladder.

4. Common Anemarrhena, Chinese Corktree Bark and Motherwort Decoction (知柏坤草汤, zhi bai kun cao tang) *Journal of the Combination of Traditional Chinese Medicine with Western Medicine* 《中西医结合杂志》

This is comprised of Chinese Corktree Bark (黄柏, Huangbai), Common Anemarrhena Rhizome (知母, Zhimu), Twotooth Achyranthes Root (牛膝, Niuxi), Motherwort Herb (益母草, Yimucao), Dan-Shen Root (丹参, Danshen) and Rhubarb (大黄, Dahuang). Its actions are activating blood circulation, inducing diuresis, clearing away heat and toxic material. It is indicated for prostatomegaly manifested as dysuria, red tongue with yellow coating, wiry and rapid pulse.

Renal Colic Decoction
(肾绞痛汤, shen jiao tong tang)

Source: *New Traditional Chinese Medicine* 《新中医》
Composition: Composition: Chinese Thorowax Root (柴胡, Chaihu)9g
Green Tangerine Peel (青皮, Qingpi)9g
Licorice Root (甘草, Gancao)9g
Red Peony Root (赤芍, Chishao)12g
Bitter Orange (枳壳, Zhiqiao)9g
Corydalis Tuber (延胡索, Yanhusuo)9g
Sandalwood (檀香, Tanxiang)6g
Szechwan Chinaberry Fruit (川楝子, Chuanlianzi)9g
Combined Spicebush Root (乌药, Wuyao)15g
Common Aucklandia Root (木香, Muxiang)12g
Ovateleaf Holly Bark (救必应, Jiubiying)15g
Twotooth Achyranthes Root (牛膝, Niuxi)15g
Actions: Activating flow of qi, relieving convulsion and alleviating pain.

Applied Syndrome: Renal colic which is manifested by sudden lumbago, difficulty in turning about, sweating, hematuria or discharge of stone, red tongue with yellow and greasy coating, wiry and tense pulse.

Renal Colic Decoction
(Qi-Activating and Pain-Alleviating Method)

Ingredients	Effects	Combined Effects	Syndrome	Chief Symptoms
Chinese Thorowax Root (柴胡, Chaihu)9g	Relieving the depressed liver-qi	Promoting flow of qi, relieving convulsion and alleviating pain	Renal colic (due to blockage of urinary calculus and stagnation of qi and blood)	Severe lumbago, difficulty in turning about, sweating, hematuria or discharging stone, red tongue with yellow and greasy coating, wiry and tense pulse
Green Tangerine Peel (青皮, Qingpi)9g Bitter Orange (枳壳, Zhiqiao)9g Common Aucklandia Root (木香, Muxiang)12g Sandalwood (檀香, Tanxiang)6g Szechwan Chinaberry Fruit (川楝子, Chuanlianzi)9g Corydalis Tuber (延胡索, Yanhusuo)9g Red Peony Root (赤芍, Chishao)12g Combined Spicebush Root (乌药, Wuyao)15g	Activating flow of qi and alleviating pain			
Twotooth Achyranthes Root (牛膝, Niuxi)15g	Conducting qi downward to promote urination			
Ovateleaf Holly Bark (救必应, Jiubiying)15g	Clearing away heat and toxic material, inducing diuresis and alleviating pain			
Licorice Root (甘草, Gancao)9g	Coordinating the actions of the above drugs, relieving muscular spasm and alleviating pain			

Points in Constitution: This formula is the modification of both the Bupleurum liver-Soothing Powder(柴胡疏肝散, chai hu shu gan san) and Sichuan Chinaberry Powder(金铃子散, jin ling zi san). The addition of Ovateleaf Holly Bark (救必应, Jiubiying) is to clear away toxic material and alleviate pain. Thus, it is applied for various pains due to qi stagnation.

Indications:
1. Urinary tract calculus, renal colic
2. Gastric spasm
3. Cholecystitis, cholelithiasis, cholecyst colic
4. Woman dysmenorrhea

Precaution: The qi-activating and pain-relieving method of this formula is only used in the emergency case to treat the incidental of the disease. After the pain is relieved, treatment of the fundamental should be immediately given.

Associated Formulas:

1. Galangal and Cyperus Pill (良附丸, liang fu wan) *Collection of Effective Formulaes* 《良方集腋》

This is comprised of Lesser Galangal Rhizome (高良姜, Gaoliangjiang) and Nutgrass Galingale Rhizome (香附, Xiangfu). Its actions are warming the middle-jiao and expelling cold. It is indicated for epigastric pain and distention, white tongue coating due to depression of the liver-qi and cold in the stomach.

2. Szechwan Chinaberry Powder (金铃子散, jin ling zi san) *Collection of Pathogenesis for Protecting Healthy Qi from Plain Question* 《素问病机气宜保命集》

This is comprised of Szechwan Chinaberry Fruit (川楝子, Chuanlianzi) and Corydalis Tuber (延胡索, Yanhusuo). Its actions are dispersing the stagnated liver-qi, purging heat, activating flow of qi and alleviating pain. It is good at treating pain in the chest, abdomen and hypochondrium due to transformation of fire resulting from stagnation of liver-qi.

Effective Formula for Impotence
(亢痿灵, kang wei ling)

Source: *Journal of Traditional Chinese Medicine* 《中医杂志》
Composition: Centipede (蜈蚣, Wugong) 3 pieces
White Peony Root (白芍药, Baishaoyao) 60g
Chinese Angelica Root (当归, Danggui) 60g
Licorice Root (甘草, Gancao) 60g
Actions: Regulating the liver and enriching blood, dredging the meridians and collaterals.
Applied Syndrome: Sexual impotence due to stagnation of the liver-qi, insufficiency of blood and deficiency of the spleen, manifested by sexual impotence, irritability, listlessness and lack of strength, lusterless lips and finger nails, pale tongue or with ecchymosis, wiry and thin or thin and unsmooth pulse.

Effective Formula for Impotence
(Method of Regulating the Liver and Spleen)

Ingredients	Effects	Combined Effects	Syndrome	Chief Symptoms
Centipede (蜈蚣, Wugong) 3 条	Dredging the meridians and collaterals	Regulating the liver and tonifying blood, dredging the meridians and collaterals	Sexual impotence (due to stagnation of the liver-qi and deficiency of blood)	Sexual impotence, irritability, listlessness and lack of strength, lusterless lips and finger nails, pale tongue or with ecchymosis, wiry and thin or thin and unsmooth pulse
White Peony Root (白芍药, Baishaoyao) 60g Chinese Angelica Root (当归, Danggui) 60g	Enriching blood and activating blood circulation			
Licorice Root (甘草, Gancao) 60g	Replenishing qi and regulating the middle-jiao			

Points in Constitution: In recent years sexual impotence is usually treated by using Centipede (蜈蚣, Wugong), which is warm and migratory in nature and attributed to the liver and spleen meridians. Sexual impotence is mostly due to kidney deficiency. In clinic, however, there are also many cases which are related to incoordination of the liver and spleen. Therefore, this formula is appropriate and twice the effect will be achieved with half the effort if Membranous Milkvetch Root (黄芪, Huangqi) which may invigorate the spleen is added to the formula.

Indications: Sexual hypoesthesia or hypogonadism.

Precaution: This formula should be cautiously used for hypertension and edema since it has a large dose of Licorice Root (甘草, Gancao).

Associated Formulas: 1. Ursine Seal Kidney-Benefiting Decoction (海狗益肾饮, hai gou yi shen yin) *Modern Practical Chinese Medicine* 《现代实用中药》
This is comprised of Testes and Penis of an Ursine Seal (海狗肾, Haigoushen), Desertliving Cistanche Herb (肉苁蓉, Roucongrong), Medicinal Indian Mulberry Root (巴戟肉, Bajirou) and Asiatic Cornelian Cherry Fruit (山茱萸, Shanzhuyu). Its actions are warming the kidney and strengthening yang, supplementing essence and tonifying marrow. It is indicated for sexual impotence and prospermia, listlessness, soreness of loins and cold feeling in the lower body due to deficiency of the kidney-qi and declination of fire from the gate of life.

2. Five Kinds of Seeds Pill for Sterility (五子衍宗丸, wu zi yan zong wan) *An Introduction to Medicine* 《医学入门》
This is comprised of Barbary Wolfberry Fruit (枸杞子, Gouqizi), Chinese Dodder Seed (菟丝子, Tusizi), Chinese Magnoliavine Fruit (五味子, Wuweizi), Palmleaf Raspberry Fruit (覆盆

子，Fupenzi) and Plantain Seed (车前子，Cheqianzi). Its actions are supplementing essence and marrow, regulating and replenishing kidney-qi. It is indicated for seminal emission, sexual impotence and prospermia due to kidney deficiency.

3. Land and Water Two Fairies Pellet (水陆二仙丹，shui lu er xian dan) *Hong's Collection of Proved Recipe*《洪氏集验方》

This is comprised of Gordon Euryale Seed (芡实，Qianshi) and Cherokee Rose Fruit (金樱子，Jinyingzi). Its actions are invigorating the kidney and inducing astringing. It is indicated for male emission and nebulous urine or female leucorrhea due to kidney deficiency.

4. Kidney-Replenishing Rehmannia Pill(补益地黄丸，bu yi di huang wan) *Imperial Benevolent Prescriptions of Taiping Period*《太平圣惠方》

This is comprised of Prepared Rehmannia Root (熟地黄，Shudihuang), Desertliving Cistanche Herb (肉苁蓉，Roucongrong), Antler (鹿角，Lujiao), Chinese Magnoliavine Fruit (五味子，Wuweizi), Thinleaf Milkwort Root (远志，Yuanzhi), Medicinal Indian Mulberry Root (巴戟天，Bajitian), Chinese Dodder Seed (菟丝子，Tusizi), Ranuculus Sceleratus Herb(石龙芮，Shilongrui), Cochinchinese Asparagus Root (天门冬，Tianmendong) and Cassia Bark (桂心，Guixin). Its actions are invigorating the kidney and supplementing essence. It is indicated for sexual impotence, soreness of the loins and listlessness due to consumptive diseases and deficiency of essence.

5. Kidney-Invigorating and Essence-Supplementing Decoction (益肾填精汤，yi shen tian jing tang) *Yang Shaohua's Medical Records*《杨少华医案》

This is comprised of Prepared Rehmannia Root (熟地黄，Shudihuang), Actinolite (阳起石，Yangqishi), Common Yam Rhizome (山药，Shanyao), East Asian Tree Fern Rhizome (狗脊，Gouji), Palmleaf Raspberry Fruit (覆盆子，Fupenzi), Shorthorned Epimedium Herb (仙灵脾，Xianlingpi), Lobed Kudzuvine Root (葛根，Gegen), Himalayan Teasel Root (川续断，Chuanxuduan), Common Clubmoss Herb (伸筋草，Shenjincao), Mantis Egg-Case (桑螵蛸，Sangpiaoxiao), Common Anemarrhena Rhizome (知母，Zhimu), Medicinal Indian Mulberry Root (巴戟天，Bajitian), Common Cnidium Fruit (蛇床子，Shechuangzi) and Thinleaf Milkwort Root (远志，Yuanzhi). Its actions are replenishing the kidney, supplementing essence and restoring yang. It is indicated for sexual impotence due to deficiency of both the liver and the kidney.

6. Mental Depression-Alleviating Decoction (达郁汤，da yu tang) *Source and Cause of Miscellaneous Diseases*《杂病源流犀烛》

This is comprised of Shunk Bugbane Rhizome (升麻，Shengma), Chinese Thorowax Root (柴胡，Chaihu), Szechwan Lovage Rhizome (川芎，Chuanxiong), Nutgrass Galingale Rhizome (香附，Xiangfu), Tribulus Fruit (白蒺藜，Baijili), White Mulberry Root-Bark (桑白皮，Sangbaipi) and Tangerine Leaf (橘叶，Juye). Its actions are relieving the depressed liver-qi and alleviating mental depression. It is indicated for acid vomiting and sexual impotence due to impairment of the liver by mental depression.

Essence-Supplementing, Kidney-Invigorating and Breeding Decoction
(填精补肾育种汤, tian jing bu shen yu zhong tang)

Source: *Jinlin Journal of Traditional Chinese Medicine*《吉林中医药》
Composition: Prepared Rehmannia Root (熟地黄, Shudihuang) 15g
Barbary Wolfberry Fruit (枸杞子, Gouqizi) 15g
Palmleaf Raspberry Fruit (覆盆子, Fupenzi) 15g
Mulberry (桑椹, Sangshen) 15g
Chinese Dodder Seed (菟丝子, Tusizi) 15g
Asiatic Cornelian Cherry Fruit (山萸肉, Shanyurou) 9g
Chinese Magnoliavine Fruit (五味子, Wuweizi) 9g
Actions: Supplementing essence, invigorating the kidney and breeding.
Applied Syndrome: Deficiency of essence and insufficiency of blood due to deficiency of both the liver and kidney, manifested by sexual hypoesthesi, sexual impotence, emission and prospermia, red tongue with little coating, thin and rapid pulse.

Essence-Supplementing, Kidney-Invigorating and Breeding Decoction
(Kidney-Invigorating and Essence-Supplementing Method)

Ingredients	Effects	Combined Effects	Syndrome	Chief Symptoms
Prepared Rehmannia Root (熟地黄, Shudihuang) 15g Barbary Wolfberry Fruit (枸杞子, Gouqizi) 15g Mulberry (桑椹, Sangshen) 15g	Tonifying the essence and nourishing the blood	Balancing and nourishing yin and yang, supplementing essence and supporting the primary qi	Deficiency of essence and insufficiency of blood due to deficiency of both the liver and kidney	Sexual hypoesthesi, sexual impotence, emission and prospermia, red tongue with little coating, thin and rapid pulse
Chinese Dodder Seed (菟丝子, Tusizi) 15g	Invigorating the kidney and strengthening yang			
Asiatic Cornelian Cherry Fruit (山萸肉, Shanyurou) 9g Chinese Magnoliavine Fruit (五味子, Wuweizi) 9g Palmleaf Raspberry Fruit (覆盆子, Fupenzi) 15g	Tonifying the liver and kidney and inducing astringency			

Points in Constitution: This formula is the modified Five Kinds of Seeds Pill for Sterility(五子衍宗丸, wu zi yan zong wan) and has the actions of tonifying five zang-organs and replenishing the essence and qi. The use of all the drugs which are mild in nature lies in slowly treating the primary aspect of the disease. It is not only applied for infertility but also used for various diseases due to weak body resistance.

Indications:
1. Inejaculation
2. Sexual hypoesthesia or hypogonadism

Associated Formulas:

1. Five Kinds of Seeds Pill for Sterility (五子衍宗丸, wu zi yan zong wan) *An Introduction to Medicine*《医学入门》

This is comprised of Barbary Wolfberry Fruit (枸杞子, Gouqizi), Chinese Dodder Seed (菟丝子, Tusizi), Chinese Magnoliavine Fruit (五味子, Wuweizi), Palmleaf Raspberry Fruit (覆盆子, Fupenzi) and Plantain Seed (车前子, Cheqianzi). Its actions are supplementing essence and marrow, regulating and replenishing kidney qi. It is indicated for seminal emission, sexual impotence and prospermia, long-time infertility, early change of the beard and hair due to kidney deficiency.

2. Interior-Replenishing Hairy Antler Pill (内补鹿茸丸, nei bu lu rong wan) *The Precious Mirror of Hygiene*《卫生宝鉴》

This is comprised of Hairy Antler (鹿茸, Lurong), Chinese Dodder Seed (菟丝子, Tusizi), Flatstem Milkvetch Seed (沙苑蒺藜, Shayuanjili), Tatarian Aster Root (紫菀, Ziyuan), Tribulus Fruit(白蒺藜, Baijili), Desertliving Cistanche Herb (肉苁蓉, Roucongrong), Cassia Bark (官桂, Guangui), Aconite Root (附子, Fuzi), Actinolite (阳起石, Yangqishi), Common Cnidium Fruit (蛇床子, Shechuangzi), Mantis Egg-Case (桑螵蛸, Sangpiaoxiao) and Membranous Milkvetch Root (黄芪, Huangqi). Its actions are warming and invigorating the kidney-yang. It is indicated for sexual impotence and seminal emission due to deficiency of the kidney yang resulting from overstrain and overthinking.

3. Human Placenta Marrow-Sealing Pellets (河车封髓丹, he che feng sui dan) *Syndrome-Cause-Pulse-Treatment*《症因脉治》

This is comprised of Cochinchinese Asparagus Root (天门冬, Tianmendong), Prepared Rehmannia Root (熟地黄, Shudihuang), Ginseng (人参, Renshen) and Dried Human Placenta (紫河车, Ziheche). Its actions are invigorating the kidney and supplementing essence. It is indicated for lumbago, seminal emission and exhausted essence due to sexual indulgence.

4. Fairy Gelatin Containing Tortoise Shell and Plastron and Antler (龟鹿二仙胶, gui lu er xian jiao) *Course and Model of Orchid Platform*《兰台规范》

This is comprised of Antler (鹿角, Lujiao), Tortoise Shell and Plastron (龟版, Guiban), Barbary Wolfberry Fruit (枸杞子, Gouqizi) and Ginseng (人参, Renshen). Its actions are greatly tonifying essence and marrow, replenishing qi and calming the mind. It is indicated for soreness in the loins and back, seminal emission and dizziness due to deficiency of kidney qi.

5. Essence-Supplementing and Infertility-Treating Pill (填精嗣续丸, tian jing ci xu wan) *Es-*

sentials of Differential Diagnosis《辨证录》

This is comprised of Ginseng (人参, Renshen), Antler Glue (鹿角胶, Lujiaojiao), Glue of Tortoise Shell and Plastron (龟版胶, Guibanjiao), Common Yam Rhizome (山药, Shanyao), Barbary Wolfberry Fruit (枸杞子, Gouqizi), Asiatic Cornelian Cherry Fruit (山茱萸, Shanzhuyu), Dwarf Lilyturf Root (麦门冬, Maimendong), Chinese Dodder Seed (菟丝子, Tusizi), Desertliving Cistanche Herb (肉苁蓉, Roucongrong), Prepared Rehmannia Root (熟地黄, Shudihuang), Fried Swimming Bladder (炒鱼鳔, Chaoyubiao), Medicinal Indian Mulberry Root (巴戟天, Bajitian), Chinese Magnoliavine Fruit (五味子, Wuweizi), Cassia Bark (肉桂, Rougui) and Chinese Arborvitae Seed (柏子仁, Baiziren). Its actions are supplementing essence and invigorating the kidney. It is indicated for female spermacrasia and infertility.

6. Innateness-Tonifying and Breeding Pill (补天育麟丹, bu tian yu lin dan) *Essentials of Differential Diagnosis*《辨证录》

This is comprised of Hairy Antler (鹿茸, Lurong), Ginseng (人参, Renshen), Asiatic Cornelian Cherry Fruit (山茱萸, Shanzhuyu), Prepared Rehmannia Root (熟地黄, Shudihuang), Desertliving Cistanche Herb (肉苁蓉, Roucongrong), Medicinal Indian Mulberry Root (巴戟天, Bajitian), Stir-Baked Largehead Atractylodes Rhizome (炒白术, Chao Baizhu), Toasted Membranous Milkvetch Root (炙黄芪, Zhi Huangqi), Shorthorned Epimedium Herb (淫羊藿, Yinyanghuo), Common Yam Rhizome (山药, Shanyao), Gordon Euryale Seed (芡实, Qianshi), Chinese Angelica Root (当归, Danggui), Common Cnidium Fruit (蛇床子, Shechuangzi), Chinese Dodder Seed (菟丝子, Tusizi), Chinese Arborvitae Seed (柏子仁, Baiziren), Cassia Bark (肉桂, Rougui), Dwarf Lilyturf Root (麦门冬, Maimendong), Chinese Magnoliavine Fruit (五味子, Wuweizi), Songaria Cynomorium Herb (锁阳, Suoyang), Dried Human Placenta (紫河车, Ziheche), Coptis Rhizome (黄连, Huanglian), Villous Amomum Fruit (砂仁, Sharen), Giant Gecko (蛤蚧, Gejie) and Penis and Testes of an Ursine Seal (腽肭脐, Wanaqi). Its actions are tonifying the liver and kidney, supplementing essence and marrow. It is indicated for prospermia and spermacrasia in man.

7. Procreation-Helping Pellet (赞育丹, zan yu dan) *Jingyue's Complete Works*《景岳全书》

This is comprised of Prepared Rehmannia Root (熟地黄, Shudihuang), Chinese Angelica Root (当归, Danggui), Eucommia Bark (杜仲, Duzhong), Medicinal Indian Mulberry Root (巴戟肉, Bajirou), Desertliving Cistanche Herb (肉苁蓉, Roucongrong), Shorthorned Epimedium Herb (淫羊藿, Yinyanghuo), Common Cnidium Fruit (蛇床子, Shechuangzi), Cassia Bark (肉桂, Rougui), Largehead Atractylodes Rhizome (白术, Baizhu), Barbary Wolfberry Fruit (枸杞子, Gouqizi), Common Curculigo Rhizome (仙茅, Xianmao), Asiatic Cornelian Cherry Fruit (山茱萸, Shanzhuyu), Tuber Onion Seed (韭子, Jiuzi), Aconite Root (附子, Fuzi), Ginseng (人参, Renshen) and Hairy Antler (鹿茸, Lurong). Its actions are invigorating the kidney and strengthening yang. It is indicated for sexual impotence, deficiency of essence and infertility due to declination of fire from the gate of life.

Formula for Immune Infertility Number One
(免疫性不育Ⅰ号方, mian yi xing bu yu yi hao fang)

Source: *Practical Prescriptions for Diseases of Urogenital System* 《泌尿生殖系病实用方》
Composition: Chinese Corktree Bark (黄柏, Huangbai) 9g
Dried Rehmannia Root (生地黄, Shengdihuang) 15g
Dan-Shen Root (丹参, Danshen) 15g
European Verbena Herb (马鞭草, Mabiancao) 15g
Stir-backed Turtle Carapace (炙鳖甲, Zhi Biejia) 9g
Silkworm Feculae (蚕沙, Cansha) 9g
Tree Peony Bark (牡丹皮, Mudanpi) 9g
Spreading Hedyotis Herb (白花蛇舌草, Baihuasheshecao) 30g
Twotooth Achyranthes Root (牛膝, Niuxi) 9g
Black Nightshade Herb (龙葵, Longkui) 15g
Actions: Clearing away heat and drying dampness, cooling blood and removing blood stasis.

Formula for Immune Infertility Number One
(Heat-Removing and Dampness-Eliminating Method)

Ingredients	Effects	Combined Effects	Syndrome	Chief Symptoms
European Verbena Herb (马鞭草, Mabiancao) 15g Spreading Hedyotis Herb (白花蛇舌草, Baihuasheshecao) 30g Chinese Corktree Bark (黄柏, Huangbai) 9g Black Nightshade Herb (龙葵, Longkui) 15g Silkworm Feculae (蚕沙, Cansha) 9g	Clearing away heat and drying dampness	Clearing away heat and drying dampness, cooling blood and removing blood stasis	Sterility (due to obstruction of accumulated damp-heat and blood stasis)	Sexual impotence, dark yellowish urine, dry mouth and throat, red tongue with yellow coating, wiry pulse
Dried Rehmannia Root (生地黄, Shengdihuang) 15g Stir-Backed Turtle Carapace (炙鳖甲, Zhi Biejia) 9g Tree Peony Bark (丹皮, danpi) 9g Dan-Shen Root (丹参, Danshen) 15g	Removing heat from the blood, nourishing yin and removing blood stasis			
Twotooth Achyranthes Root (牛膝, Niuxi) 9g	Inducing other drugs downwards			

Applied Syndrome: Immune infertility in male due to blood stasis and accumulated noxious heat in the interior, manifested by sterility, sexual impotence, dark yellowish urine, dry mouth and throat, red tongue with yellow coating, wiry pulse.

Points in Constitution: This formula is designed for infertility with syndrome of damp-heat in the lower-jiao. Thus, it mainly consists of the drugs for clearing away heat, drying dampnes and removing toxic material. Heat often impairs yin fluid, so yin-nourishing drugs are used. Heat may also cause blood stasis. Thus, blood-cooling and blood-activating drugs are added. Meanwhile, Spreading Hedyotis Herb（白花蛇舌草，Baihuasheshecao）and Black Nightshade Herb（龙葵，Longkui）are also used to exert their immunologic effect.

Indications: Immune infertility

Precaution: This formula is designed for immune infertility due to blood stasis and accumulation of noxious heat in the interior. If the infertility belongs to the case caused by deficiency of the spleen and kidney, or caused by deficiency of the kidney-yang, Formula for Immune Infertility Number Two(免疫性不育Ⅱ号方，mian yi xing bu yu er hao fang) or Formula for Immune Infertility Number Three(免疫性不育Ⅲ号方，mian yi xing bu yu san hao fang) should be respectively used.

Associated Formulas:

1. Formula for Immune Infertility Number Two (免疫性不育Ⅱ号方，mian yi xing bu yu er hao fang) *Practical Prescriptions for Diseases of Urogenital System*《泌尿生殖系病实用方》

This is comprised of Pilose Asiabell Root（党参，Dangshen），Largehead Atractylodes Rhizome（白术，Baizhu），Common Yam Rhizome（山药，Shanyao），Asiatic Cornelian Cherry Fruit（山萸肉，Shanyurou），White Peony Root（白芍药，Baishaoyao），Tuckahoe（茯苓，Fuling），Dried Rehmannia Root（生地黄，Shengdihuang）and Prepared Rehmannia Root（熟地黄，Shudihuang），Chinese Dodder Seed（菟丝子，Tusizi），Barbary Wolfberry Fruit（枸杞子，Gouqizi），Oyster Shell（牡蛎，Muli），Dragon's Bone（龙骨，Longgu），Baikal Skullcap Root（黄芩，Huangqin）and Ramie Root（苎麻根，Zhumagen）. Its actions are invigorating the spleen and benefiting the kidney. It is indicated for immune infertility in male due to deficiency of the spleen and kidney.

2. Formula for Immune Infertility Number Three (免疫性不育Ⅲ号方，mian yi xing bu yu san hao fang) *Practical Prescriptions for Diseases of Urogenital System*《泌尿生殖系病实用方》

This is comprised of Prepared Rehmannia Root（熟地黄，Shudihuang），Fleeceflower Root（何首乌，Heshouwu），Asiatic Cornelian Cherry Fruit（山萸肉，Shanyurou），Barbary Wolfberry Fruit（枸杞子，Gouqizi），Common Yam Rhizome（怀山药，Huaishanyao），Medicinal Indian Mulberry Root（巴戟肉，Bajirou），Shorthorned Epimedium Herb（淫羊藿，Yinyanghuo），Chinese Dodder Seed（菟丝子，Tusizi），Pepermulberry Fruit（楮实子，Chushizi），Dan-Shen Root（丹参，Danshen），Achyranthes Root（怀牛膝，Huainiuxi），Stir-Backed Turtle Carapace（炙鳖甲，Zhi Biejia），Giant Knotweed Rhizome（虎杖，Huzhang），Antler Glue（鹿角胶，Lujiaojiao）and Glue of Swimming Bladder（鱼鳔胶，Yubiaojiao）. Its actions are warming yang, benefiting the kidney, activating blood circulation and dredging the collaterals. It is indicated for immune infertility in male due to blockage of collaterals by blood stasis resulting from deficiency of the kidney-yang.

Chapter Five
Formulas for the Nervous and Psychogenic Diseases

According to the theory of traditional Chinese medicine the heart controls mental and emotional activities while the brain is the seat of mentality. Simultaneously spirit is closely connected with all the five zang-organs. Therefore, acute diseases of the neveous system or psychoses are usually considered as the problem of the heart and liver and those chronic ones as the problem of the heart and kidney. The occurrence of these diseases are always related to wind-fire, wind-phlegm or blood stasis. For the treatment and prevention of the difficult and complicated cases of this system such as cerebrovascular disease and its sequela, epilepsy, and senile dementia, the formula-ology of TCM has a vast prospect to explore and develop. Meanwhile, the Prescription for various neurosis, coronary heart disease and psychosis are widely used in clinic.

1. Head-Clearing and Pain-Alleviating Decoction
（清上蠲痛汤, qing shang juan tong tang）

Source: *Longevity and Life Prescription*《寿世保元》
Composition: Threeleaf Chastertree Fruit (蔓荆子, Manjingzi)6g
Chinese Ligusticum Rhizome (藁本, Gaoben)6g
Dahurican Angelica Root (白芷, Baizhi)6g
Divaricate Saposhnikovia Root (防风, Fangfeng)6g
Chrysanthemum Flower (菊花, Juhua)6g
Doubleteeth Pubescent Angelica Root (独活, Duhuo)6g
Incised Notopterygium Rhizome or Root (羌活, Qianghuo)6g
Asarum Herb (细辛, Xixin)3g
Szechwan Lovage Rhizome (川芎, Chuanxiong)6g
Chinese Angelica Root (当归, Danggui)6g
Swordlike Atractylodes Rhizome (苍术, Cangzhu)6g
Fresh Ginger (生姜, Shengjiang)3g
Dwarf Lilyturf Root (麦门冬, Maimendong)12g
Baikal Skullcap Root (黄芩, Huangqin)6g
Licorice Root (甘草, Gancao)3g
Actions: Expelling wind, opening the nasal passage and alleviating pain.
Applied Syndrome: Attack of the head by pathogenic wind, manifested by pain in the head,

dizziness, stuffy nose, toothache, sore throat, red tongue, superficial and rapid pulse.

Head-Clearing and Pain-Alleviating Decoction
(Wind-Expelling and Pain-Alleviating Method)

Ingredients	Effects	Combined Effects	Syndrome	Chief Symptoms
Incised Notopterygium Rhizome or Root (羌活, Qianghuo) 6g Doubleteeth Pubescent Angelica Root (独活, Duhuo) 6g Divaricate Saposhnikovia Root (防风, Fangfeng) 6g Dahurican Angelica Root (白芷, Baizhi) 6g Chinese Ligusticum Rhizome (藁本, Gaoben) 6g Asaru (细辛, Xixin) 3g Szechwan Lovage Rhizome (川芎, Chuanxiong) 6g Fresh Ginger (生姜, Shengjiang) 3g	Expelling wind, alleviating pain and opening the nasal passage	Expelling wind, opening the nasal passage and alleviating pain	Attack of the head by pathogenic wind	Pain in the head and face, dizziness, stuffy nose, toothache, sore throat, red tongue, superficial and rapid pulse
Chrysanthemum Flower (菊花, Juhua) 6g Threeleaf Chastertree Fruit (蔓荆子, Manjingzi) 6g Baikal Skullcap Root (黄芩, Huangqin) 6g	Clearing the head and eyes			
Swordlike Atractylodes Rhizome (苍术, Cangzhu) 6g	Expelling wind and removing dampness			
Chinese Angelica Root (当归, Danggui) 6g	Enriching blood and dredging the collaterals			
Dwarf Lilyturf Root (麦门冬, Maimendong) 12g	Clearing away heat and nourishing yin			
Licorice Root (甘草, Gancao) 3g	Coordinating the actions of the above drugs			

Points in Constitution: In the formula, there are a number of wind-dispelling and pain-stopping drugs. They are light and ascendent in nature, which corresponds to the saying that "the diseases in upper-jiao are treated with feather-light herbs". In the treatment of headache, obvious and credible effects are gained by using Szechwan Lovage Rhizome (川芎, Chuanxiong), Swordlike Atractylodes Rhizome (苍术, Cangzhu) and Dahurican Angelica Root (白芷, Baizhi). Since the wind-dispelling drugs are dry in property and tend to impair yin-blood, Chinese Angelica Root (当归, Danggui) and Dwarf Lilyturf Root (麦门冬, Maimendong) are added to avoid deflection of the potency.

Indications:
1. Headache
2. Trigeminal neuritis

Precaution: This formula is contraindicated in headache due to hyperactivity of liver yang or due to deficiency of blood.

Associated Formula: Tea-Blended Szechwan Lovage Powder(川芎茶调散, chuan xiong cha tiao san) *Prescriptions of Peaceful Benevolent Dispensary*《和剂局方》

This is comprised of Szechwan Lovage Rhizome (川芎, Chuanxiong), Fineleaf Schizonepeta Herb (荆芥, Jingjie), Divaricate Saposhnikovia Root (防风, Fangfeng), Dahurican Angelica Root (白芷, Baizhi), Incised Notopterygium Rhizome or Root (羌活, Qianghuo), Wild Mint Herb (薄荷, Bohe), Manchurian Wildginger Herb (细辛, Xixin) and Licorice Root (甘草, Gancao). Its actions are expelling wind, relieving the exterior syndrome and alleviating pain. It is indicated for faint and heaviness of the head, hemicrania and headache, stuffy nose with obvious rhinolalis, thin and white tongue coating, superficial pulse due to attack of the head by wind.

2. Tea-Blended Szechwan Lovage Powder
(川芎茶调散, chuan xiong cha tiao san)

Source: *Prescriptions of Peaceful Benevolent Dispensary*《和剂局方》
Composition: Szechwan Lovage Rhizome (川芎, Chuanxiong)9g
Fineleaf Schizonepeta Herb (荆芥, Jingjie)9g
Dahurican Angelica Root (白芷, Baizhi)6g
Incised Notopterygium Rhizome or Root (羌活, Qianghuo)6g
Licorice Root (甘草, Gancao)6g
Manchurian Wildginger Herb (细辛, Xixin)3g
Divaricate Saposhnikovia Root (防风, Fangfeng)6g
Wild Mint Herb (薄荷, Bohe)6g
Tea (茶, Cha)proper dose

Actions: Expelling wind and cold, alleviating pain.
Applied Syndrome: Headache due to exopathic wind manifested by headache, hemicrania, or pain on the top of the head, accompanied with aversion to cold, fever, dizziness and stuffy nose,

thin and white tongue coating, wiry and superficial pulse.

Tea-Blended Szechwan Lovage Powder
(Exogenous Wind-Dispelling Method)

Ingredients	Effects	Combined Effects	Syndrome	Chief Symptoms
Szechwan Lovage Rhizome (川芎, Chuanxiong) 9g	Activating qi flow and blood circulation, expelling wind and alleviating pain	Expelling wind and cold and alleviating pain	Headache due to exopathic wind	Headache, or hemicrania, or pain on the top of the head, accompanied with aversion to cold and fever, dizziness and stuffy nose, thin and white tongue coating, wiry and superficial pulse
Incised Notopterygium Rhizome or Root (羌活, Qianghuo) 6g Dahurican Angelica Root (白芷, Baizhi) 6g Fineleaf Schizonepeta Herb (荆芥, Jingjie) 9g Divaricate Saposhnikovia Root (防风, Fangfeng) 6g	Expelling wind and cold, being good at treating headache			
Manchurian Wildginger Herb (细辛, Xixin) 3g	Warming the meridian and alleviating pain			
Wild Mint Herb (薄荷, Bohe) 6g Tea (茶, Cha) proper dose	Clearing the head and eyes			
Licorice Root (甘草, Gancao) 6g	Coordinating the actions of various ingredients in the prescription			

Points in Constitution: Szechwan Lovage Rhizome (川芎, Chuanxiong) is the key drug for headache due to the problem of various meridians. In TCM, there is a saying that "only wind can attack the top of the head", thus this formula contains many wind-expelling drugs to relieve headache.

Indications:
1. Sinusitis, chronic rhinitis
2. Hemicrania, nervous headache.

Precaution: This formula is only suitable for headache due to affection of exopathogen. It is not fit for headache due to internal damage.

Associated Formulas:

1. Tea-Blended Chrysanthemum Flower Powder(菊花茶调散, ju hua cha tiao san) *Collection of Prescriptions with Exposition*《医方集解》

This consists of Chrysanthemum Flower (菊花, Juhua), Silkworm with Batrytis Larva (僵蚕, Jiangcan) and the ingredients of Tea-Blended Szechwan Lovage Powder (川芎茶调散, chuan xiong cha tiao san). Its actions are expelling wind, alleviating pain and clearing the head and the eyes. It is fit for headache due to attack of the head by wind-heat.

2. Wind-Dispersing Powder(消风散, xiao feng san) *Orthodox Manual of Surgery*《外科正宗》

This is made up of Chinese Angelica Root (当归, Danggui), Dried Rehmannia Root (生地, Shengdi), Divaricate Saposhnikovia Root (防风, Fangfeng), Cicada Slough (蝉蜕, Chantui), Common Anemarrhena Rhizome (知母, Zhimu), Lightyellow Sophora Root (苦参, Kushen), Hemp Seed (胡麻仁, Humaren), Fineleaf Schizonepeta Herb (荆芥, Jingjie), Swordlike Atractylodes Rhizome (苍术, Cangzhu), Gypsum (石膏, Shigao), Licorice Root (甘草, Gancao) and Akebia Stem (木通, Mutong). Its actions are expelling wind, enriching blood, clearing away heat and removing dampness. It is good at treating rubella and eczema marked by red rashes, itching with effusion, yellow tongue coating, superficial and rapid pulse.

3. Arctium Muscles-Relieving Decoction(牛蒡解肌汤, niu bang jie ji tang) *Experience Gained in Treating Sores*《疡科心得集》

This is comprised of Arctium fruit (牛蒡子, Niubangzi), Wild Mint Herb (薄荷, Bohe), Fineleaf Schizonepeta Herb (荆芥, Jingjie), Weeping Forsythia Capsule (连翘, Lianqiao), Cape Jasmine Fruit (山栀子, Shanzhizi), Tree Peony Bark (牡丹皮, Mudanpi), Dendrobium Herb (石斛, Shihu), Figwort Root (玄参, Xuanshen) and Common Selfheal Fruit-Spike (夏枯草, Xiakucao). The actions of this formula are expelling wind and clearing away heat, dissipating blockages and reducing swelling. It is applicable for attack of the neck, nape, head and face by heat-toxin, manifested by local redness, swelling, pain, slight aversion to cold but high fever, little sweating, thirst, yellow tongue coating and rapid pulse.

4. General Recipe for Treating Headache(头痛统治方, tou tong tong zhi fang) *Author's Experienced Prescription*(笔者经验方)

This is composed of Manchurian Wildginger Herb(细辛, Xixin), Gypsum(石膏, Shigao), Szechwan Lovage Root(川芎, Chuanxiong), Dahurian Angelica Root(白芷, Baizhi), Fineleaf Schizonepeta Herb(荆芥穗, Jingjiesui), Swordlike Atractylodes Rhizome(苍术, Cangzhu), Centipede(蜈蚣, Wugong) and Prepared Licorice Root(炙甘草, Zhigancao). It is applicable for angioneurotic headache which attacks irregularly and is unbearable. For the case accompanied with tiredness or fatigue, Ginseng(人参, Renshen) should be added.

3. Gallbladder-Warming Decoction
(温胆汤, wen dan tang)

Source: *Treatise on the Triple-Pathogenic Doctrine of Etiology*《三因极一病证方论》

Composition: Pinellia Rhizome (半夏, Banxia)6g
Bamboo Shavings (竹茹, Zhuru)6g
Immature Bitter Orange (枳实, Zhishi)6g
Tangerine Peel (橘皮, Jupi)6g
Tuckahoe (茯苓, Fuling)6g
Licorice Root (甘草, Gancao)3g
Fresh Ginger (生姜, Shengjiang)3g
Chinese Date (大枣, Dazao)3g

Actions: Drying dampness and removing phlegm, clearing away heat of the gallbladder and regulating stomach-qi.

Applied Syndrome: Syndrome of incoordination between the gallbladder and the stomach and disturbance of phlegm-heat in the interior, which is manifested by restlessness, insomnia, palpitation, indecision, or vomiting and hiccup, yellow and greasy tongue coating, smooth and rapid pulse.

Gallbladder-Warming Decoction
(Dampness-Removing and Phlegm-Resolving Method)

Ingredients	Effects	Combined Effects	Syndrome	Chief Symptoms
Pinellia Rhizome (半夏, Banxia)6g	Drying dampness and removing phlegm, regulating the stomach qi and keeping the adverse qi downwards	Drying dampness and removing phlegm, clearing away heat of the gallbladder and regulating the stomach qi	Incoordination between the gallbladder and the stomach and disturbance of phlegm-heat in the interior	Restlessness and insomnia, palpitation, vomiting and hiccup, yellow and greasy tongue coating, smooth and rapid pulse
Bamboo Shavings (竹茹, Zhuru)6g	Clearing away heat and removing phlegm, stopping vomiting and relieving restlessness			
Immature Bitter Orange (枳实, Zhishi)6g Tangerine Peel (橘皮, Jupi)6g	Regulating qi, drying dampness and removing phlegm			
Tuckahoe (茯苓, Fuling)6g	Invigorating the spleen and inducing diuresis			
Fresh Ginger (生姜, Shengjiang)3g Licorice Root (甘草, Gancao)3g Chinese Date (大枣, Dazao)3g	Invigorating the spleen and regulating the middle-jiao and coordinating the actions of various ingredients in a prescription			

Points in Constitution: This formula is comprised of Immature Bitter Orange (枳实, Zhishi) and Bamboo Shavings (竹茹, Zhuru) in addition to the ingredients of Two Vintage Herbs Decoction (二陈汤, er chen tang). It has the actions of removing dampness, clearing away heat, regulating flow of qi and resolving phlegm. Though this formula is entitled "warming the gallbladder", in fact, it is to clear away heat and resolve phlegm so as to restore the normal function of the gallbladder. This formula may be used as the basic Prescription for mental syndrome due to phlegm-heat. For the case with excessive heat, Coptis Rhizome (黄连, Huanglian) and Chinese Gentian Root (龙胆草, Longdancao) should be added. For the case with mental confusion due to phlegm, Grassleaf Sweetflag Rhizome (石菖蒲, Shichangpu) and Thinleaf Milkwort Root (远志, Yuanzhi) should be added. And for case with weak constitution, Dwarf Lilyturf Root (麦门冬, Maimendong) and Chinese Magnoliavine Fruit (五味子, Wuweizi) should be added.

Indications:
1. Vertigo
2. Epilepsy
3. Ménière's syndrome
4. Climacteric syndrome
5. Nervous vomiting
6. Vegetative nerve functional disturbance

Precaution: This formula is especially used for insomnia, vertigo and palpitation due to phlegm-heat. It is not suitable for insomnia and palpitation due to deficiency of yin and blood which is unable to nourish heart or due to hyperactivity of yang with deficiency of yin.

Associated Formulas:

1. Two Vintage Herbs Decoction (二陈汤 er chen tang) *Prescriptions of Peaceful Benevolent Dispensary*《和剂局方》

This consists of Pinellia Rhizome (半夏, Banxia), Tangerine Peel (橘皮, Jupi), Tuckahoe (茯苓, Fuling), Prepared Licorice Root (炙甘草, Zhi Gancao), Fresh Ginger (生姜, Shengjiang) and Chinese Date (大枣, Dazao). Its actions are drying dampness, removing phlegm, regulating qi and regulating the middle-jiao. This is indicated for cough due to damp-phlegm manifested as profuse and white sputum, oppressing feeling in the chest and vomiting, greasy tongue coating and smooth pulse.

2. Phlegm-Conducting Decoction (导痰汤, dao tan tang) *Complete Effective Prescriptions for Diseases of Women*《妇人良方大全》

This is comprised of Immature Bitter Orange (枳实, Zhishi) and Arisaema with Bile (胆南星, Dannanxing) in addition to the ingredients of Two Vintage Herbs Decoction (二陈汤, er chen tang). This formula can greatly remove phlegm and activate flow of qi. This is suitable for stuffiness sensation in the chest, cough, nausea, anorexia, dizziness or faint, greasy tongue coating and wiry pulse.

3. Phlegm-Dispelling Decoction (涤痰汤 di tan tang) *Prescriptions for Rescuring the Sick*《济生方》

This is comprised of ingredients of Two Vintage Herbs Decoction (二陈汤, er chen tang) plus

Grassleaf Sweetflag Rhizome (石菖蒲, Shichangpu), Immature Bitter Orange (枳实, Zhishi) and Bamboo Shavings (竹茹, Zhuru). This formula has strong actions of eliminating phlegm and inducing resuscitation. This is fit for aphasia due to wind-phlegm or stiff tongue due to mental confusion by phlegm or even coma, greasy tongue coating, wiry pulse.

4. Pinellia, Largehead Atractylodes and Tall Gastrodia Decoction (半夏白术天麻汤, ban xia bai zhu tian ma tang) *Comprehension of Medicine*《医学心悟》

This contains Pinellia Rhizome (半夏, Banxia), Tall Gastrodia Rhizome (天麻, Tianma), Tuckahoe (茯苓, Fuling), Tangerine Peel (橘红, Juhong), Largehead Atractylodes Rhizome (白术, Baizhu), Licorice Root (甘草, Gancao), Fresh Ginger (生姜, Shengjiang) and Chinese Date (大枣, Dazao). Its actions are drying dampness, removing phlegm and stopping the wind. This is good at treating vertigo, headache, oppressing feeling in the chest and vomiting due to attack of the head by wind-phlegm.

4. Bamboo Shavings Gallbladder-Warming Decoction (竹茹温胆汤, zhu ru wen dan tang)

Source: *Longevity and Life Prescription*《寿世保元》
Composition: Chinese Thorowax Root (柴胡, Chaihu)6g
Bamboo Shavings (竹茹, Zhuru)9g
Balloonflower Root (桔梗, Jiegeng)6g
Immature Bitter Orange (枳实, Zhishi)6g
Coptis Rhizome (黄连, Huanglian)6g
Ginseng (人参, Renshen)3g
Dwarf Lilyturf Root (麦门冬, Maimendong)6g
Tangerine Peel (橘皮, Jupi)6g
Pinellia Rhizome (半夏, Banxia)6g
Tuckahoe (茯苓, Fuling)6g
Licorice Root (甘草, Gancao)3g
Nutgrass Galingale Rhizome (香附, Xiangfu)6g
Fresh Ginger (生姜, Shengjiang)3g
Chinese Date (大枣, Dazao)6g

Actions: Clearing away heat and removing phlegm, regulating flow of qi and tranquilizing the mind.

Applied Syndrome: Shaoyang disease due to disturbance of phlegm-heat in the interior. The symptoms are insomnia, palpitation, low fever, irritability, trance, cough with profuse expectoration, feeling of fullness and stuffiness in the chest and hypochondrium, red tongue with white and greasy tongue coating, wiry and smooth pulse.

Bamboo Shavings Gallbladder-Warming Decoction
(Heat-Clearing and Phlegm-Resolving Method)

Ingredients	Effects	Combined Effects	Syndrome	Chief Symptoms
Bamboo Shavings (竹茹, Zhuru)9g Immature Bitter Orange (枳实, Zhishi)6g Pinellia Rhizome (半夏, Banxia)6g Tangerine Peel (橘皮, Jupi)6g Tuckahoe (茯苓, Fuling)6g Fresh Ginger (生姜, Shengjiang)3g Chinese Date (大枣, Dazao)6g Licorice Root (甘草, Gancao)3g Balloonflower Root (桔梗, Jiegeng)6g	Clearing away heat and removing phlegm	Clearing away heat and removing phlegm, regulating qi and tranquilizing the mind	Disturbance of phlegm-heat in the interior and disorder of the gallbladder	Insomnia and palpitation, irritability, trance, cough with profuse expectoration, feeling of fullness and stuffiness in the chest and hypochondrium, red tongue with white and greasy coating, wiry and smooth pulse
Coptis Rhizome (黄连, Huanglian)6g	Clearing away heart heat and tranquilizing the mind			
Chinese Thorowax Root (柴胡, Chaihu)6g Nutgrass Galingale Rhizome (香附, Xiangfu)6g	Dispersing the stagnated liver-qi			
Ginseng (人参, Renshen)3g	Replenishing qi and tranquilizing the mind			
Dwarf Lilyturf Root (麦门冬, Maimendong)6g	Nourishing yin and tranquilizing the mind			

Points in Constitution: Although it is entitled "warming gallbladder", this formula actually has the actions of clearing away heat, resolving phlegm and regulating the functions of the liver and the stomach. Phlegm is the source of the disease and is changeable, so it can't be ignored in clinical practice.

Indication: Neurosis.

Associated Formulas:

1. Coptis Gallbladder-Warming Decoction (黄连温胆汤, huang lian wen dan tang) *Analysis of Six Causes* 《六因条辨》

This is comprised of Pinellia Rhizome (半夏, Banxia), Bamboo Shavings (竹茹, Zhuru), Immature Bitter Orange (枳实, Zhishi), Tangerine Peel (橘皮, Jupi), Coptis Rhizome (黄连, Huanglian), Tuckahoe (茯苓, Fuling) and Prepared Licorice Root (炙甘草, Zhi Gancao). Both this formula and Bamboo Shaving Gallbladder-Warming Decoction (竹茹温胆汤, zhu ru wen dan tang) have the actions of regulating qi, removing phlegm, clearing away heat of the gallbladder and regulating the stomach-qi. However, the heat-clearing action of the former is better than that of the latter. Thus, the former is very suitable for incoordination between the gallbladder and the stomach accompanied with interior attack of the phlem and excessive heat.

2. Ten Drugs Decoction for Warming Gallbladder (十味温胆汤, shi wei wen dan tang) *Standard for Diagnosis and Treatment* 《证治准绳》

This is composed of Pinellia Rhizome (半夏, Banxia), Immature Bitter Orange (枳实, Zhishi), Tangerine Peel (橘皮, Jupi), Tuckahoe (茯苓, Fuling), Spine Date Seed (酸枣仁, Suanzaoren), Thinleaf Milkwort Root (远志, Yuanzhi), Chinese Magnoliavine Fruit (五味子, Wuweizi), Prepared Rehmannia Root (熟地黄, Shudihuang), Ginseng (人参, Renshen), Prepared Licorice Root (炙甘草, Zhi Gancao), Fresh Ginger (生姜, Shengjiang) and Chinese Date (大枣, Dazao). Its actions are replenishing qi, enriching blood and tranquilizing the mind. This is applicable to palpitation or severe palpitation, insomnia and irritability.

5. Liver-Inhibiting Powder
(抑肝散, yi gan san)

Source: *Essentials for the Care of Infants* 《保婴摄要》

Composition: Chinese Thorowax Root (柴胡, Chaihu) 6g

Chinese Angelica Root (当归, Danggui) 6g

Largehead Atractylodes Rhizome (白术, Baizhu) 6g

Tuckahoe (茯苓, Fuling) 6g

Gambirplant Hooked Stem and Branch (钩藤, Gouteng) 6g

Szechwan Lovage Rhizome (川芎, Chuanxiong) 6g

Licorice Root (甘草, Gancao) 3g

Actions: Calming the liver and stopping the wind, dispersing the stagnated liver-qi and invigorating the spleen.

Applied Syndrome: Fever, convulsion of eyelid, tic of the limbs, insomnia, irritability and morbid night crying of a baby due to transformation of heat by stagnation of the liver-qi.

Liver-Inhibiting Powder
(Liver-Calming and Wind-Stopping Method)

Ingredients	Effects	Combined Effects	Syndrome	Chief Symptoms
Gambirplant Hooked Stem and Branch (钩藤, Gouteng) 6g	Clearing away heat of the liver	Dispersing the stagnated liver-qi and invigorating the spleen, clearing away liver heat and stopping the wind	Incoordination between the liver and spleen and excessive liver-fire	Fever, convulsion of eyelid, tic of the limbs, irritability, insomnia and morbid night crying of a baby
Chinese Thorowax Root (柴胡, Chaihu) 6g	Dispersing the stagnated liver-qi			
Chinese Angelica Root (当归, Danggui) 6g Szechwan Lovage Rhizome (川芎, Chuanxiong) 6g	Regulating blood			
Tuckahoe (茯苓, Fuling) 6g Largehead Atractylodes Rhizome (白术, Baizhu) 6g	Invigorating the spleen			
Licorice Root (甘草, Gancao) 3g	Coordinating the actions of various ingredients in a prescription			

Points in Constitution: This formula is the modification of Merry Life Powder (逍遥散, xiao yao san) with the actions of dispersing the stagnated liver-qi and invigorating the spleen accompanied with cooling the liver and stopping the wind.

Indications:

1. Infantile neurosis.
2. Morbid night crying of a baby.

Precaution: This formula should be used cautiously for the patient with deficiency-cold of the stomach and intestines.

Associated Formulas:

1. Gambirplant Hooked Stem and Branch Decoction (钩藤饮, gou teng yin) *The Golden Mirror of Medicine* 《医宗金鉴》

This contains Ginseng (人参, Renshen), Scorpion (全蝎, Quanxie), Antelope Horn (羚羊角, Lingyangjiao), Tall Gastrodia Rhizome (天麻, Tianma), Prepared Licorice Root (炙甘草, Zhi Gancao), Gambirplant Hooked Stem and Branch (钩藤, Gouteng). Both this formula and Liver-Inhibiting Powder (抑肝散, yi gan san) have the actions of clearing away heat and stopping the wind. However, the latter also has the actions of replenishing qi and relieving convulsion and is good at treating infantile convulsions due to excessive heat with deficiency of healthy qi.

2. Antelope Horn and Gambirplant Hooked Stem and Branch Decoction(羚角钩藤汤, ling jiao gou teng tang) *Revised Popular Treatise on Exogenous Febrile Diseases* 《重订通俗伤寒论》

This consists of Antelope Horn (羚羊角, Lingyangjiao), Mulberry Leaf (桑叶, Sangye), Tendrilleaf Fritillary Bulb (川贝母, Chuan Beimu), Dried Rehmannia Root (生地黄, Shengdihuang), Gambirplant Hooked Stem and Branch (钩藤, Gouteng), Chrysanthemum Flower (菊花, Juhua), Indian Bread with Hostwood (茯神, Fushen), White Peony Root (杭芍药, Hangshaoyao), Licorice Root (甘草, Gancao) and Bamboo Shavings (淡竹茹, Danzhuru). Both this formula and Liver-Inhibiting Powder (抑肝散, yi gan san) have the actions of clearing away heat and stopping the wind. However, the actions of clearing away heat, cooling the liver and stopping the wind of this Antelope Horn and Gambirplant Hooked Stem Dicoction (羚角钩藤汤, ling jiao gou teng tang) are stronger than these of Liver-Inhibiting Powder (抑肝散, yi gan san) and it is good at treating the syndrome of wind resulting from extreme heat.

6. Miraculous Musk Powder
(妙香散, miao xiang san)

Source: *Prescriptions of Peaceful Benevolent Dispensary* 《和剂局方》
Composition: Musk (麝香, Shexiang) 0.03g (taking it directly with water)
Common Aucklandia Root (木香, Muxiang) 3g
Common Yam Rhizome (山药, Shanyao) 12g
Indian Bread With Hostwood (茯神, Fushen) 12g
Tuckahoe (茯苓, Fuling) 12g
Membranous Milkvetch Root (黄芪, Huangqi) 12g
Thinleaf Milkwort Root (远志, Yuanzhi) 12g
Ginseng (人参, Renshen) 6g
Balloonflower Root (桔梗, Jiegeng) 6g
Licorice Root (甘草, Gancao) 6g
Cinnabar (朱砂, Zhusha) 3g (taking it directly with water)
Actions: Replenishing qi and tranquilizing the mind, dispersing the stagnated qi and opening orifices.
Applied Syndrome: Insufficiency of the heart-qi manifested by trance, fright and sadness, nocturnal emission, palpitation and amnesia, restlessness and insomnia, pale tongue and feeble pulse.

Miraculous Musk Powder
(Heart-Nourishing and Mind-Tranquilizing Method)

Ingredients	Effects	Combined Effects	Syndrome	Chief Symptoms
Common Yam Rhizome (山药, Shanyao)12g Tuckahoe (茯苓, Fuling)12g Ginseng (人参, Renshen)6g Membranous Milkvetch Root (黄芪, Huangqi)12g Licorice Root (甘草, Gancao)6g	Replenishing qi and nourishing heart	Replenishing qi and tranquilizing the mind, dispersing the stagnated qi and opening orifices	Insufficiency of the heart-qi	Trance, fright and sadness, nocturnal emission, palpitation and amnesia, restlessness and insomnia, pale tongue and thin pulse
Thinleaf Milkwort Root (远志, Yuanzhi)12g Cinnabar (朱砂, Zhusha)3g Indian Bread with Hostwood (茯神, Fushen)12g	Tranquilizing the mind and relieving mental stress			
Common Aucklandia Root (木香, Muxiang)3g	Regulating qi and invigorating the spleen			
Balloonflower Root (桔梗, Jiegeng)6g	Directing other herbs to ascend			
Musk (麝香, Shexiang)0.03g	Smoothing flow of qi, restoring consciousness and increasing intelligence			

Points in Constitution: The characteristic of this formula is the good use of Musk (麝香, Shexiang) which is fragrant in flavor and has a nature of traveling around the body. It can smooth flow of qi, restore consciousness and increase intelligence. Thus, it contributes to relieving mental problems and always proves effective in clinic.

Indications:
1. Sexual neurasthenia.
2. Neurosis.

Precaution: This formula is applicable for nocturnal emission and palpitation due to insufficiency of heart-qi, thus it is not suitable for the case due to excessive prime-minister fire.

Associated Formula:

Mind-Tranquilizing and Heart-Easing Pill(安神定心丸, an shen ding xin wan) *Source and Cause of Miscellaneous Diseases*《杂病源流犀烛》

This is comprised of Ginseng (人参, Renshen), Largehead Atractylodes Rhizome (白术, Baizhu), Tuckahoe (茯苓, Fuling), Indian Bread with Hostwood (茯神, Fushen), Grassleaf Sweetflag Rhizome (石菖蒲, Shichangpu), Thinleaf Milkwort Root (远志, Yuanzhi), Dwarf Lilyturf Root (麦门冬, Maimendong), Spine Date Seed (酸枣仁, Suanzaoren), Cow-Bezoar (牛黄, Niuhuang) and Cinnabar (朱砂, Zhusha). It can calm the fright and stabilize the spirit, nourish heart and tranquilize the mind. This is suitable for the syndrome of deficiency of the heart and timidity, manifested by palpitation, fright and fear, restlessness, insomnia, dreaminess, aversion to sound, spontaneous or night sweating, shortness of breath, listlessness, pale tongue with thin coating, wiry and thin pulse.

7. Heart-Washing Decoction
(洗心汤, xi xin tang)

Source: *Essentials of Differential Diagnosis*《辨证录》
Composition: Ginseng (人参, Renshen)30g
Indian Bread with Hostwood (茯神, Fushen)30g
Spine Date Seed (生酸枣仁, Sheng Suanzaoren)30g
Pinellia Rhizome (半夏, Banxia)15g
Tangerine Peel (橘皮, Jupi)9g
Medicated Leaven (神曲, Shenqu)9g
Licorice Root (甘草, Gancao)3g
Aconite Root (附子, Fuzi)3g
Grassleaf Sweetflag Rhizome (石菖蒲, Shichangpu)3g

Actions: Warming yang and eliminating turbid evils, resolving phlegm and inducing resuscitation.

Applied Syndrome: Senile dementia due to retention of turbid phlegm in seven orifices manifested by dull or retarded expression, mental decline, amnesia, caducity of crying and laughing, mumbling or keeping silence all day, anorexia, profuse saliva, pale tongue with white and greasy coating, thin and slippery pulse.

Points in Constitution: Dementia is caused by retention of turbid phlegm in seven orifices and deficiency of yang-qi. This formula lies in removing phlegm aand inducing resuscitation in the course of restoring yang-qi, which belongs to the method of "reinforcing the fire of the gate of life to remove the turbid".

Indications:
1. Senile dementia, cerebrovascular dementia and mixed dementia.
2. Lobar atrophy.

Heart-Washing Decoction
(Phlegm-Resolving and Resuscitation-Inducing Method)

Ingredients	Effects	Combined Effects	Syndrome	Chief Symptoms
Tangerine Peel (橘皮, Jupi)9g Pinellia Rhizome (半夏, Banxia)15g	Drying dampness and removing phlegm	Warming yang and eliminating turbid evils, resolving phlegm and inducing resuscitation	Dementia (due to retention of phlegm in seven orifices)	Dull and trancing expression, mental decline, amnesia, caducity of crying and laughing, muttering or keeping silent all day, profuse saliva, pale tongue with white and greasy coating, thin and slippery pulse
Indian Bread with Hostwood (茯神, Fushen) 30g Spine Date Seed (生酸枣仁, Sheng Suanzaoren)30g	Tranquilizing the mind and relieving mental stress			
Grassleaf Sweetflag Rhizome (石菖蒲, Shichangpu)3g	Eliminating turbid evils and inducing resuscitation			
Ginseng (人参, Renshen)30g Aconite Root (附子, Fuzi)3g Licorice Root (甘草, Gancao)3g	Replenishing qi and restoring yang			
Medicated Leaven (神曲, Shenqu)9g	Strengthening the stomach and promoting digestion			

3. Metabolic encephalopathy, toxic encephalopathy.

4. Possitive pressure hydrocephalus.

Precautions:

1. This formula is forbidden for the syndrome of hyperactivity of fire due to yin deficiency or the syndrome of pure deficiency without phlegm.

2. For those with blood stasis, the blood-activating and stasis-removing drugs such as DanShen Root (丹参, Danshen) and Szechwan Lovage Rhizome (川芎, Chuanxiong) should be added.

Associated Formulas:

1. Dementia-Curing Pill(转呆丹, zhuan dai dan) *Essentials of Differential Diagnosis* 《辨证录》

This consists of Ginseng (人参, Renshen), Chinese Angelica Root (当归, Danggui), Pinellia Rhizome (半夏, Banxia), Spine Date Seed (生酸枣仁, Sheng Suanzaoren), Grassleaf Sweetflag

Rhizome (石菖蒲, Shichangpu), Indian Bread with Hostwood (茯神, Fushen), White Peony Root (白芍药, Baishaoyao), Chinese Thorowax Root (柴胡, Chaihu), Aconite Root (附子, Fuzi), Medicated Leaven (神曲, Shenqu), Chinese Arborvitae Seed (柏子仁, Baiziren) and Snakegourd Root (天花粉, Tianhuafen). Its actions are enriching blood, tranquilizing the mind, removing phlegm and inducing resuscitation. It is good at treating dementia manifestated as staying alone indoors all day, muttering and no desire for food or even anorexia.

2. Longevity Pill (寿星丸, shou xing wan) *Source and Cause of Miscellaneous Diseases* 《杂病源流犀烛》

This is composed of Thinleaf Milkwort Root (远志, Yuanzhi), Ginseng (人参, Renshen), Membranous Milkvetch Root (黄芪, Huangqi), Largehead Atractylodes Rhizome (白术, Baizhu), Licorice Root (甘草, Gancao), Chinese Angelica Root (当归, Danggui), Dried Rehmannia Root (生地黄, Shengdihuang), White Peony Root (白芍药, Baishaoyao), Tuckahoe (茯苓, Fuling), Tangerine Peel (橘皮, Jupi), Cassia Bark (肉桂, Rougui), Arisaema with Bile (胆南星, Dannanxing), Amber (琥珀, Hupo), Cinnabar (朱砂, Zhusha) and Chinese Magnoliavine Fruit (五味子, Wuweizi). Its actions are replenishing qi, enriching the blood, tranquilizing the mind, removing phlegm and eliminating turbid evils. It is applicable for senile diseases due to insufficiency of the heart-qi, deficiency of yin and blood and excessive turbid phlegm which cause deficiency of the heart and disorder of the brain, manifested as palpitation, insomnia, amnesia, slow speaking, dull expression, white and greasy tongue coating, smooth and thin pulse. In clinic, it may be applied for senile dementia, encephalatrophy and cerebral aneurysm.

8. Lucid Yang-Generating Decoction
(滋生清阳汤, zi sheng qing yang tang)

Source: *Supplement to Essence of Medicine* 《医醇賸义》
Composition: Dried Rehmannia Root (生地黄, Shengdihuang)9g
Abalone Shell (石决明, Shijueming)15g
Magnetite (磁石, Cishi)15g
Dendrobium Herb (石斛, Shihu)9g
Dwarf lilyturf Root (麦门冬, Maimendong)9g
Tree Peony Bark (牡丹皮, Mudanpi)9g
White Peony Root (白芍药, Baishaoyao)9g
Chrysanthemum Flower (菊花, Juhua)9g
Wild Mint Herb (薄荷, Bohe)3g
Chinese Thorowax Root (柴胡, Chaihu)3g
Tall Gastrodia Rhizome (天麻, Tianma)9g
Mulberry Leaf (桑叶, Sangye)3g
Actions: Nourishing yin and checking exuberance of yang, lifting clear yang and keeping the adverse qi downwards.

Applied Syndrome: Deficiency of kidney-water and stirring of wind and yang in the interior, manifestated as vertigo and distention of the head, dry mouth and tongue, flushed face, irritability, gradual appearing of involuntary shaking of the head and limbs, red tongue with thin and yellow coating, wiry and tense pulse.

Lucid Yang-Generating Decoction
(Yin-Nourishing and Exuberant Yang-Checking Method)

Ingredients	Effects	Combined Effects	Syndrome	Chief Symptoms
Dried Rehmannia Root (生地黄, Shengdihuang)9g White Peony Root (白芍药, Baishaoyao)9g Dwarf Lilyturf Root (麦门冬, Maimendong)9g Dendrobium Herb (石斛, Shihu)9g	Nourishing body fluid and liver yin, relieving muscular spasm	Nourishing yin and checking exuberance of yang, lifting clear yang and keeping the adverse qi downwards	Deficiency of kidney-water and stirring of wind and yang in the interior	Vertigo and distention of the head, dry mouth and tongue, red face and irritability, gradully appearing involuntary shake of the head and limbs, red tongue with thin and yellow coating, wiry and tense pulse
Mulberry Leaf (桑叶, Sangye)3g Chrysanthemum Flower (菊花, Juhua)9g Tree Peony Bark (牡丹皮, Mudanpi)9g	Cooling the liver and clearing away heat			
Abalone Shell (石决明, Shijueming)15g Magnetite (磁石, Cishi)15g	Calming the liver and stopping the wind			
Tall Gastrodia Rhizome (天麻, Tianma)9g	Especially treating wind-phlegm			
Chinese Thorowax Root (柴胡, Chaihu)3g Wild Mint Herb (薄荷, Bohe)3g	Raising clear yang			

Points in Constitution: The characteristic of this formula is to combine the actions of calming the liver, clearing the liver, nourishing the liver and dispersing the stagnated liver-qi together to check the exuberance of liver-yang and raise the clear yang simultaneously.

Indications:
1. Paralysis agitans.
2. Athetosis.
3. Chorea.

Associated Formulas:

1. Antelop's Horn and Gambirplant Hooked Stem and Branch Decoction(羚角钩藤汤, ling jiao gou teng tang) *Revised Popular Treatise on Exogenous Febrile Diseases* 《重订通俗伤寒论》

This is comprised of Antelope Horn (羚羊角, Lingyangjiao), Mulberry Leaf (桑叶, Sangye), Tendrilleaf Fritillary Bulb (川贝母, Chuan Beimu), Dried Rehmannia Root (生地黄, Shengdihuang), Gambirplant Hooked Stem and Branch (钩藤, Gouteng), Chrysanthemum Flower (菊花, Juhua), Indian Bread With Hostwood (茯神木, Fushenmu), White Peony Root (白芍药, Baishaoyao), Licorice Root (甘草, Gancao) and Bamboo Shavings (淡竹茹, Danzhuru). Its actions are clearing away heat and stopping the wind, nourishing yin and calming the liver. It is suitable for the syndrome of wind which results from extreme heat with impairment of yin.

2. Phlegm-Removing and Brain-Activating Pill(化痰透脑丸, hua tan tou nao wan) *Free Record on Practising Medicine* 《悬壶漫录》

This consists of Fried Jackinthepulpit Tuber (制天南星, Zhi Tiannanxing), Tabasheer (天竺黄, Tianzhuhuang), Roasting Chinese Honeylocusy Fruit (煨皂角, Wei Zaojiao), Musk (麝香, Shexiang), Amber (琥珀, Hupo), Turmeric Root-Tuber (郁金, Yujin), Pinellia Rhizome (半夏, Banxia), Snake Gallbladder (蛇胆, Shedan), Tangerine Peel (橘皮, Jupi), Thinleaf Milkwort Root (远志, Yuanzhi), Pearl (珍珠, Zhenzhu), Chinese Eaglewood Wood (沉香, Chenxiang), Agar (石花菜, Shihuacai) and Sea Hedgehog (海胆, Haidan). Its actions are stopping the wind and resolving phlegm. It is suitable for wind syndrome inside the body due to phlegm-heat and manifested by dizziness, shaking of the head trembling of the limbs, inability of the hands to hold something, or even numbness of limbs without painful and itching sensation, oppressed feeling in the chest, vomiting, or even vomiting of sputum, cough and asthma, corpulent tongue with teeth print, red tongue with white, thick and greasy or yellow tongue coating, deep and smooth pulse or deep and soft pulse. In clinic, it treats paralysis, agitans, chorea, athetosis, corpulmonale and pulmonary encephalopathy.

3. Brain-Benefiting and Spirit-Invigorating Pill(益脑强神丸, yi nao qian shen wan) *Free Record on Practising Medicine* 《悬壶漫录》

This is comprised of Musk (麝香, Shexiang), Grassleaf Sweetflag Rhizome (石菖蒲, Shichangpu), Asiatic Cornelian Cherry Fruit (山茱萸, Shanzhuyu), Common St. Paulswort Herb (豨莶草, Xiqiancao), Antler Glue (鹿角胶, Lujiaojiao), Glue of Tortoise Shell and Plastron (龟版胶, Guibanjiao), Prepared Rehmannia Root (熟地黄, Shudihuang), Barbary Wolfberry Fruit (枸杞子, Gouqizi), Fleeceflower Root (何首乌, Heshouwu), Sophora Flower-Bud (槐米, Huaimi), Sea-Horse (海马, Haima), Saliva Swallow Net (燕窝, Yanwo), Siberian Solomonseal Rhizome (黄精, Huangjing), Chinese Magnoliavine Fruit (五味子, Wuweizi), Peach Seed (桃仁, Taoren), Safflower (红花, Honghua) and Hawksbill Shell (玳瑁, Daimao). Its actions are supplementing essence and marrow, increasing intelligence and tranquilizing the mind. It is suitable for tremor due to insufficiency of the sea of marrows and manifested by shake of the head and trembling of the limbs, tinnitus and dizziness, poor memory, reversal of awake and sleep, or even dementia, corpulent tongue with teeth print, red tongue with thin and white coating, deep and weak pulse or wiry, thin and tense pulse. In clinic, it is suitable for paralysis agitans, chorea and athetosis.

9. Magnetite and Cinnabar Pill
(磁朱丸, ci zhu wan)

Source: *Prescription Worth a Thousand Gold for Emergencies*《备急千金要方》
Composition: Magnetite (磁石, Cishi)
Cinnabar (朱砂, Zhusha)
Medicated Leaven (神曲, Shenqu)
(It is a patent medicine and its preparation is omitted)
Actions: Tranquilizing mind, nourishing yin and improving acuity of sight.
Applied Syndrome: Breakdown of the normal physiological coordination between the heart and the kidney, manifested by blurred vision, tinnitus and deafness, palpitation and insomnia. It is also suitable for epilepsy.

Magnetite and Cinnabar Pill
(Method of Tranquilizing the Mind with Heavy Materials)

Ingredients	Effects	Combined Effects	Syndrome	Chief Symptoms
Magnetite (磁石, Cishi)	Tonifying the kidney and calming the liver, calming the frightened and tranquilizing the mind	Restoring the equilibrium between the heart and the kidney, tranquilizing the mind with sedative of heavy weight	Breakdown of the normal physiological coordination between the heart and the kidney	Palpitation and insomnia, tinnitus and deafness, blurring vision and epilepsy
Cinnabar (朱砂, Zhusha)	Clearing away heart heat and eliminating fire, calming the heart and tranquilizing the mind			
Medicated Leaven (神曲, Shenqu)	Promoting digestion of medicine			

Points in Constitution: The heavy mineral drugs which are often used for tranquilizing the mind can easily impair the stomach. Thus, they are always accompanied with Medicated Leaven (神曲, Shenqu) to improve absorption of the medicine by promoting digestion and regulating the stomach-qi.

Indications:
1. Neurasthenia.
2. Hypertension.
3. Epilepsy.
4. Pathogenic change of retina, optic nerve, vitreous body and lens or disorder of circulation of aqueous humor.

Precaution: This formula is designed for the syndromes of deficiency of kidney-yin, hyperactivity of heart-yang and breakdown of the normal physiological coordination between the heart and the kidney. Since the Cinnabar（朱砂, Zhusha）in the formula contains hydrargyrum, it is not suitable to be taken for a long time.

Associated Formulas:

1. Modified Magnetite and Cinnabar Pill（加味磁朱丸, jia wei ci zhu wan）*Records of Traditional Chinese and Western Medicine in Combination*《医学衷中参西录》

This is comprised of Magnetite（磁石, Cishi）, Hematite（代赭石, Daizheshi）, Pinellia Rhizome（清半夏, Qing Banxia）, Cinnabar（朱砂, Zhusha）and Distiller's Yeast（酒曲, Jiuqu）. Its actions are tranquilizing the mind and removing phlegm with heavy minerals. It is mainly used for epilepsy.

2. Epilepsy-Relieving Pill（定痫丸 ding xian wan）*Comprehension of Medicine*《医学心悟》

This is made up of Tall Gastrodia Rhizome（天麻, Tianma）, Tendrilleaf Fritillary Bulb（川贝母, Chuan Beimu）, Pinellia Rhizome（半夏, Banxia）, Tuckahoe（茯苓, Fuling）, Indian Bread with Hostwood（茯神, Fushen）, Arisaema with Bile（胆南星, Dannanxing）, Grassleaf Sweetflag Rhizome（石菖蒲, Shichangpu）, Scorpion（全蝎, Quanxie）, Silkworm with Batrytis Larva（僵蚕, Jiangcan）, Amber（琥珀, Hupo）, Tangerine Peel（橘皮, Jupi）, Thinleaf Milkwort Root（远志, Yuanzhi）, Dan-Shen Root（丹参, Danshen）, Dwarf Lilyturf Root（麦门冬, Maimendong）, Cinnabar（朱砂, Zhusha）, Bamboo Juice（竹沥, Zhuli）, Ginger Juice（姜汁, Jiangzhi）and Licorice Root（甘草, Gancao）. It has the actions of resolving phlegm, stopping the wind, dredging the collaterals and relieving convulsion. It is applicable to epilepsy due to phlegm-heat. It is also applicable to schizophrenia, hysteria and obsession

3. General Recipe for Treating Epilepsy（癫痫统治方, dian xian tong zhi fang）*Author's Experinenced Prescription*（笔者经验方）

This consists of White Mustard Seed（白芥子, Baijiezi）, Turmeric Root-Tuber（郁金, Yujin）, Wine-Fried Rhubarb（酒炒大黄, Jiuchaodahuang）, Mirabilite（芒硝, mangxiao）, Peach Seed（桃仁, Taoren）, Cassia Twig（桂枝, Guizhi）, Thinleaf Milkwort Root（远志, Yuanzhi）, Calamus Rhizome（菖蒲, Changpu）, Dried Human Placenta（紫河车 Ziheche）and Roasted Licorice（炙甘草, Zhigancao）. Its actions are resolving phlegm, removing blood stasis, benefiting primordial energy and regulating flow of qi. It is indicated for prolonged epilepsy accompanied with asthenia and blood stasis marked by dim or blackish complexion and uneven pulse.

10. Face Distortion-Treating Powder
(牵正散, qian zheng san)

Source: *Yang's Formulae Handed Down by Family* 《杨氏家藏方》
Composition: Giant Typhonium Rhizome (白附子, Baifuzi) 9g
Silkworm with Batrytis Larva (僵蚕, Jiangcan) 9g
Scorpion (全蝎, Quanxie) 9g
Actions: Expelling wind and removing phlegm, dredging the collaterals and relieving convulsion.
Applied Syndrome: Blockage of the meridians and collaterals in the head and face due to wind-phlegm, manifested by sudden deviation of the eye and mouth, or even twitch and spasm of muscles in the face, pale tongue with white coating, wiry pulse.

Face Distortion-Treating Powder
(Wind-Expelling and Spasm-Relieving Method)

Ingredients	Effects	Combined Effects	Syndrome	Chief Symptoms
Giant Typhonium Rhizome (白附子, Baifuzi) 9g	Expelling wind and removing phlegm	Expelling wind and removing phlegm, dredging the collaterals and relieving convulsion	Wind in the meridians and collaterals and wind phlegm blocking the meridians and collaterals	Sudden deviation of the eye and mouth, pale tongue with white coating and wiry pulse
Silkworm with Batrytis Larva (僵蚕, Jiangcan) 9g Scorpion (全蝎, Quanxie) 9g	Expelling wind and removing phlegm, dredging the collaterals and relieving convulsion			

Points in Constitution: The three are especially the wind-expelling, phlegm-removing, meridian-warming and collateral-dredging drugs. They are particularly applicable to blockage of the the meridians and collaterals due to phlegm or paralysis or spasm and pain.

Indications:
1. Facial nerve paralysis, sequela of wind-stroke.
2. Trigeminal neuralgia.
3. Hemicrania.

Precautions:
1. This is a common Prescription for deviation of the eyes and mouth due to attack of the wind upon the meridians and collaterals. It is applicable to blockage of collaterals due to wind-phlegm

accompanied with excessive cold. However, it is not suitable for deviation of the eye and mouth or hemiplegia due to qi deficiency and blood stasis, or stirring of liver-wind inside the body.

2. Both Giant Typhonium Rhizome (白附子, Baifuzi) and Scorpion (全蝎, Quanxie) are poisous and the dose of them should be cautiously used.

Associated Formulas:

1. Convulsion-Relieving Powder (止痉散, zhi jing san) *Formula-ology by Shanghai College of Traditional Chinese Medicine* 上海中医学院《方剂学》

This consists of Scorpion (全蝎, Quanxie) and Centipede (蜈蚣, Wugong) and has the actions of expelling wind and relieving convulsion. It is indicated for faint due to emotional upset or convulsion of the limbs. It also has a good action of alleviating pain for intractable headache and arthralgia.

2. General Recite for Treating Prosopagia (三叉神经统治方, san cha shen jing tong zhi fang) *Author's Experienced Prescription* (笔者经验方)

This is composed of Szechwan Lovage Rhizome (川芎, Chuanxiong), Gambirplant Hooked Stem and Branch (钩藤, Gouteng), Dahurian Angelica Root (白芷, Baizhi), White Peony Root (白芍药, Baishaoyao), Manchurian Angenica Herb (细辛, Xixin), Yanhusuo (延胡索, Yanhusuo), Licorice Root (甘草, Gancao) and Centipede (蜈蚣, Wugong). Its actions are soothing the liver, relieving pain, dispelling wind and removing obstruction in the channels. It is indicated for prosopallgia. If the patient is accompanied with overabundance of heat, Gypsum (生石膏, Shengshigao) and Shunk Bugbane Rhizome (升麻, Shengma) are added. If the patient is accompanied with deficiency of yin, Figwart Root (元参, Yuanshen) and Dried Rehmannia Root (生地黄, Shengdihuang) are added.

11. Minor Life-Prolonging Decoction
(小续命汤, xiao xu ming tang)

Source: *Prescription Worth a Thousand Gold for Emergencies* 《备急千金要方》

Composition: Ephedra (麻黄, Mahuang) 6g

Fourstamen Stephania Root (防己, Fangji) 6g

Ginseng (人参, Renshen) 6g

Cassia Bark (肉桂, Rougui) 6g

Baikal Skullcap Root (黄芩, Huangqin) 6g

White Peony Root (白芍药, Baishaoyao) 6g

Licorice Root (甘草, Gancao) 6g

Szechwan Lovage Rhizome (川芎, Chuanxiong) 6g

Apricot Seed (杏仁, Xingren) 6g

Divaricate Saposhnikovia Root (防风, Fangfeng) 9g

Aconite Root (附子, Fuzi) 3g

Fresh Ginger (生姜, Shengjiang) 6g

Actions: Supporting healthy qi and expelling wind, expelling cold and removing dampness.

Applied Syndrome: Attack of the meridians and collaterals by wind-cold-dampness resulting from weakness of the body resistance aand deficiency of ying and blood, manifested as deviation of the eyes and mouth, spasm of tendons and vessels, or hemiplegia, dysphasia, or accompanied with chills and fever, pale tongue with white coating, wiry and weak pulse.

Minor Life-prolonging Decoction
(Exogenous Wind-Expelling Method)

Ingredients	Effects	Combined Effects	Syndrome	Chief Symptoms
Divaricate Saposhnikovia Root (防风, Fangfeng) 9g Ephedra (麻黄, Mahuang) 6g Fourstamen Stephania Root (防己, Fangji) 6g Apricot Seed (杏仁, Xingren) 6g Fresh Ginger (生姜, Shengjiang) 6g	Expelling the exterior wind	Supporting the healthy qi and expelling wind, dispelling cold and removing dampness	Attack of the meridians and collaterals by pathogenic wind.	Deviation of the eye and mouth, spasm of tendons and vessels, hemiplegia, dysphasia, or accompanied with chills and fever, pale tongue with white coating, wiry and weak pulse
Ginseng (人参, Renshen) 6g	Replenishing the primary qi			
Cassia Bark (肉桂, Rougui) 6g Aconite Root (附子, Fuzi) 3g	Warming yang and expelling cold			
Szechwan Lovage Rhizome (川芎, Chuanxiong) 6g Peony Root (Shaoyao, 芍药) 6g	Enriching blood and activating blood circulation			
Baikal Skullcap Root (黄芩, Huangqin) 6g	Used as corrigent to modify the action of the principal ingredients			
Licorice Root (甘草, Gancao) 6g	Coordinating the actions of various ingredients in a Prescription			

Points in Constitution: Most drugs in this formula are warm and dry in nature. Thus Baikal Skullcap Root (黄芩, Huangqin), which is bitter in taste and cold in property is used to control the action of the principal ingredients so as to avoid the excessively warming and drying exertation.

Indications:
1. Cold due to wind-cold.
2. Facial nerve paralyse.
3. Facial nerve spasm.
4. Rheumatoid arthritis.

Precautions:
1. This formula is warm, dry, pungent and has a strong dispersing action. Thus, it is applicable to true wind-stroke syndrome due to attack of wind directly upon the meridians and collaterals. It is contraindicated in wind-stroke syndrome caused by hyperactivity of yang due to deficiency of yin.
2. This formula is applicable for arthralgia due to wind-cold-dampness. It is not suitable for arthralgia due to wind-heat-dampness.

Associated Formula:

Major Gentian Decoction (大秦艽汤, da qin jiao tang) *Collection of Pathogenesis for Protecting Healthy Qi from Plain Question* 《素问病机气宜保命集》

This is comprised of Largeleaf Gentian Root (秦艽, Qinjiao), Licorice Root (甘草, Gancao), Szechwan Lovage Rhizome (川芎, Chuanxiong), Chinese Angelica Root (当归, Danggui), White Peony Root (白芍药, Baishaoyao), Manchurian Wildginger Herb (细辛, Xixin), Incised Notopterygium Rhizome or Root (羌活, Qianghuo), Divaricate Saposhnikovia Root (防风, Fangfeng), Baikal Skullcap Root (黄芩, Huangqin), Gypsum (石膏, Shigao), Dahurican Angelica Root (白芷, Baizhi), Largehead Atractylodes Rhizome (白术, Baizhu), Dried Rehmannia Root (生地黄, Shengdihuang), Prepared Rehmannia Root (熟地黄, Shudihuang), Tuckahoe (白茯苓, Baifuling) and Doubleteeth Pubescent Angelica Root (独活, Duhuo). This formula can support the healthy qi and expel wind. It is applicable to deviation of the eyes and mouth, dysphasia, hemiplegia, irritability and thirst due to attack of the meridians and collaterals by wind.

12. Iron Scales Decoction
(生铁落饮, sheng tie luo yin)

Source: *Comprehension of Medicine* 《医学心悟》
Composition: Cochinchinese Asparagus Root (天门冬, Tianmendong) 9g
Dwarf Lilyturf Root (麦门冬, Maimendong) 9g
Tendrilleaf Fritillary Bulb (贝母, Beimu) 9g
Arisaema with Bile (胆南星, Dannanxing) 6g
Tangerine Peel (橘红, Juhong) 9g

Iron Scales Decoction
(Method of Tranquilizing the Mind with Heavy Materials)

Ingredients	Effects	Combined Effects	Syndrome	Chief Symptoms
Iron Scales (生铁落, Shengtieluo)30g	Calming the heart and the liver	Calming the heart and tranquilizing the mind, clearing away heat and removing phlegm	Depressive psychosis and mania (Stirring-up of phlegm-fire)	Unconsciousness, or madness, moodiness, abuse and howl regardless of relatives or strangers, red tongue with greasy coating, smooth and forceful pulse
Cinnabar (朱砂, Zhusha)3g Thinleaf Milkwort Root (远志, Yuanzhi)9g Indian Bread with Hostwood (茯神, Fushen)9g	Tranquilizing the mind and calming the spirit			
Arisaema with Bile (胆南星, Dannanxing)6g Tangerine Peel (橘红, Juhong)9g Tendrilleaf Fritillary Bulb (贝母, Beimu)9g Tuckahoe (茯苓, Fuling)9g Grassleaf Sweetflag Rhizome (石菖蒲, Shichangpu)9g	Regulating qi and removing phlegm			
Gambirplant Hooked Stem and Branch (钩藤, Gouteng)9g Weeping Forsythia Capsule (连翘, Lianqiao)9g Figwort Root (玄参, Xuanshen)9g Dan-Shen Root (丹参, Danshen)9g	Clearing away heart heat and calming the liver			
Cochinchinese Asparagus Root (天门冬, Tianmendong)9g Dwarf Lilyturf Root (麦门冬, Maimendong)9g	Nourishing yin and relieving restlessness			

Thinleaf Milkwort Root (远志, Yuanzhi)9g
Grassleaf Sweetflag Rhizome (石菖蒲, Shichangpu)9g
Weeping Forsythia Capsule (连翘, Lianqiao)9g
Tuckahoe (茯苓, Fuling)9g

Indian Bread with Hostwood (茯神, Fushen)9g
Figwort Root (玄参, Xuanshen)9g
Gambirplant Hooked Stem and Branch (钩藤, Gouteng)9g
Dan-Shen Root (丹参, Danshen)9g
Cinnabar (朱砂, Zhusha)3g(taking it separately with water)
Iron Scales (生铁落, Shengtieluo)30g

Actions: Calming the heart and tranquilizing the mind, clearing away heat and removing phlegm.

Applied Syndrome: Depressive psychosis and mania due to stirring-up of phlegm-fire and mental derangement, manifested by unconsciousness, or irritability, madness, moodiness, abuse and howl regardless of relatives or strangers, red tongue with greasy coating, and smooth and forceful pulse.

Points in Constitution: This formula mainly treats the heart disease, and also the diseases of the liver and spleen. The characteristic of this formula is to put the stress on tranquilizing the mind and nourishing the heart at the same time, which is a real good way and an effective Prescription for mental problems. Iron Scales (生铁落, Shengtieluo) is the monarch drug and has the similar actions as Hematite (代赭石, Daizheshi), which can calm the heart and liver, quiet fetch and soul and tranquilize the mind.

Indications:
1. Schizophrenia, manic psychosis.
2. Post-traumatic brain syndrome.

Precaution: It should be used cautiously for the patient with a weak body resistance.

Associated Formula:

Tangerine Leaf, Bitter Orange, Dragon's Bone and Oyster Shell Decoction(桔枳龙牡汤, jiu zhi long mu tang) *Practical Formula-ology*《实用方剂学》

This consists of Dragon's Bone (生龙骨, Sheng Longgu), Oyster Shell (生牡蛎, Sheng Muli), White Peony Root (生杭芍, Shenghangshao), Blackend Swallowwort Root (白薇, Baiwei), Dwarf Lilyturf Root (麦门冬, Maimendong), Medicinal Achyranthes Root (川牛膝, Chuan Niuxi), Dried Rehmannia Root (生地黄, Shengdihuang), Figwort Root (元参, Yuanshen), Cape Jasmine Fruit (山栀子, Shanzhizi), Bamboo Shavings (竹茹, Zhuru), Tangerine Leaf (橘叶, Juye), Bitter Orange (枳壳, Zhiqiao) and Licorice Root (甘草, Gancao). Its actions are nourishing yin, clearing away fire and tranquilizing the mind with heave materials. It is indicated for hysteria due to yin deficiency and hyperactivity of fire manifested as irritability, reversed flow of qi and feeling of fullness in the chest, sticky sputum, trance and sensitiveness.

Additional Formulas

Dawn Formula for Vascular Headache
(曙光血管头痛方, shu guang xue guan tou tong fang)

Source: *Shanghai Journal of Traditional Chinese Medicine*《上海中医药杂志》
Composition: Abalone Shell (石决明, Shijueming)30g
Szechwan Lovage Rhizome (川芎, Chuanxiong)9g
Dahurican Angelica Root (白芷, Baizhi)6g
Manchurian Wildginger Herb (细辛, Xixin)3g
Actions: Calming the liver and keeping the adverse qi downwards, activating blood circulation and relieving pain.
Applied Syndrome: Headache due to hyperactivity of liver-yang or flaming-up of wind-fire of the liver meridian, manifested by fainting, distention and pain of the head, vertigo, nausea and vomiting, or red eyes and stuffy nose, wiry and tense pulse or wiry and smooth pulse.

Dawn Formula for Vascular Headache
(Liver-Calming and Pain-Alleviating Method)

Ingredients	Effects	Combined Effects	Syndrome	Chief Symptoms
Abalone Shell (石决明, Shijueming)30g	Calming the liver and checking exuberance of yang	Calming the liver and keeping the adverse qi downwards, activating blood circulation and alleviating pain	Headache (due to hyperactivity of liver-yang or flaming-up of wind and fire)	Faint, distention and pain of the head, vertigo, nausea and vomiting, red eyes and stuffy nose, wiry and tense pulse or wiry and smooth pulse
Szechwan Lovage Rhizome (川芎, Chuanxiong)9g	Activating blood circulation and flow of qi, being good at treating headache			
Dahurican Angelica Root (白芷, Baizhi)6g	Expelling wind and alleviating pain			
Manchurian Wildginger Herb (细辛, Xixin)3g	Expelling wind and inducing resuscitation, being good at alleviating pain			

Points in Constitution: Szechwan Lovage Rhizome (川芎, Chuanxiong), Dahurican Angelica Root (白芷, Baizhi) and Manchurian Wildginger Herb (细辛, Xixin) are all good at alleviating pain. But since they are light in nature and inclined to go up, they may assist in liver-yang, leading to up-stirring of the liver. So a large dose of Abalone Shell (石决明, Shijueming) is used to calm the liver, clear away liver-heat and check exuberance of yang.

Indications:
1. Angioneurotic headache.
2. Hemicrania.

Precaution: This formula is contraindicated in headache due to blood deficiency.

Associated Formulas:

1. Formula for Qi and Fire of the Liver Meridian (肝经气火方, gan jing qi huo fang) *New Traditional Chinese Medicine*《新中医》

This is made up of Red Peony Root (赤芍, Chishao), White Peony Root (白芍药, Baishaoyao), Szechwan Lovage Rhizome (川芎, Chuanxiong), Tribulus Fruit (白蒺藜, Baijili), Chrysanthemum Flower (菊花, Juhua), Threeleaf Chastertree Fruit (蔓荆子, Manjingzi), Gambirplant Hooked Stem and Branch (钩藤, Gouteng), Oyster Shell (生牡蛎, Sheng Muli), Common Selfheal Fruit-Spike (夏枯草, Xiakucao), Akebia Stem (木通, Mutong) and Wild Mint Herb (薄荷, Bohe). Its action is clearing away or purging liver-fire. It is suitable for headache with distention of the head, irritability and vexation due to rushing-up of qi and fire of the liver meridian.

2. Gastrodian and Uncaria Decoction (天麻钩藤饮, tian ma gou teng yin) *New Explanation of Diagnosis and Treatment of Miscellaneous Disease*《杂病证治新义》

This is comprised of Tall Gastrodia Rhizome (天麻, Tianma), Gambirplant Hooked Stem and Branch (钩藤, Gouteng), Abalone Shell (石决明, Shijueming), Cape Jasmine Fruit (山栀子, Shanzhizi), Baikal Skullcap Root (黄芩, Huangqin), Medicinal Achyranthes Root (川牛膝, Chuan Niuxi), Eucommia Bark (杜仲, Duzhong), Motherwort Herb (益母草, Yimucao), Chinese Taxillus Twig (桑寄生, Sangjisheng), Fleece-Flower Stem (夜交藤, Yejiaoteng) and Indian Bread with Hostwood (茯神, Fushen). Its actions are calming the liver to stop the wind, clearing away heat and tranquilizing the mind. It is indicated for headache and vertigo due to upward attack of liver-wind resulting from hyperactivity of liver yang.

3. Tea-Blended Szechwan Lovage Powder (川芎茶调散, chuan xiong cha tiao san) *Prescriptions of Peaceful Benevolent Dispensary*《和剂局方》

This consists of Szechwan Lovage Rhizome (川芎, Chuanxiong), Fineleaf Schizonepeta Herb (荆芥, Jingjie), Dahurican Angelica Root (白芷, Baizhi), Incised Notopterygium Rhizome or Root (羌活, Qianghuo), Licorice Root (甘草, Gancao), Manchurian Wildginger Herb (细辛, Xixin), Divaricate Saposhnikovia Root (防风, Fangfeng), Wild Mint Herb (薄荷, Bohe) and Tea (清茶, Qingcha). Its actions are expelling wind and alleviating pain. It is suited to headache due to affection of exopathogen or severe intermittant headache due to wind cold.

4. Tea-Blended Chrysanthemum Flower Powder (菊花茶调散, ju hua cha tiao san) *Collection of Prescriptions with Exposition*《医方集解》

This is comprised of Szechwan Lovage Rhizome (川芎, Chuanxiong), Fineleaf Schizonepeta Herb (荆芥, Jingjie), Dahurican Angelica Root (白芷, Baizhi), Incised Notopterygium Rhizome or Root (羌活, Qianghuo), Licorice Root (甘草, Gancao), Manchurian Wildginger Herb (细辛, Xixin), Divaricate Saposhnikovia Root (防风, Fangfeng), Wild Mint Herb (薄荷, Bohe), Tea (清茶, Qingcha), Chrysanthemum Flower (菊花, Juhua) and Silkworm with Batrytis Larva (僵蚕, Jiangcan). Its actions are expelling wind, alleviating pain and clearing away heat of the head and eyes. It is indicated for headache due to upwad attack of wind-heat.

5. Szechwan Lovage Rhizome and Manchurian Wildginger Herb Powder (芎辛散, xiong xin san) *Jifeng Prescriptions for Universal Benevolence* 《鸡峰普济方》

This is comprised of Szechwan Lovage Rhizome (川芎, Chuanxiong), Swordlike Atractylodes Rhizome (苍术, Cangzhu), Licorice Root (甘草, Gancao), Manchurian Wildginger Herb (细辛, Xixin) and Tea (清茶, Qingcha). This formula can clear away heat, expel wind and alleviate pain. It is suited to headache, vertigo, fever and chills due to wind attacking yang meridians.

Brain-Benefiting and Blood-Activating Formula
(益脑活血方, yi nao huo xue fang)

Source: *Modern Internal Medicine of Traditional Chinese Medicine* 《现代中医内科学》
Composition: Grassleaf Sweetflag Rhizome (石菖蒲, Shichangpu)12g
Prepared Rehmannia Root (熟地黄, Shudihuang)12g
Fleeceflower Root (何首乌, Heshouwu)12g
Barbary Wolfberry Fruit (枸杞子, Gouqizi)12g
Giant Knotweed Rhizome (虎杖, Huzhang)12g
Dan-Shen Root (丹参, Danshen)15g
Szechwan Lovage Rhizome (川芎, Chuanxiong)9g
Hawthorn Fruit (山楂, Shanzha)9g
Sharpleaf Galangal Fruit (益智仁, Yizhiren)9g
Safflower (红花, Honghua)6g
Thinleaf Milkwort Root (远志, Yuanzhi)6g
Glossy Privet Fruit (女贞子, Nüzhenzi)12g
Actions: Nourishing the liver and kidney, dissolving blood stasis and removing phlegm.
Applied Syndrome: Mental confusion due to accumulation of phlegm and blood stasis resulting from deficiency of the liver and kidney which leads to insufficiency of essence and blood, manifested by poor memory, slow response, vertigo, palpitation, pallor, soreness of loins and legs, insomnia and dreaminess, early change of the beard and hair, pale tongue with slippery coating, thin and smooth pulse.
Points in Constitution: Generally old persons have a weak kidney-qi, which may easily bring about phlegm and dampness. Besides, as the result of the weak kidney-qi, blood may circulate slowly, leading to blood stasis. Accumulation of phlegm and blood stasis is the root of all diseases.

This formula has a mild nature and can treat both the root cause and symptoms, thus it is regarded as an effective Prescription

Brain-Benefitting and Blood-Activating Formula
(Kidney-Nourishing and Blood-Activating Method)

Ingredients	Effects	Combined Effects	Syndrome	Chief Symptoms
Prepared Rehmannia Root (熟地黄, Shudihuang)12g Fleeceflower Root (何首乌, Heshouwu)12g Barbary Wolfberry Fruit (枸杞子, Gouqizi)12g Glossy Privet Fruit (女贞子, Nüzhenzi)12g Sharpleaf Galangal Fruit (益智仁, Yizhiren)9g	Nourishing the liver and kidney	Nourishing the liver and kidney, dissolving blood stasis and removing phlegm	Deficiency of the liver and kidney, accumulation of phlegm and blood stasis in the seven orifices	Poor memory, slow response, vertigo and palpitation, pallor, soreness of loins and legs, insomnia and dreaminess, early change of the beard and hair, pale tongue with slippery coating, thin and smooth pulse
Dan-Shen Root (丹参, Danshen)15g Hawthorn Fruit (山楂, Shanzha)9g Szechwan Lovage Rhizome (川芎, Chuanxiong)9g Safflower (红花, Honghua)6g Giant Knotweed Rhizome (虎杖, Huzhang)12g	Activating blood circulation and removing blood stasis			
Grassleaf Sweetflag Rhizome (石菖蒲, Shichangpu)12g Thinleaf Milkwort Root (远志, Yuanzhi)6g	Removing phlegm and inducing resuscitation, calming the heart and tranquilizing the mind			

Indications:

1. Senile dementia.
2. Cerebral aneurysm, hyperlipemia.

Associated Formulas:

1. Seven Valuable Herbs Beard-Improving Pellet(七宝美髯丹, qi bao mei ran dan) *Prescriptions of Jishan Tang quoted from Compendium of Materia Medica* 《本草纲目》引积善堂方

This is comprised of Fleeceflower Root (何首乌, Heshouwu), Barbary Wolfberry Fruit (枸杞子, Gouqizi), Chinese Dodder Seed (菟丝子, Tusizi), Twotooth Achyranthes Root (牛膝, Niuxi), Malaytea Scurfpea Fruit (补骨脂, Buguzhi), Indian Bread Pink Epidermis (赤茯苓, Chifuling) and Tuckahoe (白茯苓, Baifuling). Its actions are nourishing the liver and kidney, blackening hair and strengthening the bone. It is indicated for cerebral aneurysm due to deficiency of the liver and kidney.

2. Capillary Wormwood Herb Fat-Lowering Formula (茵陈降脂方, yin chen jiang zhi fang) *Shanghai Journal of Traditional Chinese Medicine*《上海中医药杂志》

This consists of Capillary Wormwood Herb (茵陈, Yinchen), Hawthorn Fruit (生山楂, Sheng Shanzha) and Malt (生麦芽, Sheng Maiya), whose actions are clearing away heat in the liver and gallbladder, activating spleen-qi and lowering fat. It is suited to hyperlipemia and cerebral aneurysm due to phlegm (dampness) and heat accumulated in the liver and gallbladder

3. Efficacious Vessels-Softening Formula (软脉灵, ruan mai ling) *Modern Internal Medicine of Traditional Chinese Medicine*《现代中医内科学》

This is made up of Ginseng (人参, Renshen), Prepared Rehmannia Root (熟地黄, Shudihuang), Barbary Wolfberry Fruit (枸杞子, Gouqizi), Twotooth Achyranthes Root (牛膝, Niuxi), Fleeceflower Root (何首乌, Heshouwu), Szechwan Lovage Rhizome (川芎, Chuanxiong), Dan-Shen Root (丹参, Danshen) and Chinese Angelica Root (当归, Danggui). Its actions are invigorating the kidney and activating blood circulation. It is indicated for cerebral aneurysm, vertigo and amnesia.

Chapter Six
Formulas for Endocrine and Metabolic Diseases

Diabetes (xiaoke in TCM), hyperthyroidism (goiter in TCM) and diabetes insipidus (renal diabetes in TCM) have been known in traditional Chinese medicine for a long time and this knowledge is still practiced in the modern clinic. Since the causes of the endocrine disease, metabolic disease and diseases of the blood system are complicated and their symptoms are varied, the treatment of these illnesses based on differentiation of symptoms and signs becomes complex. Though these diseases are usually related to many systems such as five-zang and six-fu organs of the body, the major treating principle in clinic is still "treating the primary aspect of the disease based on differentiation of symptoms and signs, designing or choosing the formula in the light of different syndrome and modifying the drugs in accordance with specific symptoms".

1. Jade Liquid Decoction (Yuye Decoction)
(玉液汤, yu ye tang)

Source: *Records of Traditional Chinese and Western Medicine in Combination*《医学衷中参西录》
Composition: Common Yam Rhizome (生山药, Sheng Shanyao) 15g
Membranous Milkvetch Root (生黄芪, Sheng Huangqi) 9g
Common Anemarrhena Rhizome (知母, Zhimu) 6g
Chicken Gizzard Membrane (鸡内金, Jineijin) 3g
Lobed Kudzuvine Root (葛根, Gegen) 6
Chinese Magnoliavine Fruit (五味子, Wuweizi) 3g
Snakegourd Root (天花粉, Tianhuafen) 9g
Actions: Replenishing qi and promoting the production of body fluid, moistening dryness and quenching thirst.
Applied Syndrome: Diabetes due to deficiency of both qi and yin, manifested by thirst, desire for drinking, frequency of micturition and profuse urine, or turbid urine, tiredness, shortness of breath, thin, rapid and weak pulse.
Points in Constitution: In this formula the combination of Membranous Milkvetch Root (黄芪, Huangqi) and Lobed Kudzuvine Root (葛根, Gegen) can raise clear yang to make the body fluid ascend, which corresponds to what Zhang Xichun (张锡纯) says that diabetes can be treated "by using the raising and reinforcing drugs to promote the transformation of qi and conduct body fluid to go upward".

Jade Liquid Decoction (Yuye Decoction)
(Qi-Replenishing and Body Fluid-Producing Method)

Ingredients	Effects	Combined Effects	Syndrome	Chief Symptoms
Membranous Milkvetch Root (生黄芪, Sheng Huangqi) 9g Lobed Kudzuvine Root (葛根, Gegen) 6	Replenishing qi and raising clear yang, promoting the production of body fluid and quenching thirst	Replenishing qi and promoting the production of body fluid, moistening dryness and quenching thirst	Diabetes (due to qi and yin deficiency)	Thirst, polydipsia, polyphagia and polyuria with turbid urine, tiredness, corpulent tongue, thin, rapid and weak pulse
Snakegourd Root (天花粉, Tianhuafen) 9g Common Anemarrhena Rhizome (知母, Zhimu) 6g	Clearing away heat and promoting the production of body fluid			
Common Yam Rhizome (生山药, Sheng Shanyao) 15g Chinese Magnoliavine Fruit (五味子, Wuweizi) 3g	Uniformly reinforcing yin and yang and astringing essence and qi			
Chicken Gizzard Membrane (鸡内金, Jineijin) 3g	Assiting the spleen in transport			

Indications:
1. Diabetes.
2. Diabetes insipidus.

Precaution: The dose of Snakegourd Root Power (天花粉, Tianhuafen) may be increased. Besides, the yin-nourishing and fluid-producing dugs such as Dwarf Lilyturf Root (麦门冬, Maimendong), Dendrobium Herb (石斛, Shihu) can be appropriately added to this formula.

Associated Formula:

Diabetes-Relieving Formula (消渴方, xiao ke fang) *Danxi's Experiential Therapy* 《丹溪心法》

This is comprised of Snakegourd Root (天花粉, Tianhuafen), Juice of Rehmannia Root (生地汁, Shengdizhi), Juice of Lotus (藕汁, Ouzhi), Milk (牛乳, Niuru) and Coptis Rhizome (黄连, Huanglian). Its actions are nourishing yin, promoting the production of body fluid and clearing away heat. This is applicable to diabetes due to heat in the stomach accompanied with polyorexia.

2. Seaweed Jade Kettle Decoction
(海藻玉壶汤, hai zao yu hu tang)

Source: *Orthodox Manual of Surgery* 《外科正宗》
Composition: Seaweed (海藻, Haizao)9g
Kelp (昆布, Kunbu)9g
Thunberg Fritillary Bulb (浙贝母, Zhe Beimu)9g

Seaweed Jade Kettle Decoction
(Phlegm-Resolving and Mass-Dissipating Method)

Ingredients	Effects	Combined Effects	Syndrome	Chief Symptoms
Seaweed (海藻, Haizao)9g Kelp (昆布, Kunbu)9g	Softening hardness and removing phlegm	Removing phlegm and softening hardness, dissipating blockages and dissolving goiter	Goiter	The beginning of goiter, swelling or hardness, red or normal colour of skin, unbroken, greasy coating and wiry and slow pulse
Pinellia Rhizome (清半夏, Qing Banxia)9g Thunberg Fritillary Bulb (浙贝母, Zhe Beimu)9g	Removing phlegm and dissipating blockages			
Green Tangerine Peel (青皮, Qingpi)9g Tangerine Peel (橘皮, Jupi)9g	Dispersing the stagnated liver-qi			
Szechwan Lovage Rhizome (川芎, Chuanxiong)9g Chinese Angelica Root (当归, Danggui)9g	Activating blood circulation and dredging the collaterals			
Weeping Forsythia Capsule (连翘, Lianqiao)9g	Clearing away heat and dissipating blockages			
Doubleteeth Pubescent Angelica Root (独活, Duhuo)9g	Dispersing and dredging the meridians and collaterals			
Licorice Root (生甘草, Sheng Gancao)9g	Coordinating the actions of various ingredients in a prescription			

Pinellia Rhizome (清半夏, Qing Banxia)9g
Green Tangerine Peel (青皮, Qingpi)9g
Tangerine Peel (橘皮, Jupi)9g
Szechwan Lovage Rhizome (川芎, Chuanxiong)9g
Chinese Angelica Root (当归, Danggui)9g
Doubleteeth Pubescent Angelica Root (独活, Duhuo)9g
Weeping Forsythia Capsule (连翘, Lianqiao)9g
Licorice Root (生甘草, Sheng Gancao)9g

Actions: Removing phlegm and softening hardness, dissolving goiter and dissipating blockages.

Applied Syndrome: The beginning of goiter marked by swelling, or hardness, or redness or not redness but without rupture or ulceration.

Points in Constitution: Goiter results from accumulation of phlegm and qi in the meridians, which causes blood stasis. Thus, this formula has the actions of removing phlegm, regulating flow of qi and activating blood circulation to dissipate blockages. Seaweed (海藻, Haizao) and Kelp (昆布, Kunbu) are used as monarchs in this formula because salt drugs have the action of softening hardness. The book Shennong's Classic of Herbology(本草, ben cao) records eighteen incompatible drugs which include Seaweed (海藻, Haizao), Peking Euphorbia Root (大戟, Daji), kansui Root (甘遂, Gansui) and Lilac Daphne Flower-Bud (芫花, Yuanhua). They are incompatible with Licorice Root (甘草, Gancao). However, in this formula Seaweed (海藻, Haizao) and Licorice Root (甘草, Gancao) are used simultaneously, which shows that in ancient times the combination of drugs was not limited to "eighteen incompatible drugs".

Indications:

1. Thyroid adenom
2. Simple thyroid enlargement.
3. Hyperplasia of mammary glands.

Precaution: In the original book, this formula is mainly used to treat the beginning of goiter, while in the book of The Golden Mirror of Medicine (《医宗金鉴》, yi zong jin jian), this is used to treat "stony goiter". Now it is usually used for thyroid adenoma and thyroid enlargement. Taking this formula for a long time (3-6 months) may have an obvious effect on the above diseases if they are at the early enlargement stage.

Associated Formula:

Internally Tumour-Relieving Pill(内消肿瘤丸, nei xiao zhong liu wan) *Manual of Prescriptions and Drugs of Traditional Chinese Medicine*《中医方药手册》

This is made up of Common Selfheal Fruit-Spike (夏枯草, Xiakucao), Sinkiang Arnebia Root or Redroot Gromwell Root (紫草, Zicao), Chinese Gentian Root (龙胆草, Longdancao), Licorice Root (甘草, Gancao), Figwort Root (玄参, Xuanshen), Dan-Shen Root (丹参, Danshen), Coix Seed (薏苡仁, Yiyiren), Peach Seed (桃仁, Taoren), Snakegourd Fruit (瓜蒌, Gualou), Asiatic Cornelian Cherry Fruit (山茱萸, Shanzhuyu), Tonkin Sophora Root (山豆根, Shandougen), Solanum Lyratum(蜀羊泉, Shuyangquan), Appendiculate Cremastra Pseudobulb (山慈姑, Shancigu), Nux Vomica (番木鳖, Fanmubie), Cinnabar (朱砂, Zhusha) and Red

Orpiment (雄黄, Xionghuang). The actions of this formula are purging fire and clearing away toxic material, activating blood circulation and reducing swelling. It is suited to breast cancer, gastric cancer and tumors which are unable to be operated on or postoperative rescent tumour.

3. Internally Scrofula-Eliminating Pill
(肉消瘰疬丸, nei xiao lei li wan)

Source: *Complete Works for Treating Sores*《疡医大全》
Composition: Common Selfheal Fruit-Spike (夏枯草, Xiakucao)15g
Figwort Root (玄参, Xuanshen)9g
Black Salt (青盐, Qingyan)6g
Snakegourd Root (天花粉, Tianhuafen)3g
Licorice Root (生甘草, Sheng Gancao)3g
Japanese Ampelopsis Root (白蔹, Bailian)3g
Chinese Angelica Root (全当归, Quan Danggui)3g
Seaweed (海藻, Haizao)3g
Bitter Orange (枳壳, Zhiqiao)3g
Balloonflower Root (桔梗, Jiegeng)3g
Tendrilleaf Fritillary Bulb (川贝母, Chuan Beimu)3g
Prepared Rhubarb (制大黄, Zhi Dahuang)3g
Wild Mint Herb (薄荷, Bohe)3g
Weeping Forsythia Capsule (连翘, Lianqiao)3g
Powder of Clam Shell (海蛤粉, Haigefen)3g
Niter (硝石 Xiao Shi)3g
Dried Rehmannia Root (生地黄, Shengdihuang)3g.

Actions: Softening hardness and dissipating blockages, removing phlegm and dissolving a goiter.

Applied Syndrome: Goiter, scrofula and subcutaneous nodule due to retention of heat-toxin in the interior, stagnation of qi and blood and accumulation of phlegm and dampness.

Points in Constitution: Scrofula is usually caused by stagnation of qi and retention of phlegm in the shaoyang meridian, which originates first from qi and then from phlegm. Thus, this formula first emphasizes removing phlegm and dissipating blockages, then emphasizes soothing the liver and regulating circulation of qi.

Indications:
1. Simple thyroid enlargement.
2. Hyperparathyroidism.
3. Thyroidtis.
4. Thyroid adenoma.
5. Tuberculosis of cervical lymph nodes.

Internally Scrofula-Eliminating Pill
(Phlegm-Resolving and Mass-Dissipating Method)

Ingredients	Effects	Combined Effects	Syndrome	Chief Symptoms
Common Selfheal Fruit-Spike (夏枯草, Xiakucao) 15g	Clearing away liver heat and dissipating blockages; especial drug for eliminating scrofula	Removing phlegm and dissipating blockages, softening hardness and dissolving a goiter	Goiter, scrofula and subcutaneous nodule (due to heat of the liver, stagnation of qi and retention of phlegm)	Thyroid enlargement, thyroidtis, tuberculosis of cervical lymph nodes, red tongue with yellow and greasy coating and wiry and rapid pulse
Figwort Root (玄参, Xuanshen)9g Tendrilleaf Fritillary Bulb (川贝母, Chuan Beimu)3g Seaweed (海藻, Haizao)3g Powder of Clam Shell (海蛤粉, Haigefen)3g Japanese Ampelopsis Root (白蔹, Bailian)3g Snakegourd Root (天花粉, Tianhuafen)3g	Removing phlegm and softening hardness			
Bitter Orange (枳壳, Zhiqiao)3g Balloonflower Root (桔梗, Jiegeng)3g	Regulating flow of qi			
Chinese Angelica Root (全当归, Quan Danggui)3g Dried Rehmannia Root (生地黄, Shengdihuang)3g.	Regulating circulation of blood			
Weeping Forsythia Capsule (连翘, Lianqiao)3g Wild Mint Herb (薄荷, Bohe)3g	Dispersing the stagnated liver-qi and dissipating blockages			
Black Salt (青盐, Qingyan)6g Niter(硝石, Xiaoshi)3g Prepared Rhubarb (制大黄, Zhi Dahuang)3g Licorice Root (生甘草, Sheng Gancao)3g	Clearing away and purging liver-fire			

Precaution: This is a mild formula for scrofula and should be taken for a long period of time, during which the condition of the patient should be observed.

Associated Formulas:

1. Scrofula-Dispelling Pill(消瘰丸, xiao lei wan) *Comprehension of Medicine* 《医学心悟》

This is comprised of Figwort Root (玄参, Xuanshen), Oyster Shell (牡蛎, Muli) and Tendrilleaf Fritillary Bulb (贝母, Beimu). Its actions are dispelling scrofula, nourishing yin, removing phlegm and softening hardness. It is applicable to scrofula and subcutaneous nodule.

2. Five Seafoods Goiter-Dissolving Pill (消瘿五海丸, xiao ying wu hai wan) *National Selected Prescriptions of Chinese Patent Medicine* 《全国中成药处方集》

This is composed of Seaweed (海藻, Haizao), Cuttlefish Bone (海螵蛸, Haipiaoxiao), Clam Shell (海蛤壳, Haigeqiao), Kelp (昆布, Kunbu), Tendrilleaf Fritillary Bulb (贝母, Beimu) and Common Aucklandia Root (木香, Muxiang), whose actions are softening hardness, reducing swelling, removing phlegm and treating goiter. It is suited to goiter, scrofula and nodule in breast with distention and pain.

4. Ten Strong Tonic Herbs Pill
(十全大补丸, shi quan da bu wan)

Source: *Prescriptions of Peaceful Benevolent Dispensary* 《和剂局方》

Composition: Toasted Membranous Milkvetch Root (炙黄芪, Zhi Huangqi)15

Cassia Bark (肉桂, Rougui)6g

Ginseng (人参, Renshen)9g

Szechwan Lovage Rhizome (川芎, Chuanxiong)6g

Prepared Rehmannia Root (熟地黄, Shudihuang)15g

Tuckahoe (茯苓, Fuling)9g

Stir-baked Largehead Atractylodes Rhizome (炒白术, Chao Baizhu)9g

Prepared Licorice Root (炙甘草, Zhi Gancao)6g

Chinese Angelica Root (当归, Danggui)9g

White Peony Root (白芍药, Baishaoyao)9g

Actions: Warming and replenishing qi and blood.

Applied Syndrome: Syndrome of deficiency of both qi and blood, manifested by cough due to comsuptive diseases, dizziness, emission, tiredness of the loin and knees, shortness of breath, reluctance to speak, poor appetite, palpitation, lusterless complexion, cold limbs, unhealing ulcer, metrorrhagia and metrostaxis, pale tongue, thin and feeble pulse.

Points in Constitution: This formula is composed of the ingredients of Four Gentalmem Decoction(四君子汤, si jun zi tang) and Four Herbs Decoction(四物汤, si wu tang) plus the drugs of Membranous Milkvetch Root (黄芪, Huangqi) and Cassia Bark (肉桂, Rougui). The main action of it is to warm and replenish qi and blood and it is applicable to syndrome of deficiency of qi and blood accompanying with cold of deficient type. Among the drugs in this formula. Cassia

Bark (肉桂, Rougui) is connected with blood system to warm and activate yang in the blood so as to attain the purpose of promoting the production and transformation of blood.

Ten Strong Tonic Herbs Pill
(Method of Replenishing both Qi and Blood)

Ingredients	Effects	Combined Effects	Syndrome	Chief Symptoms
Toasted Membranous Milkvetch Root (炙黄芪, Zhi Huangqi)15g	Replenishing qi and lifting yang	Warming and replenishing qi and blood	Deficiency of qi and blood	Weak body due to long-time illness, sallow complexion, listlessness, cold limbs, anorexia, unhealed ulcer, or metrorrhagia and metrostaxis, pale tongue, thin and feeble pulse
Cassia Bark (肉桂, Rougui)6g	Restoring the transformation of yang			
Ginseng (人参, Renshen)9g Stir-Baked Largehead Atractylodes Rhizome (炒白术, Chao Baizhu)9g Tuckahoe (茯苓, Fuling)9g Prepared Licorice Root (炙甘草, Zhi Gancao)6g	Replenishing qi and invigorating the spleen			
Chinese Angelica Root (当归, Danggui)9g Szechwan Lovage Rhizome (川芎, Chuanxiong)6g White Peony Root (白芍药, Baishaoyao)9g Prepared Rehmannia Root (熟地黄, Shudihuang)15g	Enriching and regulating blood			

Indications:

1. Patient with deficiency of both qi and blood after severe or prolonged diseases, post operation or post partum.

2. Senity and weakness with deficiency of qi and blood.

3. Late pulmonary tuberculosis.

4. Emission, prospermia, female infertility.

5. Metrorrhagia and metrostaxis, habitual abortion.

6. Long-time or stubborn sores and ulcer.

Precaution: This is a Prescription for warming and replenishing qi and blood. Thus it is forbidden for excess syndrome without deficiency.

Associated Formulas:

1. Chinese Angelica Blood-Tonifying Decoction (当归补血汤, dang gui bu xue tang) *Differentiation on Endogenous and Exogenous Diseases* 《内外伤辨惑论》

This is made up of Membranous Milkvetch Root (黄芪, Huangqi) and Chinese Angelica Root (当归, Danggui) and its actions are invigorating qi and promoting production of blood. It is mainly used to treat internal damage due to overstrain, weakness of qi and deficiency of blood manifested as flushed face, irritability, thirst with desire to drink, fever during menstruation or postpartum fever, stubborn or long-time unhealed sores and ulcers.

2. Back to the Spleen Decoction(归脾汤, gui pi tang) *Prescriptions for Rescuring the Sick* 《济生方》

This is comprised of Largehead Atractylodes Rhizome (白术, Baizhu), Tuckahoe (茯苓, Fuling), Membranous Milkvetch Root (黄芪, Huangqi), Longan Aril (龙眼肉, Longyanrou), Spine Date Seed (枣仁, Zaoren), Ginseng (人参, Renshen), Common Aucklandia Root (木香, Muxiang), Licorice Root (甘草, Gancao), Chinese Angelica Root (当归, Danggui) and Thinleaf Milkwort Root (远志, Yuanzhi). Its actions are replenishing qi, enriching the blood, invigorating the spleen and nourishing the heart. It is suited to palpitation or severe palpitation, amnesia, insomnia, anorexia, tiredness, hematochezia, metrorrhagia and metrostaxis, advanced menstrual period with profuse and light blood due to failure of the spleen to control blood resulting from deficiency of the heart and spleen.

3. Prepared Licorice Decoction(炙甘草汤, zhi gan cao tang) *Treatise on Exogenous Febrile Diseases* 《伤寒论》

This is comprised of Prepared Licorice Root (炙甘草, Zhi Gancao), Fresh Ginger (生姜, Shengjiang), Ginseng (人参, Renshen), Dried Rehmannia Root (生地黄, Shengdihuang), Cassia Twig (桂枝, Guizhi), Ass-hide Glue (阿胶, Ejiao), Dwarf Lilyturf Root (麦门冬, Maimendong), Hemp Seed (火麻仁, Huomaren) and Chinese Date (大枣, Dazao). Its actions are replenishing qi and nourishing yin, enriching the blood and restoring regular pulsation. It is suited to severe palpitation, knotted and intermittent pulse due to deficiency of qi and insufficiency of blood or dry cough without expectoratin or with bloody sputum, tiredness, shortness of breath, spontaneous sweating or night sweating, dry throat and constipation, feeble and rapid pulse due to consumptive lung disease.

5. Ginseng Nutrition Decoction
(人参养荣汤, ren shen yang rong tang)

Source: *Prescriptions of Peaceful Benevolent Dispensary* 《和剂局方》
Composition: White Peony Root (白芍药, Baishaoyao)9g
Chinese Angelica Root (当归, Danggui)9g

Ginseng Nutrition Decoction
(Method of Replenishing both Qi and Blood)

Ingredients	Effects	Combined Effects	Syndrome	Chief Symptoms
Toasted Membranous Milkvetch Root (炙黄芪, Zhi Huangqi)9g Ginseng (人参, Renshen)9g Largehead Atractylodes Rhizome (白术, Baizhu)9g Tuckahoe (茯苓, Fuling)6g	Replenishing qi and invigorating the spleen	Replenishing qi and enriching blood, nourishing heart and tranquilizing the mind	Deficiency of qi and blood	Shortness of breath, asthma on Movement, palpitation, insomnia, vertigo, dry throat and lips, tiredness, poor appetite, anaemia, pale tongue with white coating and little fluid, deep, thin and rapid pulse or large feeble pulse
White Peony Root (白芍药, Baishaoyao)9g Chinese Angelica Root (当归, Danggui)9g Prepared Rehmannia Root (熟地黄, Shudihuang)9g	Enriching blood and regulating blood			
Cassia Bark (肉桂, Rougui)3g	Restoring yang to promote the functional activities of qi			
Tangerine Peel (橘皮, Jupi)6g	Activating flow of qi and invigorating the spleen			
Chinese Magnoliavine Fruit (五味子, Wuweizi)6g Thinleaf Milkwort Root (远志, Yuanzhi)6g	Astringing qi and promoting the production of body fluid, calming the heart and tranquilizing the mind			
Fresh Ginger (生姜, Shengjiang)3g Chinese Date (大枣, Dazao)3g Prepared Licorice Root (炙甘草, Zhi Gancao)9g	Warming the middle-jiao and invigorating the spleen			

Tangerine Peel (橘皮, Jupi) 6g
Toasted Membranous Milkvetch Root (炙黄芪, Zhi Huangqi) 9g
Cassia Bark (肉桂, Rougui) 3g
Ginseng (人参, Renshen) 9g
Largehead Atractylodes Rhizome (白术, Baizhu) 9g
Prepared Licorice Root (炙甘草, Zhi Gancao) 9g
Prepared Rehmannia Root (熟地黄, Shudihuang) 9g
Chinese Magnoliavine Fruit (五味子, Wuweizi) 6g
Tuckahoe (茯苓, Fuling) 6g
Thinleaf Milkwort Root (远志, Yuanzhi) 6g
Fresh Ginger (生姜, Shengjiang) 3g
Chinese Date (大枣, Dazao) 3g

Actions: Replenishing qi and enriching blood, nourishing the heart and tranquilizing the mind.

Applied Syndrome: Syndrome of deficiency of both qi and blood due to constant overstrain, manifested by shortness of breath, asthma on movement, palpitation, dry throat and lips, insomnia and dreaminess, tiredness, poor appetite, pale tongue with white coating and little fluid, deep, thin and rapid pulse or large, feeble pulse.

Points in Constitution: This formula is the modification of Eight Treasures Decoction (八珍汤, ba zhen tang,) and Ten Strong Tonic Herbs Decoction (十全大补汤, shi quan da bu tang). Thus, it has the actions of warming and replenishing qi and blood, tranquilizing the mind and calming the spirit.

Indications:

1. Syndrome of deficiency of qi and blood due to severe disease, long-time illness, old age or post operation and after childbirth.
2. Climacteric syndrome.
3. Vegetative nerve functional disturbance.
4. Lleukocytogenesis caused by radiotherapy and chemotherapy.

Precaution: This formula is designed for consumptive disease due to deficiency of qi and blood. It should not be used singly for the syndrome of deficiency of qi and blood accompanied with heat of deficiency type.

Associated Formulas:

1. Pulse-Activating Powder(生脉散, sheng mai san) *Differentiation on Endogenous and Exogenous Diseases* 《内外伤辨惑论》

This is comprised of Ginseng (人参, Renshen), Dwarf Lilyturf Root (麦门冬, Maimendong) and Chinese Magnoliavine Fruit (五味子, Wuweizi). Its actions are astringing yin and arresting perspiration. It is suited to profuse sweating, thirst, shortness of breath, reluctance to speak, dry throat and tongue, weak pulse due to impairment of both qi and body fluid resulting from damage of the lung by pathogenic heat.

2. Four Herbs Decoction (四物汤, si wu tang) *Prescriptions of Peaceful Benevolent Dispensary* 《和剂局方》

This is comprised of Chinese Angelica Root（当归, Danggui）, Szechwan Lovage Rhizome（川芎, Chuanxiong）, Prepared Rehmannia Root（熟地黄, Shudihuang）and White Peony Root（白芍药, Baishaoyao）. Its actions are enriching blood and regulating the circulation of blood. It is good at treating palpitation, vertigo, tinnitus, irregular menstruation or amenorrhea due to deficiency and stagnation of ying-blood.

3. Holy Disease-Curing Decoction（圣愈汤, sheng yu tang） *The Golden Mirror of Medicine* 《医宗金鉴》

This consists of Prepared Rehmannia Root（熟地黄, Shudihuang）, White Peony Root（白芍药, Baishaoyao）, Szechwan Lovage Rhizome（川芎, Chuanxiong）, Chinese Angelica Root（当归, Danggui）, Ginseng（人参, Renshen）and Membranous Milkvetch Root（黄芪, Huangqi）. Its actions are replenishing qi, enriching and controlling the blood. It is mainly used to treat advanced menstrual periods with profuse and pink menses, tiredness and listlessness due to failure of controling blood resulting from deficiency of qi.

Additional Formulas

Blood Sugar-Reducing Decoction
(降糖汤, jian tang tang)

Source: *Fujian Journal of Traditional Chinese Medicine*《福建中医药》
Composition: Membranous Milkvetch Root (生黄芪, Sheng Huangqi)30g
Lobed Kudzuvine Root (葛根, Gegen)30g
Common Yam Rhizome (生山药, Sheng Shanyao)30g
Swordlike Atractylodes Rhizome (苍术, Cangzhu)9g
Largehead Atractylodes Rhizome (白术, Baizhu)9g

Blood Sugar-Reducing Decoction
(Qi-Replenishing and Spleen-Invigorating Method)

Ingredients	Effects	Combined Effects	Syndrome	Chief Symptoms
Membranous Milkvetch Root (生黄芪, Sheng Huangqi)30g	Replenishing qi and lifting yang, replenishing the lung and spleen potently	Replenishing qi, invigorating the spleen and nourishing yin	Diabetes (excessive dampness due to deficiency of the spleen and impairment of fluid in the lung and stomach)	Fatness, polyorexia, thirst, polydipsia, diuresis, listlessness and heaviness sensation of the limbs, pale tongue, white and greasy coating, soft and slow pulse
Largehead Atractylodes Rhizome (白术, Baizhu)9g Common Yam Rhizome (生山药, Sheng Shanyao)30g Tuckahoe (茯苓, Fuling)9g	Replenishing qi and invigorating the spleen			
Swordlike Atractylodes Rhizome (苍术, Cangzhu)9g	Drying dampness and invigorating the spleen			
Lobed Kudzuvine Root (葛根, Gegen)30g Snakegourd Root (天花粉, Tianhuafen)60g Figwort Root (玄参, Xuanshen)15g	Clearing away heat and nourishing yin and promoting the production of body fluid			

Figwort Root (玄参, Xuanshen)15g
Snakegourd Root (天花粉, Tianhuafen)60g
Tuckahoe (茯苓, Fuling)9g

Actions: Replenishing qi, invigorating the spleen and nourishing yin.

Applied Syndrome: Diabetes due to deficiency of yin accompanying with heat in the interior resulting from excessive dampness and deficiency of the spleen, manifested by fatness, polyorexia, thirst, polydipsia, diuresis, listlessness, heaviness sensation of the limbs, pale tongue with white and greasy coating, soft and slow pulse.

Points in Constitution: Swordlike Atractylodes Rhizome (苍术, Cangzhu) has the actions of removing dampness and invigorating the spleen. When it is combined with the drugs for nourishing yin and moistening dryness such as Snakegourd Root (天花粉, Tianhuafen), and Figwort Root (元参, Yuanshen), it can prevent impairment of spleen yang, which are opposite and complementary to each other. In addition, Swordlike Atractylodes Rhizome (苍术, Cangzhu) can treat blindness and prevent the complication of the eye dieases due to diabetes.

Indication: Diabetes (type II).

Precaution: This formula is applied to diabetes both with dampness and impairment of body fluid which is manifested as polyphagia and polyuria. It is not suitable for excessive eating, erosion of mucous membrane of the oral cavity, dry mouth and thirst due to simple excessive heat in the stomach, or loose stool due to deficiency of the spleen and excessive dampness.

Associated Formulas:

1. Diabetes-Relieving Formula(消渴方, xiao ke fang) *Danxi's Experiential Therapy*《丹溪心法》

This is comprised of Snakegourd Root (天花粉, Tianhuafen), Coptis Rhizome (黄连, Huanglian), Dried Rehmannia Root (生地黄, Shengdihuang) and Juice of Lotus (藕汁, Ouzhi). Its actions are clearing away lung-heat and nourishing yin-fluid. It is mainly used to treat diabetes involving the upper-jiao manifested as thirst, polydipsia, yellow tongue coating, forceful, bounding and rapid pulse.

2. Jade Maid Decoction (玉女煎, yu nu jian) *Jingyue's Complete Works*《景岳全书》

This consists of Gypsum (生石膏, Sheng Shigao), Common Anemarrhena Rhizome (知母, Zhimu), Dwarf Lilyturf Root (麦门冬, Maimendong), Prepared Rehmannia Root (熟地, Shudi) and Twotooth Achyranthes Root (牛膝, Niuxi). Both this formula and Decoction for Reducing Blood Sugar(降糖汤, jiang tang tang) have the actions of clearing away stomach-fire and promoting the production of body fluid for diabetes. However, the main action of Jade Maid Decoction (玉女煎, yu nu jian) is clearing away stomach-heat and nourishing yin. It is good at treating diabetes involving the middle-jiao manifested as polyorexia, emaciated body, constipation, yellow and dry tongue coating, smooth and forceful pulse compared with Decoction for Reducing Blood Sugar(降糖汤, jiang tang tang) which does not have the actions of invigorating the spleen and promoting diuresis.

3. Anemarrhena, Phellodendron and Rehmannia Pill (知柏地黄丸, zhi bai di huang wan) *Syndrome-Cause-Pulse-Treatment*《症因脉治》

This is comprised of the ingredients of Rehmanniae Pill with Six Herbs(六味地黄丸, liu wei di huang wan) plus Common Anemarrhena Rhizome (知母, Zhimu) and Chinese Corktree Bark (黄柏, Huangbai). Its actions are clearing away heat and nourishing yin. It is applicable to diabetes, especially to diabetes involving the lower-jiao manifested as polyuria, or turbid urine, or greasy urine, dry mouth and throat, red tongue, thin and rapid pulse caused by deficiency of kidney-yin, interior heat due to deficiency of yin and unconsolidation of the kidney-qi.

4. Diabetes-Relieving Formula(消渴方, xiao ke fang) *Elite of Effective Prescriptions of Contemporary Famous Doctors of China* 《中华当代名医妙方精华》

This consists of Common Yam Rhizome (山药, Shanyao), Dragon's Bone (龙骨, Longgu), Calcined Oyster Shell (煅牡蛎, Duan Muli), Pilose Asiabell Root (党参, Dangshen), Figwort Root (玄参, Xuanshen), Dwarf Lilyturf Root (麦门冬, Maimendong), Common Anemarrhena Rhizome (知母, Zhimu) and Snakegourd Root (天花粉, Tianhuafen). Its actions are replenishing qi, promoting the production of body fluid, quenching thirst and decreasing urination. It is suited to diabetes involving the lower-jiao due to deficiency of both qi and yin, manifested by profuse and clear urine, frequency of urination, soreness of loins and tiredness, palpitation, shortness of breath, light red tongue, thin and weak pulse.

5. Blood Sugar-Reducing Formula (降糖方, jiang tang fang) *Elite of Effective Prescriptions of Contemporary Famous Doctors of China* 《中华当代名医妙方精华》

This is comprised of Membranous Milkvetch Root (生黄芪, Sheng Huangqi), Dried Rehmannia Root (生地, Shengdi), Swordlike Atractylodes Rhizome (苍术, Cangzhu), Figwort Root (元参, Yuanshen), Lobed Kudzuvine Root (葛根, Gegen) and Dan-Shen Root (丹参, Danshen). Its actions are replenishing qi, nourishing yin and activating blood circulation. It is used for diabetes due to deficiency of qi and yin.

Goiter-Curing Decoction
(平甲汤, ping jia tang)

Source: *Elite of Effective Prescriptions of Contemporary Famous Doctors of China* 《中华当代名医妙方精华》

Composition: Seaweed (海藻, Haizao)30g

Chinese Gentian Root (龙胆草, Longdancao)3g

Oyster Shell (生牡蛎, Sheng Muli)30g

Nacre (珍珠母, Zhenzhumu)30g

Thunberg Fritillary Bulb (浙贝母, Zhe Beimu)9g

Common Selfheal Fruit-Spike (夏枯草, Xiakucao)30g

Baikal Skullcap Root (黄芩, Huangqin)3g

Licorice Root (生甘草, Sheng Gancao)3g

Red Peony Root (赤芍, Chishao)9g

Natural Indigo (青黛, Qingdai)3g

Clam Shell (海蛤壳, Haigeqiao) 12g
Plantainseed (车前子, Cheqianzi) 12g

Actions: Clearing away heat from the liver and regulating flow of qi, softening hardness and dissipating blockages.

Applied Syndrome: Goiter due to accumulation of phlegm and blood stasis resulting from transformation of fire by stagnation of the liver-qi, manifested by mass over the neck, exophthalmos, palpitation and insomnia, irritability, polyorexia, or emaciated body, flushed face, profuse sweating, tremor of the hands, red tongue, wiry and rapid pulse.

Goiter-Curing Decoction
(Hardness-Softening and Mass-Dissipating Method)

Ingredients	Effects	Combined Effects	Syndrome	Chief Symptoms
Seaweed (海藻, Haizao) 30g Thunberg Fritillary Bulb (浙贝母, Zhe Beimu) 9g Oyster Shell (生牡蛎, Sheng Muli) 30g	Softening hardness and dissipating blockages	Clearing away liver-heat and regulating qi, softening hardness and dissipating blockages	Goiter	Mass over the neck, exophthalmos, palpitation and insomnia, polyorexia, profuse sweating, red tongue, wiry and rapid pulse
Natural Indigo (青黛, Qingdai) 3g Clam Shell (海蛤壳, Haigeqiao) 12g	Clearing away heat and removing phlegm			
Common Selfheal Fruit-Spike (夏枯草, Xiakucao) 30g Chinese Gentian Root (龙胆草, Longdancao) 3g Baikal Skullcap Root (黄芩, Huangqin) 3g Plantain Seed (车前子, Cheqianzi) 12g	Clearing away heat of the liver meridian, promoting urination and removing phlegm			
Red Peony Root (赤芍, Chishao) 9g	Activating blood circulation and dissipating blockages			
Nacre (珍珠母, Zhenzhumu) 30g	Tranquilizing the mind and checking exuberance of yang			
Licorice Root (生甘草, Sheng Gancao) 3g	Coordinating the actions of various ingredients in a Prescription			

Points in Constitution: This formula is similar to Jade Kettle Decoction of Seaweed (海藻玉壶汤, hai zao yu hu tang) in action. Though the ingredients of the two Prescription are different, the treating principle is same. In comparision, this formula has a strong heat-removing action because the liver-heat is severe.

Indication: Hyperparathyroidism.

Precaution: Adding Stir-Backed Pangolin Scales (炮山甲, Paoshanjia), Peach Seed (桃仁, Taoren) and Honeysuckle Stem (忍冬藤, Rendongteng) for the case accompanied with nodes; adding Scorpion (全蝎, Quanxie) and Gambirplant Hooked Stem and Branch (钩藤, Gouteng) for the case with tremor of hands.

Associated Formula:

Hyperparathyroidism-Treating Decoction with Five Methods (五法合一甲亢汤, wu fa he yi jia kang tang) *Elite of Effective Prescriptions of Contemporary Famous Doctors of China* 《中华当代名医妙方精华》

This consists of White Peony Root (白芍药, Baishaoyao), Smoked Plum (乌梅, Wumei), Common Floweringquince Fruit (木瓜, Mugua), Chinese Thorowax Root (柴胡, Chaihu), Coastal Glehnia Root and Fourleaf Ladybell Root (沙参, Shashen), Dwarf Lilyturf Root (麦门冬, Maimendong), Dendrobium Herb (石斛, Shihu), Largehead Atractylodes Rhizome (白术, Baizhu), Lotus Seed (莲子, Lianzi), Mulberry Leaf (桑叶, Sangye) and Cape Jasmine Fruit (山栀子, Shanzhizi). Its main action is purging heat of the liver with sour drugs. Besides, it has the actions of nourishing yin, invigorating the spleen, removing phlegm and clearing away heat. It is suited to hyperparathyroidism.

An Obesity-Reducing Formula
(轻身一方, qing shen yi fang)

Source: *Journal of Traditional Chinese Medicine* 《中医杂志》
Composition: Membranous Milkvetch Root (黄芪, Huangqi)15g
Fourstamen Stephania Root (汉防己, Han Fangji)15g
Largehead Atractylodes Rhizome (白术, Baizhu)15g
Szechwan Lovage Rhizome (川芎, Chuanxiong)15g
Prepared Tuber Fleeceflower Root (制何首乌, Zhiheshouwu)15g
Oriental Waterplantain Rhizome (泽泻, Zexie)30g
Hawthorn Fruit (山楂, Shanzha)30g
Dan-Shen Root (丹参, Danshen)30g
Capillary Wormwood Herb (茵陈, Yinchen)30g
Buffalo Horn (水牛角, Shuiniujiao)30g
Rhubarb (大黄, Dahuang)6g
Shorthorned Epimedium Herb (淫羊藿, Yinyanghuo)9g

Actions: Invigorating the spleen and expelling dampness, eliminating turbid evils and reducing blood lipid.

An Obesity-Reducing Formula
(Spleen-Strengthening and Dampness-Removing Method)

Ingredients	Effects	Combined Effects	Syndrome	Chief Symptoms
Membranous Milkvetch Root (黄芪, Huangqi) 15g	Replenishing qi and lifting yang, promoting urination and reducing swelling	Invigorating the spleen and expelling dampness, eliminating turbid evils and reducing blood lipid	Simple obesity (due to deficiency of the spleen and kidney-yang, accumulation of phlegm and dampness in the interior)	Fatness or corpulence, listlessness, tiredness, lumbago, loose stool, pale tongue with greasy coating, deep and thin pulse
Fourstamen Stephania Root (汉防己, Han Fangji) 15g	Expelling wind-dampness, promoting urination and removing dampness			
Shorthorned Epimedium Herb (淫羊藿, Yinyanghuo) 9g Largehead Atractylodes Rhizome (白术, Baizhu) 15g Oriental Waterplantain Rhizome (泽泻, Zexie) 30g	Invigorating the spleen, drying dampness and promoting diuresis			
Prepared Tuber Fleeceflower Root (制何首乌, Zhiheshouwu) 15g Rhubarb (大黄, Dahuang) 6g	Relaxing the bowels and purging turbid material			
Szechwan Lovage Rhizome (川芎, Chuanxiong) 15g Dan-Shen Root (丹参, Danshen) 30g	Activating blood circulation and dissolving blood stasis			
Hawthorn Fruit (山楂, Shanzha) 30g Capillary Wormwood Herb (茵陈, Yinchen) 30g Buffalo Horn (水牛角, Shuiniujiao) 30g	Normalizing the secretion of gallbladder and reducing blood lipid			

Applied Syndrome: Simple obesity. Deficiency of the spleen and kidney yang may cause retention of fluid in the body which may then transform into phlegm, leading to accumulation of phlegm and dampness in the interior, manifested by fatness or corpulence, listlessness and tiredness, oppressing feeling in the chest and tachypnea, lumbago, loose stool, edema, or irregular menstruation, pale tongue with greasy coating, deep and thin pulse.

Points in Constitution: This formula is the modification of Fourstamen Stephania and Membranous Decoction (防己黄芪汤, fang ji huang qi tang). The ancients said: "Corpulent persons usually have dampness". They also said: "Fat persons are usually in the condition of qi deficiency". Obesity is mostly due to deficiency of qi which fails to transport the body fluid and causes body fluid accumulating in the interior, and then transforming into phlegm. If the phlegm accumulates outside the vessels, the striae is full of it and if it accumulates within the vessels, the blood stagnation may be brought about. Fourstamen Stephania and Membranous Decoction (防己黄芪汤, fang ji huang qi tang) has the actions of improving transformation of qi and promoting the flow of body fluid which just corresponds to the pathogenesis. This formula also contains the drugs for regulating flow of blood and removing blood stasis. Thus, it can eliminate dampness and dredge vessels. This formula not only treats the secondary aspect but also the primary aspect of the illness.

Indications:
1. Simple obesity.
2. Hyperlipemia.

Precautions:
1. This formula is not suitable for obesity without excessive phlegm and dampness.
2. This formula should be forbidden for pregnant women.

Associated Formulas:

1. Capillary Wormwood Lipid-Reducing Formula (茵陈降脂方, yin chen jiang zhi fang) *Shanghai Journal of Traditional Chinese Medicine* 《上海中医药杂志》

This is comprised of Capillary Wormwood Herb (茵陈, Yinchen), Hawthorn Fruit (山楂, Shanzha) and Malt (麦芽, Maiya). Its actions are clearing away heat and resolving dampness, activating the spleen-qi and eliminating turbids. It is applicable to hyperlipemia.

2. General Recipe for Treating Fatigue (疲劳统治方, pi lao tong zhi fang) *Author's Experienced Prescription* (笔者经验方)

This is comprised of Chinese Magnolia Vine (五味子, Wuweizi), Smoked Plum (乌梅, Wumei), Dogwood Fruit (山茱萸, Shanzhuyu), Common Floweringguince Fruit (木瓜, Mugua), Cherokee Rose Fruit (金樱子, Jinyingzi), Barbary Woltberry Fruit (枸杞子, Goqizi), Common Yam (山药, Shanyao) and Hairyvein Agrimonia Herb (仙鹤草, Xianhecao). Its actions are enriching blood and nourishing the liver. It is indicated for a person's sub-health condition marked by physical and mental fatigue.

Hemocyte-Increasing Mixture
(升血合剂, sheng xue he ji)

Source: *Zhejiang Journal of Traditional Chinese Medicine*《浙江中医杂志》
Composition: Prepared Fleeceflower Root (制何首乌, Zhi Heshouwu) 15g
Asiatic Cornelian Cherry Fruit (山茱萸, Shanzhuyu) 9g
Glossy Privet Fruit (女贞子, Nüzhenzi) 9g
Shorthorned Epimedium Herb (淫羊藿, Yinyanghuo) 9g
Dan-Shen Root (丹参, Danshen) 9g
Officinal Magnolia Bark (厚朴, Houpo) 9g
Stir-Backed Pangolin Scales (炮山甲, Pao shanjia) 9g
Suberect Spatholobus Stem (鸡血藤, Jixueteng) 30g
Prepared Licorice Root (炙甘草, Zhi Gancao) 6g

Actions: Enriching the blood, activating blood circulation and dissolving blood stasis.

Applied Syndrome: Leukocytopenia after chemotherapy which is manifested by vertigo, tinnitus, brittle and sparse hair, sallow complexion, listlessness and reluctance to speak, reddish tongue, thin and weak pulse.

Points in Constitution: It is said that prolonged illness surely results in deficiency, prolonged illness will affect the collaterals and then cause blood stasis, which can't be ignored in the treatment. This formula uses the blood stasis-removing drugs in the course of tonifying essence and blood so as to eliminate the blood stasis and promote the generation of blood simultaneously.

Indications:
1. Leukocytopenia after chemotherapy for malignancy.
2. Anaemia due to a severe disease, a prolonged disease or after childbirth.

Precaution: This formula is designed to vertigo due to blood stasis in the interior resulting from deficiency of qi and blood. Thus, it is not suitable for vertigo due to hyperactivity of liver-yang which attacks upwards the clear orifices, or the vertigo due to upward floating of yang in deficiency condition resulting from deficiency of liver-yin and kidney-yin.

Associated Formulas:

1. Ginseng Decoction (人参汤, ren shen tang) *Female Branch of Standards for Diagnosis and Treatment*《证治准绳女科》

This is comprised of Ginseng (人参, Renshen), Dwarf Lilyturf Root (麦门冬, Maimendong), Prepared Rehmannia Root (熟地黄, Shudihuang), Main Part of Chinese Angelica Root (当归身, Dangguishen), White Peony Root (白芍药, Baishaoyao), Toasted Membranous Milkvetch Root (炙黄芪, Zhi Huangqi), Tuckahoe (茯苓, Fuling) and Prepared Licorice Root (炙甘草, Zhi Gancao). Its actions are replenishing qi, nourishing yin and enriching the blood. It is suited to vertigo and palpitation due to postpartum hemorrhage.

2. Ginseng Blood-tonitfying Decoction (人参养血汤, ren shen yang xue tang) *Prescriptions*

Hemocyte-Increasing Mixture
(Blood-Enriching and Circulation-Activating Method)

Ingredients	Effects	Combined Effects	Syndrome	Chief Symptoms
Prepared Fleeceflower Root (制何首乌, Zhi Heshouwu)15g Asiatic Cornelian Cherry Fruit (山茱萸, Shanzhuyu)9g Shorthorned Epimedium Herb (淫羊藿, Yinyanghuo)9g Glossy Privet Fruit (女贞子, Nüzhenzi)9g	Replenishing the liver and kidney and nourishing essence and blood	Enriching the blood and nourishing yin, activating blood circulation and dissolving blood stasis	Qi deficiency with blood stasis	Vertigo, tinnitus, brittle and sparse hair, sallow complexion, listlessness and reluctance to speak, pale tongue, thin and weak pulse
Suberect Spatholobus Stem (鸡血藤, Jixueteng)30g Dan-Shen Root (丹参, Danshen)9g Stir-Backed Pangolin Scales (炮山甲, Pao shanjia)9g	Dissolving blood stasis and producing new blood			
Officinal Magnolia Bark (厚朴, Houpo)9g	Regulating flow of qi and regulating the middle-jiao			
Prepared Licorice Root (炙甘草, Zhi Gancao)6g	Coordinating the actions of various ingredients in a Prescription			

of Peaceful Benevolent Dispensary《和剂局方》

This is made up of Smoked Plum (乌梅, Wumei), Prepared Rehmannia Root (熟地黄, Shudihuang), Main Part of Chinese Angelica Root (当归身, Dangguishen), Ginseng (人参, Renshen), Szechwan Lovage Rhizome (川芎, Chuanxiong), Red Peony Root (赤芍, Chishao) and Grassleaf Sweetflag Rhizome (石菖蒲, Shichangpu). Its actions are tonifying Chong and Ren Meridians, regulating the blood circulation, removing heat evil and relieving arthralgia due to cold. It is applicable to metrorrhagia, vertigo, postpartum and emaciated body due to weak body resistance and deficiency of blood and qi.

3. Ginseng Nutrition Decoction (人参养荣汤, ren shen yang rong tang) *Prescriptions of*

Peaceful Benevolent Dispensary《和剂局方》

This consists of White Peony Root（白芍药，Baishaoyao）, Chinese Angelica Root（当归，Danggui）, Tangerine Peel（橘皮，Jupi）, Toasted Membranous Milkvetch Root（炙黄芪，Zhi Huangqi）, Cassia Bark（肉桂心，Rouguixin）, Ginseng（人参，Renshen）, Largehead Atractylodes Rhizome（白术，Baizhu）, Prepared Licorice Root（炙甘草，Zhi Gancao）, Prepared Rehmannia Root（熟地黄，Shudihuang）, Chinese Magnoliavine Fruit（五味子，Wuweizi）, Tuckahoe（茯苓，Fuling）and Thinleaf Milkwort Root（远志，Yuanzhi）. Its actions are replenishing qi, enriching the blood and tranquilizing the mind. It is suited to palpitation, vertigo, shortness of breath and asthma due to overstrain or consumptive disease.

4. Chinese Angelica Blood-Tonifying Decoction(当归补血汤, dang gui bu xue tang) *Differentiation on Endogenous and Exogenous Diseases*《内外伤辨惑论》

This is comprised of only two herbs, Membranous Milkvetch Root（黄芪，Huangqi）and Chinese Angelica Root（当归，Danggui）. Its actions are invigorating qi and promoting the production of blood. It is suited to fever, irritability, thirst, forceful, large and feeble pulse due to internal damage resulting from overstrain, weakness of qi and deficiency of blood.

5. Eight Treasures Decoction(八珍汤, ba zhen tang) *Classification and Treatment of Traumatic Diseases*《正体类要》

This is made up of Chinese Angelica Root（当归，Danggui）, Szechwan Lovage Rhizome（川芎，Chuanxiong）, White Peony Root（白芍药，Baishaoyao）, Prepared Rehmannia Root（熟地黄，Shudihuang）, Ginseng（人参，Renshen）, Largehead Atractylodes Rhizome（白术，Baizhu）, Tuckahoe（茯苓，Fuling）, Prepared Licorice Root（炙甘草，Zhi Gancao）, Fresh Ginger（生姜，Shengjiang）and Chinese Date（大枣，Dazao）. Its actions are replenishing qi and blood. It is suited to the syndrome of deficiency of both qi and blood.

6. Back to the Spleen Decoction(归脾汤, gui pi tang) *Prescriptions for Rescuring the Sick*《济生方》

This is comprised of Largehead Atractylodes Rhizome（白术，Baizhu）, Indian Bread with Hostwood（茯神，Fushen）, Toasted Membranous Milkvetch Root（炙黄芪，Zhi Huangqi）, Longan Aril（龙眼肉，Longyanrou）, Spine Date Seed（酸枣仁，Suanzaoren）, Ginseng（人参，Renshen）, Common Aucklandia Root（木香，Muxiang）, Prepared Licorice Root（炙甘草，Zhi Gancao）, Chinese Angelica Root（当归，Danggui）and Thinleaf Milkwort Root（远志，Yuanzhi）. Its actions are replenishing qi, enriching the blood, invigorating the spleen and nourishing heart. It is suited to the syndrome of deficiency of qi and blood or failure of the spleen in controlling blood resulting from deficiency of both the heart and spleen.

7. Blood-Producing Powder(生血散, shen xue san) *Lianning Journal of Traditional Chinese Medicine*《辽宁中医》

This is comprised of Dried Human Placenta（紫河车，Ziheche）, Malachite Ore（皂矾，Zaofan）, Cassia Bark（肉桂，Rougui）, Cuttlefish Bone（海螵蛸，Haipiaoxiao）and Ass-hide Glue（阿胶，Ejiao）. Its actions are tonifying marrow and invigorating the kidney, promoting the production of blood and arresting bleeding. It is applicable to anaemia.

8. Dan-Shen and Tuber Fleeceflower Blood-Producing Panacea(丹首生血灵, dan shou sheng

xue ling) *Experimental Prescriptions of Pediatrics of Combining Traditional Chinese with Western Medicine* 《中西医结合儿科试用新方》

This consists of Dan-Shen Root (丹参, Danshen), Prepared Tuber Fleeceflower Root (制首乌, Zhishouwu), Suberect Spatholobus Stem (鸡血藤, Jixueteng), Shorthorned Epimedium Herb (仙灵脾, Xianlingpi), Toasted Membranous Milkvetch Root (炙黄芪, Zhi Huangqi), Barbary Wolfberry Fruit (枸杞, Gouqi), Desertliving Cistanche Herb (肉苁蓉, Roucongrong), Madder Root (茜草, Qiancao) and Red Ginseng (红参, Hongshen). Its actions are replenishing qi and blood. It is suited to alopecia and leukocytopenia due to deficiency of qi and blood.

Qi-Replenishing and Rash-Dissipating Decoction
(益气化斑汤, yi qi hua ban tang)

Source: *Famous Prescriptions of the Past and Present* 《古今名方》
Composition: Toasted Membranous Milkvetch Root (炙黄芪, Zhi Huangqi)15g
Pilose Asiabell Root (党参, Dangshen)15g
Stir-Baked Largehead Atractylodes Rhizome (炒白术, Chao Baizhu)9g
Chinese Angelica Root (当归, Danggui)9g
Red Peony Root (赤芍药, Chishaoyao) 15g
White Peony Root (白芍药, Baishaoyao) 15g
Ass-hide Glue (阿胶, Ejiao)9g
Charred Human Hair (血余炭, Xueyutan)6g
Charred Tangerine Peel (橘皮炭, Jupitan)9g
Calcined Dragon's Bone (煅龙骨, Duan Longgu)15g
Calcined Oyster Shell (煅牡蛎, Duan Muli)15g
Suberect Spatholobus Stem (鸡血藤, Jixueteng)30g
Powder of Sanchi Root (三七粉, Sanqifen)3g (taking it with water)
Actions: Replenishing qi, enriching blood, dissolving blood stasis and arresting bleeding.

Applied Syndrome: Purpura, mostly due to deficiency of qi in the middle-jiao which fails to control blood and causes blood tp flow outside the vessels, manifested by subcutaneous hemorrhage, dark purplish spots, or accompanied with epistaxis, bleeding from the gum, pallor, listlessness and tiredness, dizziness, tinnitus, palpitation, anorexia, irregular defecation, dark and pale tongue with thin and white coating, thin and feeble pulse.

Points in Constitution: In this formula, the choice of drugs is based on the consideration of replenishing qi, dissolving blood stasis and inducing astringency, but the main purpose is to stop bleeding, which is a good example of attaining the same goal by taking different routes.

Indications:
1. Anaphylactoid purpura.
2. Thrombocytopenic purpura.
3. Thrombocytopenia after chemotherapy and radiotheraphy.

Qi-Replenishing and Rash-Dissipating Decoction
(Qi-Benefiting and Blood-Controlling Method)

Ingredients	Effects	Combined Effects	Syndrome	Chief Symptoms
Toasted Membranous Milkvetch Root (炙黄芪, Zhi Huangqi) 15g Pilose Asiabell Root (党参, Dangshen) 15g Stir-Baked Largehead Atractylodes Rhizome (炒白术, Chao Baizhu) 9g	Replenishing qi to control blood	Replenishing qi and enriching blood, dissolving blood stasis and arresting bleeding	Purpura (due to deficiency of qi in the middle-jiao which fails to control blood)	Subcutaneous hemorrhage, dark purplish spots, epistaxis, bleeding from the gum, pallor, listlessness and tiredness, palpitation and dizziness, dark pale tongue, thin and white coating, thin and feeble pulse
Chinese Angelica Root (当归, Danggui) 9g Ass-hide Glue (阿胶, Ejiao) 9g White Peony Root (白芍药, Baishaoyao) 15g	Nourishing yin and enriching blood			
Powder of Sanchi Root (三七粉, Sanqifen) 3g Red Peony Root (赤芍药, Chishaoyao) 15g Suberect Spatholobus Stem (鸡血藤, Jixueteng) 30g	Dissolving blood stasis and arresting bleeding			
Charred Human Hair (血余炭, Xueyutan) 6g Calcined Dragon's Bone (煅龙骨, Duan Longgu) 15g Calcined Oyster Shell (煅牡蛎, Duan Muli) 15g	Inducing astringency and arresting bleeding			
Charred Tangerine Peel (橘皮炭, Jupitan) 9g	Regulating qi and regulating the middle-jiao			

Precaution: This formula is not suitable for purpura due to blood-heat.
Associated Formulas:

1. Back to the Spleen Decoction(归脾汤, gui pi tang) *Prescriptions for Rescuing the Sick* 《济生方》

This consists of Largehead Atractylodes Rhizome(白术, Baizhu), Indian Bread with Hostwood(茯神, Fushen), Toasted Membranous Milkvetch Root(炙黄芪, Zhi Huangqi), Longan Aril(龙眼肉, Longyanrou), Spine Date Seed(酸枣仁, Suanzaoren), Ginseng(人参, Renshen), Common Aucklandia Root(木香, Muxiang), Licorice Root(甘草, Gancao), Chinese Angelica Root(当归, Danggui) and Thinleaf Milkwort Root(远志, Yuanzhi). Its actions are replenishing qi, enriching the blood, invigorating the spleen and nourishing the heart. It is suited to various hemorrhage due to deficiency of spleen-qi which fails to control blood.

2. Two Organs-Replenishing Decoction(双补汤, shuang bu tang) *Detailed Analysis of Epidemic Febrile Diseases* 《温病条辨》

This is comprised of Ginseng(人参, Renshen), Fried Common Yam Rhizome(炒山药, Chao Shanyao), Tuckahoe(茯苓, Fuling), Lotus Seed(莲子, Lianzi), Gordon Euryale Seed(芡实, Qianshi), Malaytea Scurfpea Fruit(补骨脂, Buguzhi), Desertliving Cistanche Herb(肉苁蓉, Roucongrong), Asiatic Cornelian Cherry Fruit(山茱萸, Shanzhuyu), Chinese Magnoliavine Fruit(五味子, Wuweizi), Medicinal Indian Mulberry Root(巴戟天, Bajitian), Chinese Dodder Seed(菟丝子, Tusizi) and Palmleaf Raspberry Fruit(覆盆子, Fupenzi). Its actions are warming and tonifying the spleen and kidney. It is suited to purpura with dark spots, listlessness, lassitude, anorexia, pale tongue with white coating, deep, thin and weak pulse due to deficiency of the spleen and kidney yang.

3. Purpura-Relieving Decoction(消癜汤, xiao dian tang) *Zhejiang Journal of Traditional Chinese Medicine* 《浙江中医杂志》

This consists of Pokeberry Root(商陆, Shanglu), Hairyvein Agrimonia Herb(仙鹤草, Xianhecao), Sanguisorba Root(生地榆, Sheng Diyu), Pilose Asiabell Root(党参, Dangshen), Largehead Atractylodes Rhizome(白术, Baizhu), Asiatic Cornelian Cherry Fruit(山萸肉, Shanyurou), Dan-Shen Root(丹参, Danshen), Toasted Membranous Milkvetch Root(炙黄芪, Zhi Huangqi), Prepared Tuber Fleeceflower Root(制首乌, Zhishouwu), Figwort Root(玄参, Xuanshen), Prepared Rehmannia Root(熟地黄, Shudihuang) and Licorice Root(生甘草, Sheng Gancao). Its actions are replenishing qi, activating blood circulation, invigorating the spleen and benefiting the kidney. It is suited to thrombocytopenic purpura due to deficiency of qi and stagnation of blood resulting from deficiency of the spleen and kidney.

Chapter Seven
Formulas for Gynecological Diseases

There is a long history and remarkable achievements in the prevention and treatment of gynopathy with Chinese Prescription. The theory of traditional Chinese medicine holds that woman is dominated by the liver, but tiangui (Generally referring to sexual function of both sexes, here referring to menstruation) after all is stored in the kidney from which Chong and Ren Meridians originated. Thus, the treatment of woman's diseases mostly begins with the liver and kidney. However, it should be pointed out that the diseases of anemia, hemorrhage and leucorrhea are always related to the spleen and usually due to deficiency of the spleen, which can't be ignored in the determination of treatment based on differenciation of syndromes. There are many corresponding Prescription for irregular menstruation, dysfunctional uterine bleeding, adnexitis, endometriosis, old exfetation, habitual abortion and sterility. For the diseases of ectopic pregnancy, hysteromyoma and gynecologic tumor, much clinical research has equally been done for many years by combining traditional with western medicine.

1. Szechwan Lovage and Chinese Angelica Decoction for Regulating Blood Flow
(芎归调血饮, xiong gui tiao xue yin)

Source: *Curative Measures for Diseases*《万病回春》
Composition: Chinese Angelica Root (当归, Danggui)6g
Szechwan Lovage Rhizome (川芎, Chuanxiong)6g
Prepared Rehmannia Root (熟地黄, Shudihuang)6g
Largehead Atractylodes Rhizome (白术, Baizhu)6g
Tuckahoe (茯苓, Fuling)6g
Dried Ginger (干姜, Ganjiang)3g
Nutgrass Galingale Rhizome (香附, Xiangfu)6g
Commbined Spicebush Root (乌药, Wuyao)6g
Tangerine Peel (橘皮, Jupi)6g
Tree Peony Bark (牡丹皮, Mudanpi)6g
Motherwort Herb (益母草, Yimucao)6g
Fresh Ginger (生姜, Shengjiang)3g
Chinese Date (大枣, Dazao)6g
Licorice Root (生甘草, Sheng Gancao)3g
Actions: Activating blood circulation and dissolving blood stasis, expelling cold and alleviating

pain.

Applied Syndrome: Lower abdominal pain after childbirth or during menstruation due to deficiency of qi and blood accompanying with blood stasis, manifested as lower abdominal pain with tenderness, hemorrhage, dark purple blood with clot, dripping bleeding, blue and white complexion, dark purplish tongue, wiry and unsmooth pulse.

Szechwan Lovage and Chinese Angelica Decoction for Regulating Blood Flow
(Blood-Activating and Stasis-Removing Method)

Ingredients	Effects	Combined Effects	Syndrome	Chief Symptoms
Chinese Angelica Root (当归, Danggui)6g Szechwan Lovage Rhizome (川芎, Chuanxiong)6g Prepared Rehmannia Root (熟地黄, Shudihuang)6g	Enriching and regulating blood	Activating blood circulation and dissolving blood stasis, expelling cold and alleviating pain	Lower abdominal pain (due to blood deficiency with blood stasis)	Postpartum abdominal pain and tenderness, or lochiorrhea after childbirth, dysmenorrhea, dark purple blood with clot, dark purplish tongue, wiry and unsmooth pulse
Motherwort Herb (益母草, Yimucao)6g Tree Peony Bark (牡丹皮, Mudanpi)6g	Activating blood circulation and removing blood stasis			
Nutgrass Galingale Rhizome (香附, Xiangfu)6g Commbined Spicebush Root (乌药, Wuyao)6g	Activating flow of qi and alleviating pain			
Largehead Atractylodes Rhizome (白术, Baizhu)6g Tuckahoe (茯苓, Fuling)6g	Replenishing qi and invigorating the spleen			
Dried Ginger (干姜, Ganjiang)3g	Warming the meridian and expelling cold			
Tangerine Peel (橘皮, Jupi)6g	Regulating the stomach-qi			
Fresh Ginger (生姜, Shengjiang)3g Chinese Date (大枣, Dazao)6g Licorice Root (生甘草, Sheng Gancao)3g	Warming the middle-jiao and replenishing the healthy qi			

Points in Constitution: The disease, after childbirth, is prone to change because of the patient's weakness and stagnation of blood. This formula has a replenishing action. It can strengthen the body resistance but does not bring about stagnation of blood; it can dispel stasis but does not consume the healthy qi. The characteristic of this formula is that it can invigorate qi, tonify blood, promote circulation of qi and activate flow of blood at the same time, which is aimed at treating the primary aspect to relieve various symptoms after childbirth.

Indications:

1. Postpartum abdominal pain, lochiorrhea.
2. Postpartum neurasthenia.
3. Irregular menstruation.

Precaution: This formula is contraindicated in postpartum infection and attack of the uterus due to pathogenic heat, dampness and toxic material.

Associated Formulas:

1. Ten Strong Tonic Herbs Decoction (十全大补汤, shi quan da bu tang) *Prescriptions of Peaceful Benevolent Dispensary*《和剂局方》

This consists of Ginseng (人参, Renshen), Cassia Bark (肉桂, Rougui), Szechwan Lovage Rhizome (川芎, Chuanxiong), Prepared Rehmannia Root (熟地黄, Shudihuang), Tuckahoe (茯苓, Fuling), Largehead Atractylodes Rhizome (白术, Baizhu), Licorice Root (甘草, Gancao), Membranous Milkvetch Root (黄芪, Huangqi), Chinese Angelica Root (当归, Danggui) and White Peony Root (白芍药, Baishaoyao). Its actions are warming and replenishing qi and blood. It is indicated for emission, blood loss, female metrorrhagia and metrostaxis, irregular menstruation, comsuptive diseases with asthma and cough due to deficiency of both qi and blood.

2. Szechwan Lovage Rhizome, Chinese Angelica Root, Ass-hide Glue and Argy Wormwood Leaf Decoction (芎归胶艾汤, xiong gui jiao ai tang) *Synopsis of Golden Cabinet*《金匮要略》

This is comprised of Szechwan Lovage Rhizome (川芎, Chuanxiong), Ass-hide Glue (阿胶, Ejiao), Licorice Root (生甘草, Sheng Gancao), Argy Wormwood Leaf (艾叶, Aiye), Chinese Angelica Root (当归, Danggui), White Peony Root (白芍药, Baishaoyao) and Prepared Rehmannia Root (干地黄, Gandihuang). Its actions are enriching blood and regulating menstruation, arresting bleeding and preventing miscarriage. It is applicable for deficiency and damage of the Chong and Ren Meridians in woman manifested by metrorrhagia and metrostaxis, menorrhagia, continuous bleeding, or miscarriage with continuous bleeding, or bleeding during pregnancy with abdominal pain.

2. Zhechong Decoction
(折冲饮, zhe chong yin)

Source: *Treatise on Delivery*《产论》
Composition: Chinese Angelica Root (当归, Danggui) 6g
Szechwan Lovage Rhizome (川芎, Chuanxiong) 6g

White Peony Root (白芍药, Baishaoyao)6g
Tree Peony Bark (牡丹皮, Mudanpi)6g
Peach Seed (桃仁, Taoren)6g
Safflower (红花, Honghua)3g
Corydalis Tuber (延胡索, Yanhusuo)3g
Cassia Twig (桂枝, Guizhi)3g
Twotooth Achyranthes Root (牛膝, Niuxi)6g

Actions: Activating blood circulation and removing blood stasis, warming the meridian and alleviating pain.

Applied Syndrome: Female abdominal pain due to blood stasis, manifested as pain in the lower abdomen with tenderness which is relieved by warming, impediment of menstrual flow, purple blood clots, dark purplish tongue, unsmooth pulse.

Zhechong Decoction
(Blood-Activating and Stasis-Removing Method)

Ingredients	Effects	Combined Effects	Syndrome	Chief Symptoms
Chinese Angelica Root (当归, Danggui)6g White Peony Root (白芍药, Baishaoyao)6g Szechwan Lovage Rhizome (川芎, Chuanxiong)6g Peach Seed (桃仁, Taoren)6g Safflower (红花, Honghua)3g Tree Peony Bark (牡丹皮, Mudanpi)6g Corydalis Tuber (延胡索, Yanhusuo)3g	Activating blood circulation and dissolving blood stasis, restoring menstrual flow and alleviating pain	Activating blood circulation and removing blood stasis, warming the meridian and alleviating pain	Stagnation of blood	Pain in the lower abdomen with tenderness which is relieved by warming, impediment of menstrual flow, purple blood clots, dark purplish tongue, unsmooth pulse
Cassia Twig (桂枝, Guizhi)3g	Warming the meridian and alleviating pain			
Twotooth Achyranthes Root (牛膝, Niuxi)6g	Activating blood circulation, dissipating blood stasis and conducting the effect of drugs downward			

Points in Constitution: This formula is the modified Four Herbs Decoction (四物汤, si wu tang) without Prepared Rehmannia Root (熟地黄, Shudihuang). The so-called Zhechong in fact means activating blood circulation. The characteristic of this formula lies in the good use of the

Cassia Twig (桂枝, Guizhi), which can warm the meridian and aid in pomoting blood circulation, and Twotooth Achyranthes Root (牛膝, Niuxi), which can conduct the effect of the other drugs downward and remove blood stasis in the lower-jiao.

Indications:
1. Chronic adnexitis.
2. Irregular menstruation, dysmenorrhea.
3. Postpartum lochiostasis, or lochiorrhea.
4. Lumbago.

Precaution: This formula is forbidden for abdominal pain due to deficiency of blood or menorrhagia.

Associated Formulas:

1. Twotooth Achyranthes Root Powder (牛膝散, niu qi san) *Effective Prescription for Diseases of Women* 《妇人良方》

This is the Zhechong Decoction (折冲饮, zhe chong yin) without Szechwan Lovage Rhizome (川芎, Chuanxiong) and Safflower (红花, Honghua) but plus Common Aucklandia Root (木香, Muxiang). Its actions are activating flow of qi and circulation of blood, regulating menstruation and alleviating pain. It is suited to dysmenorrhea due to blood stasis manifested as impediment of menstrual flow, abdominal pain or the pain radiating to the chest, hypochondrium and the lumbaosacral region. It is also indicated for lochiorrhea after childbirth with abdominal pain.

2. Cassia Twig and Tuckahoe Pill (桂枝茯苓丸, gui zhi fu ling wan) *Synopsis of Golden Cabinet* 《金匮要略》

It is comprised of Cassia Twig (桂枝, Guizhi), Tuckahoe (茯苓, Fuling), Tree Peony Bark (牡丹皮, Mudanpi), Peach Seed (桃仁, Taoren) and White Peony Root (白芍药, Baishaoyao). Its actions are activating blood circulation, removing blood stasis and gradually resolving mass. It is suited to mass in the lower abdomen of women, metrostaxis, or difficulty of menstrual flow, or distention and pain in the abdomen during menstruation, or retention of placenta, or missed labor, or lochiorrhea after childbirth with abdominal pain and tenderness.

3. Lower Abdomen Blood Stasis-Dispelling Decoction (少腹逐瘀汤, shao fu zhu yu tang) *Correction of Medical Classics* 《医林改错》

This is comprised of Fennel Fruit (小茴香, Xiaohuixiang), Dried Ginger (干姜, Ganjiang), Trogopterus Dung (五灵脂, Wulingzhi), Chinese Angelica Root (当归, Danggui), Szechwan Lovage Rhizome (川芎, Chuanxiong), Cassia Bark (肉桂, Rougui), Myrrh (没药, Moyao), Red Peony Root (赤芍, Chishao), Cattail Pollen (生蒲黄, Sheng Puhuang), Corydalis Tuber (延胡索, Yanhusuo). Its actions are activating blood circulation and dissolving blood stasis, warming the meridian and alleviating pain. It is suited to mass in the lower abdomen with pain or without pain, or pain in the lower abdomen without mass, or feeling of distention and fullness in the lower abdomen, or soreness of the loins during menstruation, or three to five times of menstruation per month, continuous bleeding, purple or dark blood, or with clots, or metrorrhagia or metrostaxis, accompanying with lower abdominal pain, or leucorrhea with pink discharge.

3. Liver-Clearing and Depression-Alleviating Decoction
(清肝达郁饮, qing gan da yu yin)

Source: *Treatise onPopular Treatise on Exogenous Febrile Diseases* 《通俗伤寒论》

Composition: Charred Cape Jasmine Fruit (焦山栀, Jiaoshanzhi)9g

White Peony Root (白芍药, Baishaoyao)6g

Chinese Angelica Root (当归, Danggui)3g

Chinese Thorowax Root (柴胡, Chaihu)3g

Tree Peony Bark (牡丹皮, Mudanpi)6g

Prepared Licorice Root (炙甘草, Zhi Gancao)3g

Tangerine Peel (橘皮, Jupi)3g

Wild Mint Herb (薄荷, Bohe)3g

Chrysanthemum Flower (菊花, Juhua)6g

Tangerine Leaf (青橘叶, Qing Juye)6g

Actions: Dispersing constrained liver-qi and alleviating mental depression, clearing away heat and purging fire.

Applied Syndrome: Fire-syndrome due to stagnation of the liver-qi, manifested by fullness feeling in the chest and pain in the hypochondrium, irritability, bitter taste in the mouth, restlessness, or irregular menstruation, or alternating episodes of chills and fever, yellow tongue coating, wiry and rapid pulse.

Points in Constitution: This formula is the modified Tree Peony Bark and Cape Jasmine Fruit Plus Merry Life Powder(丹栀逍遥散, dan zhi xiao yao san)by removing such spleen-replenising drugs as Tuckahoe (茯苓, Fuling) and Largehead Atractylodes Rhizome (白术, Baizhu) but adding Tangerine Peel (橘皮, Jupi) and Tangerine Leaf (橘叶, Juye) to sooth the liver and relieve the depressed-qi. It is especially designed for the fire-syndrome due to stagnation of qi, and is applicable to irregular menstruation due to mental depression and stagnation of qi.

Indications:

1. Irregular menstruation.
2. Climacteric syndrome.
3. Vegetative nerve functional disturbance.
4. Adnexitis.
5. Cholecystitis.

Associated Formulas:

1. Merry Life Powder(逍遥散, xiao yao san) *Treatise on Prescriptions of Peaceful Benevolent Dispensary*《和剂局方》

This is comprised of Chinese Thorowax Root (柴胡, Chaihu), Chinese Angelica Root (当归, Danggui), White Peony Root (白芍药, Baishaoyao), Largehead Atractylodes Rhizome (白术, Baizhu), Tuckahoe (茯苓, Fuling), Wild Mint Herb (薄荷, Bohe), Prepared Licorice Root (炙

甘草, Zhi Gancao) and Roasted Ginger (煨姜, Weijiang). Its actions are soothing the liver and alleviating depressed-qi, invigorating the spleen and enriching blood. It is indicated for irregular menstruation due to deficiency of blood, stagnation of liver-qi and deficiency of the spleen.

Liver-Clearing and Depression-Alleviating Decoction
(Liver-Dispersing and Fire-Purging Method)

Ingredients	Effects	Combined Effects	Syndrome	Chief Symptoms
Chinese Thorowax Root (柴胡, Chaihu) 3g	Dispersing constrained liver-qi and alleviating mental depression	Dispersing constrained liver-qi and alleviating mental depression and purging liver fire	Fire derived from stagnation of the liver-qi	Pain in the hypochondrium and feeling of fullness in the chest, irritability and bitter taste in the mouth, or irregular menstruation, or alternating episodes of chills and fever, yellow tongue coating, wiry and rapid pulse
Charred Cape Jasmine Fruit (焦山栀, Jiaoshanzhi) 9g Tree Peony Bark (牡丹皮, Mudanpi) 6g	Purging heat of the liver and removing heat from the blood and activating blood circulation			
White Peony Root (白芍药, Baishaoyao) 6g Chinese Angelica Root (当归, Danggui) 3g	Enriching blood and nourishing liver yin			
Tangerine Peel (橘皮, Jupi) 3g 青 Tangerine Leaf (橘叶, Juye) 6g	Activating qi flow and alleviating pain			
Wild Mint Herb (薄荷, Bohe) 3g Chrysanthemum Flower (菊花, Juhua) 6g	Dispersing stagnated heat			
Prepared Licorice Root (炙甘草, Zhi Gancao) 3g	Coordinating the actions of various ingredients in a Prescription			

2. Bupleurum Liver-Soothing Powder (柴胡舒肝散, chai hu shu gan san) *Treatise on Jingyue's Complete Works* 《景岳全书》

This is comprised of Tangerine Peel (橘皮, Jupi), Chinese Thorowax Root (柴胡, Chaihu), Szechwan Lovage Rhizome (川芎, Chuanxiong), Nutgrass Galingale Rhizome (香附, Xiangfu), Bitter Orange (枳壳, Zhiqiao), White Peony Root (白芍药, Baishaoyao) and Licorice Root (甘草, Gancao). Its actions are activating flow of qi and alleviating pain. It is suited to pain in the hypochondrium due to stagnation of liver-qi.

3. Three Herbs Baikal Skullcap Decoction (三物黄芩汤, san wu huang qin tang) *Synopsis of Golden Cabinet* 《金匮要略》

This is comprised of Baikal Skullcap Root (黄芩, Huangqin), Lightyellow Sophora Root (苦参, Kushen) and Dried Rehmannia Root (生地黄, Shengdihuang). Its actions are nourishing yin and clearing away heat. It is suited to postpartum fever and climacteric syndrome due to deficiency of yin and blood heat. It is also indicated for tinea and cutaneous pruritus.

4. Motherwort Gold-Exceeding Pill
(益母胜金丹, yi mu sheng jin dan)

Source: *Treatise on Comprehension of Medicine* 《医学心悟》
Composition: Motherwort Herb (益母草, Yimucao) 9g
Motherwort Fruit (茺蔚子, Chongweizi) 6g
Chinese Angelica Root (当归, Danggui) 6g
Prepared Rehmannia Root (熟地黄, Shudihuang) 9g
White Peony Root (白芍药, Baishaoyao) 6g
Szechwan Lovage Rhizome (川芎, Chuanxiong) 3g
Dan-Shen Root (丹参, Danshen) 9g
Largehead Atractylodes Rhizome (白术, Baizhu) 6g
Nutgrass Galingale Rhizome (香附, Xiangfu) 6g
Actions: Enriching blood, activating blood circulation and regulating menstruation.
Applied Syndrome: Irregular menstruation due to blood stasis manifested as irregular menstrual period, abdominal pain during menstruation, impediment of menstrual flow with blood clots, or scanty menstruation, or amenorrhea, lusterless complexin, dizziness, pale tongue or with ecchymosis, deep, thin and unsmooth pulse.
Points in Constitution: This formula is based on Four Herbs Decoction (四物汤, si wu tang) and modified by adding Motherwort Fruit (茺蔚子, Chongweizi), Motherwort Herb (益母草, Yimucao) and Dan-Shen Root (丹参, Danshen) which have the action of activating blood circulation to treat irregular menstruation due to deficiency of blood and blood stasis. Nutgrass Galingale Rhizome (香附, Xiangfu) was regarded by ancient physician as the "monarch drug for diseases due to qi disorder and Commanding drug for all women diseases" and it is often used for irregular menstruation.

Indications:
1. Irregular menstruation.
2. Dysmenorrhea.

Associated Formulas:

1. Motherwort Herb Ointment (益母草膏, yi mu cao gao) *Treatise on Shanghai Standard for Materia Medica* 《上海市药品标准》

This is made up of Motherwort Herb (益母草, Yimucao) and Red Sugar (赤砂糖, Chishatang). Its actions are activating blood circulation and regulating menstruation. It is suited to irregular menstruation and postpartum abdominal pain due to blood stasis.

2. Four-Processed Nutgrass Galingale Pill (四制香附丸, si zhi xiang fu wan) *Complete Collection of Jingyue's Treatise* 《景岳全书》

This is comprised of Nutgrass Galingale Rhizome (香附, Xiangfu), Prepared Rehmannia Root (熟地黄, Shudihuang), White Peony Root (白芍药, Baishaoyao), Chinese Angelica Root (当归, Danggui), Szechwan Lovage Rhizome (川芎, Chuanxiong), Tangerine Peel (橘皮, Jupi), Largehead Atractylodes Rhizome (白术, Baizhu), Licorice Root (生甘草, Sheng Gancao), Chinese Corktree Bark (黄柏, Huangbai) and Hirsute Shiny Bugleweed Herb (泽兰叶, Zelanye). Its actions are enriching blood, regulating menstruation, activating flow of qi and alleviating depressed qi. It is indicated for irregular menstruation and abdominal pain during menstruation due to stagnation of qi.

Motherwort Gold-Exceeding Pill
(Blood-Tonifying and Circulation-Activating Method)

Ingredients	Effects	Combined Effects	Syndrome	Chief Symptoms
Chinese Angelica Root (当归, Danggui)6g Prepared Rehmannia Root (熟地黄, Shudihuang)9g White Peony Root (白芍药, Baishaoyao)6g Szechwan Lovage Rhizome (川芎, Chuanxiong)3g	Enriching and regulating the blood	Enriching the blood and activating blood circulation, regulating menstruation and relieving pain	Irregular menstruation due to blood stasis	Irregular menstrual period, abdominal pain during menstruation, blood clots, or amenorrhea, or scanty menstruation, lusterless complexin, dizziness, pale tongue, deep, thin and unsmooth pulse
Motherwort Herb (益母草, Yimucao)9g Motherwort Fruit (茺蔚子, Chongweizi)6g Dan-Shen Root (丹参, Danshen)9g	Activating blood circulation and dissolving blood stasis			
Nutgrass Galingale Rhizome (香附, Xiangfu)6g	Regulating flow of qi and alleviating pain			
Largehead Atractylodes Rhizome (白术, Baizhu)6g	Replenishing qi and invigorating the spleen			

3. Goddess Powder(女神散, nu sheng san) *Letters on Eerroneous Use of Prescriptions* 《勿误药室方函》

This is composed of Nutgrass Galingale Rhizome (香附, Xiangfu), Common Aucklandia Root (木香, Muxiang), Areca Seed (槟榔, Binglang), Chinese Angelica Root (当归, Danggui), Szechwan Lovage Rhizome (川芎, Chuanxiong), Ginseng (人参, Renshen), Swordlike Atractylodes Rhizome (苍术, Cangzhu), Licorice Root (甘草, Gancao), Cassia Twig (桂枝, Guizhi),

Clove Flower-Bud (丁香, Dingxiang), Coptis Rhizome (黄连, Huanglian) and Baikal Skullcap Root (黄芩, Huangqin). Its actions are regulating flow of qi, activating blood circulation, keeping the adverse qi downwards and alleviating pain. It is applicable for various female syndromes due to qi stagnation and blood stasis, manifested by stuffiness feeling in the chest, dizziness, tension, insomnia, irregular menstruation, dysmenorrhea, postpartum abdominal pain, lochiostasis, deep and forceful pulse. It is also suited to chronic abdominal pain and climacteric syndrome in women.

4. Meridian-Warming Decoction(温经汤, wen jing tang) *Synopsis of Golden Cabinet* 《金匮要略》

This is comprised of Medicinal Evodia Fruit (吴茱萸, Wuzhuyu), Chinese Angelica Root (当归, Danggui), White Peony Root (白芍药, Baishaoyao), Szechwan Lovage Rhizome (川芎, Chuanxiong), Ginseng (人参, Renshen), Cassia Twig (桂枝, Guizhi), Ass-hide Glue (阿胶, Ejiao), Tree Peony Bark (牡丹皮, Mudanpi), Fresh Ginger (生姜, Shengjiang), Prepared Licorice Root (炙甘草, Zhi Gancao), Pinellia Rhizome (半夏, Banxia) and Dwarf Lilyturf Root (麦门冬, Maimendong). Its actions are warming the meridian and expelling cold, enriching blood and dissolving blood stasis. It is indicated for irregular menstruation due to blood stasis resulting from deficiency-cold of Chong and Ren Meridians.

5. Menstruation-Normalizing Decoction
(顺经汤, shun jing tang)

Source: *Treatise on Fu Qingzhu's Obstetrics and Gynecology* 《傅青主女科》
Composition: Chinese Angelica Root (当归, Danggui)6g
Prepared Rehmannia Root (熟地黄, Shudihuang)9g
White Peony Root (白芍药, Baishaoyao)9g
Tuckahoe (茯苓, Fuling)6g
Coastal Glehnia Root and Fourleaf Ladybell Root (沙参, Shashen)9g
Carbonized Spike of Fineleaf Schizonepeta Herb (黑芥穗, Heijiesui)6g
Tree Peonybark (牡丹皮, Mudanpi)9g

Actions: Nourishing the kidney and clearing away liver heat, eliminating fire and arresting bleeding.

Applied Syndrome: Retrograde menstruation due to deficiency of kidney-yin and upward invasion of the hyperactive liver-qi manifested by sudden onset of hematemesis and apostaxis in small amount and red bright color one or two days before menstruation, often accompanied with dizziness, tinnitus, feverish sensation over the palm and sole, hectic fever, dry cough, flushed cheeks and red lips, crimson tongue, lingua geographica or without coating, thin and rapid pulse.

Points in Constitution: This formula not only has the actions of enriching blood and nourishing yin but also can clear away liver-heat and moisten the lung to promote descent of the lung-qi, thus menses will be in order and retrograde menstruation be cured. Besides, Sichuan Achyranthes Root

(川牛膝, Chuanniuxi) can be added to induce the blood to run downward.

Indication: Vicarious menstruation.

Precaution: Pungent and peppery food should be avoided while taking this formula. This formula is forbidden for hemorrhage without heat.

Menstruation-Normalizing Decoction
(Kidney-Nourishing and Liver-Clearing Method)

Ingredients	Effects	Combined Effects	Syndrome	Chief Symptoms
Prepared Rehmannia Root (熟地黄, Shudihuang)9g White Peony Root (白芍药, Baishaoyao)9g Chinese Angelica Root (当归, Danggui)6g	Nourishing the liver and kidney, enriching blood and regulating menstruation	Nourishing yin, clearing away heat and arresting bleeding	Retrograde menstruation (caused by interior heat due to yin deficiency)	Hematemesis and apostaxis before menstruation, scanty and bright red blood, hectic fever and flushed face, dizziness and tinnitus, crimson tongue, lingua geographica or without coating, thin and rapid pulse
Tree Peony Bark (牡丹皮, Mudanpi)9g Carbonized Spike of Fineleaf Schizonepeta Herb (黑芥穗, Heijiesui)6g	Nourishing yin and eliminating fire, removing heat from the blood and arresting bleeding			
Coastal Glehnia Root and Fourleaf Ladybell Root (沙参, Shashen)9g	Nourishing yin and moistening the lung			
Tuckahoe (茯苓, Fuling)6g	Invigorating the spleen and the lung			

Associated Formula:

Menstruation-Normalizing Decoction(顺经汤, shuen jing tang) *Essentials of Ophthalmology*《银海精微》

This is comprised of Ending Part of Chinese Angelica Root (当归尾, Dangguiwei), Szechwan Lovage Rhizome (川芎, Chuanxiong), Bitter Orange (枳壳, Zhiqiao), Fennel Fruit (小茴香, Xiaohuixiang), Chinese Thorowax Root (柴胡, Chaihu), Tangerine Peel (橘皮, Jupi), Corydalis Tuber (延胡索, Yanhusuo), White Peony Root (白芍药, Baishaoyao), Green Tangerine Peel (青皮, Qingpi), Nutgrass Galingale Rhizome (香附, Xiangfu), Apricot Seed (杏仁, Xingren), Safflower (红花, Honghua) and Cassia Bark (肉桂, Rougui). Its actions are activating flow of menses and relieving pain. It is suited to retrograde menstruation.

6. Pregnancy-Promoting Pearl
(毓麟珠, yu lin zhu)

Source: *Jingyue's Complete Works* 《景岳全书》
Composition: Ginseng (人参, Renshen)6g
Tuckahoe (茯苓, Fuling)6g
Largehead Atractylodes Rhizome (白术, Baizhu)6g
White Peony Root (白芍药, Baishaoyao)6g
Eucommia Bark (杜仲, Duzhong)6g
Deglued Antler Powder (鹿角霜, Lujiaoshuang)6g
Pricklyash Peel (川椒, Chuanjiao)6g
Szechwan Lovage Rhizome (川芎, Chuanxiong)3g
Prepared Licorice Root (炙甘草, Zhi Gancao)3g
Chinese Angelica Root (当归, Danggui)12g
Prepared Rehmannia Root (熟地黄, Shudihuang)12g
Chinese Dodder Seed (菟丝子, Tusizi)12g

Actions: Replenishing qi and nourishing blood, warming the kidney and tonifying the liver.

Applied Syndrome: Female sterility due to insufficiency of the liver and kidney resulting from deficiency of both qi and blood, manifested by retarded menstruation with scanty amount and pale color, lassitude of the loins and legs, cold feeling in the lower abdomen, sexual hypoesthesia, anorexia, tiredness, profuse clear urine, pale tongue with white coating, deep and thin pulse.

Points in Constitution: Since qi and blood are the origin of the growth, it is difficult for women to become pregnant with the condition of deficiency of qi and blood. Meanwhile declination of fire from the gate of life gives no chance for the uterus to develop an embryo. This formula has the actions of warming the uterus, replenishing qi and enriching blood to promote pregnancy and give birth to a child.

Indication: Ovulation impediment sterility.

Precaution: This formula is designed for sterility due to insufficiency of qi and blood resulting from deficiency of both the liver and kidney, thus it is not suitable for sterility due to damp-phlegm and stagnation of the liver-qi.

Associated Formulas:

1. Uterus-Warming Powder (温胞散, wen bao san) *Essentials of Differential Diagnosis* 《辨证录》

This consists of Ginseng (人参, Renshen), Largehead Atractylodes Rhizome (白术, Baizhu), Medicinal Indian Mulberry Root (巴戟天, Bajitian), Malaytea Scurfpea Fruit (破故纸, Poguzhi), Eucommia Bark (杜仲, Duzhong), Chinese Dodder Seed (菟丝子, Tusizi), Gordon Euryale Seed (芡实, Qianshi), Fried Common Yam Rhizome (炒山药, Chao Shanyao), Cassia

Bark (肉桂, Rougui) and Prepared Aconite Root (炮附子, Pao Fuzi). Its actions are warming the kidney and the uterus, regualting and replenishing Chong and Ren Meridians. It is suited to female sterility due to cold of the uterus.

Pregnancy-Promoting Pill

(Method of Replenishing both Qi and Blood)

Ingredients	Effects	Combined Effects	Syndrome	Chief Symptoms
Ginseng (人参, Renshen)6g Tuckahoe (茯苓, Fuling)6g Largehead Atractylodes Rhizome (白术, Baizhu)6g White Peony Root (白芍药, Baishaoyao)6g Chinese Angelica Root (当归, Danggui)12g Prepared Rehmannia Root (熟地黄, Shudihuang)12g Prepared Licorice Root (炙甘草, Zhi Gancao)3g	Replenishing qi and enriching blood	Replenishing qi and nourishing blood, warming the kidney and tonifying the liver	Sterility (due to insufficiency of the liver and kidney and deficiency of both qi and blood)	Prolonged sterility after marriage, retarded menstruation, scanty in amount and pink in color, lassitude of the loins and legs, cold feeling in the lower abdomen, sexual hypoesthesia, pale tongue with white coating, deep and thin pulse
Chinese Dodder Seed (菟丝子, Tusizi)12g Eucommia Bark (杜仲, Duzhong)6g	Warming the kidney and tonifying the liver			
Deglued Antler Powder (鹿角霜, Lujiaoshuang)6g Sichuan Pricklyash Peel(川椒, Chuanjiao)6g	Warming uterus			

2. Essence-Nourishing and Pregnancy-Promoting Decoction(养精种玉汤, yang jing zhong yu tang) *Fu Qingzhu's Obstetrics and Gynecology*《傅青主女科》

This is comprised of Prepared Rehmannia Root (熟地黄, Shudihuang), Chinese Angelica Root (当归, Danggui), White Peony Root (白芍药, Baishaoyao) and Asiatic Cornelian Cherry Fruit (山茱萸, Shanzhuyu). Its actions are enriching blood and nourishing essence. It is suitable for sterility and irregular menstruation due to deficiency of essence and blood.

3. Blood-Enriching and Heart-Replenishing Decoction(养血补心汤, yang xue bu xin tang) *Essentials of Differential Diagnosis*《辨证录》

This is composed of Prepared Rehmannia Root (熟地黄, Shudihuang), White Peony Root (白芍药, Baishaoyao), Chinese Angelica Root (当归, Danggui), Tuckahoe (茯苓, Fuling), Asiatic Cornelian Cherry Fruit (山茱萸, Shanzhuyu), Chrysanthemum Flower (菊花, Juhua), Tree Peony Bark (牡丹皮, Mudanpi), Common Yam Rhizome (山药, Shanyao), Eucommia Bark (杜仲, Duzhong) and Achyranthes Root (怀牛膝, Huainiuxi). Its actions are enriching blood, nourishing essence, clearing away liver-heat and invigorating the spleen. It is indicated for prolonged sterility due to latent stirring of liver-fire resulting from deficiency of blood and essence.

4. Eight Treasures Motherwort Pill（八珍益母丸, ba zhen yi mu wan）*Jingyue's Complete Works*《景岳全书》

This is comprised of Motherwort Herb（益母草, Yimucao）, Ginseng（人参, Renshen）, Stir-Baked Largehead Atractylodes Rhizome（炒白术, Chao Baizhu）, White Peony Root（白芍药, Baishaoyao）, Szechwan Lovage Rhizome（川芎, Chuanxiong）, Prepared Rehmannia Root（熟地黄, Shudihuang）, Chinese Angelica Root（当归, Danggui）and Prepared Licorice Root（炙甘草, Zhi Gancao）. Its actions are enriching blood and replenishing qi. It is suitable for prolonged sterility or threatened abortion or irregular menstruation due to deficiency of qi and blood.

5. Silky Fowl Black-Bone Chicken Bolus（乌鸡丸, wu ji wan）*Jade Ruler for Gynecology*《妇科玉尺》

This is made up of Male Silky Fowl with White Fur（白毛乌骨雄鸡, Baimaowuguxiongji）, Rehmannia Root（生地黄, Shengdihuang）, Prepared Rehmannia Root（熟地黄, Shudihuang）, Cochinchinese Asparagus Root（天门冬, Tianmendong）, Dwarf Lilyturf Root（麦门冬, Maimendong）, Eucommia Bark（杜仲, Duzhong）, Chinese Angelica Root（当归, Danggui）, Szechwan Lovage Rhizome（川芎, Chuanxiong）, Largehead Atractylodes Rhizome（白术, Baizhu）, Dan-Shen Root（丹参, Danshen）, Tuckahoe（茯苓, Fuling）, Malaytea Scurfpea Fruit（补骨脂, Buguzhi）, Ginseng（人参, Renshen）, Prepared Licorice Root（炙甘草, Zhi Gancao）, Desertliving Cistanche Herb（肉苁蓉, Roucongrong）, Fried Fennel Fruit（炒小茴香, Chao Xiaohuixiang）, Villous Amomum Fruit（砂仁, Sharen）and Nutgrass Galingale Rhizome（香附, Xiangfu）. Its actions are replenishing qi, enriching blood and regulating menstruation. It is fit for irregular menstruation, dizziness, tiredness and sterility due to deficiency of qi and blood resulting from weakness of the spleen and stomach.

7. Miscarriage-Preventing Pill
（寿胎丸, shou tai wan）

Source: *Records of Traditional Chinese and Western Medicine in Combination*《医学衷中参西录》

Composition: Chinese Dodder Seed（菟丝子, Tusizi）12g
Chinese Taxillus Twig（桑寄生, Sangjisheng）6g
Himalayan Teasel Root（续断, Xuduan）6g
Ass-hide Glue（阿胶, Ejiao）6g（melting in decoction）

Actions: Invigorating the kidney and preventing miscarriage.

Applied Syndrome: Habitual abortion due to deficiency of the liver and kidney which causes inablity of blood to nourish embryo and dysfunction of fetal qi, often accompanied with ache in the loins and knees, pink-coloured bleeding during pregnancy, listlessness and tiredness, pale tongue and thin pulse

Points in Constitution: The kidney is the origin of congenital constitution. It dominates reproduction and stores the essence. If the kidney is deficient, the original qi of the fetus will not be consolidated and if the blood is insufficient, the habitual abortion will be brought about. This formula is especially designed for habitual abortion due to deficiency of the kidney and insufficiency of blood.

Indications:

1. Threatened abortion, habitual abortion.
2. Sterility
3. Sexual hypoesthesia.

Miscarriage-Preventing Pill
(Kidney-Invigorating and Abortion-Preventing Method)

Ingredients	Effects	Combined Effects	Syndrome	Chief Symptoms
Chinese Dodder Seed (菟丝子, Tusizi)12g Chinese Taxillus Twig (桑寄生, Sangjisheng)6g	Invigorating the kidney, nourishing essence and preventing miscarriage	Invigorating the kidney and preventing miscarriage	Habitual abortion (due to deficiency of the liver and kidney and failuree of blood to nourish embryo)	Threatened abortion, repeatedly habitual abortion, ache in the loins, pink bleeding during pregnancy, listlessness and tiredness, pale tongue and thin pulse
Himalayan Teasel Root (续断, Xuduan) 6g	Arresting bleeding and preventing miscarriage			
Ass-hide Glue (阿胶, Ejiao)6g	Enriching blood and arresting bleeding			

Precaution: This formula is contraindicated in threatened abortion due to blood heat or blood stasis.

Associated Formulas:

1. Miscarriage-Preventing Decoction(安胎饮, an tai yin) *Longevity and Life Prescription*《寿世保元》

This is comprised of Chinese Angelica Root (当归, Danggui), White Peony Root (白芍药, Baishaoyao), Tangerine Peel (橘皮, Jupi), Prepared Rehmannia Root (熟地黄, Shudihuang), Szechwan Lovage Rhizome (川芎, Chuanxiong), Perilla Stem (苏梗, Sugeng), Baikal Skullcap Root (黄芩, Huangqin), Stir-Baked Largehead Atractylodes Rhizome (炒白术, Chaobaizhu), Villous Amomum Fruit (砂仁, Sharen) and Licorice Root (甘草, Gancao). Its actions are enriching blood and preventing miscarriage. It is fit for inability to nourish fetus during pregnancy due to deficiency of both qi and blood.

2. Miscarriage-Preventing Decoction(安胎饮, an tai yin) *Collection of Experiences Derived from Conjecture*《揣摩有得集》

This consists of Hirsute Shiny Bugleweed Herb (泽兰叶, Zelanye), Fried Baikal Skullcap Root (炒黄芩, Chao Huangqin), Coastal Glehnia Root and Fourleaf Ladybell Root (沙参, Shashen),

White Peony Root（白芍药，Baishaoyao）, Licorice Root（生甘草，Sheng Gancao）, Fried Villous Amomum Fruit（炒砂仁，Chaosharen）, Chinese Wolfberry Root-Bark（地骨皮，Digupi）, Dwarf Lilyturf Root（麦门冬，Maimendong）, Tophatherum Leaf（竹叶，Zhuye）and Common Rush Pith（灯心草，Dengxincao）. Its action is removing heat from the blood to prevent miscarriage. It is fit for threatened abortion due to blood-heat during pregnancy.

3. Largehead Atractylodes Miscarriage-Preventing Powder（安胎白术散，an tai bai zhu san）*Standard for Diagnosis and Treatment*《证治准绳》

This is comprised of Largehead Atractylodes Rhizome（白术，Baizhu）, Szechwan Lovage Rhizome（川芎，Chuanxiong）, Medicinal Evodia Fruit（吴茱萸，Wuzhuyu）and Prepared Licorice Root（炙甘草，Zhi Gancao）. Its actions are replenishing rong and wei to pretect fetal qi. It is fit for retardation of growth of fetus or habitual abortion due to cold uterus.

4. Chinese Taxillus Twig Miscarriage-Preventing Decoction（安胎寄生汤，an tai ji sheng tang）*The Medical Secrets of An Offical*《外台秘要》

This is comprised of Chinese Taxillus Twig（桑寄生，Sangjisheng）, Largehead Atractylodes Rhizome（白术，Baizhu）, Tuckahoe（茯苓，Fuling）and Prepared Licorice Root（炙甘草，Zhi Gancao）. Its actions are replenishing qi and preventing miscarriage. It is fit for threatened abortion with vaginal bleeding during pregnancy.

5. Rong-Soothing Decoction（安荣汤，an rong tang）*Jade Ruler for Gynecology*《妇科玉尺》

This is composed of Prepared Rehmannia Root（熟地黄，Shudihuang）, White Peony Root（白芍药，Baishaoyao）, Szechwan Lovage Rhizome（川芎，Chuanxiong）, Chinese Taxillus Twig（桑寄生，Sangjisheng）, Chinese Angelica Root（当归，Danggui）, Ass-hide Glue（阿胶，Ejiao）, Nutgrass Galingale Rhizome（香附，Xiangfu）, Largehead Atractylodes Rhizome（白术，Baizhu）, Villous Amomum Fruit（砂仁，Sharen）, Baikal Skullcap Root（黄芩，Huangqin）and Sticky Rice（糯米，Nuomi）. Its actions are clearing away heat, enriching blood and preventing miscarriage. It is fit for threatened abortion with heat.

6. Major Miscarriage-Preventing Decoction（大安胎如胜饮，da an tai ru sheng yin）*Jade Ruler for Gynecology*《妇科玉尺》

This is made up of Chinese Angelica Root（当归，Danggui）, Charred Largehead Atractylodes Rhizome（焦白术，Jiao Baizhu）, Wine-Prepared Baikal Skullcap Root（酒黄芩，Jiu Huangqin）, Wine-Prepared White Peony Root（酒白芍，Jiu Baishao）, Fried Villous Amomum Fruit（炒砂仁，Chao Sharen）, Tuckahoe（茯苓，Fuling）, Himalayan Teasel Root（续断，Xuduan）and Prepared Licorice Root（炙甘草，Zhi Gancao）. Its actions are enriching blood, invigorating the kidney and preventing miscarriage. It is fit for dysfunction of fetal qi, or gradual distending pain and threatened abortion.

7. Kidney-Invigorating and Chong Meridian-Consolidating Pill（补肾固冲丸，bu shen gu chong wan）*Gynecology*《妇产科学》

This is comprised of Chinese Dodder Seed（菟丝子，Tusizi）, Himalayan Teasel Root（续断，Xuduan）, Deglued Antler Powder（鹿角霜，Lujiaoshuang）, Medicinal Indian Mulberry Root（巴戟天，Bajitian）, Eucommia Bark（杜仲，Duzhong）, Barbary Wolfberry Fruit（枸杞子，Gouqizi）, Largehead Atractylodes Rhizome（白术，Baizhu）, Chinese Angelica Root（当归，Danggui）,

Ass-hide Glue (阿胶, Ejiao), Pilose Asiabell Root (党参, Dangshen), Villous Amomum Fruit (砂仁, Sharen), Chinese Date (大枣, Dazao) and Prepared Rehmannia Root (熟地黄, Shudihuang). Its actions are invigorating the kidney, strengthening yang and preventing miscarriage. It is fit for habitual abortion due to deficiency of kidney-qi and unconsolidation of Chong and Ren Meridians.

8. Taishan Rock Powder
(泰山盘石散, tai shan pan shi san)

Source: *Jingyue's Complete Works*《景岳全书》
Composition: Ginseng (人参, Renshen)6g
Toasted Membranous Milkvetch Root (炙黄芪, Zhi Huangqi)15g
Chinese Angelica Root (当归, Danggui)9g
Himalayan Teasel Root (续断, Xuduan)6g
Baikal Skullcap Root (黄芩, Huangqin)6g
Largehead Atractylodes Rhizome (白术, Baizhu)9g
Szechwan Lovage Rhizome (川芎, Chuanxiong)3g
White Peony Root (白芍药, Baishaoyao)6g
Prepared Rehmannia Root (熟地黄, Shudihuang)9g
Villous Amomum Fruit (砂仁, Sharen)3g
Prepared Licorice Root (炙甘草, Zhi Gancao)3g
Sticky Rice (糯米, Nuomi)6g

Actions: Replenishing qi and invigorating the spleen, enriching blood and preventing miscarriage.

Applied Syndrome: Threatened abortion due to deficiency of both qi and blood which brings about malnutrition of fetus during pregnancy, manifested as pale or sallow complexion, tiredness, poor appetite or anorexia, pale tongue with white coating, smooth and weak pulse or deep and feeble pulse.

Points in Constitution: This formula uses the ingredients of Four Herbs Decoction (四物汤, si wu tang) to enrich blood and those of Four Gentlemen Decoction (四君子汤, si jun zi tang) which excludes Tuckahoe (茯苓, Fuling) but adds Membranous Milkvetch Root (黄芪, Huangqi) to replenish qi. By nourishing both qi and blood, the fetus can be developed. The combination of Himalayan Teasel Root (续断, Xuduan) with Prepared Rehmannia Root (熟地黄, Shudihuang) is to invigorate the kidney and prevent miscarriage while the cooperation of Largehead Atractylodes Rhizome (白术, Baizhu) and Baikal Skullcap Root (黄芩, Huangqin) is to invigorate the spleen, clear away heat and prevent miscarriage.

Indications:
1. Habitual abortion.
2. Dysfunctional uterine bleeding.

3. Climacteric syndrome.

Taishan Rock Powder
(Method of Replenishing both Qi and Blood)

Ingredients	Effects	Combined Effects	Syndrome	Chief Symptoms
Ginseng (人参, Renshen)6g Toasted Membranous Milkvetch Root (炙黄芪, Zhi Huangqi)15g Largehead Atractylodes Rhizome (白术, Baizhu)9g	Replenishing qi and invigorating the spleen	Replenishing qi and invigorating the spleen, enriching blood and preveting miscarriage	Threatened abortion due to deficiency of qi and blood	Threatened abortion or repeated habitual abortion, pale or sallow complexion, tiredness, poor appetite or anorexia, paletongue with white coating, smooth and weak pulse or deep and feeble pulse
Villous Amomum Fruit (砂仁, Sharen) 3g	Regulating qi and preventing miscarriage			
Chinese Angelica Root (当归, Danggui)9g Prepared Rehmannia Root (熟地黄, Shudihuang)9g White Peony Root (白芍药, Baishaoyao)6g Szechwan Lovage Rhizome (川芎, Chuanxiong)3g	Enriching and regulating blood			
Himalayan Teasel Root (续断, Xuduan) 6g	Arresting bleeding and preventing miscarriage			
Baikal Skullcap Root (黄芩, Huangqin)6g	Clearing away heat and preventing miscarriage			
Sticky Rice (糯米, Nuomi)6g Prepared Licorice Root (炙甘草, Zhi Gancao)3g	Replenishing the spleen and stomach			

Precaution: This formula is contraindicated in threatened abortion due to blood-heat.
Associated Formulas:
1. Eight Treasures Decoction (八珍汤, ba zhen tang) *Classification and Treatment of*

Traumatic Diseases《正体类要》

This is the combination of Four Gentlemen Decoction (四君子汤, si jun zi tang) and Four Herbs Decoction (四物汤, si wu tang). It is a Prescription to uniform the replenishment of qi and blood. However, compared with Taishan Rock Powder (泰山磐石散, tai san pan shi san), this formula has a weak action for preventing miscarriage.

2. Ten Strong Tonic Herbs Decoction (十全大补汤, shi quan da bu tang) *Prescriptions of Peaceful Benevolent Dispensary*《和剂局方》

This is the Eight Treasures Decoction (八珍汤, ba zhen tang) plus Toasted Membranous Milkvetch Root (炙黄芪, Zhihuangqi) and Cassia Bark (肉桂, Rougui). Its actions are warming and replenishing qi and blood. It is fit for consumptive diseases with cough, poor appetite, emission, soreness and weakness of the loins and knees, unhealed ulcer, metrorrhagia and metrostaxis due to deficiency of qi and blood.

9. Blood Stasis-Removing Decoction
(通瘀煎, tong yu jian)

Source: *Jingyue's Complete Works*《景岳全书》
Composition: Ending Part of Chinese Angelica Root (当归尾, Dangguiwei) 9g
Safflower (红花, Honghua) 6g
Hawthorn Fruit (山楂, Shanzha) 9g
Nutgrass Galingale Rhizome (香附, Xiangfu) 6g
Commbined Spicebush Root (乌药, Wuyao) 6g
Green Tangerine Peel (青皮, Qingpi) 6g
Common Aucklandia Root (木香, Muxiang) 3g
Oriental Waterplantain Rhizome (泽泻, Zexie) 6g

Actions: Activating flow of qi and circulation of blood.

Applied Syndrome: Blockage of meridians due to stagnation of qi and blood stasis manifested by impediment of menstrual flow, abdominal pain with tenderness, postpartum abdominal pain due to blood stasis. It is also fit for puerperant contrary blood flow, syncope due to blood disorders, dark tongue, deep and forceful pulse.

Points in Constitution: The characteristic of this formula is that among the qi-activating and stasis-removing drugs, Oriental Waterplantain Rhizome (泽泻, Zexie) is added to induce water downward.

Indications:
1. Dysmenorrhea.
2. Postpartum abdominal pain.

Precaution: This formula is designed for excess syndrome due to stagnation of qi and blood stasis. Thus, it is not suitable for those with blood deficiency.

Associated Formulas:

1. Peach Kernel and Chinese Angelica Decoction (桃仁当归汤, tao ren dang gui tang) *Syndrome-Cause-Pulse-Treatment*《症因脉治》

This is comprised of Peach Seed (桃仁, Taoren), Chinese Angelica Root (当归, Danggui), Tree Peony Bark (牡丹皮, Mudanpi), Turmeric Root-Tuber (郁金, Yujin), Hirsute Shiny Bugleweed Herb (泽兰, Zelan), Hawthorn Fruit (山楂肉, Shanzharou), Safflower (红花, Honghua), Cape Jasmine Fruit (山栀子, Shanzhizi) and Red Peony Root (赤芍, Chishao). Its actions are activating blood circulation and removing blood stasis. It is fit for blood stasis, abdominal pain without distention, hiccup while drinking, severe localized pain in the night which is relieved by warming, usually hollow and unsmooth pulse.

Blood Stasis-Removing Decoction

(Method of Activating Flow of Qi and Circulation of Blood)

Ingredients	Effects	Combined Effects	Syndrome	Chief Symptoms
Ending Part of Chinese Angelica Root (当归尾, Dangguiwei)9g Safflower (红花, Honghua)6g Hawthorn Fruit (山楂, Shanzha)9g	Activating blood circulation and dissipating blood stasis	Activating flow of qi and blood circulation	Qi stagnation and blood stasis	Impediment of menstrual flow, distention and pain in the lower abdomen with tenderness, dark tongue, deep and forceful pulse
Commbined Spicebush Root (乌药, Wuyao)6g Green Tangerine Peel (青皮, Qingpi)6g Common Aucklandia Root (木香, Muxiang)3g Nutgrass Galingale Rhizome (香附, Xiangfu)6g	Activating flow of qi and alleviating pain			
Oriental Waterplantain Rhizome (泽泻, Zexie)6g	Promoting urination and restoring menstrual flow			

2. Intestines-Calming Decoction(肠宁汤, chang ning tang) *Fu Qingzhu's Obstetrics and Gynecology*《傅青主女科》

This is composed of Chinese Angelica Root (当归, Danggui), Prepared Rehmannia Root (熟地黄, Shudihuang), Ginseng (人参, Renshen), Dwarf Lilyturf Root (麦门冬, Maimendong), Ass-hide Glue (阿胶, Ejiao), Common Yam Rhizome (山药, Shanyao), Himalayan Teasel Root (续断, Xuduan), Prepared Licorice Root (炙甘草, Zhi Gancao) and Cassia Bark (肉桂,

Rougui). Its actions are enriching blood, replenishing qi, regulating ying and alleviating pain. It is fit for postpartum abdominal pain due to deficiency and stagnation of qi and blood manifested as postpartum dull pain in the lower abdomen, pink and scanty lochia, pale and red tongue, feeble and thin pulse.

3. Largehead Atractylodes, Chinese Angelica, Cassia Bark and Licorice Decoction (术归桂草汤, zhu gui gui cao tang) *Essentials of Differential Diagnosis* 《辨证录》

This is comprised of Largehead Atractylodes Rhizome (白术, Baizhu), Chinese Angelica Root (当归, Danggui), Cassia Bark (肉桂, Rougui) and Prepared Licorice Root (炙甘草, Zhi Gancao). Its actions are invigorating the spleen and enriching the blood, warming yang and relieving pain. It is fit for women postpartum abdominal pain due to blood deficiency and invasion of cold.

10. Liver-Clearing and Stranguria-Treating Decoction
(清肝止淋汤, qin gan zhi lin tang)

Source: *Fu Qingzhu's Obstetrics and Gynecology* 《傅青主女科》
Composition: White Peony Root (白芍药, Baishaoyao)9g
Chinese Angelica Root (当归, Danggui)9g
Dried Rehmannia Root (生地黄, Shengdihuang)12g
Tree Peony Bark (牡丹皮, Mudanpi)9g
Chinese Corktree Bark (黄柏, Huangbai)9g
Medicinal Achyranthes Root (川牛膝, Chuan Niuxi)9g
Nutgrass Galingale Rhizome (香附, Xiangfu)12g
Black Soy Bean (黑豆, Heidou)9g
Ass-hide Glue (阿胶, Ejiao)9g

Actions: Clearing away heat from the liver, removing dampness and stopping leukorrhea.

Applied Syndrome: Leucorrhea due to attack of damp-heat on the lower-jiao resulting from transformation of fire by depressed liver, manifested by continuous leukorrhea with bloody, sticky and thick discharge, foul and sour in odor, red tongue with yellow and greasy coating, smooth and rapid pulse.

Points in Constitution: Leucorrhea with reddish discharge is the manifestation of syndrome of invasion of damp-heat into blood system. Thus, more drugs for blood system are used than the drugs for removing damp-heat in this formula. The so-called "liver-clearing" is, in fact, to remove heat from blood or ying system.

Indications:
1. Cervicitis, cervical erosion.
2. Carcinoma of uterine cervix.
3. Vaginitis.

Precaution: There are many causes for pruritus of vulva in woman. So, besides taking internal medicine orally, external treatment should be given to the local part.

Associated Formula:

Formula for Cervicitis Number Two (宫颈炎Ⅱ号, gong jing yan er hao) *Clinical Manual of Gynecology of Traditional Chinese Medicine*《中医妇科临床手册》

This is composed of Tokyo Violet Herb (紫花地丁, Zihuadiding), Indian Dendranthema Flower (野菊花, Yejuhua), Barbed Skullcap Herb (半枝莲, Banzhilian) and Chinese Corktree Bark (黄柏, Huangbai). Its actions are clearing away heat, removing toxic material and drying dampness. It is applicable to acute cervicitis. This decoction should be used externally by washing the vagina or putting the cotton ball into the vagina after it is soaked with the decoction.

Liver-Clearing and Stranguria-Treating Decoction
(Heat-Removing and Blood-Cooling Method)

Ingredients	Effects	Combined Effects	Syndrome	Chief Symptoms
Chinese Corktree Bark (黄柏, Huangbai)9g	Clearing away heat and drying dampness			
Tree Peony Bark (牡丹皮, Mudanpi)9g Dried Rehmannia Root (生地黄, Shengdihuang)12g	Removing heat from the blood			
Chinese Angelica Root (当归, Danggui)9g White Peony Root (白芍药, Baishaoyao)9g Black Soya Bean (黑豆, Heidou)9g Ass-hide Glue (阿胶, Ejiao)9g	Nourishing yin and enriching blood	Clearing away liver- heat and removing heat from the blood, drying dampness and stopping leukorrhea	Leucorrhea (due to fire derived from stagnation of the liver-qi and downward attack of the lower-jiao by damp-heat)	Continuous leukorrhea with reddish discharge which is sticky and thick, foul and sour in odor, red tongue, yellow and greasy coating, smooth and rapid pulse
Nutgrass Galingale Rhizome (香附, Xiangfu)12g	Dispersing the stagnated liver-qi			
Medicinal Achyranthes Root (川牛膝, Chuan Niuxi)9g	Conducting the effect of drugs downward			

11. Postmenopausal Bleeding-Preventing Decoction
(安老汤, an lao tang)

Source: *Fu Qingzhu's Obstetrics and Gynecology*《傅青主女科》

Composition: Ginseng（人参，Renshen）30g
Membranous Milkvetch Root（生黄芪，Shenghuangqi）30g
Prepared Rehmannia Root（熟地黄，Shudihuang）30g
Stir-Baked Largehead Atractylodes Rhizome（炒白术，Chao Baizhu）15g
Chinese Angelica Root（当归，Danggui）15g
Asiatic Cornelian Cherry Fruit（山茱萸，Shanzhuyu）15g
Ass-Hide Glue（阿胶，Ejiao）9g
Carbonized Spike of Fineleaf Schizonepeta Herb（黑芥穗，Heijiesui）6g
Licorice Root（生甘草，Sheng Gancao）3g
Nutgrass Galingale Rhizome（香附，Xiangfu）6g
Charred Agaric（木耳炭，Muertan）6g

Actions: Invigorating the spleen and replenishing the liver, nourishing yin and stopping metrostaxis.

Applied Syndrome: Postmenopausal bleeding due to insufficiency of kidney-water resulting from deficiency of the liver and the spleen, manifested by purple blood clots, or stranguria complicated by hematuria and metrostaxis, profuse or scanty blood, like normal menstruation but actually not menstruation, sallow complexion, shortness of breath and reluctance to speak, dizziness, oppressing feeling in the chest, groan, thin and white tongue coating, red tongue, thin, wiry and rapid pulse.

Points in Constitution: This formula emphasizes replenishing qi and blood, nourishing the spleen and regulating the liver to treat the primary aspect of the illness. Thus it may be not strong enough for acute diseases with excessive pathogens.

Indication: Postmenopausal bleeding.

Precaution: This formula is designed for postmenopausal bleeding due to insufficiency of kidney-water and deficiency of both the liver and spleen. Thus, it is not suitable for postmenopausal bleeding due to damp-heat and blood stasis with toxic material.

Associated Formulas:

1. Membranous Milkvetch and Largehead Atractylodes Powder for Regulating Menstruation（芪术调经散 qin zhu tiao jing san）*Essentials of Differential Diagnosis*《辨证录》

This is comprised of Ginseng（人参，Renshen）, Sanchi Root（三七，Sanqi）, Largehead Atractylodes Rhizome（白术，Baizhu）, Chinese Angelica Root（当归，Danggui）, Membranous Milkvetch Root（生黄芪，Sheng Huangqi）and Dried Rehmannia Root（生地黄，Shengdihuang）. Its actions are invigorating the spleen, replenishing qi, nourishing yin and regulating the liver. It is applicable to postmenopausal bleeding in woman.

2. Interior-Replenishing Pill（内补丸，nei bu wan）*Key of Obstetrics and Gynecology*《女科切要》

This is made up of Hairy Antler（鹿茸，Lurong）, Chinese Dodder Seed（菟丝子，Tusizi）, Flatstem Milkvetch Seed（潼蒺藜，Tongjili）, Membranous Milkvetch Root（黄芪，Huangqi）, Tribulus Fruit（白蒺藜，Baijili）, Tatarian Aster Root（紫菀，Ziyuan）, Cassia Bark（肉桂，Rougui）, Mantis Egg-Case（桑螵蛸，Sangpiaoxiao）, Desertliving Cistanche Herb（肉苁蓉，

Roucongrong) and Prepared Aconite Root (制附子, Zhi Fuzi). Its actions are warming the kidney, restoring yang, astringing the essence and stopping leukorrhea. It is applicable to leucorrhea due to deficiency of kidney-yang, manifested by profuse leucorrhea with white, clear and watery discharge, dizziness, tinnitus, lumbago as if broken, intolerance of cold, cold limbs, discomfort in the lower abdomen which can be relieved by warming, frequency of urination in the night, loose stool, pale tongue with thin and white coating, deep, slow and thin pulse.

Postmenopausal Bleeding-Preventing Decoction
(Spleen-Replenishing, Liver-Regulating and yin-Nourishing Method)

Ingredients	Effects	Combined Effects	Syndrome	Chief Symptoms
Ginseng (人参, Renshen)30g Membranous Milkvetch Root (生黄芪, Sheng Huangqi) 30g Stir-Baked Largehead Atractylodes Rhizome (炒白术, Chao Baizhu)15g	Replenishing qi and invigorating the spleen	Invigorating the spleen and regulating the liver, nourishing yin and stopping metrostaxis	Deficiency of all the liver, spleen and kidney	Metrostaxis, profuse or scanty blood, purple or bright blood, sallow complexion, shortness of breath and reluctance to speak, oppressing feeling in the chest and groan, thin and white coating, red tongue, thin, wiry and rapid pulse
Chinese Angelica Root (当归, Danggui)15g Prepared Rehmannia Root (熟地黄, Shudihuang)30g Ass-hide Glue (阿胶, Ejiao)9g Asiatic Cornelian Cherry Fruit (山茱萸, Shanzhuyu)15g	Enriching blood and replenishing the liver			
Nutgrass Galingale Rhizome (香附, Xiangfu)6g	Dispersing constrained liver qi and alleviating mental depression			
Carbonized Spike of Fineleaf Schizonepeta Herb (黑芥穗, Heijiesui)6g Charred Agaric (木耳炭, Muertan)6g	Arresting bleeding			
Licorice Root (生甘草, Sheng Gancao)3g	Coordinating the actions of various ingredients in a Prescription			

3. Essence-Astringing Pill (固精丸, gu jing wan) *Compendium of the Therapy for Women's Diseases* 《济阴纲目》

This is comprised of Mantis Egg-Case (桑螵蛸, Sangpiaoxiao), Calcined Dragon's Bone (煅龙骨, Duan Longgu), White Halloysite (白石脂, Baishizhi), Tuckahoe (茯苓, Fuling), Chinese Magnoliavine Fruit (五味子, Wuweizi), Chinese Dodder Seed (菟丝子, Tusizi) and Tuber Onion Seed (韭子, Jiuzi). Its actions are replenishing the spleen and kidney, astringing the essence and stopping leukorrhea. It is applicable to "leukorrhea with whitish discharge" manifested as sudden, profuse discharge of white and thin fluid from vagina due to deficiency of the kidney which is unable to control body fluid.

12. Springing like Lactation-Promoting Powder (下乳涌泉散, xia ru yong quan san)

Source: *Formulae of Imperial Physician in the Qing Dynasty* 《清太医院配方》
Composition: Chinese Angelica Root (当归, Danggui)6g
White Peony Root (白芍药, Baishaoyao)6g
Szechwan Lovage Rhizome (川芎, Chuanxiong)6g
Dried Rehmannia Root (生地黄, Shengdihuang)6g
Chinese Thorowax Root (柴胡, Chaihu)6g
Green Tangerine Peel (青皮, Qingpi)6g
Snakegourd Root (天花粉, Tianhuafen)6g
Globethistle Root (漏芦, Loulu)3g
Akebia Stem (木通, Mutong)3g
Balloonflower Root (桔梗, Jiegeng)3g
Ricepaperplant Pith (通草, Tongcao)3g
Dahurican Angelica Root (白芷, Baizhi)3g
Pangolin Scales (穿山甲, Chuanshanjia)9g
Cowherb Seed (王不留行, Wangbuliuxing)9g
Licorice Root (甘草, Gancao)3g

Actions: Soothing the liver and regulating the circulation of qi, dredging the collaterals and inducing and promoting lactation.

Applied Syndrome: Postpartum lack of lactation due to stagnation of liver qi which causes deficiency of yin and blood, dysfunction of the liver and obstruction of the meridians and collaterals, manifested by postpartum lack of lactation, or no lactation, feeling of distention and fullness or pain in the breast, feeling of distention and stuffiness in the chest and hypochondrium, mental depression, or low fever, poor appetite, anorexia, thin and yellow tongue coating; wiry and thin or rapid pulse.

Points in Constitution: This formula contains a large dose of meridian-dredging drugs, thus it is applicable to lack of lactation due to obstruction in the meridians and collaterals but not suitable for the case due to deficiency of qi and blood.

Indication: Postpartum lack of lactation.

Springing like Lactation-Promoting Powder
(Liver-Soothing and Collaterals-Dredging Method)

Ingredients	Effects	Combined Effects	Syndrome	Chief Symptoms
Chinese Angelica Root (当归, Danggui)6g White Peony Root (白芍药, Baishaoyao)6g Szechwan Lovage Rhizome (川芎, Chuanxiong)6g Dried Rehmannia Root (生地黄, Shengdihuang)6g	Enriching and regulating blood	Dispersing constrained liver qi and alleviating depression, dredging the collaterals and inducing and promoting lactation	Lack of lactation (due to stagnation of liver qi)	Postpartum lack of lactation, feeling of distention and fullness or pain in the breast, feeling of distention and stuffiness in the chest and hypochondrium, mental depression, or low fever, thin and yellow tongue coating, wiry and thin or rapid pulse
Snakegourd Root (天花粉, Tianhuafen)6g	Nourishing yin and promoting the production of body fluid			
Green Tangerine Peel (青皮, Qingpi)6g Chinese Thorowax Root (柴胡, Chaihu)6g	Dispersing constrained liver-qi and alleviating mental depression			
Ricepaperplant Pith (通草, Tongcao)3g Akebia Stem (木通, Mutong)3g Dahurican Angelica Root (白芷, Baizhi)3g Globethistle Root (漏芦, Loulu)3g Pangolin Scales (穿山甲, Chuanshanjia)9g Cowherb Seed (王不留行, Wangbuliuxing)9g	Dredging the collaterals and inducing lactation			
Balloonflower Root (桔梗, Jiegeng)3g	Inducing the effect of drugs ascending			
Licorice Root (甘草, Gancao)3g	Coordinating the actions of various ingredients in a Prescription			

Precautions:

1. This formula is designed for lack of lactation with feeling of distention, fullness and pain in the breast caused by depressed liver-qi and internal damage by emotional stress after delivery. For the case with severe distention, Towel Gourd Vegetable Sponge (丝瓜络, Sigualuo) and Beautiful Sweetgum Fruit (路路通, Lulutong) may be added to aid in dredging the meridian and collateral. For the case with enlargement of the nodules with erythema and feeling of slight hot sensation, appropriate amount of Dandelion (蒲公英, Pugongying), Snakegourd Fruit (全瓜蒌, Quangualou) and Common Selfheal Fruit-Spike (夏枯草, Xiakucao) may be added to clear away heat and dissipate blockages.

2. This formula is not suitable for lack of lactation due to deficiency of qi and blood.

Associated Formula:

Lactation-Inducing Pill (通乳丹, tong ru dan) *Fu Qingzhu's Obstetrics and Gynecology* 《傅青主女科》

This is comprised of Ginseng (人参, Renshen), Membranous Milkvetch Root (生黄芪, Sheng Huangqi), Chinese Angelica Root (当归, Danggui), Dwarf Lilyturf Root (麦门冬, Maimendong), Akebia Stem (木通, Mutong) [or Ricepaperplant Pith (通草, Tongcao)] and Balloonflower Root (桔梗, Jiegeng), which should be decocted with the soup of pork hoof or meat soup. Its actions are replenishing qi, enriching blood and promoting lactation. It is applicable to lack of lactation after delivery manifested as watery latex, soft breast, pallor, listlessness, poor appetite or anorexia, pale tongue with little coating, feeble and thin pulse.

Additional Formulas:

Charred Fortune Windmillpalm Petiole and Charred Cattail Pollen Powder
(棕蒲散, zong pu san)

Source: *Supplement on Explanation of Chen Suan's Gynecology*《陈素庵妇科补解》
Composition: Charred Fortune Windmillpalm Petiole (棕榈炭, Zonglütan) 9g
Charred Cattail Pollen (蒲黄炭, Puhuangtan) 9g
Hirsute Shiny Bugleweed Herb (泽兰, Zelan) 6g
Tree Peony Bark (牡丹皮, Mudanpi) 9g
Eucommia Bark (杜仲, Duzhong) 15g
Largeleaf Gentian Root (秦艽, Qinjiao) 6g
Chinese Angelica Root (当归, Danggui) 6g
White Peony Root (白芍药, Baishaoyao) 9g
Szechwan Lovage Rhizome (川芎, Chuanxiong) 6g
Dried Rehmannia Root (生地黄, Shengdihuang) 9g

Actions: Activating blood circulation and removing blood stasis, consolidating Chong Meridian and regulating menstruation.

Applied Syndrome: Metrorrhagia and metrostaxis due to blood stasis in uterus which causes failure of blood to circulate within vessels, manifested by continuous menstruation with profuse or scanty menses which are dark purple and in the form of blood clot, pain in the lower abdomen with tenderness, petechia in the tongue, unsmooth and forceful pulse.

Points in Constitution: This formula contains the ingredients of Four Herbs Decoction (四物汤, si wu tang) and other blood-cooling, stasis-removing, astringency-inducing and bleeding-arresting drugs. The characteristic of this formula is to combine the dispersing method with the astringing one so that the blood stasis may be resolved and bleeding arrested without leaving any blood stasis.

Indication: Menostaxis due to pelvic inflammation, endometritis or incomplete atrophy of corpus luteum.

Precaution: This formula is not suitable for those without blood stasis.

Associated Formulas:

1. Blood Stasis-Removing and Bleeding-Arresting Decoction (逐瘀止血汤, zhu yu zhi xue tang) *Fu Qingzhu's Obstetrics and Gynecology*《傅青主女科》

This is comprised of Dried Rehmannia Root (生地黄, Shengdihuang), Rhubarb (大黄, Dahuang), Red Peony Root (赤芍, Chishao), Tree Peony Bark (牡丹皮, Mudanpi), Ending Part of Chinese Angelica Root (当归尾, Dangguiwei), Bitter Orange (枳壳, Zhiqiao), Peach Seed (桃仁, Taoren) and Tortoise Shell and Plastron (龟版, Guiban). Its actions are activating blood circulation, removing blood stasis, regulating blood and keeping blood circulating in vessels. It is applicable to irregular menstruation and intermenstrual bleeding due to blood stasis in the interior and disorder of qi.

Charred Fortune Windmillpalm Petiole and Charred Cattail Pollen Powder
(Blood-Activating and Stasis-Removing Method)

Ingredients	Effects	Combined Effects	Syndrome	Chief Symptoms
Chinese Angelica Root (当归, Danggui)6g Szechwan Lovage Rhizome (川芎, Chuanxiong)6g Dried Rehmannia Root (生地黄, Shengdihuang)9g White Peony Root (白芍药, Baishaoyao)9g	Enriching and regulating blood	Activating blood circulation and dissolving blood stasis, consolidating Chong Meridian and regulating menstruation	Metrorrhagia and metrostaxis (due to blood stasis)	Prolonged menstruation, continuous bleeding with profuse or scanty menses which are dark purple in color and blood clots, pain in the lower abdomen with tenderness, petechia in the tongue, unsmooth and forceful pulse
Tree Peony Bark (牡丹皮, Mudanpi)9g Hirsute Shiny Bugleweed Herb (泽兰, Zelan)6g Largeleaf Gentian Root (秦艽, Qinjiao)6g	Removing heat from the blood, dissipating blood stasis and arresting bleeding			
Eucommia Bark (杜仲, Duzhong)15g	Consolidating Chong Meridian and arresting bleeding			
Charred Cattail Pollen (蒲黄炭, Puhuangtan)9g Charred Fortune Windmillpalm Petiole (棕榈炭, Zonglütan)9g	Arresting bleeding by astringent			

2. Blood Stasis-Removing and Metrorrhagia-Stopping Decoction(逐瘀止崩汤, zhu yu zhi beng tang) Selections of *Proved Prescriptions of Traditional Chinese Medicine in Anhui* 《安徽中医验方选集》

This is made up of Chinese Angelica Root (当归, Danggui), Szechwan Lovage Rhizome (川芎, Chuanxiong), Sanchi Root (三七, Sanqi), Myrrh (没药, Moyao), Trogopterus Dung (五灵脂, Wulingzhi), Charred Tree Peony Bark (牡丹皮炭, Mudanpitan), Fried Dan-Shen Root (炒丹参, Chao Danshen), Fried Argy Wormwood Leaf (炒艾叶, Chao Aiye), Ass-hide Glue (阿胶, Ejiao) which is fried with Cattail Pollen (蒲黄, Puhuang), Calcined Drago's Bone (煅龙骨, Duan Longgu), Calcined Oyster Shell (煅牡蛎, Duan Muli) and Cuttlefish Bone (乌贼骨,

Wuzeigu). Its actions are activating blood circulation and dissolving blood stasis, consolidating Chong Meridian and arresting bleeding. It is suited to metrorrhagia and metrostaxis due to blood stasis in the Chong and Ren Meridians.

3. Blood Stasis-Resolving and Metrorrhagia-Stopping Decoction (化瘀止崩汤, hua yu zhi beng tang) *Gynecology of Traditional Chinese Medicine* 《中医妇科学》

This is comprised of Carbonized Cattail Pollen (炒蒲黄, Chao Puhuang), Trogopterus Dung (五灵脂, Wulingzhi), Motherwort Herb (益母草, Yimucao), Fourleaf Ladybell Root (南沙参, Nan Shashen), Chinese Angelica Root (当归, Danggui), Szechwan Lovage Rhizome (川芎, Chuanxiong) and Powder of Sanchi Root (三七粉, Sanqifen). Its actions are activating blood circulation, dissolving blood stasis and alleviating pain. It is indicated for postpartum metrorrhagia.

4. Bleeding-Arresting Panacea (止血灵, zhi xue ling) *Hubei Journal of Traditional Chinese Medicine* 《湖北中医杂志》

This consists of Purslane Herb (马齿苋, Machixian), Motherwort Herb (益母草, Yimucao), Sanguisorba Root (地榆, Diyu), Cattail Pollen (生蒲黄, Sheng Puhuang), India Madder Root (茜草根, Qiancaogen) and Shunk Bugbane Rhizome (升麻, Shengma). Its actions are removing heat from the blood, dissolving blood stasis and arresting bleeding. It is indicated for hemorrhagic diseases in gynecology such as metrorrhagia, metrostaxis, menorrhagia and lochiorrhea due to attack of blood-heat. It is also used for hematemesis and apostaxis due to blood-heat.

5. General Recipe for Treating Metrorrhagia and Metrostaxis(血崩统治方, xue beng tong zhi fang) *Author's Experienced Prescription* (笔者经验方)

This is composed of Chinese Wolfberry Root(地骨皮, Digupi), Motherwort Herb(益母草, Yimucao), India Madder Root(茜草, Qiancao), Hairyvein Agrimonia Herb(仙鹤草, Xianhecao) and Prepared Licorice(炙甘草, Zhigancao). Its actions are cooling blood, removing stasis and stopping bleeding. It is indicated for acute and unceasing metrorrhagia with large amount of fresh blood. For the case of exhaustion of qi resulting from hemorrhea, Membranous Milkvetch Root(黄芪, Huangqi) and Chinese Angelica Root(当归, Danggui) are added.

Formula for Exfetation Number Two
(宫外孕Ⅱ号方, gong wai yun er hao Fang)

Source: The First Hospital Affiliated to Shanxi Medical College 山西医学院附属第一医院
Composition: Red Peony Root (赤芍, Chishao)15g
Dan-Shen Root (丹参, Danshen)15g
Peach Seed (桃仁, Taoren)9g
Kwangsi Turmeric Rhizome (莪术, Ezhu)6g
Common Burreed Rhizome (三棱, Sanleng)6g
Actions: Activating blood circulation and removing blood stasis, eliminating mass and killing embryo.
Applied Syndrome: Exfetation due to blood stasis in the lower abdomen manifested by dull pain

in the lower abdomen, bearing-down and distention sensation, soft mass in the affected side with tenderness, wiry and smooth pulse.

Formula for Exfetation Number Two
(Blood-Activating and Stasis-Removing Method)

Ingredients	Effects	Combined Effects	Syndrome	Chief Symptoms
Dan-Shen Root (丹参, Danshen)15g Red Peony Root (赤芍, Chishao)15g Peach Seed (桃仁, Taoren)9g	Activating blood circulation and removing blood stasis	Activating blood circulation and removing blood stasis, eliminating mass and killing embryo	Exfetation (due to abdominal mass resulting from blood stasis)	Dull pain in the lower abdomen, bearing-down sensation and distention, mass in the abdomen with tenderness, wiry and smooth pulse
Common Burreed Rhizome (三棱, Sanleng) 6g Kwangsi Turmeric Rhizome (莪术, Ezhu)6g	Eliminating mass and dissipating blockages			

Points in Constitution: This formula is especially used for activating blood circulation and removing blood stasis drastically, which is aimed to eliminate mass quickly to avoid diseases. Common Burreed Rhizome (三棱, Sanleng) and Kwangsi Turmeric Rhizome (莪术, Ezhu), whose actions are removing blood stasis and activating flow of qi, are the commonly used drugs to eliminate mass.

Indication: Exfetation (tubal pregnancy without rupture).

Precaution: Since exfetation is a complicated disease, it is very important to treat it reasonably by combining traditional Chinese medicine with western medicine.

Associated Formulas:

1. Formula for Exfetation Number One (宫外孕Ⅰ号方, gong wai yun yi hao fang) The First Hospital Affiliated to Shanxi Medical College 山西医学院附属第一医院

This consists of Dan-Shen Root (丹参, Danshen), Red Peony Root (赤芍, Chishao) and Peach Seed (桃仁, Taoren). Its actions are activating blood circulation and removing blood stasis to elilminate mass. It is suited to abortion or rupture of tubal pregnancy.

2. Mass-Eliminating Powder (消癥散, xiao zheng san) *Gynecology of Traditional Chinese Medicine* 《中医妇科学》

This is made up of Obscured Homalomena Rhizome (千年健, Qiannianjian), Himalayan Teasel Root (川断, Chuanduan), Moghaniae Root (追地风, Zhuidifeng), Bunge Pricklysh (花椒, Huajiao), Slenderstyle Acanthopanax Root-Bark (五加皮, Wujiapi), Dahurican Angelica Root (白芷, Baizhi), Chinese Taxillus Twig (桑寄生, Sangjisheng), Argy Wormwood Leaf (艾叶, Aiye), Tuberculate Speranskia Herb (透骨草, Tougucao), Incised Notopterygium Rhizome or Root (羌活, Qianghuo), Doubleteeth Pubescent Angelica Root (独活, Duhuo), Red Peony

Root (赤芍, Chishao), Ending Part of Chinese Angelica Root (当归尾, Dangguiwei), Dragon's Blood (血竭, Xuejie), Olibanum (乳香, Ruxiang) and Myrrh (没药, Moyao). Its actions are removing blood stasis drastically and eliminating mass. It is applicable for rupture of exfetation manifested as haematoma in the abdomen, relief of pain, bearing-down and distention sensation in the lower abdomen or with desire to discharge stool, gradual disappearing of vaginal bleeding, thin and unsmooth pulse.

Two Immortals Powder
(二仙汤, er xian tang)

Source: Prescriptions of Shuguan Hospital Affiliated to Shanghai Traditional Chinese Medicine College 上海中医学院附属曙光医院处方

Composition: Common Curculigo Rhizome (仙茅, Xianmao)6g

Shorthorned Epimedium Herb (淫羊藿, Yinyanghuo)9g

Chinese Angelica Root (当归, Danggui)9g

Medicinal Indian Mulberry Root (巴戟天, Bajitian)6g

Chinese Corktree Bark (黄柏, Huangbai)6g

Common Anemarrhena Rhizome (知母, Zhimu)6g

Actions: Simultaneously reinforcing yin and yang and regulating Chong and Ren Meridians.

Applied Syndrome: Syndrome of heat in the upper-jiao and cold in the lower-jiao which is manifested as vertigo and tinnitus, hot sensation, flushed face, restlessness, irritability, soreness and weakness of the loin and knees, cold limbs, profuse watery and white leucorrhea, pale tongue, wiry and thin pulse.

Points in Constitution: This formula lays equal stress on warming and invigorating the kidney yang and clearing away fire of deficient type to regulate yin and yang and Chong and Ren Meridians.

Indications:

1. Climacteric syndrome, climacteric hypertension.
2. Senile vaginitis, chronic pelvic inflammation.

Precautions: It is forbidden for those with deficiency of yin and excessive liver-fire.

Associated Formulas:

1. Pill for Balancing the Heart and the Kidney (交泰丸, jiao tai wan) *Han's Treatise on General Medicine* 《韩氏医通》

This is made up of Cassia Bark (桂心, Guixin) and Coptis Rhizome (黄连, Huanglian). Its actions are restoring the equilibrium between the heart and the kidney. It is indicated for severe palpitation or insomnia due to deficiency of kidney water and hyperactivity of heart fire resulting from breakdown of the normal physiological coordination between the heart and the kidney.

Two Immortals Powder
(Method of Uniformly Nourishing Yin and Yang)

Ingredients	Effects	Combined Effects	Syndrome	Chief Symptoms
Common Curculigo Rhizome (仙茅, Xianmao) 6g Shorthorned Epimedium Herb (淫羊藿, Yinyanghuo) 9g Medicinal Indian Mulberry Root (巴戟天, Bajitian) 6g	Invigorating the kidney and strengthening yang	Uniformly reinforcing yin and yang and regulating Chong and Ren Meridians	Climacterid syndrome (due to heat in the upper-jiao and cold in the lower-jiao)	Vertigo, tinnitus, flushed face, hot sensation, irritability, soreness and weakness of the loins and knees, cold limbs, profuse watery and white leucorrhea, pale tongue, wiry and thin pulse
Chinese Corktree Bark (黄柏, Huangbai) 6g Common Anemarrhena Rhizome (知母, Zhimu) 6g	Purging fire and keeping yin			
Chinese Angelica Root (当归, Danggui) 9g	Enriching blood and regulating Chong Meridian			

2. General Recipe for Treating Climacterium (更年期统治方, geng nian qi tong zhi fang) *Author's Experienced Prescription* (笔者经验方)

This is composed of Lily Bulb (百合, Baihe), Silktree Albiziae Bark (合欢皮, Hehuanpi), Common Anemarrhea Rhizomme (知母, Zhimu), Dried Rehmannia Root (生地黄, Shengdihuang), Light Wheat (浮小麦, Fuxiaomai), Prepared Licorice Root (炙甘草, Zhigancao), Chinese Date (大枣, Dazao), Dragon Teeth (龙齿, Longchi), Coptis Rhizome (黄连, Huanglian) and Cassia Bark (肉桂, Rougui). Its actions are uniformly nourishing yin and yang and restoring normal coordination between the heart and kidney. It is indicated to woman's climacteric syndrome, manifested as hot feeling, sweating, irritability and restlessness.

Chapter Eight
Formulas for Pediatric Diseases

With the development of Pediatric of TCM, effective formulas adapted for children's *diseases* have emerged one after another since the book *Key to Therapeutics of Children's Diseases* 《小儿药证直诀》was published in Song Dynasty. The characteristics of these formulas mainly present as: 1. Pay enough attention to the physiological and pathological particularity of the children that they are not adequately developed and are very susceptible to the syndrome of deficiency or excess. 2. Drugs are used mildly and flexibly and they are mostly prepared into pill or powder form so as to be taken easily and conveniently. And 3. Place special emphasis on strengthening the spleen, nourishing the stomach and promoting digestion.

For the treatment of diseases such as upper respiratory tract infection, pulmonary infection, asthma, acute and chronic nephritis, indigestion, malnutrition and neurosism in children, the Chinese formulas have proved extremely effective without side-effects. Thus, they are widely used in clinic.

1. Spleen-Invigorating Pill
（启脾丸, qi pi wan）

Source: *A Prescription Selected from One Hundred Prescriptionss* 《百一选方》
Composition: Ginseng（人参, Renshen）6g
Largehead Atractylodes Rhizome（白术, Baizhu）6g
Green Tangerine Peel（青皮, Qingpi）6g
Fried Medicated Leaven（炒神曲, Chao Shenqu）9g
Fried Malt（炒麦芽, Chao Maiya）9g
Tangerine Peel（陈皮, Chenpi）6g
Officinal Magnolia Bark（厚朴, Houpo）6g
Villous Amomum Fruit（砂仁, Sharen）6g
Dried Ginger（干姜, Ganjiang）3g
Prepared Licorice Root（炙甘草, Zhi Gancao）3g
Actions: Invigorating spleen-qi and pomoting digestion.
Applied Syndrome: Syndrome of food retention due to spleen deficiency manifested as stiffness and fullness sensation in the chest, abdominal distention, diarrhea with borborygmus, poor appetite, shortness of breath, tiredness, sickly complexion, slightly greasy tongue coating and feeble pulse.

Spleen-Invigorating Pill

(Spleen-Strengthening and Digestion-Promoting Method)

Ingredients	Effects	Combined Effects	Syndrome	Chief Symptoms
Ginseng (人参, Renshen) 6g Largehead Atractylodes Rhizome (白术, Baizhu) 6g Fried Licorice Root (炙甘草, Zhi Gancao) 3g	Invigorating spleen-qi	Replenishing qi, strengthening the spleen, alleviating stagnation in the middle-jiao and promoting digestion	Food retention due to spleen deficiency	Feeling of distention and fullness in the gastric cavity and abdomen, borborygmus and diarrhea, poor appetite, the shortness of breath and tiredness, slightly greasy tongue coating and weak pulse
Tangerine Peel (陈皮, Chenpi) 6g Green Tangerine Peel (青皮, Qingpi) 6g Villous Amomum Fruit (砂仁, Sharen) 6g Officinal Magnolia Bark (厚朴, Houpo) 6g	Activating flow of qi to relieve stagnation in the middle-jiao			
Dried Ginger (干姜, Ganjiang) 3g	Warming middle-jiao and regulating stomach-qi			
Fried Medicated Leaven (炒神曲, Chao Shenqu) 9g Fried Malt (炒麦芽, Chao Maiya) 9g	Removing retained food			

Points in Constitution: This formula is the Aucklandia and Amomum, Six Gentlemen Decoction (香砂六君子汤, xiang sha liu jun zi tang) without Tuckahoe (茯苓, Fuling), Pinellia Rhizome (半夏, Banxia) and Common Aucklandia Root (木香, Muxiang) but plus Medicated Leaven (神曲, Shenqu) and Fried Malt (炒麦芽, Chao Maiya) which can promote digestion and Green Tangerine Peel (青皮, Qingpi), Officinal Magnolia Bark (厚朴, Houpo) and Dried Ginger (干姜, Ganjiang) which can regulate flow of qi and warm middle-jiao. This formula has both the dispelling and tonifying actions and emphasizes warming the middle-jiao and invigorating the spleen. Besides, it also has the actions of activating flow of qi and eliminating food stagnation.

Indications:
1. Chronic gastritis or enteritis
2. Chronic hepatitis
3. Indigestion, postoperative dyspepsia or dyspepsia in the stage of recovery

Precaution: This formula is not suitable for heat syndrome of food retention.

Associated Formulas:
1. Spleen-Strengthening Pill (健脾丸, jian pi wan) *Standard for Diagnosis and Treatment*

《证治准绳》

This consists of Largehead Atractylodes Rhizome (白术, Baizhu), Common Aucklandia Root (木香, Muxiang), Coptis Rhizome (黄连, Huanglian), Prepared Licorice Root (炙甘草, Zhi Gancao), Tuckahoe (茯苓, Fuling), Ginseng (人参, Renshen), Medicated Leaven (神曲, Shenqu), Tangerine Peel (陈皮, Chenpi), Villous Amomum Fruit (砂仁, Sharen), Malt (麦芽, Maiya), Hawthorn Fruit (山楂, Shanzha), Common Yam Rhizome (山药, Shanyao) and Nutmeg Seed (肉豆蔻, Roudonkou). Its actions are invigorating the spleen, regulating the stomach, promoting digestion and stopping diarrhea. It is indicated for the syndrome of the heat-dampness due to spleen deficiency and food retention.

2. Powder for Sallow Complexion (益黄散, yi huang san) *Key to Therapeutics of Children's Diseases*《小儿药证直诀》

This is composed of Tangerine Peel (陈皮, Chenpi), Green Tangerine Peel (青皮, Qingpi), Roasted Medicine Terminalia Fruit (诃子, Hezi), Prepared Licorice Root (炙甘草, Zhi Gancao) and Clove Flower-Bud (丁香, Dingxiang). It is good at regulating stomach-qi, warming middle-jiao and stopping diarrhea. It is applicable for retention of food due to failure in transformation and transportation of food resulting from deficiency and cold of the spleen and stomach.

3. Spleen-Invigorating Body-Nouirishing Powder (健脾肥儿散, jian pi fei er san) *Practical Formula-ology*《实用方剂学》

This consists of Fried Common Yam Rhizome (炒山药, Chao Shanyao), Largehead Atractylodes Rhizome (白术, Baizhu) and Fried Chicken Gizzard Membrane (炒鸡内金, Chao Jineijin). Its actions are invigorating the spleen and stomach to stop diarrhea. It is suited to indigestion in children due to injury of the spleen and stomach by improper diet.

2. Largehead Atractylodes Powder with Seven Herbs
(七味白术散, qi wei bai zhu san)

Source: *Key to Therapeutics of Children's Diseases*《小儿药证直诀》
Composition: Largehead Atractylodes Rhizome (白术, Baizhu) 3g,
Tuckahoe (茯苓, Fuling) 3g,
Ginseng (人参, Renshen) 3g,
Licorice Root (甘草, Gancao) 1g,
Lobed Kudzuvine Root (葛根, Gegen) 3g,
Common Aucklandia Root (木香, Muxiang) 1g,
Wrinkled Gianthyssop Herb (藿香, Huoxiang) 1g

Actions: Invigorating the spleen to stop diarrhea, regulating the stomach to generate body fluid

Applied Syndromes: Vomiting and diarrhea due to spleen deficiency or infantile malnutrition manifested by emaciated body, indigestion, malnutrition, loose stool, irritability, thirst, excessive drinking or eating, or poor appetite, pale tongue and weak pulse.

Largehead Atractylodes Powder with Seven Herbs

(Spleen-Strengthening and Stomach-Regulating Method)

Ingredients	Effects	Combined Effects	Syndrome	Chief Symptoms
Ginseng（人参, Renshen）3g Largehead Atractylodes Rhizome（白术, Baizhu）3g Tuckahoe（茯苓, Fuling）3g Licorice Root（甘草, Gancao）1g	Invigorating the spleen and benefiting qi	Invigorating the spleen to stop diarrhea and regulating the stomach to generate body fluid	Indigestion due to a long-time deficiency of the stomach and the spleen	Emaciated body, indigestion, loose stool, irritation and thirst with excessive drinking or eating, hunger or poor appetite, pale tongue and weak pulse
Lobed Kudzuvine Root（葛根, Gegen）3g	Lifting yang to stop diarrhea and dispelling heat to generate body fluid			
Wrinkled Gianthyssop Herb（藿香, Huoxiang）1g	Warming middle-jiao to regulate qi and activating spleen-qi with aromatic in odor			
Common Aucklandia Root（木香, Muxiang）1g	Regulating qi in the middle-jiao			

Points in Constitution: This formula uses the ingredients of Four Gentlemen Decoction(四君子汤, si jun zi tang) to invigorate the spleen so as to treat the primary aspect, and the other drugs such as Lobed Kudzuvine Root（葛根, Gegen）, Wrinkled Gianthyssop Herb（藿香, Huoxiang）and Common Aucklandia Root（木香, Muxiang）to promote the transporting and transforming functions of the spleen, thus, tonifying the spleen without formation of qi stagnation.

Indications:

1. Infantile dyspepsia
2. Common cold with gastrointestinal symptoms
3. Diabetes with sweet taste

Precautions: 1. This formula is contraindicated in diarrhea of heat-dampness type.

2. If it is used for diabetes with sweet taste, the dose should be enlarged appropriately.

Associated Formula:

Spleen-Invigorating Pill(启脾丸, qi pi wan) *An Introduction to Medicine*《医学入门》

This is comprised of Ginseng（人参, Renshen）, Fried Largehead Atractylodes Rhizome（炒白术, Chao Baizhu）, Hawthorn Fruit（山楂, Shanzha）, Tangerine Peel（陈皮, Chenpi）, Oriental Waterplantain Rhizome（泽泻, Zexie）, Licorice Root（甘草, Gancao）, Tuckahoe（茯苓, Fuling), Common Yam Rhizome (山药, Shanyao) and Lotus Seed (莲子, Lianzi). Its actions are invigorating spleen to resolve dampness and regulating the stomach to remove food stagnation. It is suited to food stagnation due to deficiency in middle-jiao manifested as emaciated body, poor appetite, belching with fetid odour, loose stool, greasy or turbid tongue coating, and weak and soft pulse.

3. Cold-Expelling and Convulsion-Relieving Decoction
(逐寒荡惊汤, zhu han dang jing tang)

Source: *Compilation of Prescriptions for Benefiting the Children* 《福幼编》
Composition: Clove Flower-bud (丁香, Dingxiang) 3g
Cassia Bark (肉桂, Rougui) 3g
Black Pepper Fruit (胡椒, Hujiao) 3g
Dried Ginger (干姜, Ganjiang) 3g
Burnt Clay-lining of Kitchen Range (灶心土, Zaoxintu) 60g
Actions: Eliminating pathogenic cold and relieving convulsion
Applied syndrome: Chronic infantile convulsion due to deficiency and cold of middle-jiao and insufficient kidney-yang manifested as blue and pale complexion, cold feeling in the mouth and nose, cold limbs and convulsion, coma with opening eyes, vomiting, loose stool or fluid stools containing undigested food, frequent urination or oliguria, pale tongue with white coating, slow and deep pulse or feeble, thin and deep pulse.

Cold-Expelling and Convulsion-Relieving Decoction
(Interior-Warming and Cold-Dispelling Method)

Ingredients	Effects	Combined Effects	Syndrome	Chief Symptoms
Clove Flower-Bud (丁香, Dingxiang) 3g Cassia Bark (肉桂, Rougui) 3g Black Pepper Fruit (胡椒, Hujiao) 3g Dried Ginger (干姜, Ganjiang) 3g	Warming the kidney and strengthening yang, warming the middle-jiao to expel pathogenic cold	Warming the middle-jiao and strengthening yang, keeping the adverse qi downwards and stopping diarrhea	Chronic infantile convulsion due to deficiency of the spleen-yang and kidney-yang	Vomiting, fluid stools with undigested food, oliguria or frequent urination, pale complexion, cold limbs and clonic convulsion, pale tongue with white coating, slow and deep pulse or thin and deep and weak pulse
Burnt Clay-lining of Kitchen Range (灶心土, Zaoxintu) 60g	Using scorched earth to tonify the earth (spleen), stopping vomiting and diarrhea			

Points in Constitution: The function of this formula is to reinforce the spleen by warming and supplementing the fire of the gate of life. Burnt Clay-Lining of the Kitchen Range(灶心土, Zaoxintu) is used to directly supplement the earth(the spleen).

Indications:
1. Infantile diarrhea (virus type or non-infection type)
2. Infantile dehydration caused by a long period of illness and weak body
3. Chronic convulsion due to erroneously taking cold-natured drugs after pox and rash diseases
4. Nephritis and nephrotic syndrome

Precautions:
1. This formula is forbidden for convulsion due to extreme pathogenic heat or yin-deficiency.
2. This formula is contraindicated in diarrhea due to pathogenic heat.

Associated formulas:

1. Powder for Sallow Complexion (益黄散, yi huang san) *Key to Therapeutics of Children's Diseases* 《小儿药证直诀》

This formula is comprised of Clove Flower-Bud (丁香, Dingxiang), Toasted Medicine Terminalia Fruit (诃子, Hezi), Tangerine Peel (陈皮, Chenpi), Green Tangerine Peel (青皮, Qingpi) and Licorice Root (甘草, Gancao). Its actions are regulating the stomach, normalizing the flow of qi and warming the middle-jiao to stop diarrhea. It is suited to infantile dysfunction of the spleen and stomach manifested as emaciated body with a large abdomen, vomiting and diarrhea.

2. Middle-Regulating Pill (理中丸, li zhong wan) *Treatise on Exogenous Febrile Diseases*《伤寒论》

This formula consists of Ginseng (人参, Renshen), Dried Ginger (干姜, Ganjiang), Largehead Atractylodes Rhizome (白术, Baizhu) and Prepared Licorice Root (炙甘草, Zhi Gancao). Its actions are warming the middle-jiao to disperse pathogenic cold, benefiting qi and invigorating the spleen. It is suited to chronic infantile convulsion due to spleen deficiency or infantile diarrhea and vomiting due to deficiency of spleen-yang.

4. Viscera-Benefiting and Consciousness-Restoring Decoction (可保立苏汤, ke bao li su tang)

Source: *Correction on the Errors of Medical Works*《医林改错》
Composition: Toasted Membranous Milkvetch Root (炙黄芪, Zhi Huangqi)6g
Pilose Asiabell Root (党参, Dangshen) 9g
Largehead Atractylodes Rhizome (白术, Baizhu) 6g
Prepared Licorice Root (炙甘草, Zhi Gancao) 6g
Chinese Angelica Root (当归, Danggui) 6g
White Peony Root (白芍药, Baishaoyao) 6g
Spine Date Seed (酸枣仁, Suanzaoren) 9g
Asiatic Cornelian Cherry Fruit (山萸肉, Shanyurou) 3g
Barbary Wolfberry Fruit (枸杞子, Gouqizi) 6g

Malaytea Scurfpea Fruit (破故纸, Poguzhi) 3g

English Walnut (核桃, Hetao) (ground into powder with peel) 1piece

Actions: Drastically replenishing the primodial qi, warming and tonifying the spleen and kidney

Applied syndrome: Chronic infantile convulsion caused by exogenous febrile diseases, pestilence, pox and rash diseases, vomiting, diarrhea and deficiency of qi due to prolonged illness manifested by frequent onset of slow tic of the limbs with spitting out of saliva, coma, pale complexion, pale tongue and deep and thin pulse.

Viscera-Benefiting and Consciousness-Restoring Decoction
(Method of Warming and Tonifying the Spleen and Kidney)

Ingredients	Effects	Combined Effects	Syndrome	Chief Symptoms
Prepared Membranous Milkvetch Root (黄芪, Huangqi) 6g	Replenishing the primary qi			
Pilose Asiabell Root (党参, Dangshen) 9g Largehead Atractylodes Rhizome (白术, Baizhu) 6g Prepared Licorice Root (炙甘草, Zhi Gancao) 6g	Benefiting qi and invigorating the spleen			
Chinese Angelica Root (当归, Danggui) 6g White Peony Root (白芍药, Baishaoyao) 6g Asiatic Cornelian Cherry Fruit (山萸肉, Shanyurou) 3g Barbary Wolfberry Fruit (枸杞子, Gouqizi) 6g Malaytea Scurfpea Fruit (破故纸, Poguzhi) 3g English Walnut (核桃, Hetao) 1	Tonifying the liver and kidney	Benefiting qi and nourishing blood, warming and tonifying the spleen and kidney	Chronic infantile convulsion due to deficiency and cold of the spleen and kidney	Slow tic of the limbs, tiredness and listlessness, pale complexion, somnolence, pale tongue and deep and thin pulse
Spine Date Seed (酸枣仁, Suanzaoren) 9g	Tranquilizing the mind by nourishing the heart			

Points in Constitution: This formula lays equal stress on reinforcing the five zang-organs and replenishing both qi and blood. So it is very suitable for chronic infantile convulsion caused by malnutrition and indigestion.

Indications:
1. Malnutrition
2. Minor epilepsy
3. Tetany

Precautions:

1. This formula is designed for chronic infantile convulsion due to deficiency and cold of the spleen and kidney. It should be forbidden for excessive or heat syndrome.

2. Crude and cold food should be avoided while taking this decoction.

Associated formula:

Vital Qi-Consolidating Decoction(固真汤, gu zhen tang) *Standard for Diagnosis and Treatment*《证治准绳》

This is composed of Ginseng (人参, Renshen), Daughter Root of Common Monkshood (附子, Fuzi), Tuckahoe (茯苓, Fuling), Largehead Atractylodes Rhizome (白术, Baizhu), Common Yam Rhizome (山药, Shanyao), Membranous Milkvetch Root (黄芪, Huangqi), Cassia Bark (肉桂, Rougui) and Prepared Licorice Root (炙甘草, Zhi Gancao). Its actions are supplementing yang, benefiting qi, warming and tonifying the spleen and stomach. It is indicated for chronic convulsion due to deficiency of the spleen after vomiting and diarrhea, marked by a cold feeling in the mouth, nose and limbs or even coma.

5. Primary Qi-Regulating Powder
(调元散, tiao yuan san)

Source: *Personal Experience for Saving Children*《活幼心书》
Composition: Common Yam Rhizome (山药, Shanyao)12g
Ginseng (人参, Renshen) 6g
Tuckahoe (茯苓, Fuling) 6g
Indian Bread with Hostwood (茯神, Fushen) 6g
Largehead Atractylodes Rhizome (白术, Baizhu) 6g
White Peony Root (白芍药, Baishaoyao) 6g
Prepared Rehmannia Root (熟地黄, Shudihuang) 6g
Chinese Angelica Root (当归, Danggui)6g
Toasted Membranous Milkvetch Root (炙黄芪, Zhi Huangqi)6g
Szechwan Lovage Rhizome (川芎, Chuanxiong)6g
Prepared Licorice Root (炙甘草, Zhi Gancao) 6g
Grassleaf Sweetflag Rhizome (石菖蒲, Shichangpu) 6g
Fresh Ginger (生姜, Shengjiang) 3g
Chinese Date (大枣, Dazao) 3g
Actions: Benefiting qi and nourishing blood, invigorating the spleen and tonifying the kidney
Applied syndrome: Five kinds of flaccidity and metopism in children due to congenital deficien-

cy manifested as fontanel open, emaciated body, weak and thin limbs, dementia, pale complexion, being slow in speaking, walking and teeth growth, pale tongue with little coating, weak and thin pulse, light red fingerprint.

Viscera-Benefiting and Consciousness-Restoring Decoction
(Spleen-Invigorating and Kidney-Reinforcing Method)

Ingredients	Effects	Combined Effects	Syndrome	Chief Symptoms
Common Yam Rhizome (山药, Shanyao)12g	Invigorating the spleen and tonifying the kidney	Invigorating the spleen and tonifying the kidney, benefiting qi and nourishing blood	Five kinds of maldevelopment and flabbiness due to congenital deficiency	Metopism, tardiness in learning to speak and walk, emaciated body, whitish complexion, pale tongue with little coating, weak and thin pulse, light red superficial venule of the index finger
Ginseng (人参, Renshen) 6g Toasted Membranous Milkvetch Root (炙黄芪, Zhi Huangqi) 6g Largehead Atractylodes Rhizome (白术, Baizhu) 6g Tuckahoe (茯苓, Fuling) 6g	Invigorating the spleen and benefiting qi			
Chinese Angelica Root (当归, Danggui)6g Prepared Rehmannia Root (熟地黄, Shudihuang) 6g Szechwan Lovage Rhizome (川芎, Chuanxiong)6g White Peony Root (白芍, Baishao)6g	Tonifying blood and nourishing yin			
Indian Bread with Hostwood (茯神, Fushen) 6g Grassleaf Sweetflag Rhizome (石菖蒲, Shichangpu) 6g	Tranquilizing the mind and inducing resuscitation			
Fresh Ginger (生姜, Shengjiang) 3g Chinese Date (大枣, Dazao) 3g Prepared Licorice Root (炙甘草, Zhi Gancao) 6g	Regulating ying and wei			

Points in Constitution: The composition of this formula is similar to that of Ten Strong Tonic

Herbs Pill (十全大补丸, shi quan da bu wan) though Common Yam Rhizome (山药, Shanyao) is used instead of Cassia Bark (肉桂, Rougui) in this formula. Common Yam Rhizome (山药, Shanyao) can invigorate the spleen and the kidney and has a most mild nature while Cassia Bark (肉桂, Rougui) may benefit the fire in the gate of life and has a warm and hot nature. Since the body of infant belongs to yang, the drugs for tonification should be mild in nature. That is why Common Yam Rhizome (山药, Shanyao) is used instead of Cassia Bark (肉桂, Rougui).

Indications:
1. Rickets
2. Infantile malnutrition

Precaution: This formula emphasizes the warming and invigorating actions, so it is forbidden for the case of yin deficiency with hyperactivity of pathogenic fire.

Associated formula:

Grassleaf Sweetflag Rhizome Pill (菖蒲丸, chang pu wan) *Longevity and Life Prescription* 《寿世保元》

This formula consists of Grassleaf Sweetflag Rhizome (石菖蒲, Shichangpu), Ginseng (人参, Renshen), Dwarf Lilyturf Root (麦门冬, Maimendong), Szechwan Lovage Rhizome (川芎, Chuanxiong), Thinleaf Milkwort Root (远志, Yuanzhi), Chinese Angelica Root (当归, Danggui), Olibanum (乳香, Ruxiang) and Cinnabar (朱砂, Zhusha). Its actions are tonifying the heart and increasing intelligence. It is suited to tardiness in learning to speak in infants due to deficiency of heart-qi.

6. Silk Pouch Pill
(布袋丸, bu dai wan)

Source: *Modified Pocket Treatise on Pediatric Formulae* 《补要袖珍小儿方论》

Composition: Bat Dung (夜明砂, Yemingsha) 6g

Bigfruit Elm Fruit (芜荑, Wuyi) 6g

Rangooncreeper Fruit (使君子, Shijunzi) 6g

Tuckahoe (茯苓, Fuling) 3g

Largehead Atractylodes Rhizome (白术, Baizhu) 3g

Ginseng (人参, Renshen) 3g

Licorice Root (甘草, Gancao) 3g

Aloes (芦荟, Luhui) 3g

Actions: Expelling ascarides and treating infantile malnutrition, tonifying the spleen and stomach

Applied syndrome: Infantile malnutrition due to parasitic infestation and deficiency of the spleen and stomach manifested as fever, yellow complexion, thin limbs with big abdomen, dry skin, brittle hairs and photophobia, or low fever.

Silk Pouch Pill
(Spleen-Strengthening and Parasites-Destroying Method)

Ingredients	Effects	Combined Effects	Syndrome	Chief Symptoms
Ginseng (人参, Renshen) 3g Tuckahoe (茯苓, Fuling) 3g Largehead Atractylodes Rhizome (白术, Baizhu) 3g Licorice Root (甘草, Gancao) 3g	Invigorating the spleen and benefiting qi	Invigorating the spleen and destroying intestinal parasites	Ascariasis and infantile malnutrition caused by parasites	Intestinal roundworm in the abdomen, emaciation, abdominal distention, dry and brittle hair and poor vision
Bigfruit Elm Fruit (芫荑, Wuyi) 6g Rangooncreeper Fruit (使君子, Shijunzi) 6g Aloes (芦荟, Luhui) 3g	Poisoning and expelling the intestinal parasites			
Bat Dung (夜明砂, Yemingsha) 6g	Improving eyesight and curing infantile malnutrition			

Points in Constitution: This formula is indicted for infantile malnutrition caused by parasite infection. Bigfruit Elm Fruit (芫荑, Wuyi), Rangooncreeper Fruit (使君子, Shijunzi) and Aloes (芦荟, Luhui) can destroy and expel the intestinal parasites or roundworms. When they are combined with the ingredients of Four Gentlemen Decoction (四君子汤, si jun zi tang), they can replenish qi, invigorate the spleen, and conduct the elimination and replenishment simultaneously, thus, treating the malnutrition due to parasitic infestation.

Indication: Intestinal parasites accompanied with indigestion and malnutritionPrecaution: This formula is not suitable for infantile malnutrition with roundworm

Associated formulas:

1. Chicken's Liver Powder(鸡肝散, ji gan san) *ChinesePatent Medicines in common use* 《常用中成药》

This consists of Rangooncreeper Fruit (使君子, Shijunzi), Stone-like Omphalia (雷丸, Leiwan) and Fresh Chicken's Liver(鲜鸡肝, Xianjigan). Its actions are curing infantile malnutrition, killing parasites and improving acuity of sight. It is suited to infantile malnutrition manifested as parasitic infection, abdominal pain, poor appetite, diarrhea, yellow complexion, emaciated body and blurring of vision.

2. Baby-Nourishing Pill (肥儿丸, fei er wan) *Prescriptions of Peaceful Benevolent Dispensary* 《和剂局方》

This is composed of Medicated Leaven (神曲, Shenqu), Coptis Rhizome (黄连, Huanglian), Nutmeg Seed (肉豆蔻, Roudoukou), Rangooncreeper Fruit (使君子, Shijunzi), fried Malt (麦

芽, Maiya), Areca Seed（槟榔, Binglang）, Common Aucklandia Root（木香, Muxiang）and Pig's Bile（猪胆汁, Zhudanzhi）. Its actions are killing parasites and curing infantile malnutrition, invigorating the spleen and clearing away pathogenic heat. It is suited to infantile parasitic infection due to spleen deficiency and liver-heat.

3. Parasite-Eliminating Pill（化虫丸, hua chong wan） *Prescriptions of Peaceful Benevolent Dispensary*《和剂局方》

This consists of Minium Powder（铅粉, Qianfen）, Common Carpesium Fruit（鹤虱, Heshi）, Areca Seed（槟榔, Binglang）, Szechwan Chinaberry Bark（苦楝皮, Kulianpi）and Alum（白矾, Baifan）. It can expel and destroy many kinds of parasites in the intestinal tract such as roundworm, pinworm and tapeworm. It is used for parasites in the intestines.

7. Shen's Pill for Enuresis
（沈氏閟泉丸, shen shi men quan wan）

Source: *Source and Cause of Miscellaneous Diseases*《杂病源流犀烛》
Composition: Sharpleaf Galangal Fruit（益智仁, Yizhiren）9g
Tuckahoe（茯苓, Fuling）6g
Largehead Atractylodes Rhizome（白术, Baizhu）6g
Japanese Ampelopsis Root（白蔹, Bailian）6g
Cape Jasmine Fruit（山栀子, Shanzhizi）6g
White Peony Root（白芍药, Baishaoyao）6g
Actions: Arresting enuresis and clearing away pathogenic heat in three-jiao
Applied syndrome: Enuresis caused by stagnant heat in the three-jiaos manifested as involuntary discharge of scanty amount of yellow urine with stinking and foul smell when sleeping at night, irritability, or ulttered words with teeth grinding during sleeping, red tongue with yellow coating, thin and wiry pulse.
Points in Constitution: The characteristic of this formula is to induce astringency and remove damp-heat at the same time so as to be indicated for infantile enuresis with retention of damp-heat.
Indications: Infantile enuresis
Precaution: This formula is contraindicated in enuresis caused by kidney deficiency without heat symptoms.
Associated formula:
Urination-Decreasing Pill（缩泉丸, suo quan wan） *The Complete Effective Prescriptions for Women Diseases*《妇人良方大全》

This consists of Chinese Yam（Shanyao, 山药）, Commbined Spicebush Root（乌药, Wuyao）and Sharpleaf Galangal Fruit（益智仁, Yizhiren）. Its actions are warming the kidney, dispelling cold and arresting enuresis. It is suited to frequent urination or enuresis caused by deficiency and cold of the urinary bladder.

Shen's Pill for Enuresis
(Heart-Removing, Liver-Soothing and Astringency-Inducing Method)

Ingredients	Effects	Combined Effects	Syndrome	Chief symptom
Japanese Ampelopsis Root (白蔹, Bailian) 6g Sharpleaf Galangal Fruit (益智仁, Yizhiren) 9g	Arresting enuresis	Clearing away heat, regulating the liver-qi and arresting enuresis	Enuresis caused by stagnant heat in three-jiao	Involuntary discharging scanty amount of yellow urine in sleeping, irritability, red tongue with yellow coating, thin and wiry pulse
White Peeony Root (白芍药, Baishaoyao) 6g	Retaining body fluid with astringent			
Largehead Atractylodes Rhizome (白术, Baizhu) 6g Tuckahoe (茯苓, Fuling) 6g	Invigorating the spleen to eliminate dampness			
Cape Jasmine Fruit (山栀子, Shanzhizi) 6g	Clearing heat in three-jiao			

8. Hang Xie Pellet
(沆瀣丹, hang xie dan)

Source: *A Collection of Pediatrics* 《幼幼集成》
Composition: Szechwan Lovage Rhizome (川芎, Chuanxiong) 3g
Rhubarb (大黄, Dahuang) 3g
Baikal Skullcap Root (黄芩, Huangqin) 3g
Chinese Corktree Bark (黄柏, Huangbai) 3g
Pharbitis Seed (牵牛子, Qianniuzi) 1.5g
Wild Mint Herb (薄荷, Bohe) 1.5g
Talc (滑石, Huashi) 3g
Areca Seed (槟榔, Binglang) 3g
Bitter Orange (枳壳, Zhiqiao) 3g
Weeping Forsythia Capsule (连翘, Lianqiao) 3g
Red Peony Root (赤芍药, Chishaoyao) 3g
Actions: Clearing away heat and toxic material, expelling fire and removing retained food
Applied syndrome: Fetal toxicosis, heat-syndrome of the newborn, icterus neonatorum, thrush, sublingual swelling and stiff tongue, sorethroat or inflammation of the throat, measles, wandering edema, tinea and scabies, erysipelas and urticaria, flushed face with closed eyes, re-

tention of phlegm and food with pathogenic wind-heat, mumps with swollen face and all kinds of convulsion caused by accumulated heat of excess type in the three-jiaos.

Hang Xie Pellet
(Heat-Clearing and Fire-Purging Method)

Ingredients	Effects	Combined Effects	Syndrome	Chief symptom
Baikal Skullcap Root(黄芩, Huangqin) 3g Chinese Corktree Bark (黄柏, Huangbai) 3g Weeping Forsythia Capsule (连翘, Lianqiao) 3g	Clearing away heat and toxic material	Clearing away heat and toxic material, and expelling fire and removing retained food	Stagnation of heat and toxin	Heat-syndrome of the newborn, fetal toxicosis, icterus neonatorum, thrush, sublingual swelling and stiff tongue, sorethroat, acute tonsillitis, erysipelas, mumps, constipation, scanty dark urine, red tongue with yellow coating and rapid pulse
Rhubarb (大黄, Dahuang) 3g Pharbitis Seed (牵牛子, Qianniuzi) 1.5g Areca Seed (槟榔, Binglang) 3g	Eliminating retained food and expelling heat			
Bitter Orange (枳壳, Zhiqiao) 3g Szechwan Lovage Rhizome (川芎, Chuanxiong) 3g Red Peony Root (赤芍药, Chishaoyao) 3g	Regulating flow of qi and blood			
Talc (滑石, Huashi) 3g	Clearing away heat and promoting diuresis			
Wild Mint Herb (薄荷, Bohe) 1.5g	Relieving the exterior syndrome and expelling heat			

Points in Constitution: This formula uses the heat-clearing, purgative, diaphoresis and dispelling methods altogether to clear away the stagnated heat and toxic material as soon as possible. All the drugs of Pharbitis Seed (牵牛子, Qianniuzi), Areca Seed (槟榔, Binglang) and Talc (滑石, Huashi) have the actions of purging water retention and promoting diuresis. Thus, they are especially suitable for the heat syndrome due to restention of water.

Indications:
1. Infantile upper respiratory tract infection
2. Pharyngitis, acute tonsillitis and thrush
3. Scarlet fever

4. Skin pyogenic infection
5. Parotitis
6. Hydrocephalus

Precaution: This formula is only suitable for the heat syndrome of excessive type and not for other ones.

Associated formulas:

1. Diaphiagm-Cooling Powder (凉膈散, liang ge san) *Prescriptions of Peaceful Benevolent Dispensary*《和剂局方》

This consists of Rhubarb (大黄, Dahuang), Mirabilite (芒硝, Mangxiao), Licorice Root (甘草, Gancao), Cape Jasmine Fruit (山栀子, Shanzhizi), Wild Mint Herb (薄荷, Bohe), Baikal Skullcap Root (黄芩, Huangqin) and Weeping Forsythia Capsule (连翘, Lianqiao). Its action is expelling fire to loosen the bowels by clearing away heat in the upper and purging the fire in the lower. It is suited to restlessness, irritability, thirst, flushed face and dry lips, constipation, red tongue with yellow coating, rapid and smooth pulse due to excessive fire in the upper-jiao and middle-jiao.

2. Coptis Detoxificating Decoction (黄连解毒汤, huang lian jie du tang) *The Medical Secrets of An Offical*《外台秘要》

This consists of Baikal Skullcap Root (黄芩, Huangqin), Coptis Rhizome (黄连, Huanglian), Chinese Corktree Bark (黄柏, Huangbai) and Cape Jasmine Fruit (山栀子, Shanzhizi). Its actions are expelling fire and clearing away toxic material. It is indicated to high fever, irritability, dry mouth and throat, delirium and insomnia caused by excessive fire in three jiaos.

Additional Formulas

Infantile Convulsion-Relieving Pill
(小儿回春丹, xiao er hui chun dan)

Source: *Shanghai Standard for Preparation of Chinese Patent Medicine*《上海市中药成药制剂规范》

Composition: Cow-Bezoar (牛黄, Niuhuang)
Borneol (冰片, Bingpian)
Cinnabar (朱砂, Zhusha)
Incised Notopterygium Rhizome or Root (羌活, Qianghuo)
Silkworm with Batrytis Larva (僵蚕, Jiangcan)
Tall Gastrodia Rhizome (天麻, Tianma)
Divaricate Saposhnikovia Root (防风, Fangfeng)
Scorpion (全蝎, Quanxie)
Giant Typhonium Rhizome (白附子, Baifuzi)
Red Orpiment (雄黄, Xionghuang)
Tabasheer (天竺黄, Tianzhuhuang)
Tendrilleaf Fritillary Bulb (川贝母, Chuan Beimu)
Licorice Root (生甘草, Sheng Gancao)
Arisaema with Bile (胆南星, Dannanxing)
Gambirplant Hooked Stem and Branch (钩藤, Gouteng)
Limonitum (蛇含石, Shehanshi)
Musk (麝香, Shexiang)
(It is a patent medicine and its preparation is omitted)

Actions: Restoring consciousness and relieving convulsion, clearing away heat and eliminating phlegm.

Applied syndromes: Infantile convulsion due to mental confusion by phlegm-heat manifested as fever, irritability, coma, convulsion, cough and asthma with shortness of breath.

Points in Constitution: This formula is based on Peaceful Palace Bovine Gall-Stone Bolus (安宫牛黄丸, an gong niu huang wan). Its main actions are clearing away heat, inducing resuscitation, calming the liver, expelling wind, eliminating phlegm and relieving convulsion.

Indications:
1. Convulsion with high fever
2. Convulsion caused by intracranial infection

Precaution: This formula is not suitable for chronic infantile convulsion due to cold and deficiency of the kidney and spleen.

Infantile Convulsion-Relieving Pill
(Heat-Clearing and Convulsion-Stooping Method)

Ingredients	Effects	Combined Effects	Syndrome	Chief symptom
Cow-Bezoar (牛黄, Niuhuang)	Clearing away heat and eliminating phlegm, restoring consciousness and relieving convulsion	Clearing away heat, restoring consciousness, calming the liver and relieving convulsion	Infantile convulsion due to heat and phlegm confusing the heart	High fever, convulsion, unconsciousness, purplish face, rale, difficult urination, constipation, purplish superficial venule of the index finger
Borneol (冰片, Bingpian) Musk (麝香, Shexiang)	Restoring consciousness and inducing resuscitation			
Cinnabar (朱砂, Zhusha)	Tranquilizing the mind and relieving convulsion			
Gambirplant Hooked Stem and Branch (钩藤, Gouteng) Silkworm with Batrytis Larva (僵蚕, Jiangchan) Tall Gastrodia Rhizome (天麻, Tianma) Scorpion (全蝎, Quanxie) Giant Typhonium Rhizome (白附子, Baifuzi) Arisaema with Bile (胆南星, Dannanxing)	Calming the liver and dispelling wind			
Tabasheer (天竺黄, Tianzhuhuang) Tendril-leaf Fritillary Bulb (川贝母, Chuan Beimu) Limonitum (蛇含石, Shehanshi) Licorice Root (生甘草, Sheng Gancao)	Clearing away heat and eliminating phlegm			
Red Orpiment (雄黄, Xionghuang)	Clearing away toxic material and calming the mind			
Incised Notopterygium Rhizome or Root (羌活, Qianghuo) Divaricate Saposhnikovia Root (防风, Fangfeng)	Expelling wind and relieving the exterior syndrome			

Associated formulas:

1. Cow Bezoar Embracing Dragon Pill (牛黄抱龙丸, niu huang bao long wan) *Collection of Experience of Famous Physicians in Ming Dynasty*《明医杂著》

This consists of Cow-Bezoar (牛黄, Niuhuang), Red Orpiment (雄黄, Xionghuang), Cinnabar (朱砂, Zhusha), Arisaema with Bile (胆南星, Dannanxing), Tabasheer (天竺黄, Tianzhuhuang), Licorice Root (甘草, Gancao) and Musk (麝香, Shexiang). Its actions are relieving convulsion, dispelling wind, eliminating phlegm and restoring consciousness. It is suitable for acute infantile convulsion, or cough and asthma with more sputum.

2. Amber Embracing Dragon Pill (琥珀抱龙丸, hu bo bao long wan) *Personal Experience for Saving Children*《活幼心书》

This consists of Amber (琥珀, Hupo), Tabasheer (天竺黄, Tianzhuhuang), Sandalwood (檀香, Tanxiang), Ginseng (人参, Renshen), Tuckahoe (茯苓, Fuling), Licorice Root (甘草, Gancao), Immature Bitter Orange (枳实, Zhishi), Bitter Orange (枳壳, Zhiqiao), Common Yam Rhizome (山药, Shanyao), Cinnabar (朱砂, Zhusha), Arisaema with Bile (胆南星, Dannanxing) and Gold (金箔, Jinbo). Its actions are resolving phlegm and relieving convulsion. Besides, it also restores qi. It is indicated for infantile convulsion, common cold, fever, productive cough with shortness of breath and accumulation of phlegm.

Cormorant Saliva Pill
(鸬鹚涎丸, lu ci xian wan)

Source: *Collection of National Prescriptions of Chinese Patent Medicine*《全国中药成药处方集》

Composition: Cormorant Saliva (鸬鹚涎, Lucixian)
Great Burdock Achene (牛蒡子, Niubangzi)
Gypsum (石膏, Shigao)
Cape Jasmine Fruit (山栀子, Shanzhizi)
Snakegourd Root (天花粉, Tianhuafen)
Clam Shell (海蛤壳, Haigeqiao)
Blackberrylily Rhizome (射干, Shegan)
Natural Indigo (青黛, Qingdai)
Ephedra (麻黄, Mahuang)
Apricot Seed (杏仁, Xingren)
Manchurian Wildginger Herb (细辛, Xixin)
Licorice Root (甘草, Gancao)
(Ground into powder and prepared into bolus. Taken two or three times a day, one or two pieces each time. Or dissolved with boiling water or decocted after wrapped with a piece of cloth for oral use.)

Actions: Clearing away heat and eliminating phlegm to relieve a cough

Applied syndromes: Spasmodic cough due to excessive phlegm resulting from lung-heat manifested as paroxysmal spasmodic cough like cockcrow, irritability, shortness of breath, celostomia and hoarseness, flushed face and swollen eyes, dry throat and scanty sputum, dry mouth and thirst, yellow and greasy tongue coating, rapid and smooth pulse.

Cormorant Saliva Pill
(Heat-Clearing and Phlegm-Resolving Method)

Ingredients	Effects	Combined Effects	Syndrome	Chief symptom
Cormorant Saliva (鸬鹚涎, Lucixian)	Clearing away heat and removing phlegm	Clearing away heat and promoting the dispersing function of the lung, removing phlegm and relieving cough	Infantile spasmodic cough (whooping cough)	Spasmodic cough, celostomia and hoarseness, flushed face and swollen eyes, yellow and greasy coating, rapid and smooth pulse
Ephedra (麻黄, Mahuang) Apricot Seed (杏仁, Xingren) Gypsum (石膏, Shigao) Licorice Root (生甘草, Sheng Gancao)	Clearing away heat and promoting the dispersing function of the lung, relieving cough and asthma			
Blackberrylily Rhizome (射干, Shegan)	Clearing away heat and toxic material, relieving wheezing sound			
Clam Shell (海蛤壳, Haigeqiao) Natural Indigo (青黛, Qingdai) Great Burdock Achene (牛蒡子, Niubangzi) Snakegourd Root (天花粉, Tianhuafen) Cape Jasmine Fruit (山栀子, Shanzhizi)	Clearing away heat of the lung and toxic material, removing phlegm and relieving cough			
Manchurian Wildginger Herb (细辛, Xixin)	Removing phlegm and relieving cough			

Points in Constitution: In this formula Cormorant Saliva(鸬鹚涎, Lucixian) is the key drug for whooping cough. When it is combined with the ingredients of Ephedra, Apricot Seed, Gypsum and Licorice Decoction(麻杏石甘汤, ma xing shi gan tang), it has actions of clearing away heat and promoting the dispersing function of the lung. The addition of the drugs of Natural Indigo and Giant Gecko Powder(黛蛤散, dai ge san) to the formula is to cool blood, resolve phlegm and relieve cough. The drug of Great Burdock Achene(牛蒡子, Niubangzi) is to remove heat, eliminate toxic material and relieve sore throat, and a small dosage of Manchurian Wildginger Herb

(细辛, Xixin) is used to avoid excessive cold.

Indications:
1. Whooping cough
2. Bronchiolitis
3. Asthma

Precautions: For the case of severe whooping cough, it is important for the patient to tranquilize the mind and drink enough water so as to promote the elimination of sputum. Besides, to give the patient a good nursing is also necessary.

Associated formula:

Sessile Stemona Syrup for Relieving Cough (百部止咳糖浆, bai bu zhi ke tang jiang) *Manual of Preparation of Chinese Medicine* 《中药制剂手册》

This syrup, taken orally for 2~3 times one day and 10~20ml each time, consists of Sessile Stemona Root (百部, Baibu), Apricot Seed (杏仁, Xingren), Baikal Skullcap Root (黄芩, Huangqin), Tangerine Peel (陈皮, Chenpi), Prepared Jackinthepulpit Tuber (南星, Nanxing), Balloonflower Root (桔梗, Jiegeng), White Mulberry Root-Bark (桑白皮, Sangbaipi), Bitter Orange (枳壳, Zhiqiao), Dwarf Lilyturf Root (麦门冬, Maimendong), Common Anemarrhena Rhizome (知母, Zhimu), Licorice Root (生甘草, Sheng Gancao) and White Sugar (白糖, Baitang). Its actions are clearing away heat from the lung and relieving cough. It is suited to cough with much sputum and shortness of breath due to lung-heat and also suited to whooping cough.

Infantile Four Symptoms Pill
(小儿四症丸, xiao er si zhen wan)

Source: *Selected Prescriptions of National Chinese Patent Medicines* 《全国中药成药处方集》

Composition: Common Aucklandia Root (木香, Muxiang),
Perilla Leaf (苏叶, Suye),
Tangerine Peel (陈皮, Chenpi),
Officinal Magnolia Bark (厚朴, Houpo),
Wrinkled Giantshyssop Herb (藿香, Huoxiang),
Largehead Atractylodes Rhizome (白术, Baizhu),
Tuckahoe (茯苓, Fuling),
Fried Malt (炒麦芽, Chao Maiya),
Swordlike Atractylodes Rhizome (苍术, Cangzhu),
Snakegourd Root (天花粉, Tianhuafen),
Oriental Waterplantain Rhizome (泽泻, Zexie),
Fried Hawthorn Fruit (炒山楂, Chao Shanzha),
Umbellate Pore Fungus (猪苓, Zhuling),
Pinellia Rhizome (半夏, Banxia),
Medicated Leaven (神曲, Shenqu),

Dahurican Angelica Root (白芷, Baizhi),
Balloonflower Root (桔梗, Jiegeng),
Talc (滑石, Huashi),
Villous Amomum Fruit (砂仁, Sharen),
Amber (琥珀, Hupo),
Cinnabar (朱砂, Zhusha)

(Prepared into honeyed pills which is 3g for each. One piece each time and taken after it is dissolved in the boiling water. It is a patent medicine and its preparation is omitted.)

Actions: Invigorating the spleen, promoting digestion, regulating qi and dispersing cold

Applied syndromes: Infantile indigestion with food retention due to stagnation of wetness or dyspepsia due to attack of pathogenic wind and cold, manifested as indigestion, pain and distention in gastric and abdominal area, vomiting, diarrhea, dysuria, or fever, headache, abdominal pain, diarrhea and irritability.

Points in Constitution: This formula is similar to Wrinkled Gianthyssop Healthy-Restoring Powder(藿香正气散, huo xiang zheng qi san) in action. Pathogenic wind, fire, phelgm and food retention are the four symptoms for infantile illness. This formula treats all of them. But comparatively it emphasizes removing dampness and resolving phlegm.

Indications:

1. Infantile malnutrition
2. Acute gastroenteritis
3. Common cold of gastrointestinal type

Precautions:

1. This formula is not suitable for diarrhea due to retention of heat and dampness.
2. Crude and cold food should be avoided during the medication.

Associated Formula:

Wrinkled Gianthyssop Health-Restoring Decoction(藿香正气散, huo xiang zheng qi san) *Prescriptions of Peaceful Benevolent Dispensary*《和剂局方》

This consists of Areca Peel (大腹皮, Dafupi), Dahurican Angelica Root (白芷, Baizhi), Perilla Leaf (紫苏, Zisu), Tuckahoe (茯苓, Fuling), Fermented Pinellia Rhizome (半夏曲, Banxiaqu), Largehead Atractylodes Rhizome (白术, Baizhu), Tangerine Peel (陈皮, Chenpi), Officinal Magnolia Bark (厚朴, Houpo), Balloonflower Root (桔梗, Jiegeng), Wrinkled Gianthyssop Herb (藿香, Huoxiang) and Licorice Root (甘草, Gancao). Its actions are relieving exterior syndrome, removing dampness and regulating qi of the middle-jiao. It is suited to the syndrome of outward attack by wind and cold and inward damage by stagnation of dampness manifested as vomiting, diarrhea, aversion to cold, fever, headache, gastric and abdominal pain and white and greasy coating.

Infantile Four Symptoms Pill
(Digestion-Promoting and Retention-Removing Method)

Ingredients	Effects	Combined Effects	Syndrome	Chief symptom
Tangerine Peel (陈皮, Chenpi) Pinellia Rhizome (半夏, Banxia)	Regulating flow of qi and normalizing the function of the stomach, removing dampness of the middle-jiao	Invigorating the spleen and promoting digestion, regulating qi and dispersing cold, promoting diuresis and removing dampness	Retention of food and dampness or accompanied with attack of exopathic cold	Indigestion, pain and distention in the gastric and abdominal area, vomiting, diarrhea, fever and headache
Largehead Atractylodes Rhizome (白术, Baizhu) Swordlike Atractylodes Rhizome (苍术, Cangzhu) Tuckahoe (茯苓, Fuling)	Removing dampness and invigorating the spleen			
Perilla Leaf (苏叶, Suye) Wrinkled Gianthyssop Herb (藿香, Huoxiang) Dahurican Angelica Root (白芷, Baizhi)	Relieving the exterior syndrome and dispersing cold			
Fried Malt (炒麦芽, Chao Maiya) Fried Hawthorn fruit (炒山楂, Chao Shanzha) Medicated Leaven (神曲, Shenqu)	Promoting digestion and regulating the stomach			
Common Aucklandia Root (木香, Muxiang) Villous Amomum Fruit (砂仁, Sharen)	Regulating flow of qi to stop vomiting			
Oriental Waterplantain Rhizome (泽泻, Zexie) Talc (滑石, Huashi) Umbellate Pore Fungus (猪苓, Zhuling)	Inducing diuresis and removing dampness			
Snakegourd Root (天花粉, Tianhuafen)	Clearing away heat and generating body fluid			
Amber (琥珀, Hupo) Cinnabar (朱砂, Zhusha)	Inducing sedation and tranquilizing the mind			
Balloonflower Root (桔梗, Jiegeng)	Promoting the dispersing function of the lung and benefiting diaphragm			

Lower-Warming and Upper-Clearing Decoction
（温下清上汤，wen xia qing shang tang）

Source：*Pediatrics*《儿科学》

Composition：Daughter Root of Common Monkshood（附子，Fuzi）3g

Coptis Rhizome（黄连，Huanglian）3g

Magnetite（磁石，Cishi）6g

Powder of Clam Shell（蛤粉，Gefen）6g

Snakegourd Root（天花粉，Tianhuafen）6g

Malaytea Scurfpea Fruit（补骨脂，Buguzhi）3g

Palmleaf Raspberry Fruit（覆盆子，Fupenzi）3g

Chinese Dodder Seed（菟丝子，Tusizi）3g

Mantis Egg-case（桑螵蛸，Sangpiaoxiao）3g

Lotus Stamen（白莲须，Bailianxu）3g

Actions：Warming the lower-jiao and clearing away heat in the upper-jiao, restoring normal co-ordination between the heart and kidney

Applied Syndromes：Infantile summer-heat syndrome characterized by protracted fever in summer, thirst with desire to drink, polyuria and anhidrosis. It is manifested by chronic fever which is high in the morning and low at dusk, thirst with desire to drink, polyuria with watery urine, asthenia-type restlessness, listlessness, somnolence, pale complexion, cold feeling in the limbs, loose stool, pale tongue with thin coating, deep and thready pulse.

Points in Constitution：Infantile summer-heat syndrome is caused by the imbalance between kidney-water and heart-fire which ressults from excessive heart-fire and deficiency of kidney-qi, manifested by polyuria, anhidrosis, change of body temperature with the different times in the day. Therefore warming the kidney and clearing heat from the heart is the proper treatment. According to the mechanism of this disease, Coptis Rhizome（黄连，Huanglian）is used with Prepared Daughter Root of Common Monkshood（附子，Fuzi）which are both opposite and complementary each other.

Indication：Infantile summer-heat syndrome

Precaution：This formula is not suitable for heat syndrome of excessive type.

Associated formula：

Summer heat-Clearing and Qi-Benefiting Decoction（清暑益气汤，qing shu yi qi tang）*Compendium on Seasonal Febrile Diseases*《温热经纬》

This consists of American Ginseng（西洋参，Xiyangshen）, Dendrobium Herb（石斛，Shihu）, Dwarf Lilyturf Root（麦门冬，Maimendong）, Coptis Rhizome（黄连，Huanglian）, Tophatherum Leaf（竹叶，Zhuye）, Lotus Petiole（荷梗，Hegeng）, Common Anemarrhena Rhizome（知母，Zhimu）, Licorice Root（甘草，Gancao）and Watermelon Peel（西瓜翠衣，Xiguacuiyi）. Its actions are clearing away summer-heat and benefiting qi, and nourishing yin and generating body fluid. It is suited to infantile summer-heat syndrome due to outward attack by summer-heat and inward damage to body fluid and qi.

Lower-Warming and Upper-Clearing Decoction
(Kidney-Warming and Heart-Clearing Method)

Ingredients	Effects	Combined Effects	Syndrome	Chief symptom
Prepared Daughter Root of Common Monkshood (附子, Fuzi) 3g Coptis Rhizome (黄连, Huanglian) 3g	Warming the kidney and clearing away heat from the heart	Warming the kidney and clearing away heat of the heart	Infantile summer-heat syndrome which is excessive in the upper-jiao and deficient in the lower-jiao	Prolonged fever which is high in the morning and low at dusk, thirst with desire to drink water, polyuria, anhidrosis, asthenia-type restlessness, fatigue, pale complexion, cold feeling in the limbs, loose stool, pale tongue with thin coating and deep and thin pulse.
Magnetite (磁石, Cishi) 6g	Checking exuberance of yang and tranquilizing the mind			
Chinese Dodder Seed (菟丝子, Tusizi) 3g Malaytea Scurfpea Fruit (补骨脂, Buguzhi) 3g Mantis Egg-Case (桑螵蛸, Sangpiaoxiao) 3g Lotus Stamen (白莲须, Bailianxu) 3g Palmleaf Raspberry Fruit (覆盆子, Fupenzi) 3g	Warming the kidney and astringent			
Snakegourd Root (天花粉, Tianhuafen) 6g Powder of Clam Shell (蛤粉, Gefen) 6g	Clearing away heat and generating body fluid			

Caloglossa Leprieurii Decoction
(鹧鸪菜汤, zhe gu cai tang)

Source: *Brief Points of Prescriptions* 《撮要方函》
Composition: Caloglossa Leprieurii (鹧鸪菜, Zhegucai) 3~15g, Rhubarb (大黄, Dahuang) 1~1.5g, Licorice Root (甘草, Gancao) 1~1.5g
Actions: Expelling and destroyinng ascaris

Applied Syndromes: Ascariasis manifested as intermittent abdominal pain, or heterorexia, vomiting of saliva, exfoliative tongue coating, sudden or abrupt change of pulse condition.

Caloglossa Leprieurii Decoction
(Ascarid-Expelling and Parasites-Poisoning Method)

IngredientsEffects	Combined Effects	Syndrome	Chief symptom	
Caloglossa Leprieurii (鷓鴣菜, Zhegucai) 3~15g	Expelling and destroying ascaris	Poisoning and expelling ascaris	Ascariasis	Intestinal ascaris with intermittent abdominal pain, or heterorexia, exfoliative tongue coating and sudden change of pulse condition
Rhubarb (生大黄, Sheng Dahuang) 1~1.5g	Purging and removing the retention of food			
Licorice Root (甘草, Gancao) 1~1.5g	Relieving spasm and coordinating the actions of various ingredients in a Prescription			

Points in Constitution: Caloglossa Leprieurii (鷓鴣菜, Zhegucai) is the tender sprout of Hairy Vein Agrimony(仙鶴草, xianhecao). Recent researches has shown that it can paralyze ascaris and expel them out of the body.

Indications:
1. Ascariasis
2. Oxyuriasis

Precaution: This decoction should be taken in the morning or evening on an empty stomach. This formula can also be used for prevention of ascarisis.

Associated formulas:

Stomach-Clearing and Ascaris-Calming Decoction(清肌安蛔汤, qing ji an hui tang) *Record of Mannan*《蔓难录》

This is the Minor Chinese Thorowax Decoction(小柴胡汤, xiao chai hu tang) modified by removing Chinese Date (大枣, Dazao) but adding Caloglossa Leprieurii (鷓鴣菜, Zhegucai) and Dwarf Lilyturf Root (麦门冬, Maimendong). It is used for ascarisis accompanied with alternating episodes of chills and fever, dry skin, vomiting and weakness in the stomach.

Chapter Nine
Formulas for Orthopaedic and Surgical Diseases

Chinese Prescription have an unique effect in alleviating pain, resisting inflammation and promoting regeneration of tissues. Many new advances have been obtained in the combined treatment of the traditional and western medicine in osteopathy and surgical diseases.

Most of the surgical diseases which are accompanied with pain in the joints, muscles and nerves such as rheumatic arthritis, rheumatoid arthritis, deforming arthritis, gout, prolapse of lumbar intervertebral disc and sciatic belong to the category of Bi-syndrome(arthralgia-syndrome) in traditional Chinese medicine. From ancient times till now, there are many Chinese Prescription for Bi syndrome. Successful treatment of acute abdomen by combining traditional Chinese with western medicine is one of the remarkable achievements in the medical field in the past 40 years., which fully prove that Chinese Prescription are scientific and effective.

Chinese Prescription can also be widely applied to the prevention and treatment of various complications and the secondary disease after surgical operations.

1. Notopterygium Dampness-Expelling Decoction
（羌活胜湿汤, jiang huo sheng shi tang）

Source: *Differentiation on Endogenous and Exogenous Diseases*《内外伤辨惑论》
Composition: Incised Notopterygium Rhizome or Root（羌活, Qianghuo）6g
Doubleteeth Pubescent Angelica Root（独活, Duhuo）6g
Divaricate Saposhnikovia Root（防风, Fangfeng）3g
Chinese Ligusticum Rhizome（藁本, Gaoben）3g
Threeleaf Castertree Fruit（蔓荆子, Manjingzi）3g
Szechwan Lovage Rhizome（川芎, Chuanxiong）3g
Prepared Licorice Root（炙甘草, Zhi Gancao）3g
Actions: Expelling wind and dampness.
Applied Syndrome: Exterior syndrome due to wind-dampness manifested as pain in the shoulder and back which causes inability to look back, headache, heaviness sensation of the body, or pain along the the spinal cord and in the loins which causes inability to turn around, white and greasy tongue coating and superficial pulse.

Notopterygium Dampness-Expelling Decoction
(Wind-Expelling and Dampness-Removing Method)

Ingredients	Effects	Combined Effects	Syndrome	Chief Symptoms
Incised Notopterygium Rhizome or Root (羌活, Qianghuo) 6g Doubleteeth Pubescent Angelica Root (独活, Duhuo) 6g Divaricate Saposhnikovia Root (防风, Fangfeng) 3g Chinese Ligusticum Rhizome (藁本, Gaoben) 3g	Expelling wind and cold	Expelling wind and dampness, dredging the collaterals and alleviating pain	Exterior syndrome due to wind-dampness	Pain of shoulder and back which causes inability to look back, headache, heaviness of the body, or pain along the spinal cord and in the loin which causes inability to turn around, white and greasy tongue coating, superficial pulse
Threeleaf Chastertree Fruit (蔓荆子, Manjingzi) 3g	Alleviating pain			
Szechwan Lovage Rhizome (川芎, Chuanxiong) 3g	Activating blood circulation and dredging the collaterals			
Prepared Licorice Root (炙甘草, Zhi Gancao) 3g	Invigorating the spleen and regulating the middle-jiao, relieving muscular spasm and alleviating pain			

Points in Constitution: The drugs of Incised Notopterygium Rhizome or Root (羌活, Qianghuo), Doubleteeth Pubescent Angelica Root (独活, Duhuo), Divaricate Saposhnikovia Root (防风, Fangfeng) and Chinese Ligusticum Rhizome (藁本, Gaoben) can not only expel wind-cold but also remove dampness and alleviate pain. Thus they are very suitable for arthralgia at the intial stage of Bi-syndrome due to wind-cold-dampness. It is wonderful to use Szechwan Lovage Rhizome (川芎, Chuanxiong) which has an action on all the exterior, interior, qi and blood, making the whole formula work effectively.

Indications:

1. Acute rheumatic arthritis.
2. Rheumatoid arthritis.
3. Upper respiratory tract infection.

Precaution: This formula is contraindicated in arthralgia with heat.

Associated Formulas:

1. Fourstamen Stephania and Membranous Milkvetch Decoction (防己黄芪汤, fang ji huang qi

tang) *Synopsis of Golden Cabinet*《金匮要略》

This is comprised of Fourstamen Stephania Root (汉防己, Han Fangji), Toasted Membranous Milkvetch Root (炙黄芪, Zhi Huangqi), Prepared Licorice Root (炙甘草, Zhi Gancao) and Largehead Atractylodes Rhizome (白术, Baizhu). Its actions are replenishing qi and expelling wind, invigorating the spleen and promoting urination. It is fit for edema caused by wind-dampness and failure of superficial qi to protect the body, manifested as sweat, aversion to wind, heaviness sensation of the body, dysuria, white tongue coating and superficial pulse.

2. Fourstamen Stephania and Tuckahoe Decoction (防己茯苓汤, fang ji fu ling tang) *Synopsis of Golden Cabinet*《金匮要略》

This consists of Fourstamen Stephania Root (汉防己, Han Fangji), Toasted Membranous Milkvetch Root (炙黄芪, Zhi Huangqi), Cassia Twig (桂枝, Guizhi), Tuckahoe (茯苓, Fuling) and Prepared Licorice Root (炙甘草, Zhi Gancao). Its actions are replenishing qi, relieving the obstruction of yang-qi and promoting urination. It is applicable to subcutaneous edema manifested as edema of the limbs, water in the skin, cold limbs with tremor.

3. Modified Incised Notopterygium Decoction (加味羌活汤, jia wei qiang huo tang) *Medical Problems*《此事难知》

This is made up of Incised Notopterygium Rhizome or Root (羌活, Qianghuo), Divaricate Saposhnikovia Root (防风, Fangfeng), Szechwan Lovage Rhizome (川芎, Chuanxiong), Manchurian Wildginger Herb (细辛, Xixin), Licorice Root (生甘草, Sheng Gancao), Swordlike Atractylodes Rhizome (苍术, Cangzhu), Dahurican Angelica Root (白芷, Baizhi), Baikal Skullcap Root (黄芩, Huangqin) and Dried Rehmannia Root (生地黄, Shengdihuang). Its actions are inducing diaphoresis, expelling dampness and clearing away heat in the interior. It is suited to common cold in four seasons manifested as headache, anhidrosis, fever and superficial pulse.

2. Major Divaricate Saposhuikovia Decoction (大防风汤, da fang feng tang)

Source: *Prescriptions of Peaceful Benevolent Dispensary*《和剂局方》
Composition: Prepared Rehmannia Root (熟地黄, Shudihuang)6g
Divaricate Saposhnikovia Root (防风, Fangfeng)6g
Eucommia Bark (杜仲, Duzhong)9g
Chinese Angelica Root (当归, Danggui)6g
Szechwan Lovage Rhizome (川芎, Chuanxiong)6g
White Peony Root (白芍药, Baishaoyao)6g
Largehead Atractylodes Rhizome (白术, Baizhu)6g
Membranous Milkvetch Root (生黄芪, Sheng Huangqi)6g
Incised Notopterygium Rhizome or Root (羌活, Qianghuo)6g
Medicinal Achyranthes Root (川牛膝, Chuan Niuxi)9g

Ginseng（人参，Renshen）6g
Licorice Root（生甘草，Sheng Gancao）6g
Chinese Date（大枣，Dazao）6g
Prepared Aconite Root（炮附子，Pao Fuzi）3g
Dried Ginger（干姜，Ganjiang）3g

Actions: Benefiting the liver and kidney, replenishing qi and blood and expelling wind-dampness.

Applied Syndrome: Syndrome of deficiency of both qi and blood due to prolonged arthralgia resulting from wind-cold-dampness, manifested by aching pain and numbness of the joints, swelling of the joints, difficulty in walking, sweating and intolerance of cold, or accompanied with palpitation, anorexia, weakenedd limbs, pale tongue with thin and white coating, deep, slow and weak pulse.

Points in Constitution: This formula is the modified Eight Treasures Decoction（八珍汤，ba zhen tang）plus Baked Aconite Root（炮附子，Pao Fuzi）and Dried Ginger（干姜，Ganjiang）to warm the interior and expel cold. Although it has the two actions of reinforcing and expelling wind-dampness, it is mainly used for replenishing qi and blood and benefiting the liver and kidney. Thus it is very suitable for prolonged arthralgia with deficiency of healthy qi and insuffuciency of yang with cold.

Indications:
1. Rheumatic arthritis.
2. Arthralgia, lumbago.
3. Sciatica.

Precaution: This formula is applicable to prolonged arthralgia of wind-cold-dampness with deficiency of qi and blood. Thus, it is not suitable for the beginning of arthralgia without deficiency of the healthy qi.

Associated Formulas:

1. Qi-Invigorating, Blood-Replenishing and Tendons-Nourishing Decoction（气血并补荣筋汤，qi xue bing bu rong jin tang）*Internal Medicine of Traditional Chinese Medicine by Wang Yongyan*《中医内科学》王永炎

This is comprised of Coix Seed（薏苡仁，Yiyiren）, Tuckahoe（茯苓，Fuling）, Largehead Atractylodes Rhizome（白术，Baizhu）, Fleeceflower Root（何首乌，Heshouwu）, Chinese Angelica Root（当归，Danggui）, Villous Amomum Fruit（砂仁，Sharen）, Prepared Rehmannia Root（熟地黄，Shudihuang）, Siberian Solomonseal Rhizome（黄精，Huangjing）, Wasps Nest（蜂房，Fengfang）, Garter Snake（乌蛇，Wushe）, Common St. Paulswort Herb（豨莶草，Xiqiancao）, Chinese Starjasmine Stem（络石藤，Luoshiteng）, East Asian Tree Fern Rhizome（狗脊，Gouji）, Largeleaf Gentian Root（秦艽，Qinjiao）and Chinese Dodder Seed（菟丝子，Tusizi）. Its actions are replenishing the liver and kidney, dredging the collaterals and alleviating pain. It is fit to prolonged arthralgia with swelling and pain of the joints.

2. Doubleteeth Pubescent Angelica and Chinese Taxillus Twig Decoction（独活寄生汤，du huo ji sheng tang）*Prescriptions Worth a Thousand Gold for Emergencies*《备急千金要方》

Major Divaricate Saposhuikovia Decoction
(Qi-Resotoring and Arthralgia-Relieving Method)

Ingredients	Effects	Combined Effects	Syndrome	Chief Symptoms
Membranous Milkvetch Root (生黄芪, Sheng Huangqi) 6g Ginseng (人参, Renshen) 6g Largehead Atractylodes Rhizome (白术, Baizhu) 6g Chinese Date (大枣, Dazao) 6g Licorice Root (生甘草, Sheng Gancao) 6g	Invigorating qi	Benefiting the liver and kidney, replenishing qi and blood and expelling wind-dampness	Prolonged arthralgia (due to deficieny of qi and blood and deficiency of the liver and kidney)	Aching pain or swelling of the joints, numbness and difficulty in walking, sweating and intolerance of cold, palpitation, anorexia, weakness, tiredness, pale tongue, thin and white coating, deep, slow and weak pulse
Prepared Rehmannia Root (熟地黄, Shudihuang) 6g Szechwan Lovage Rhizome (川芎, Chuanxiong) 6g White Peony Root (白芍药, Baishaoyao) 6g Chinese Angelica Root (当归, Danggui) 6g	Nourishing blood			
Prepared Aconite Root (炮附子, Pao Fuzi) 3g Dried Ginger (干姜, Ganjiang) 3g	Warming yang and expelling cold			
Incised Notopterygium Rhizome or Root (羌活, Qianghuo) 6g Divaricate Saposhnikovia Root (防风, Fangfeng) 6g	Expelling wind and dampness			
Eucommia Bark (杜仲, Duzhong) 9g Medicinal Achyranthes Root (川牛膝, Chuan Niuxi) 9	Replenishing the liver and kidney and strengthening tendons and bones			

This is comprised of Doubleteeth Pubescent Angelica Root (独活, Duhuo), Chinese Taxillus

Twig (桑寄生, Sangjisheng), Largeleaf Gentian Root (秦艽, Qinjiao), Divaricate Saposhnikovia Root (防风, Fangfeng), Chinese Angelica Root (当归, Danggui), Red Peony Root (赤芍, Chishao), Eucommia Bark (杜仲, Duzhong), Twotooth Achyranthes Root (牛膝, Niuxi), Tuckahoe (茯苓, Fuling), Pilose Asiabell Root (党参, Dangshen), Manchurian Wildginger Herb (细辛, Xixin), Cassia Bark (肉桂, Rougui), Szechwan Lovage Rhizome (川芎, Chuanxiong), Prepared Rehmannia Root (熟地黄, Shudihuang) and Prepared Licorice Root (炙甘草, Zhi Gancao). Its actions are expelling wind-dampness, relieving arthralgia, benefitting the liver and kidney, replenishing qi and blood. It is indicated for prolonged wind-cold-dampness arthralgia due to deficiency of the liver and kidney and insufficiency of both qi and blood.

3. Decoction for Wind-Cold-Dampness Arthralgia (三痹汤, san bi tang) *The Complete Effective Prescriptions for Women Diseases*《妇人良方大全》

This is made up of Doubleteeth Pubescent Angelica Root (独活, Duhuo), Largeleaf Gentian Root (秦艽, Qinjiao), Divaricate Saposhnikovia Root (防风, Fangfeng), Chinese Angelica Root (当归, Danggui), Red Peony Root (赤芍, Chishao), Eucommia Bark (杜仲, Duzhong), Twotooth Achyranthes Root (牛膝, Niuxi), Tuckahoe (茯苓, Fuling), Pilose Asiabell Root (党参, Dangshen), Manchurian Wildginger Herb (细辛, Xixin), Cassia Bark (肉桂, Rougui), Szechwan Lovage Rhizome (川芎, Chuanxiong), Prepared Rehmannia Root (熟地黄, Shudihuang), Prepared Licorice Root (炙甘草, Zhi Gancao), Membranous Milkvetch Root (生黄芪, Sheng Huangqi), Szechwan Lovage Rhizome (川芎, Chuanxiong) and Fresh Ginger (生姜, Shengjiang). The action of this formula is similar to that of Major Divaricate Saposhnikovia Decoction (大防风汤, da fang feng tang).

3. Coix Seed Decoction
(薏苡仁汤, yi yi ren tang)

Source: *Guidance of Famous Physician*《明医指掌》
Composition: Chinese Angelica Root (当归, Danggui)9g
White Peony Root (白芍药, Baishaoyao)15g
Coix seed (薏苡仁, Yiyiren)15g
Swordlike Atractylodes Rhizome (苍术, Cangzhu)9g
Ephedra (麻黄, Mahuang)6g
Cassia twig (桂枝, Guizhi)6g
Prepared Licorice Root (炙甘草, Zhi Gancao)9g
Actions: Expelling wind and removing dampness, clearing away cold and alleviating pain.
Applied Syndrome: Arthralgia of dampness-type, manifested by swelling and pain of the joints, limited movement, tiredness, numbness of the limbs, or accompanied with edema, white and greasy tongue coating, deep and wiry pulse or soft and slow pulse.
Points in Constitution: This formula contains large dose of Coix Seed (薏苡仁, Yiyiren) and Swordlike Atractylodes Rhizome (苍术, Cangzhu), which are good at expelling dampness to re-

lieve arthralgia and are the key drugs for arthralgia of dampness type.

Coix Seed Decoction
(Wind-Dispelling and Dampness-Removing Method)

Ingredients	Effects	Combined Effects	Syndrome	Chief Symptoms
Coix Seed (薏苡仁, Yiyiren)15g Swordlike Atractylodes Rhizome (苍术, Cangzhu)9g	Removing dampness and relieving arthralgia	Expelling wind-dampness, expelling cold and alleviating pain	Arthralgia of dampness-type	Swelling and pain of the joints, tiredness and limited movement, numbness, or accompanied with edema, white and greasy tongue coating, deep and wiry pulse or soft and slow pulse
Ephedra (麻黄, Mahuang)6g Cassia Twig (桂枝, Guizhi)6g	Expelling wind-cold-dampness			
Chinese Angelica Root (当归, Danggui)9g White Peony Root (白芍药, Baishaoyao)15g	Regulating blood and alleviating pain			
Prepared Licorice Root (炙甘草, Zhi Gancao)9g	Relieving muscular spasm and alleviating pain			

Indications: Rheumatic arthritis or rheumatic myocarditis.

Precaution: This formula is applicable to arthralgia of dampness type without obvious heat syndrome, thus it is not suitable for arthralgia due to heat-dampness.

Associated Formulas:

1. Major Divaricate Saposhnikovia Decoction(大防风汤, da fang feng tang) *Prescriptions of Peaceful Benevolent Dispensary*《和剂局方》

This is comprised of Prepared Rehmannia Root (熟地黄, Shudihuang), Divaricate Saposhnikovia Root (防风, Fangfeng), Eucommia Bark (杜仲, Duzhong), Chinese Angelica Root (当归, Danggui), Szechwan Lovage Rhizome (川芎, Chuanxiong), White Peony Root (白芍药, Baishaoyao), Largehead Atractylodes Rhizome (白术, Baizhu), Toasted Membranous Milkvetch Root (炙黄芪, Zhi Huangqi), Incised Notopterygium Rhizome or Root (羌活, Qianghuo), Twotooth Achyranthes Root (牛膝, Niuxi), Ginseng (人参, Renshen), Licorice Root (生甘草, Sheng Gancao), Chinese Date (大枣, Dazao), Prepared Aconite Root (炮附子, Pao Fuzi) and Dried Ginger (干姜, Ganjiang). Its actions are benefiting the liver and kidney, replenishing qi and blood and expelling wind-dampness. It is indicated for prolonged wind-cold-dampness arthralgia due to deficiency of the liver and kidney, yang inssufficiency and interior cold.

2. Swordlike Atractylodes and Largehead Atractylodes Decoction (二术汤, er zhu tang) *Curative Measures for Diseases* 《万病回春》

This is made up of Swordlike Atractylodes Rhizome (苍术, Cangzhu), Largehead Atractylodes Rhizome (白术, Baizhu), Jackinthepulpit Tuber (天南星, Tiannanxing), Tangerine Peel (橘皮, Jupi), Tuckahoe (茯苓, Fuling), Nutgrass Galingale Rhizome (香附, Xiangfu), Baikal Skullcap Root (黄芩, Huangqin), Chinese Clematis Root (威灵仙, Weilingxian), Incised Notopterygium Rhizome or Root (羌活, Qianghuo), Licorice Root (生甘草, Sheng Gancao) and Pinellia Rhizome which is prepared with Fresh Ginger (姜半夏, Jiangbanxia). Its actions are expelling wind-dampness, removing phlegm, dredging the collaterals and alleviating pain. It is indicated for arthralgia due to blockage of the meridians and collaterals by wind-cold-dampness-phlegm.

3. Dampness-Removing Decoction (胜湿汤, shen shi tang) *Practical Formula-ology* 《实用方剂学》

This is comprised of Coix Seed (薏苡仁, Yiyiren), Swordlike Atractylodes Rhizome (苍术, Cangzhu), Fourstamen Stephania Root (汉防己, Han Fangji), Divaricate Saposhnikovia Root (防风, Fangfeng), Incised Notopterygium Rhizome or Root (羌活, Qianghuo), Doubleteeth Pubescent Angelica Root (独活, Duhuo), Chinese Clematis Root (威灵仙, Weilingxian) and Slenderstyle Acanthopanax Root-Bark (五加皮, Wujiapi). Its actions are expelling wind, drying dampness, dredging the collaterals and alleviating pain. It is suited to arthralgia due to dampness manifested as heaviness and pain of the joints, numbness of the skin, heaviness sensation of the hands and feet, white and greasy tongue coating, soft and slow pulse.

4. Proven Recipes for Arthralgia of Damp type (着痹验方, zhuo bi yan fang) *Manual of Barefoot Doctors* 《赤脚医生手册》

This consists of Centipede (蜈蚣, Wugong), Scorpion (全蝎, Quanxie), Dung Beetle (蜣螂, Tanglang), Long-Nosed Pit Viper Snake (蕲蛇, Qishe), Ground Bettle (地鳖虫, Dibiechong), Prepared Licorice Root (炙甘草, Zhi Gancao), Roasted Wasps Nest (炙蜂房, Zhi Fengfang), Tiger Bone (虎骨, Hugu) [it can be replaced by Antler (鹿角, Lujiao)], Hairy Birth Wort (寻骨风, Xungufeng), Common Clubmoss Herb (伸筋草, Shenjincao), schizoophraagma Integrifolium (钻地风, Zuandifeng), Chinese Pyrola Herb (鹿衔草, Luxiancao), Chinese Angelica Root (当归, Danggui) and Wilfword Cranesbill Herb (老鹳草, Laohecao). Its actions are expelling pathogens, dredging the collaterals, activating blood circulation and dissolving blood stasis, strengthening tendons and bones, relieving arthralgia and alleviating pain. It is indicated for arthralgia of dampness type manifested as repeated swelling and pain of the joints which can not be cured after a long-time, or even malformation and rigidity of the joints, dyskinesia of the limbs.

4. Cassia Twig, White Peony and Common Anemarrhena Decoction
(桂枝芍药知母汤, gui zhi shao yao zhi mu tang)

Source: *Synopsis of Golden Cabinet*《金匮要略》
Composition: Cassia Twig (桂枝, Guizhi) 9g
White Peony Root (白芍药, Baishaoyao) 9g
Prepared Licorice Root (炙甘草, Zhi Gancao) 6g
Ephedra (麻黄, Mahuang) 6g
Fresh Ginger (生姜, Shengjiang) 9g
Largehead Atractylodes Rhizome (白术, Baizhu) 12g
Common Anemarrhena Rhizome (知母, Zhimu) 9g
Divaricate Saposhnikovia Root (防风, Fangfeng) 9g
Prepared Aconite Root (制附子, Zhi Fuzi) 9g

Actions: Warming the channels and expelling cold, expelling wind and removing dampness, also nourishing yin and clearing away heat.

Applied Syndrome: Acute arthritis due to wind-dampness. When wind-dampness invades tendons and joints, qi and blood will not circulate normally, causing the pathogens to transform into heat which damages yin fluid. It is manifested by swelling and pain of the joints all over the body, often accompanied with hot sensation in the swollen area, emaciation, faint and blindness, edema of the feet, shortness of breath, vomiting, thin, yellow and greasy tongue coating, rapid or soft, rapid pulse.

Points in Constitution: This formula is the modified Ephedra Decoction (麻黄汤, ma huang tang) and Cassia Twig and Prepared Aconite Decoction (桂枝附子汤, gui zhi fu zi tang). The addition of Common Anemarrhena Rhizome (知母, Zhimu), which has the action of clearing away heat, to the fomula is to adapt to the pathogenesis of prolonged arthralgia which has transformed into heat.

Indications:
1. Rheumatic arthritis.
2. Rheumatoid arthritis.
3. Sciatica.

Precaution: This formula is applicable for swelling and pain in the joints with hot sensation rather than the heat syndrome. It is not suitable for heat syndrome of excessive type due to noxious heat.

Associated Formulas:

1. Common Monkshood's Mother Decoction (乌头汤, wu tou tang) *Synopsis of Golden Cabinet*《金匮要略》

This consists of Common Monkshood's Mother Root (川乌头, Chuanwutou), Ephedra (麻黄, Mahuang), White Peony Root (白芍药, Baishaoyao), Membranous Milkvetch Root (黄芪,

Huangqi) and Prepared Licorice Root (炙甘草, Zhi Gancao). Both this formula and Cassia Twig, White Peony and Common Anemarrhena Decoction(桂枝芍药知母汤, gui zhi shao yao zhi mu tang) have the actions of expelling wind-dampness and relieving arthralgia and are applicable for acute arthritis. However, Cassia Twig, White Peony and Common Anemarrhena Decoction (桂枝芍药知母汤, gui zhi shao yao zhi mu tang) is applicable for acute arthritis due to wind-dampness, mainly manifested as swelling and pain of the joints and fever, thus its treatment is to expel wind, remove dampness, relieving arthralgia and clear away heat. This Common Monkshood's Mother Root Decoction (乌头汤, wu tou tang) is applicable for acute arthritis due to cold-dampness, mainly manifested as pain of the joints and dyskinesia of the limbs, thus its treatment is to warm the meridian, expelg cold, remove dampness and relieveg pain.

Cassia Twig, White Peony and Common Anemarrhena Decoction
(Wind-Expelling and Dampness-Removing Method)

Ingredients	Effects	Combined Effects	Syndrome	Chief Symptoms
Ephedra (麻黄, Mahuang) 6g Cassia Twig (桂枝, Guizhi) 9g White Peony Root (白芍药) 9g Fresh Ginger (生姜, Shengjiang) 9g Prepared Licorice Root (炙甘草, Zhi Gancao) 6g	Relieving the exterior syndrome with drugs acrid in flavor and warm in nature, expelling cold and alleviating pain	Warming the meridian and expelling cold, expelling wind and removing dampness, nourishing yin and clearing away heat	Heat syndrome due to wind-dampness attacking the joints for a long time	Pain and swelling of the joints, emaciation, edema and numbness of the feet, dizziness, shortness of breath, vomiting, thin, yellow and greasy tongue coating, rapid pulse or soft rapid pulse
Prepared Aconite Root (制附子, Zhi Fuzi) 9g	Warming yang and expelling cold, relieving arthralgia and alleviating pain			
Largehead Atractylodes Rhizome (白术, Baizhu) 12g	Invigorating the spleen and expelling dampness			
Divaricate Saposhnikovia Root (防风, Fangfeng) 9g	Expelling wind and alleviating pain			
Common Anemarrhena Rhizome (知母, Zhimu) 9g	Clearing away heat and keeping yin			

2. Fourstamen Stephania and Membranous Milkvetch Decoction(防己黄芪汤, fang ji huang qi tang) *Synopsis of Golden Cabinet* 《金匮要略》

This is comprised of Fourstamen Stephania Root (汉防己, Han Fangji), Toasted Membranous Milkvetch Root (炙黄芪, Zhi Huangqi), Largehead Atractylodes Rhizome (白术, Baizhu), Fresh Ginger (生姜, Shengjiang), Licorice Root (生甘草, Sheng Gancao) and Chinese Date (大枣, Dazao). Both this formula and Cassia Twig, White Peony and Common Anemarrhena Decoction (桂枝芍药知母汤, gui zhi shao yao zhi mu tang) have the same actions of expelling wind, removing dampness, dispersing wind and clearing the obstruction of yang-qi. However, Cassia Twig, White Peony Root and Common Anemarrhena Decoction(桂枝芍药知母汤, gui zhi shao yao zhi mu tang) is indicated for wind-cold-dampness arthralgia due to weak body with deficiency of qi and blood while this Fourstamen Stephania and Membranous Milkvetch Decoction(防己黄芪汤, fang ji huang qi tang) is indicated for edema caused by exogenous wind and stagnation of dampness in the superficial resulting from failure of the superficial qi in protecting the healthy qi in the body.

3. Cassia Twig and Aconite Decoction (桂枝附子汤, gui zhi fu zi tang) *Synopsis of Golden Cabinet* 《金匮要略》

This is made up of Cassia Twig Decoction(桂枝汤, gui zhi tang) without White Peony Root (白芍药, Baishaoyao) but adding Aconite Root (附子, Fuzi). Both this formula and Cassia Twig, White Peony and Common Anemarrhena Decoction (桂枝芍药知母汤, gui zhi shao yao zhi mu tang) have the actions of warming the meridian, removing obstruction of yang-qi and expelling wind and dampness. But this Cassia Twig and Aconite Decoction(桂枝附子汤, gui zhi fu zi tang) contains a large dose of Cassia Twig (桂枝, Guizhi) to expel wind in the superficies. The use of Aconite Root (附子, Fuzi) is to warm the meridian and restore yang. Thus it is good at treating deficiency of yang in the exterior with excessive wind.

4. Cassia Twig plus White Tiger Decoction (白虎加桂枝汤, bai hu jia gui zhi tang) *Synopsis of Golden Cabinet* 《金匮要略》

This is the White Tiger Decoction (白虎汤, bai hu tang) plus Cassia Twig (桂枝, Guizhi). Its actions are clearing away heat, regulating ying, alleviating pain and preventing attack or recurrence of malaria. It is indicated for malaria of warm type malaria and arthralgia of heat type with pain of the joints.

5. General Recipe for Treating Mogratory Arthralgia(痛风统治方, tong feng tong zhi fang) *Author's Experienced Prescription* (笔者经验方)

This is composed of Hypoglauca Yam or Seven-Lobed Yam(萆薢, Bixie), Oriental Waterplantain Rhizome(泽泻, Zexie), Swordlike Atractylodes Rhizome(苍术, Cangzhu), Fourstamen Stephania Root(防己, Fangji), Suberect Spatholobus Stem(鸡血藤, Jixueteng), Chinese Corktree Bark(黄柏, Huangbai), Coix Seed(薏苡仁, Yiyiren), Membranous Milkvetch Root(黄芪, Huangqi), Licorice Root(甘草, Gancao) and Common St. Paulwort(豨莶草, Xixiancao). Its actions are clearing away heat, removing dampness, relieving arthralgia and alleviating pain. It is indicated for migratory arthragia manifested as reddish swelling and sharp pain of the toe joints, local hot feeling and difficulty in walking.

5. Doubleteeth Pubescent Angelica and Chinese Taxillus Twig Decoction
(独活寄生汤, du huo ji sheng tang)

Source: *Prescription Worth a Thousand Gold for Emergencies* 《备急千金要方》
Composition: Doubleteeth Pubescent Angelica Root (独活, Duhuo)6g
Manchurian Wildginger Herb (细辛, Xixin)3g
Largeleaf Gentian Root (秦艽, Qinjiao)6g
Divaricate Saposhnikovia Root (防风, Fangfeng)6g
Chinese Taxillus Twig (桑寄生, Sangjisheng)9g
Eucommia Bark (杜仲, Duzhong)9g
Medicinal Achyranthes Root (川牛膝, Chuan Niuxi)9g
Szechwan Lovage Rhizome (川芎, Chuanxiong)6g
Dried Rehmannia Root (干地黄, Gandihuang)6g
Chinese Angelica Root (当归, Danggui)6g
White Peony Root (白芍药, Baishaoyao)6g
Ginseng (人参, Renshen)6g
Tuckahoe (茯苓, Fuling)6g
Licorice Root (甘草, Gancao)6g
Cassia Bark (肉桂, Rougui)3g

Actions: Tonifying the liver and kidney, replenishing qi and blood, expelling wind-dampness and relieving arthralgia.

Applied Syndrome: Bi-syndrome, also known as prolonged arthralgia of wind-cold-dampness, caused by deficiency of the liver and kidney and insufficiency of qi and blood which is manifested by cold and pain in the loins and knees, dyskinesia, numbness, chills which can be relieved by warming, palpitation, shortness of breath, anorexia, tiredness, pallor, pale tongue with white coating, thin and weak pulse.

Points in Constitution: This formula can both nourish the liver, kidney, qi and blood and expelling wind-cold-dampness simultaneously so as to support the healthy qi and eliminate pathogenic factors. It treats both the primary and secondary aspects of the disease.

Indications:
1. Rheumatic arthritis.
2. Sciatica.
3. Lumbago.
4. Rheumatoid arthritis.

Precaution: Owing to the warm nature of the herbs, this formula should be cautiously used for the patient with yin deficiency or blood deficiency with heat, or the pregnant women.

Doubleteeth Pubescent Angelica and Chinese Taxillus Twig Decoction
(Qi-Restoring and Arthralgia-Relieving Method)

Ingredients	Effects	Combined Effects	Syndrome	Chief Symptoms
Doubleteeth Pubescent Angelica Root (独活, Duhuo) 6g Divaricate Saposhnikovia Root (防风, Fangfeng) 6g Manchurian Wildginger Herb (细辛, Xixin) 3g Largeleaf Gentian Root (秦艽, Qinjiao) 6g	Expelling wind-cold-dampness, relaxing muscles and tendons and alleviating pain	Tonifying the liver and kidney, replenishing qi and blood, expelling wind-dampness and relieving arthralgia	Arthralgia of wind-cold-dampness, deficiency of the liver and kidney and insufficiency of qi and blood	Cold and pain in the loins and knees, dyskinesia, numbness, chills which can be relieved by warming, palpitation, shortness of breath, pale tongue with white coating, thin and weak pulse
Chinese Angelica Root (当归, Danggui) 6g Szechwan Lovage Rhizome (川芎, Chuanxiong) 6g Cassia Bark (肉桂, Rougui) 3g	Warming the meridian, expelling cold and dredging blood vessels			
Chinese Taxillus Twig (桑寄生, Sangjisheng) 9g Eucommia Bark (杜仲, Duzhong) 9g Medicinal Achyranthes Root (川牛膝, Chuan Niuxi) 9g	Replenishing the liver and kidney, expelling wind and dampness			
Ginseng (人参, Renshen) 6g Tuckahoe (茯苓, Fuling) 6g White Peony Root (白芍药, Baishaoyao) 6g Dried Rehmannia Root (干地黄, Gandihuang) 6g Licorice Root (甘草, Gancao) 6g	Replenishing qi and blood and supporting the healthy qi to eliminate pathogenic factors			

Associated Formulas:

1. Doubleteeth Pubescent Angelica and Largeleaf Gentian Decoction (独活秦艽汤, du huo qin jiao tang) *Syndrome-Cause-Pulse-Treatment* 《症因脉治》

This is composed of Doubleteeth Pubescent Angelica Root (独活, Duhuo), Largeleaf Gentian Root (秦艽, Qinjiao), Divaricate Saposhnikovia Root (防风, Fangfeng), Szechwan Lovage Rhizome (川芎, Chuanxiong) and Swordlike Atractylodes Rhizome (苍术, Cangzhu). Its action is expelling wind and dampness. It is suited to lumbago due to attack of wind-dampness.

2. Doubleteeth Pubescent Angelica Decoction (独活汤, du huo tang) *Standard for Diagnosis and Treatment* 《证治准绳》

This is comprised of Doubleteeth Pubescent Angelica Root (独活, Duhuo), Chinese Taxillus Twig (桑寄生, Sangjisheng), Medicinal Achyranthes Root (川牛膝, Chuan Niuxi), Largeleaf Gentian Root (秦艽, Qinjiao), Indian Bread Pink Epidermis (赤茯苓, Chifuling), Cassia Bark (桂心, Guixin), Divaricate Saposhnikovia Root (防风, Fangfeng), Baked Aconite Root (炮附子, Pao Fuzi), Chinese Angelica Root (当归, Danggui), Dried Rehmannia Root (生地黄, Shengdihuang), Eucommia Bark (杜仲, Duzhong), Manchurian Wildginger Herb (细辛, Xixin), Szechwan Lovage Rhizome (川芎, Chuanxiong), Red Peony Root (赤芍, Chishao) and Prepared Licorice Root (炙甘草, Zhi Gancao). Its actions are expelling wind, removing dampness and relieving pain. It is indicated for arthralgia manifested as dyskinesia of extremities or pain of the body.

3. Arthralgia-Relieving Decoction (蠲痹汤, juan bi tang) *Yang's Formulae Handed Down by Family* 《杨氏家藏方》

This is comprised of Chinese Angelica Root (当归, Danggui), Incised Notopterygium Rhizome or Root (羌活, Qianghuo), Turmeric Rhizome (姜黄, Jianghuang), White Peony Root (白芍药, Baishaoyao), Toasted Membranous Milkvetch Root (炙黄芪, Zhi Huangqi), Divaricate Saposhnikovia Root (防风, Fangfeng), Prepared Licorice Root (炙甘草, Zhi Gancao) and Fresh Ginger (生姜, Shengjiang). Its actions are replenishing qi, regulating ying, expelling wind and removing dampness. It is indicated for irritability, pain of the body and heaviness sensation of the loins and legs due to accumulation of wind and dampness resulting from deficiency of both ying and wei.

4. Arthralgia-Relieving Decoction (蠲痹汤, juan bi tang) *Comprehension of Medicine* 《医学心悟》

This consists of Incised Notopterygium Rhizome or Root (羌活, Qianghuo), Largeleaf Gentian Root (秦艽, Qinjiao), Doubleteeth Pubescent Angelica Root (独活, Duhuo), Mulberry Twigs (桑枝, Sangzhi), Chinese Angelica Root (当归, Danggui), Szechwan Lovage Rhizome (川芎, Chuanxiong), Prepared Licorice Root (炙甘草, Zhi Gancao), Cassia Bark (桂心, Guixin), Kadsura Pepper Stem (海风藤, Haifengteng), Olibanum (乳香, Ruxiang) and Common Aucklandia Root (木香, Muxiang). Its actions are expelling wind and dampness, dispelling cold and alleviating pain. It is indicated for arthralgia due to wind, cold and dampness.

5. Dampness-Removing and Arthralgia-Relieving Decoction (除湿蠲痹汤, chu shi juan bi tang) *Differential Diagnosis and Treatment of Diseases* 《类证治裁》

This is comprised of Swordlike Atractylodes Rhizome (苍术, Cangzhu), Largehead Atractylodes Rhizome (白术, Baizhu), Tuckahoe (茯苓, Fuling), Incised Notopterygium Rhizome or Root (羌活, Qianghuo), Oriental Waterplantain Rhizome (泽泻, Zexie), Tangerine Peel (橘皮, Jupi), Prepared Licorice Root (炙甘草, Zhi Gancao) and Bamboo Juice (竹沥, Zhuli). Its actions are removing dampness and relieving arthralgia. It is indicated for arthralgia of dampness type manifested as pain, soreness and heaviness sensation of the body.

6. General Recipe for Treating Sciatica(坐骨神经统治方, zuo gu shen jing tong zhi fang) *Author's Experienced Prescription* (笔者经验方)

This is made up of Doubleteeth Pulbescent Angelica Root(独活, Duhuo), Loranthus Mulberry Mistletoe(桑寄生, Sangjisheng), Drynaria Rhizome(骨碎补, Gusuibu), Aconiite Root(附子, Fuzi), Manchurian Wildginger Herb(细辛, Xixin), Ephedra(麻黄, Mahuang), Centipede(蜈蚣, Wugong) and Prepared Licorice(炙甘草, Zhigancao). Its actions are warming the channels, removing coldness and eliminating the obstructions in the channels to stop pain. It is indicated for sciatica. For those accompanied with a weak body, Membranous Milkvetch Root (黄芪, Huangqi) and Chinese Angrlica Root(当归, Danggui) are added. For those with fever, Common St. Paulwort(豨莶草, Xixiancao) is added. And for those with deformed lumbar vertebra, Anter(鹿角, Lujiao) is added.

6. Channels-Dredging and Blood-Activating Decoction (疏经活血汤, shu jing huo xue tang)

Source: *Curative Measures for Diseases* 《万病回春》
Composition: Chinese Angelica Root (当归, Danggui)9g
White Peony Root (白芍药, Baishaoyao)9g
Prepared Rehmannia Root (熟地黄, Shudihuang)9g
Swordlike Atractylodes Rhizome (苍术, Cangzhu)9g
Medicinal Achyranthes Root (川牛膝, Chuan Niuxi)9g
Tangerine Peel (橘皮, Jupi)9g
Peach Seed (桃仁, Taoren)9g
Chinese Clematis Root (威灵仙, Weilingxian)9g
Szechwan Lovage Rhizome (川芎, Chuanxiong)9g
Root of Dutchman-Spipe (木防己, Mu Fangji)9g
Incised Notopterygium Rhizome or Root (羌活, Qianghuo)9g
Divaricate Saposhnikovia Root (防风, Fangfeng)9g
Dahurican Angelica Root (白芷, Baizhi)9g
Chinese Gentian Root (龙胆草, Longdancao)6g
Tuckahoe (茯苓, Fuling)9g
Licorice Root (生甘草, Sheng Gancao)6g
Actions: Expelling wind and removing dampness, regulating blood and relieving arthralgia.
Applied Syndrome: Bi-syndrome(prolonged arthralgia due to wind-cold-dampness accompanied with deficiency of blood) manifested by pain of all over the body, pain of the tendons, muscles and joints which causes limited movement of the limbs, or lumbago, tiredness, lusterless complexion, or accompanied with palpitation and shortness of breath, pale tongue with thin and white coating, wiry and unsmooth pulse.

Channels-Dredging and Blood-Activating Decoction
(Wind-Dispelling and Dampness-Removing Method)

Ingredients	Effects	Combined Effects	Syndrome	Chief Symptoms
Chinese Angelica Root (当归, Danggui)9g Szechwan Lovage Rhizome (川芎, Chuanxiong)9g Prepared Rehmannia Root (熟地黄, Shudihuang)9g White Peony Root (白芍药, Baishaoyao)9g	Enriching and regulating blood	Expelling wind and removing dampness, regulating blood and relieving arthralgia	Prolonged arthralgia of wind-cold-dampness with deficiency of blood	Pain of the body, pain of the tendons, muscles and joints, dyskinesia, lusterless complexion, or accompanied with palpitation, pale tongue with thin and white coating, wiry and unsmooth pulse
Divaricate Saposhnikovia Root (防风, Fangfeng)9g Root of Dutchman-Spipe (木防己, Mu Fangji)9g Incised Notopterygium Rhizome or Root (羌活, Qianghuo)9g Chinese Clematis Root (威灵仙, Weilingxian)9g Dahurican Angelica Root (白芷, Baizhi)9g	Expelling wind and removing dampness, dredging meridians and activating the flow of qi and blood in the meridian and collateral			
Swordlike Atractylodes Rhizome (苍术, Cangzhu)9g Tuckahoe (茯苓, Fuling)9g Tangerine Peel (橘皮, Jupi)9g Licorice Root (生甘草, Sheng Gancao)6g	Invigorating the spleen and drying dampness			
Medicinal Achyranthes Root (川牛膝, Chuan Niuxi)9g Peach Seed (桃仁, Taoren)9g	Activating blood circulation and alleviating pain			
Chinese Gentian Root (龙胆草, Longdancao)6g	Clearing away heat by using corrigent			

Points in Constitution: This formula emphasizes expelling wind-dampness, enriching blood and dredging the collaterals. However, its actions of activating blood circulation and removing blood stasis are not strong. In the clinic, drugs for activating blood circulation can be added according to different conditions.

Indications:

1. Rheumatic arthrit
2. Rheumatoid arthritis.
3. Soft tissue injury.
4. Lumbago.

Precaution: This formula is not suitable for the initial stage of arthralgia of wind-cold-dampness type without blood deficiency.

Associated Formulas:

1. Qi-Invigorating, Blood-Replenishing and Tendons-Nourishing Decoction（气血并补荣筋汤, qi xue bing bu rong jin tang） *Internal Medicine of Traditional Chinese Medicine* by Wang Yongyan《中医内科学》王永炎著

This consists of Coix Seed（生薏苡仁, Sheng Yiyiren）, Tuckahoe（茯苓, Fuling）, Largehead Atractylodes Rhizome（白术, Baizhu）, Fleeceflower Root（何首乌, Heshouwu）, Chinese Angelica Root（当归, Danggui）, Villous Amomum Fruit（砂仁, Sharen）, Prepared Rehmannia Root（熟地黄, Shudihuang）, Siberian Solomonseal Rhizome（黄精, Huangjing）, Wasps Nest（蜂房, Fengfang）, Garter Snake（乌梢蛇, Wushaoshe）, Common St. Paulswort Herb（豨莶草, Xiqiancao）, Chinese Starjasmine Stem（络石藤, Luoshiteng）, East Asian Tree Fern Rhizome（狗脊, Gouji）, Largeleaf Gentian Root（秦艽, Qinjiao） and Chinese Dodder Seed（菟丝子, Tusizi）. The main actions of this formula are replenishing qi, activating blood circulation and dredging the collaterals. It is indicated for prolonged arthralgia with deficiency of qi and blood.

2. Kidney-Invigorating, Cold-Expelling and Arthralgia-Relieving Decoction（补肾祛寒治痹汤, bu shen qu han zhi bi tang） *Internal Medicine of Traditional Chinese Medicine* by Wang Yongyan《中医内科学》王永炎著

This is comprised of Himalayan Teasel Root（川续断, Chuanxuduan）, Malaytea Scurfpea Fruit（补骨脂, Buguzhi）, Prepared Aconite Root（制附子, Zhi Fuzi）, Prepared Rehmannia Root（熟地黄, Shudihuang）, Fortune's Drynaria Rhizome（骨碎补, Gusuibu）, Shorthorned Epimedium Herb（淫羊藿, Yinyanghuo）, Cassia Twig（桂枝, Guizhi）, Doubleteeth Pubescent Angelica Root（独活, Duhuo）, Chinese Clematis Root（威灵仙, Weilingxian） and White Peony Root（白芍药, Baishaoyao）. This formula mainly invigorates the kidney and expels cold. Besides, it can also activate blood circulation and dredging collaterals. It is suited to prolonged arthralgia with deficiency of kidney-yang.

7. Dreging and Dissipating Powder
(通导散, tong dao san)

Source: *Curative Measures for Diseases* 《万病回春》
Composition: Chinese Angelica Root (当归, Danggui) 9g
Safflower (红花, Honghua) 9g
Sappan Wood (苏木, Sumu) 9g
Immature Bitter Orange (枳实, Zhishi) 9g
Officinal Magnolia Bark (厚朴, Houpo) 9g
Rhubarb (生大黄, Sheng Dahuang) 6g
Mirabilite (芒硝, Mangxiao) 6
Licorice Root (生甘草; Sheng Gancao) 6g
Tangerine Peel (橘皮, Jupi) 6g
Akebia Stem (木通, Mutong) 6g

Actions: Activating blood circulation and purging blood stasis, regulating qi and alleviating pain.

Applied Syndromes:

1. Blood stasis in the lower-jiao in women manifested as pain, tenderness, distention and fullness feeling in the lower abdomen or amenorrhea, constipation, dry mouth and thirst, red tongue with thick, yellow and greasy coating, deep and rapid pulse.

2. Blood stasis and obstruction of qi in the abdomen due to traumatic injury manifested as local swelling and pain, constipation, enuresis, oppressed feeling in the chest, distention or expansion of abdomen which may radiates to the pericardium and chest, even extreme dysphoria or irritability, red tongue, deep and unsmooth pulse.

Points in Constitution: This formula is based on Major Purgative Decoction (大承气汤, da cheng qi tang) plus some blood-activating and stasis-removing drugs. It has a similar function of Peach Kernel Purgative Decoction (桃核承气汤, tao he cheng qi tang) designed by the famous ancient physician Zhang zhongjing (张仲景). They can treat syndrome of blood stasis with a strong body and constipation.

Indications:

1. Internal hemorrhage and cerebral contusion due to trauma.
2. Acute intestinal obstruction and intestinal adhesion.
3. Acute pelvic inflammation.
4. Retained placenta.

Precaution: This formula is contraindicated in pregnant woman.

Associated Formulas:

1. Decoction for Recovery and Activating Blood Circulation (复元活血汤, fu yuan huo xue tang) *Invention of Medicine* 《医学发明》

This is composed of Chinese Thorowax Root (柴胡, Chaihu), Snakegourd Root (瓜蒌根, Gualougen), Safflower (红花, Honghua), Licorice Root (甘草, Gancao), Pangolin Scales (穿山甲, Chuanshanjia), Rhubarb (大黄, Dahuang), Peach Seed (桃仁, Taoren) and Chinese Angelica Root (当归, Danggui). Its actions are activating blood circulation and dissolving blood stasis, dispersing the stagnated liver-qi and dredging the collaterals. It is indicated for traumatic injury with unbearable pain due to blood stasis in the hypochondrium.

Dreging and Dissipating Powder
(Qi-Regulating and Blood-Activating Method)

Ingredients	Effects	Combined Effects	Syndrome	Chief Symptoms
Chinese Angelica Root (当归, Danggui)9g Safflower (红花, Honghua)9g Sappan Wood (苏木, Sumu)9g	Activating blood circulation and removing blood stasis	Activating blood circulation and purging blood stasis, regulating flow of qi and relaxing the bowel	Blood retention in the lower-jiao	Women blood stasis in the lower-jiao, pain and tenderness in the lower abdomen, or amenorrhea, or traumatic injury, local swelling and pain, constipation and enuresis, expansion of abdomen which radiates to the pericardium and chest, red tongue, deep and unsmooth pulse
Immature Bitter Orange (枳实, Zhishi)9g Officinal Magnolia Bark (厚朴, Houpo)9g Rhubarb (生大黄, Sheng Dahuang)6g Mirabilite (芒硝, Mangxiao)6g Licorice Root (生甘草, Sheng Gancao)6g	Purging heat and relaxing the bowel			
Tangerine Peel (橘皮, Jupi)6g	Regulating qi and removing phlegm			
Akebia Stem (木通, Mutong)6g	Dredging the meridians			

2. Peach Kernel Purgative Decoction(桃核承气汤, tao he cheng qi tang) *Treatise on Exogenous Febrile Diseases* 《伤寒论》

This is comprised of Peach Seed (桃仁, Taoren), Rhubarb (大黄, Dahuang), Cassia Twig (桂枝, Guizhi), Prepared Licorice Root (炙甘草, Zhi Gancao) and Mirabilite (芒硝, Mangxiao). Its actions are removing blood stasis drastically and purging heat. It is indicated for accumulation of blood in the lower-jiao, manifested as feeling of distention, fullness and pain with tenderness in the lower abdomen.

3. Wounds-Healing and Pain-Relieving Pill(和伤拈痛丹, he shang nian tong dan) *Book for Saving Life*《活人书》

This is comprised of Rhubarb (大黄, Dahuang), Weathered Sodium Sulfate (玄明粉, Yuanmingfen), Ending Part of Chinese Angelica Root (当归尾, Dangguiwei), Safflower (红花, Honghua), Turtle Carapace (鳖甲, Biejia), Bitter Orange (枳壳, Zhiqiao), Corydalis Tuber (延胡索, Yanhusuo), Cassia Twig (桂枝, Guizhi) and Akebia Stem (木通, Mutong). Its actions are activating blood circulation, removing blood stasis and relaxing the bowel. It is indicated for blood stasis in the interior due to traumatic injury manifested as constipation, anuresis, expansion of the abdomen, irritability, vomiting, nausia, swelling of the head and eyes.

8. Miraculous Collateral-Activating Pill
(活络效灵丹, huo luo xiao ling dan)

Source: *Records of Traditional Chinese and Western Medicine in Combination*《医学衷中参西录》

Composition: Chinese Angelica Root (当归, Danggui)15g

Dan-shen Root (丹参, Danshen)15g

Olibanum (乳香, Ruxiang)15g

Myrrh (没药, Moyao)15g

Actions: Activating blood circulation and dissolving blood stasis, dredging the collaterals and alleviating pain.

Applied Syndrome: Mass in the abdomen and various pain due to qi stagnation and blood stasis, manifested by various pericardial and abdominal pain, pain of the limbs, traumatic injury and sore in the interior or in the superficies, blue purple tongue, wiry, thin and unsmooth pulse or wiry and tense pulse.

Points in Constitution: Pain results from obstruction and if the obstruction is removed, the pain is of course relieved. This formula is especially used for activating blood circulation and dredging channels and colleterals.

Indications:

1. Coronary heart disease, angina pectoris.
2. Cerebral infarction and sequela.
3. Exfetation.
4. Sciatica.

Precautions: This formula should be cautiously used for the case of deficiency of qi and blood and those who are susceptible to hemorrhage.

Associated Formulas:

1. Blood-Activating and Pain-Alleviating Decoction (活血止痛汤, huo xue zhi tong tang) *A*

Comprehensive Summary of Traumatology《伤科大成》

Miraculous Collateral-Activating Pill

(Blood-Activating and Stasis-Removing Method)

Ingredients	Effects	Combined Effects	Syndrome	Chief Symptoms
Chinese Angelica Root（当归, Danggui）15g Dan-Shen Root（丹参, Danshen）15g	Activating blood circulation and enriching blood	Activating blood circulation and dissolving blood stasis, dredging the collaterals and alleviating pain	Pain due to qi stagnation and blood stasis	Pericardial and abdominal pain, pain of the limbs, traumatic injury and sore, mass in the abdomen, blue purple tongue, wiry, thin and unsmooth pulse
Olibanum（乳香, Ruxiang）15g Myrrh（没药, Moyao）15g	Activating blood circulation and dissolving blood stasis, activating flow of qi and alleviating pain			

    This is made up of Chinese Angelica Root（当归, Danggui）, Sappan Wood（苏木, Sumu）, Centalla（落得打, Luodeda）, Szechwan Lovage Rhizome（川芎, Chuanxiong）, Safflower（红花, Honghua）, Olibanum（乳香, Ruxiang）, Myrrh（没药, Moyao）, Sanchi Root（三七, Sanqi）, Red Peony Root（赤芍, Chishao）, Tangerine Peel（橘皮, Jupi）, Vine of Cercis（紫荆藤, Zijingteng）and Ground Bettle（地鳖虫, Dibiechong）. Its actions are activating blood circulation, removing blood stasis and alleviating pain. It is indicated for redness, swelling and pain due to blood stasis of trauma.

    2. Blood-Activating Decoction（活血汤, huo xue tang）*Longevity and Life Prescription*《寿世保元》

    This is comprised of Chinese Angelica Root（当归, Danggui）, Red Peony Root（赤芍, Chishao）, Peach Seed（桃仁, Taoren）, Tree Peony Bark（牡丹皮, Mudanpi）, Yanhusuo（元胡, Yuanhu）, Commbined Spicebush Root（乌药, Wuyao）, Nutgrass Galingale Rhizome（香附, Xiangfu）, Bitter Orange（枳壳, Zhiqiao）, Safflower（红花, Honghua）, Cassia Bark（官桂, Guangui）, Common Aucklandia Root（木香, Muxiang）, Szechwan Lovage Rhizome（川芎, Chuanxiong）, Licorice Root（甘草, Gancao）and Fresh Ginger（生姜, Shengjiang）. Its actions are activating blood circulation and dissolving blood stasis, regulating flow of qi and alleviating pain. It is suited to localized pain in the abdomen due to blood stasis.

    3. Decoction for Recovery and Activating Blood Circulation（复元活血汤, fu yuan huo xue tang）*Invention of Medicine*《医学发明》

    This consists of Chinese Thorowax Root（柴胡, Chaihu）, Turmeric Rhizome（姜黄, Jianghuang）, Chinese Angelica Root（当归, Danggui）, Rhubarb（生大黄, Sheng Dahuang）, Safflower（红花, Honghua）, Licorice Root（生甘草, Sheng Gancao）, Pangolin Scales（穿山甲,

Chuanshanjia) and Peach Seed (桃仁, Taoren). Its actions are activating blood circulation and dissolving blood stasis, dispersing the stagnated liver-qi and dredging the collaterals. It is indicated for traumatic injury with unbearable pain due to blood stasis in the hypochondrium.

4. Anti-Bruise Powder (七厘散, qi li san) *Collection of Effective Formulae*《良方集腋》

This is comprised of Dragon's Blood (血竭, Xuejie), Musk (麝香, Shexiang), Borneol (冰片, Bingpian), Olibanum (乳香, Ruxiang), Myrrh (没药, Moyao), Safflower (红花, Honghua), Cinnabar (朱砂, Zhusha) and Catechu (儿茶, Ercha). Its actions are activating blood circulation and dissipating blood stasis, alleviating pain and arresting bleeding. This is indicated for stasis of blood, swelling and pain of traumatic injury with fracture and broken of tendons, or hemorrhage of sword injury.

5. Pantalgia-Relieving and Blood Stasis-Dispelling Decoction (身痛逐瘀汤, shen tong zhu yu tang) *Correction of Medical Classics*《医林改错》

This is comprised of Largeleaf Gentian Root (秦艽, Qinjiao), Szechwan Lovage Rhizome (川芎, Chuanxiong), Peach Seed (桃仁, Taoren), Safflower (红花, Honghua), Licorice Root (生甘草, Sheng Gancao), Incised Notopterygium Rhizome or Root (羌活, Qianghuo), Myrrh (没药, Moyao), Chinese Angelica Root (当归, Danggui), Trogopterus Dung (五灵脂, Wulingzhi), Nutgrass Galingale Rhizome (香附, Xiangfu), Medicinal Achyranthes Root (川牛膝, Chuan Niuxi) and Earth Worm (地龙, Dilong). Its actions are activating blood circulation and flow of qi, dissolving blood stasis, dredging the collaterals, relieving arthralgia and alleviating pain. This is indicated for prolonged pain due to stagnation of qi and blood in the meridian and collaterals.

9. Anti-Bruise Powder
(七厘散, qi li san)

Source: *Collection of Effective Formulae*《良方集腋》
Composition: Dragon's Blood (血竭, Xuejie)
Musk (麝香, Shexiang)
Borneol (冰片, Bingpian)
Olibanum (乳香, Ruxiang)
Myrrh (没药, Moyao)
Safflower (红花, Honghua)
Cinnabar (朱砂, Zhusha)
Catechu (儿茶, Ercha)
(It is a patent medicine and its preparation is omitted)
Actions: Activating blood circulation and dissipating blood stasis, alleviating pain and arresting bleeding.
Applied Syndrome: Swelling and pain due to blood stasis resulting from traumatic injury with fracture and broken tendons, or hemorrhage of sword injury.

Anti-Bruise Powder
(Blood-Activating and Stasis-Removing Method)

Ingredients	Effects	Combined Effects	Syndrome	Chief Symptoms
Dragon's Blood (血竭, Xuejie) Safflower (红花, Honghua)	Activating blood circulation and dissolving blood stasis	Activating blood circulation and dissipating blood stasis, alleviating pain and arresting bleeding	Pain syndrome due to blood stasis	Traumatic injury, fracture and broken tendons, stasis of blood, swelling and pain
Olibanum (乳香, Ruxiang) Myrrh (没药, Moyao)	Dissolving blood stasis and activating flow of qi, reducing swelling and alleviating pain			
Musk (麝香, Shexiang) Borneol (冰片, Bingpian)	Activating blood circulation and dredging the collaterals, dissipating blood stasis and alleviating pain			
Cinnabar (朱砂, Zhusha)	Calming the heart and tranquilizing the mind			
Catechu (儿茶, Ercha)	Clearing away heat and arresting bleeding			

Points in Constitution: This formula pays equal attention to the blood-activating and stasis-removing drugs and the drugs with fragrance which have the action of traveling around the body. The drugs with fragrance can promote circulation of qi and blood to improve the pain-alleviating action.

Indications:

1. Traumatic injury and hemorrhage of cut.
2. All kinds of inflammation of soft tissues of unknown origin.
3. Burn and scald.
4. Herpes zoster.
5. Intercostal neuralgia, hepatitis with pain in the hypochondrium, remote pain in the chest and hypochondrium.
6. Lumbodorsal soft tissue of injury.
7. Viral myocharditis.
8. Coronary Heart Disease.

Precaution: This formula, which can both be taken orally or applied externally, is a commonly-used Prescription for traumatology. Since the drugs have a fragrant smell and the property of traveling around the body, they may consum qi and cause abortion. Thus, this formula is forbidden for pregnant women.

Associated Formula:

Ten Treasures Powder(十宝散, shi bao san) *Complete Works of Diagnosis and Treatment for Surgical Diseases* 《外科证治全生集》

This is made up of Dragon's Blood (血竭, Xuejie), Red Orpiment (雄黄, Xionghuang), Safflower (红花, Honghua), Catechu (儿茶, Ercha), Cinnabar (朱砂, Zhusha), Olibanum (乳香, Ruxiang), Myrrh (没药, Moyao), Ending Part of Chinese Angelica Root (当归尾, Dangguiwei), Musk (麝香, Shexiang) and Borneol (冰片, Bingpian). Its actions are removing blood stasis and arresting bleeding, relieving pain and inducing resuscitation. This is applicable for coma due to cuts, injury by sword, fracture, traumatic injury and all kinds of pain.

10. Blood-Activating and Hardness-Removing Decoction (活血化坚汤, huo xue hua jian tang)

Source: *Orthodox Manual of Surgery* 《外科正宗》
Composition: Divaricate Saposhnikovia Root (防风, Fangfeng)9g
Red Peony Root (赤芍, Chishao)9g
Ending Part of Chinese Angelica Root (当归尾, Dangguiwei)9g
Snakegourd Root (天花粉, Tianhuafen)9g
Honeysuckle Flower (金银花, Jinyinhua)15g
Thunberg Fritillary Bulb (浙贝母, Zhe Beimu)9g
Szechwan Lovage Rhizome (川芎, Chuanxiong)9g
Balloonflower Root (桔梗, Jiegeng)9g
Chinese Honeylocust Spine (皂角刺, Zaojiaoci)9g
Silkworm with Batrytis Larva (僵蚕, Jiangcan)9g
Officinal Magnolia Bark (厚朴, Houpo)9g
Trogopterus Dung (五灵脂, Wulingzhi)15g
Tangerine Peel (橘皮, Jupi)9g
Licorice Root (甘草, Gancao)9g
Olibanum (乳香, Ruxiang)9g
Dahurican Angelica Root (白芷, Baizhi)9g

Actions: Activating blood circulation and resolving phlegm, dissipating blockages and reducing swelling.

Applied Syndrome: The beginning of unbroken scrofula, goiter and subcutaneous nodule.

Points in Constitution: Removing phlegm, activating blood circulation and dissipating blockages are the common methods used for dissolving a goiter and scrofula. For the case of tuberculosis, Common Selfheal Fruit-Spike (夏枯草, Xiakucao), Weeping Forsythia Capsule (连翘, Lianqiao) and Centipede (蜈蚣, Wugong) can be appropriately added.

Blood-Activating and Hardness-Removing Decoction
(Blood-Activating and Phlegm-Removing Method)

Ingredients	Effects	Combined Effects	Syndrome	Chief Symptoms
Honeysuckle Flower (金银花, Jinyinhua) 15g	Clearing away heat and toxic material	Activating blood circulation and removing phlegm, dissipating blockages and reducing swelling	Accumulation of phlegm and blood stasis	Scrofula, goiter and subcutaneous nodule which have not suppurated.
Ending Part of Chinese Angelica Root (当归尾, Dangguiwei) 9g Red Peony Root (赤芍, Chishao) 9g Trogopterus Dung (五灵脂, Wulingzhi) 15g Olibanum (乳香, Ruxiang) 9g Szechwan Lovage Rhizome (川芎, Chuanxiong) 9g	Activating blood circulation and dissipating blood stasis			
Thunberg Fritillary Bulb (浙贝母, Zhe Beimu) 9g Snakegourd Root (天花粉, Tianhuafen) 9g Chinese Honeylocust Spine (皂角刺, Zaojiaoci) 9g Silkworm with Batrytis Larva (僵蚕, Jiangcan) 9g	Dissipating blockages and reducing swelling			
Tangerine Peel (橘皮, Jupi) 9g Officinal Magnolia Bark (厚朴, Houpo) 9g	Regulating qi and dissipating blockages			
Divaricate Saposhnikovia Root (防风, Fangfeng) 9g Dahurican Angelica Root (白芷, Baizhi) 9g	Expelling wind and dissipating blockages			
Balloonflower Root (桔梗, Jiegeng) 9g	Inducing the effect of drugs ascending			
Licorice Root (甘草, Gancao) 9g	Coordinating the actions of various ingredients in the Prescription			

Indications:

1. Scrofula, manifested by enlargement of lymph nodes in cluster on the neck, in the armpit and on the hip, hardness which can move about when pushed, no hot and painful sensation or only slight painful sensation (lymphadenitis or tuberculous lymphadenitis).

2. Goiter, manifested by free swelling over the neck with undistinct margin, normal color and softness when pressed (thyroid enlargement or cyst).

3. Mammary nodule, manifested by mammary hard lump which is neither red nor hot, smooth surface and movable when pushed (hyperplasia of mammary glands).

4. Subcutaneous nodule, manifested by mass under the skin which shows various sizes and is neither red nor hot, nor pain but soft and movable (lipoma).

Precaution: This formula is not suitable for scrofula which is suppurative.

Associated Formulas:

1. Minor Gold Tablet（小金片, xiao jin pian）*Surgery* by Guangzhou College of Traditional Chinese Medicine 广州中医学院《外科学》

This is comprised of Prepared Nux Vomica（制马钱子, Zhi Maqianzi）, Earth Worm（地龙, Dilong）, Scorpion（全蝎, Quanxie）, Prepared Aconite Root（制附子, Zhi Fuzi）, Ginger-Prepared Pinellia Rhizome（姜半夏, Jiangbanxia）, Trogopterus Dung（五灵脂, Wulingzhi）, Prepared Myrrh（制没药, Zhi Moyao）and Prepared Olibanum（制乳香, Zhi Ruxiang）. Its actions are removing blood stasis drastically and dredging the collaterals, expelling dampness and removing phlegm, reducing swelling and alleviating pain. It is indicated for subcutaneous nodule, scrofula, goiter, epididymis tuberculosis and tumor.

2. Asiatic Rhinoceros Bezoar Pill（犀黄丸, xi huang wan）*Surgery Life-Saving Collection*《外科全生集》

This consists of Asiatic Rhinoceros Bezoar（犀牛黄, Xiniuhuang）, Musk（麝香, Shexiang）, Myrrh（没药, Moyao）, Olibanum（乳香, Ruxiang）and Cooked Glutinous Millet（黄米饭, Huangmifan）. Its actions are clearing away heat and toxic material, removing phlegm and dissipating blockages, activating blood circulation and dissolving blood stasis. It is suited to scrofula, subcutaneous nodule and multiple abscess.

11. Four Powerful Herbs Decoction
（四妙勇安汤, si miao yong an tang）

Source: *New Compilation of Proved Recipe*《验方新编》

Composition: Honeysuckle Flower（金银花, Jinyinhua）9g

Figwort Root（玄参, Xuanshen）30g

Chinese Angelica Root（当归, Danggui）15g

Licorice Root（生甘草, Sheng Gancao）9g

Actions: Clearing away heat and toxic material, activating blood circulation and alleviating pain.

Applied Syndrome: Gangrene of finger or toe due to excessive heat-toxin, manifested by putrescence or suppuration and pain in the limbs, especially the extremities of the lower limbs, with dripping of purulence, dysphoria with smothery sensation, thirst, red tongue with yellow coating, rapid pulse.

Four Powerful Herbs Decoction
(Heat-Clearing and Toxin-Removing Method)

Ingredients	Effects	Combined Effects	Syndrome	Chief Symptoms
Honeysuckle Flower (金银花, Jinyinhua)9g	Clearing away heat and toxic material, removing heat from the blood	Clearing away heat and toxic material, activating blood circulation and alleviating pain	Gangrene of finger or toe (due to excessive heat-toxin)	Putrescence and pain in the extremities of the lower limbs, dripping of purulent, dysphoria with smothery sensation, thirst, red tongue with yellow coating, and rapid pulse
Figwort Root (玄参, Xuanshen)30g	Removing heat from the blood and clearing away toxic material			
Chinese Angelica Root (当归, Danggui)15g	Activating blood circulation and alleviating pain			
Licorice Root (生甘草, Sheng Gancao)9g	Clearing away heat and toxic material			

Points in Constitution: This formula only contains four drugs and they can directly reach the affected parts, enabling the illness to be controlled quick. In clinic, the dosage can be incresed two or three times according to different syndromes.

Indications:
1. Thromboangiitis obliterans.
2. Arterial embolic gangrene.
3. Embolic phlebitis(Embolic inflammation of large veins).
4. Unhealed carbuncle and gangrene.

Precautions: This formula contains only a few drugs, but the actions are obvious. Thus in clinic, it should be used with a large dose for a long time. In addition, the patients must avoid scratching the affected place.

Associated Formula:

Foot-Minding Decoction (顾步汤, gu bu tang) *Genuine Exposition on Externaal Diseases* 《外科真诠》

This is comprised of Membranous Milkvetch Root (黄芪, Huangqi), Ginseng (人参, Renshen), Dendrobium Herb (石斛, Shihu), Chinese Angelica Root (当归, Danggui), Honeysuckle

Flower (金银花, Jinyinhua), Medicinal Achyranthes Root (川牛膝, Chuan Niuxi), Chrysanthemum Flower (菊花, Juhua), Licorice Root (生甘草, Sheng Gancao), Dandelion (蒲公英, Pugongying) and Tokyo Violet Herb (紫花地丁, Zihuadiding). This formula has the actions of replenishing qi, nourishing yin, clearing away heat and regulating ying. This is indicated for gangrene of the finger or toe due to deficiency of qi and blood and excessive noxious heat.

12. Snakegourd and Great Burdock Achene Decoction (瓜蒌牛蒡汤, gua lou niu bang tang)

Source: *The Golden Mirror of Medicine* 《医宗金鉴》
Composition: Snakegourd Seed (瓜蒌仁, Gualouren)15g
Great Burdock Achene (牛蒡子, Niubangzi)12g
Snakegourd Root (天花粉, Tianhuafen)12g
Baikal Skullcap Root (黄芩, Huangqin)12g
Cape Jasmine Fruit (山栀子, Shanzhizi)12g
Honeysuckle Flower (金银花, Jinyinhua)12g
Weeping Forsythia Capsule (连翘, Lianqiao)12g
Chinese Honeylocust Spine (皂角刺, Zaojiaoci)12g
Green Tangerine Peel (青皮, Qingpi)6g
Tangerine Peel (橘皮, Jupi)6g
Chinese Thorowax Root (柴胡, Chaihu)6g
Licorice Root (生甘草, Sheng Gancao)6g

Actions: Clearing away heat and toxic material, reducing swelling and dissipating blockages.

Applied Syndrome: The beginning of mammary abscess, manifested by local redness, swelling and indurated nodules, hot sensation, severe pain, chills and fever, red tongue with thin and yellow coating, superficial and rapid pulse.

Points in Constitution: This formula is comprised of a large dose of drugs for clearing away heat and toxic material and reducing swelling. The use of Chinese Thorowax Root (柴胡, Chaihu) is to reduce fever and Chinese Honeylocust Spine (皂角刺, Zaojiaoci) is to promote pus discharge.

Indication: The beginning of mastitis without purulency.

Precaution: This formula is also called Great Burdock Achene Decoction (牛蒡子汤, niu bang zi tang) and has a dissipating action for the beginning of mammary abscess.

Associated Formulas:

1. Swelling-Reducing and Detoxicificating Decoction (消肿解毒汤, xiao zhong jie du tang) *Elite of Effective Prescriptions of Contemporary Famous Doctors of China* 《中华当代名医妙方精华》

Snakegourd and Great Burdock Achene Decoction
(Heat-Clearing and Swelling-Reducing Method)

Ingredients	Effects	Combined Effects	Syndrome	Chief Symptoms
Snakegourd Seed (瓜蒌仁, Gualouren) 15g Great Burdock Achene (牛蒡子, Niubangzi) 12g Snakegourd Root (天花粉, Tianhuafen) 12g	Clearing away heat and evacuating pus	Clearing away heat and toxic material, reducing swelling and dissipating blockages	The beginning of mammary abscess	Local redness, swelling and indurated nodules, heat sensation, severe pain, aversion to cold and fever, red tongue with thin and yellow coating, superficial and rapid pulse
Chinese Honeylocust Spine (皂角刺, Zaojiaoci) 12g	Promoting pus discharge			
Baikal Skullcap Root (黄芩, Huangqin) 12g Cape Jasmine Fruit (山栀子, Shanzhizi) 12g Honeysuckle Flower (金银花, Jinyinhua) 12g Weeping Forsythia Capsule (连翘, Lianqiao) 12g	Clearing away heat and toxic material			
Green Tangerine Peel (青皮, Qingpi) 6g Tangerine Peel (橘皮, Jupi) 6g	Regulating the stomach qi			
Chinese Thorowax Root (柴胡, Chaihu) 6g	Dispersing the stagnated liver-qi, reducing fever and directing the effect of drugs to its meridian			
Licorice Root (生甘草, Sheng Gancao) 6g	Detoxification and coordinating the actions of various ingredients in the Prescription			

This is made up of Dandelion (蒲公英, Pugongying), Tokyo Violet Herb (紫花地丁, Zihuadiding), Honeysuckle Flower (金银花, Jinyinhua), Chinese Thorowax Root (柴胡, Chaihu), Tangerine Peel (橘皮, Jupi), Paniculate Bolbostemma Rhizome (土贝母, Tubeimu) and Muskroot-like Semiaquilegia Root (天葵, Tiankui). Its actions are clearing away heat and toxic material, inducing lactation and evacuating pus. It is suited to acute mastitis.

2. Modified Snakegourd Fruit and Great Burdock Achene Decoction(加减瓜蒌牛蒡汤, jia jian gua lou niu bang tang) *Elite of Effective Prescriptions of Contemporary Famous Doctors of China*《中华当代名医妙方精华》

This is comprised of Snakegourd Fruit (瓜蒌, Gualou), Great Burdock Achene (牛蒡子, Niubangzi), Green Tangerine Peel (青皮, Qingpi), Snakegourd Root (天花粉, Tianhuafen), Red Peony Root (赤芍, Chishao), Honeysuckle Flower (金银花, Jinyinhua), Weeping Forsythia Capsule (连翘, Lianqiao), Baikal Skullcap Root (黄芩, Huangqin), Cowherb Seed (王不留行, Wangbuliuxing), Beautiful Sweetgum Fruit (路路通, Lulutong) and Licorice Root (生甘草, Sheng Gancao). This formula has the actions of dispersing the stagnated liver-qi, clearing away heat, regulating ying and inducing or promoting lactation. It is indicated for mammary abscess manifested as red, painful and distending mammary with undistinct boundary, hardness and tenderness, chills and fever, dry mouth and thirst, red tongue with yellow coating, wiry and rapid pulse.

3. Snakegourd Fruit Powder(瓜蒌散, gua lou san) *Fu Qingzhu's Obstetrics and Gynecology*《傅青主女科》

This is comprised of Snakegourd Fruit (瓜蒌, Gualou), Licorice Root (生甘草, Sheng Gancao), Chinese Angelica Root (当归, Danggui), Olibanum (乳香, Ruxiang), Myrrh (没药, Moyao), Honeysuckle Flower (金银花, Jinyinhua), Dahurican Angelica Root (白芷, Baizhi) and Green Tangerine Peel (青皮, Qingpi). Its actions are clearing away heat and toxic material, activating qi flow and blood circulation. It is applicable for mammary abscess or carbuncle due to excessive heat-toxin.

Additional Formula

Formula for Craniocerebral Contusion Number Two
(头伤Ⅱ号, tou shang er hao)

Source: Guangzhou College of Traditional Chinese Medicine, Cai Rong 广州中医学院 蔡荣
Composition: Pilose Asiabell Root (党参, Dangshen)12g
Fleeceflower Root (何首乌, Heshouwu)24g
White Peony Root (白芍药, Baishaoyao)9g
Indian Bread with Hostwood (茯神, Fushen)15g
Szechwan Lovage Rhizome (川芎, Chuanxiong)6g
Tribulus Fruit〔Tribulus Fruit(白蒺藜, Baijili)〕9g
Chinese Angelica Root (当归, Danggui)12g
Prepared Licorice Root (炙甘草, Zhi Gancao)6g
Dragon's Teeth (生龙齿, Sheng Longchi)30g
Actions: Replenishing qi and blood, tranquilizing the mind and soothing the nerves.
Applied Syndrome: The middle and later stages of craniocerebral contusion manifested as dizziness, headache, listlessness, palpitation, amnesia, dark red tongue with white coating, wiry pulse.
Points in Constitution: In addition to the drugs for replenishing qi and blood, this formula also contains Szechwan Lovage Rhizome (川芎, Chuanxiong) which can regulate flow of qi, activating blood circulation and induce the actions to ascend to the top of the head. The use of Indian Bread with Hostwood (茯神, Fushen) and Dragon's Teeth (龙齿, Longchi) is to sooth the nerves and tranquilize the mind.
Indications:
1. Vertigo and headache due to cerebral contusion.
2. Vegetative nerve functional disturbance.
Precaution: This formula is designed for vertigo and headache due to blood stasis resulting from deficiency of qi and blood. Thus, it should be cautiously used for vertigo due to hyperactivity of liver-yang or upward attack of yang in deficiency condition resulting from yin deficiency of the liver and kidney.
Associated Formulas:

1. Back to the Spleen Decoction (归脾汤, gui pi tang) *Prescriptions for Rescuing the Sick* 《济生方》
This is comprised of Ginseng (人参, Renshen), Largehead Atractylodes Rhizome (白术, Baizhu), Indian Bread with Hostwood (茯神, Fushen), Toasted Membranous Milkvetch Root (炙黄芪, Zhi Huangqi), Longan Aril (龙眼肉, Longyanrou), Fried Spine Date Seed (炒酸枣仁, Chao Suanzaoren), Common Aucklandia Root (木香, Muxiang), Chinese Angelica Root (当

归, Danggui), Prepared Licorice Root (炙甘草, Zhi Gancao) and Thinleaf Milkwort Root (远志, Yuanzhi). Its actions are replenishing qi, enriching blood, calming the heart and tranquilizing the mind. It is indicated for vertigo, palpitation and insomnia due to deficiency of qi and blood.

Formula for Craniocerebral Contusion Number Two
(Heart-Nourishing and Mind-Tranquilizing Method)

Ingredients	Effects	Combined Effects	Syndrome	Chief Symptoms
Pilose Asiabell Root (党参, Dangshen) 12g	Replenishing qi of the middle-jiao	Replenishing qi and blood, sedation and tranquilizing the mind	Cerebral contusion (due to deficiency of qi and blood and blood stasis in the interior)	Dizziness, headache, listlessness, palpitation and amnesia, dark red tongue with white coating, wiry pulse
Fleeceflower Root (何首乌, Heshouwu) 24g Chinese Angelica Root (当归, Danggui) 12g White Peony Root (白芍药, Baishaoyao) 9g	Nourishing yin and blood			
Indian Bread with Hostwood (茯神, Fushen) 15g Dragon's Teeth (生龙齿, Sheng Longchi) 30g Tribulus Fruit (白蒺藜, Baijili) 9g	Sedation and tranquilizing the mind			
Szechwan Lovage Rhizome (川芎, Chuanxiong) 6g	Activating blood circulation and activating flow of qi and alleviating pain			
Prepared Licorice Root (炙甘草, Zhi Gancao) 6g	Coordinating the actions of various ingredients in the Prescription			

2. Qi-Replenishing and Vertigo-Relieving Decoction (补气解晕汤, bu qi jie yun tang) *Fu Qingzhu's Obstetrics and Gynecology* 《傅青主女科》

This is comprised of Ginseng (人参, Renshen), Toasted Membranous Milkvetch Root (炙黄芪, Zhi Huangqi), Chinese Angelica Root (当归, Danggui), Carbonized Spike of Fineleaf Schizonepeta Herb (炒荆芥穗, Chao Jingjiesui) and Charred Ginger (姜炭, Jiangtan). Its actions are replenishing qi and blood. It is indicated for postpartum faint due to deficiency of qi.

Chapter Ten
Formulas for Dermatoses

The effects of the Chinese formulas on the prevention and treatment of various skin diseases have undergone a gradual course, during which further explorations have been made. It has been proved in clinic that many skin diseases such as skin infection, urticaria, ecaema, dermatitis, ulcer, psoriasis, pigmentation, verruca vulgaris and skin cancer can be treated with formulas, which have been widely reported.

1. Bupleurum Liver-Clearing Decoction
(柴胡清肝饮, chai hu qing gan yin)

Source: Syndrome-Cause-Pulse-Treatment 《症因脉治》
Composition: Chinese Angelica Root (当归, Danggui)6g
Szechwan Lovage Rhizome (川芎, Chuanxiong)6g
White Peony Root (白芍药, Baishaoyao)9g
Prepared Rehmannia Root (熟地黄, Shudihuang)6g
Chinese Corktree Bark (黄柏, Huangbai)6g
Baikal Skullcap Root (黄芩, Huangqin)6g
Coptis Rhizome (黄连, Huanglian)6g
Cape Jasmine Fruit (山栀子, Shanzhizi)6g
Bupleurum(柴胡, Chaihu)6g
Wild Mint Herb (薄荷, Bohe)6g
Balloonflower Root (桔梗, Jiegeng)6g
Great Burdock Achene (牛蒡子, Niubangzi)9g
Snakegourd Root (天花粉, Tianhuafen)9g
Weeping Forsythia Capsule (连翘, Lianqiao)6g
Licorice Root (甘草, Gancao)6g

Actions: Clearing away heat and dispersing stagnated liver-qi, expelling wind and clearing away toxic material.

Applied Syndrome: Syndrome of wind-heat of the liver channel manifested as redness, swelling and itching in the skin, fever, irritability, sore throat, red tongue and rapid pulse.

Points in Constitution: This formula uses the ingredients of Warming and Clearing Decoction (温清饮, wen qing yin) which is the combination of Four Herbs Decoction (四物汤, si wu tang) and Coptis Detoxicating Decoction (黄连解毒汤, huanglian jie du tang) to remove heat from the blood and clear away toxic material. Besides, Bupleurum (柴胡, Chaihu), Wild Mint Herb (薄

荷, Bohe), Great Burdock Achene (牛蒡子, Niubangzi), Snakegourd Root (天花粉, Tianhuafen) and Balloonflower Root (桔梗, Jiegeng) are added not only to disperse the stagnated liver-qi and clear away liver heat, but also to clear away the heat in the lung and remove phlegm. Thus, this formula is indicated for various syndromes due to stagnation of heat in the liver, lung, blood and qi.

Bupleurum Liver-Clearing Decoction
(Heat-Clearing and Liver-Dispersing Method)

Ingredients	Effects	Combined Effects	Syndrome	Chief Symptoms
Chinese Angelica Root (当归, Danggui)6g Szechwan Lovage Rhizome (川芎, Chuanxiong)6g White Peony Root (白芍药, Baishaoyao)9g Prepared Rehmannia (熟地黄, Shudihuang)6g	Enriching and regulating the blood	Clearing away liver heat, enriching blood and removing heat and toxic material	Wind-heat of the liver meridian	Redness, swelling and itching of the skin, irritability, fever and bitter taste in the mouth, sore throat, red tongue and rapid pulse
Chinese Corktree Bark (黄柏, Huangbai)6g Coptis Rhizome (黄连, Huanglian)6g Baikal Skullcap Root (黄芩, Huangqin)6g Cape Jasmine Fruit (山栀子, Shanzhizi)6g Weeping Forsythia Capsule (连翘, Lianqiao)6g	Clearing away heat and toxic material			
Bupleurum(柴胡, Chaihu)6g Wild Mint Herb (薄荷, Bohe)6g	Dispersing the stagnated liver-qi and reducing fever			
Balloonflower Root (桔梗, Jiegeng)6g Great Burdock Achene (牛蒡子, Niubangzi)9g Snakegourd Root (天花粉, Tianhuafen)9g	Clearing away lung heat and removing phlegm			

Indications:
1. Dermatitis, chronic eczema.
2. Tonsillitis.

Associated Formula:
Tree Peony Bark and Cape Jasmine Merry Life Power (丹栀逍遥散, dan zhi xiao yao san)

Prescriptions of Peaceful Benevolent Dispensary《和剂局方》

This is composed of Merry Life Powder (逍遥散, xiao yao san) plus Tree Peony Bark (牡丹皮, Mudanpi) and Cape Jasmine Fruit (山栀子, Shanzhizi). Its actions are dispersing the stagnated liver-qi and invigorating the spleen, regulating blood and regulating menstruation. It is applied for irritability, distending pain in the chest and hypochondrium and irregular menstruation due to transformation of fire resulted from the deficiency of the blood in the liver and spleen.

2. Head-Clearing Divaricate Saposhnikovia Decoction (清上防风汤, qing shang fang feng tang)

Source: *Curative Measures for Diseases*《万病回春》
Composition: Fineleaf Schizonepeta Herb (荆芥, Jingjie)3g
Divaricate Saposhnikovia Root (防风, Fangfeng)3g
Wild Mint Herb (薄荷, Bohe)3g
Dahurican Angelica Root (白芷, Baizhi)6g
Coptis Rhizome (黄连, Huanglian)6g
Baikal Skullcap Root (黄芩, Huangqin)6g
Cape Jasmine Fruit (山栀子, Shanzhizi)6g
Weeping Forsythia Capsule (连翘, Lianqiao)6g
Szechwan Lovage Rhizome (川芎, Chuanxiong)6g
Balloonflower Root (桔梗, Jiegeng)3g
Immature Bitter Orange (枳实, Zhishi)3g
Licorice Root (甘草, Gancao)3g

Actions: Relieving the exterior syndrome and expelling wind, clearing away heat and removing toxic material.

Applied Syndrome: Sores and rashes on the head and face due to upward attack of wind-heat.

Points in Constitution: Diseases on the face won't be cured if the wind-expelling drugs are not used. Thus, this formula is composed of the drugs for clearing away heat and toxic material and also the drugs for expelling wind and relieving the exterior syndrome.

Indications:
1. Acne.
2. Eczema of the face.
3. Brandy nose, tympanitis and gingivitis.
4. Furuncle, nail-like boil, sore and rash.

Precautions:
1. This formula is not suitable for the syndrome without excessive heat.
2. Peppery, pungent and other irritant food should be avoided while taking this formula.

Head-Clearing Divaricate Saposhnikovia Decoction
(Exterior-Relieving, Wind-Expelling, Heat-Clearing and Toxin-Removing Method)

Ingredients	Effects	Combined Effects	Syndrome	Chief Symptoms
Szechwan Lovage Rhizome (川芎, Chuanxiong) 6g Dahurican Angelica Root (白芷, Baizhi) 6g Fineleaf Schizonepeta Herb (荆芥, Jingjie) 3g Divaricate Saposhnikovia Root (防风, Fangfeng) 3g Wild Mint Herb (薄荷, Bohe) 3g	Expelling wind and relieving the exterior syndrome	Expelling wind, clearing away heat and toxic material	Upward attack of wind-heat	Sores and rashes on the head and face, dry throat and mouth, red tongue and rapid pulse
Baikal Skullcap Root (黄芩, Huangqin) 6g Coptis Rhizome (黄连, Huanglian) 6g Cape Jasmine Fruit (山栀子, Shanzhizi) 6g Weeping Forsythia Capsule (连翘, Lianqiao) 6g	Clearing away heat and toxic material and purging excessive heat of three-jiao			
Licorice Root (甘草, Gancao) 3g Balloonflower Root (桔梗, Jiegeng) 3g	Clearing away heat and relieving sore throat			
Immature Bitter Orange (枳实, Zhishi) 3g	Regulating flow of qi and dissipating blockages			

Associated Formulas:

1. Fineleaf Schizonepeta and Ledehouriella Antiphlogistic Powder (荆防败毒散 jin fang bai du san) *Theory and Examples of Surgery* 《外科理例》

This is composed of Fineleaf Schizonepeta Herb (荆芥, Jingjie), Ledehouriella (防风, Fangfeng), Ginseng (人参, Renshen), Incised Notopterygium Rhizome or Root (羌活, Qianghuo), Doubleteeth Pubescent Angelica Root (独活, Duhuo), Whiteflower Hogfennel Root (前胡, Qianhu), Chinese Thorowax Root (柴胡, Chaihu), Balloonflower Root (桔梗, Jiegeng), Bitter Orange (枳壳, Zhiqiao), Tuckahoe (茯苓, Fuling), Szechwan Lovage Rhizome (川芎, Chuanxiong) and Licorice Root (甘草, Gancao). Its actions are expelling wind, relieving the exterior syndrome, detoxicating and reducing swelling. It is indicated for all kinds of sores and seasonal noxious agents, manifested as swelling, pain and fever, superficial and rapid pulse of the left hand.

2. Divaricate Saposhnikovia Miraculous Powder (防风通圣散, fang feng tong sheng san) *Formulae and Expositions* 《宣明论方》

This is composed of Divaricate Saposhnikovia Root (防风, Fangfeng), Szechwan Lovage Rhizome (川芎, Chuanxiong), Chinese Angelica Root (当归, Danggui), White Peony Root (白芍药, Baishaoyao), Rhubarb (大黄, Dahuang), Leaf of Wild Mint Herb (薄荷叶, Boheye), Ephedra (麻黄, Mahuang), Weeping Forsythia Capsule (连翘, Lianqiao), Mirabilite (芒硝, Mangxiao), Gypsum (石膏, Shigao), Baikal Skullcap Root (黄芩, Huangqin), Balloonflower Root (桔梗, Jiegeng), Talc (滑石, Huashi), Licorice Root (甘草, Gancao), Fineleaf Schizonepeta Herb (荆芥, Jingjie), Largehead Atractylodes Rhizome (白术, Baizhu) and Cape Jasmine Fruit (山栀子, Shanzhizi). Its actions are expelling wind and relieving the exterior syndrome, clearing away heat and relaxing the bowels. It is indicated for the excess syndrome of both exterior and interior due to attack of pathogenic wind in the exterior and accumulation of heat in the interior which is manifested as aversion to cold and high fever, dizziness, red eyes with pain, bitter mouth and dry throat, constipation, dysuria with dark urine, carbuncles and sores, hematochezia and piles, mania and delirium, clonic convulsion of the extremities, red macula and urticaria, greasy and slight yellow tongue coating, rapid pulse.

3. Major Weeping Forsythia Capsule Decoction
(大连翘汤, da lian qiao tang)

Source: *One Hundred Questions in Pediatrics* 《婴童百问》
Composition: Weeping Forsythia Capsule (连翘, Lianqiao)6g
Divaricate Saposhnikovia Root (防风, Fangfeng)6g
Lilac Pink Herb (瞿麦, Qumai)6g
Spike of Fineleaf Schizonepeta Herb (荆芥穗, Jingjiesui)6g
Akebia Stem (木通, Mutong)6g
Plantain Seed (车前子, Cheqianzi)6g
Chinese Angelica Root (当归, Danggui)6g
Chinese Thorowax Root (柴胡, Chaihu)6g
Red Peony Root (赤芍药, Chishaoyao)6g
Talc (滑石, Huashi)9g
Cicada Slough (蝉蜕, Chantui)6g
Baikal Skullcap Root (黄芩, Huangqin)6g
Cape Jasmine Fruit (山栀子, Shanzhizi)6g
Licorice Root (甘草, Gancao)6g
Sinkiang Arnebia Root or Redroot Gromwell Root (紫草, Zicao)6g
Actions: Expelling wind and clearing away heat, inducing diuresis and removing toxic material.
Applied Syndrome: Smallpox due to dampness and noxious heat manifested as scattered smallpox, fever, stuffy nose, cough, thin and white tongue coating, superficial and rapid pulse.

Major Weeping Forsythia Capsule Decoction
(Wind-Expelling, Heat-Clearing, Diuresis-Inducing and Toxin-Removing Method)

Ingredients	Effects	Combined Effects	Syndrome	Chief Symptoms
Weeping Forsythia Capsule (连翘, Lianqiao)6g Baikal Skullcap Root (黄芩, Huangqin)6g Cape Jasmine Fruit (山栀子, Shanzhizi)6g	Clearing away heat and toxic material	Expelling wind and clearing heat, promoting diuresis and removing toxic material	Smallpox due to pathogens in the lung	Scattered smallpox, fever, stuffy nose, cough, thin and white tongue coating, superficial and rapid pulse
Spike of Fineleaf Schizonepeta Herb (荆芥穗, Jingjiesui)6g Divaricate Saposhnikovia Root (防风, Fangfeng)6g Chinese Thorowax Root (柴胡, Chaihu)6g	Expelling wind and relieving the exterior syndrome			
Lilac Pink Herb (瞿麦, Qumai)6g Akebia Stem (木通, Mutong)6g Talc (滑石, Huashi)9g Plantain Seed (车前子, Cheqianzi)6g	Promoting urination and dispelling dampness			
Chinese Angelica Root (当归, Danggui)6g Red Peony Root (赤芍药, Chishaoyao)6g Sinkiang Arnebia Root or Redroot Gromwell Root (紫草, Zicao)6g	Activating blood circulation and removing heat from ying			
Cicada Slough (蝉蜕, Chantui)6g	Expelling wind and alleviating itching			
Licorice Root (甘草, Gancao)6g	Coordinating the actions of various ingredients in the prescription			

Points in Constitution: Smallpox is caused by accumulation of heat and dampness in the superficies. However, the exterior syndrome is mostly based on internal factors. Thus, this formula contains many kinds of diuresis-inducing drugs such as Lilac Pink Herb (瞿麦, Qumai) and Plantain Seed (车前子, Cheqianzi) to eliminate the heat and dampness in the superficies. Fineleaf Schizonepeta Herb (荆芥, Jingjie), Divaricate Saposhnikovia Root (防风, Fangfeng), Sinkiang Arnebia Root, Redroot Gromwell Root (紫草, Zicao) and Cicada Slough (蝉蜕, Chantui) are commonly drugs for treating dermatosis.

Indications:

1. Chicken pox.
2. Herpes zoster.
3. Acute eczema, contact dermatitis.
4. Pemphigus.

Precaution: Pungent, peppery, fat and sweet food should be avoided during the medication.

Associated Formulas:

Wind-Dispersing Powder (消风散, xiao feng san) *Orthodox Manual of Surgery*《外科正宗》

This is composed of Fineleaf Schizonepeta Herb (荆芥, Jingjie), Divaricate Saposhnikovia Root (防风, Fangfeng), Great Burdock Achene (牛蒡子, Niubangzi), Cicada Slough (蝉蜕, Chantui), Swordlike Atractylodes Rhizome (苍术, Cangzhu), Lightyellow Sophora Root (苦参, Kushen), Gypsum (石膏, Shigao), Common Anemarrhena Rhizome (知母, Zhimu), Chinese Angelica Root (当归, Danggui), Hemp Seed (胡麻仁, Humaren), Dried Rehmannia Root (生地黄, Shengdihuang), Akebia Stem (木通, Mutong) and Licorice Root (甘草, Gancao). Its actions are expelling wind and enriching blood, clearing away heat and removing dampness. It is indicated for rubella and eczema caused by attack of wind-heat and damp-heat on the human body.

4. Cow Bezoar Toxin-Removing and Swelling-Reducing Pill (牛黄醒消丸, niu huang xin xiao wan)

Source: *Surgery Life-Saving Collection*《外科全生集》

Composition: Cow-Bezoar (牛黄, Niuhuang)

Musk (麝香, Shexiang)

Olibanum (乳香, Ruxiang)

Myrrh (没药, Moyao)

Cooked Glutinous Millet (黄米饭, Huangmifan)

(It is a patent medicine and its preparation is omitted.)

Actions: Clearing away toxic material and dissipating blockages, reducing swelling and alleviating pain.

Applied Syndrome: Breast cancer, carbuncle, gangrene, scrofula, subcutaneous nodule, multiple abscess and inflammation of soft tissues of unknown origin due to blood stasis and retention of phlegm manifested as located hard lump or distending pain which is lingering for a long time, dark red tongue, deep and unsmooth pulse.

Points in Constitution: In surgery of TCM, obstinate sores and carbuncles are often treated by combining the drugs for activating blood circulation and removing blood stasis with Cow-Bezoar (牛黄, Niuhuang) and Musk (麝香, Shexiang). They can dredge the circulation of qi and blood of twelve meridians to alleviate pain, clear away toxic material and reduce swelling.

Indications:

1. Lymphadenitis.

2. Hyperplasia of mammary glands.
3. Multiple abscess.
4. Osteomyelitis.
5. Malignancy.

Cow Bezoar Toxin-Removing and Swelling-Reducing Pill
(Toxin-Clearing and Swelling-Reducing Method)

Ingredients	Effects	Combined Effects	Syndrome	Chief Symptoms
Cow-Bezoar (牛黄, Niuhuang)	Clearig away toxic material and treating sore	Clearing away toxic material and dissipating blockages, reducing swelling and alleviating pain	Sore and inflammation of soft tissues	Breast cancer, unmovable hard lump, or scrofula and subcutaneous nodule, or carbuncle and gangrene, multiple abscess, distention and pain which are lingering on for a long time, dark red tongue, deep and unsmooth pulse
Musk (麝香, Shexiang)	Being fragrant in smell and travelling around the body, warming and activating qi and blood, reducing swelling and relieving pain			
Olibanum (乳香, Ruxiang) Myrrh (没药, Moyao)	Activating blood circulation and alleviating pain, reducing swelling and dissipating blockages			
Cooked Glutinous Millet (黄米饭, Huangmifan)	Adjuvant for regulating the stomach-qi			

Precaution: It is forbidden for pregnant women or the patients with hyperactivity of fire due to yin deficiency.

Associated Formulas:

1. Toxin-Clearing and Swelling-Reducing Pill (醒消丸, xin xiao wan) *Surgery Life-Saving Collection*《外科全生集》

This is made up of Olibanum (乳香, Ruxiang), Myrrh (没药, Moyao), Red Orpiment (雄黄, Xionghuang), Musk (麝香, Shexiang) and Cooked Glutinous Millet (黄米饭, Huangmifan). Its actions are clearing away toxic material and reducing swelling, activating blood circulation and alleviating pain. It is indicated for carbuncle and gangrene which are hard and painful.

2. Five Treasures Powder (五宝散, wu bao san) *Orthodox Manual of Surgery*《外科正宗》

This is made up of Stalactite (钟乳石, Zhongrushi), Cinnabar (朱砂, Zhusha), Pearl (珍珠, Zhenzhu), Borneol (冰片, Bingpian), Glabrous Greenbrier Rhizome (土茯苓, Tufuling) and Amber (琥珀, Hupo). Its action is removing heat and toxic material and is indicated for syphilitic skin diseases.

5. Sevenlobed Yam Diuresis-Inducing Decoction
(萆薢渗湿汤, bi xie shen shi tang)

Source: *Experience Gained in Treating Sores* 《疡科心得集》
Composition: Sevenlobed Yam Rhizome (萆薢, Bixie) 9g
Coix Seed (薏苡仁, Yiyiren) 15g
Chinese Corktree Bark (黄柏, Huangbai) 9g
Indian Bread Pink Epidermis (赤茯苓, Chifuling) 9g
Tree Peony Bark (牡丹皮, Mudanpi) 9g
Oriental Waterplantain Rhizome (泽泻, Zexie) 9g
Talc (滑石, Huashi) 9g
Ricepaperplant Pith (通草, Tongcao) 6g
Actions: Clearing away heat and inducing diuresis, removing toxic material and activating blood circulation.
Applied Syndrome: Ulcus cruris or ecthyma due to downward attack of dampness-heat in the lower-jiao, manifested as ulcer on the shins with discharge of pus, unbearable itching and pain which attacks alternately for a long time, yellow urine, white and greasy or yellow and greasy tongue coating, soft and rapid pulse.

Sevenlobed Yam Diuresis-Inducing Decoction
(Heat-Clearing and Diuresis-Inducing Method)

Ingredients	Effects	Combined Effects	Syndrome	Chief Symptoms
Sevenlobed Yam Rhizome (萆薢, Bixie) 9g Coix Seed (薏苡仁, Yiyiren) 15g Talc (滑石, Huashi) 9g Ricepaperplant Pith (通草, Tongcao) 6g	Clearing away heat, inducing diuresis and detoxification	Clearing away heat and inducing diuresis, removing toxic material and activating blood circulation	Ulcus cruris due to heat dampness attacking the lower-jiao	Eczema in the lower limbs, ulcer on the shins, itching, pain and oozing in the affected part which is hard to head for a long time, dark urine, yellow and greasy tongue coating, soft and rapid pulse
Indian Bread Pink Epidermis (赤茯苓, Chifuling) 9g Oriental Waterplantain Rhizome (泽泻, Zexie) 9g	Promoting urination to dispel excessive dampness			
Chinese Corktree Bark (黄柏, Huangbai) 9g	Clearing away heat and toxic material and drying dampness in the lower-jiao			
Tree Peony Bark (牡丹皮, Mudanpi) 9g	Removing heat from the blood and activating blood circulation			

Points in Constitution: In TCM, the method of eliminating pathogenic factors lies in the principle of "adroitly guiding action according to circumstancess". Thus, the method of inducing diuresis is used for the case of dampness accumulating in the lower limbs. In this formula, Sevenlobed Yam Rhizome (萆薢, Bixie) has the actions of promoting diuresis, keeping the clear and eliminating the turbid. Besides, it can also benefit the kidney.

Indications:
1. Ulcus cruris.
2. Pruritus vulvae due to damp-heat.
3. Eczema and drug rash in the lower limbs.
4. Secondary suppurative infection due to tinea on the foot.

Precaution: Fat, meat, sweet and roasted food should be avoided during medication.

Associated Formula:

Five Miraculous Drugs Decoction(五神汤, wu shen tang) *Genuine Exposition on External Diseases* 《外科真诠》

This consists of Honeysuckle Flower (金银花, Jinyinhua), Tokyo Violet Herb (紫花地丁, Zihuadiding), Tuckahoe (茯苓, Fuling), Plantain Seed (车前子, Cheqianzi) and Twotooth Achyranthes Root (牛膝, Niuxi). Its actions are clearing away heat, removing toxic material and promoting diuresis. It is indicated for perianal abscess, pyogenic infection of bone and acute pyogenic infection of popliteal fossa due to accumulation of dampness and heat.

6. Chinese Angelica Decoction
(当归饮子, dang gui yin zi)

Source: *Prescriptions for Rescuring the Sick* 《济生方》
Composition: Chinese Angelica Root (当归, Danggui) 6g
Szechwan Lovage Rhizome (川芎, Chuanxiong) 6g
White Peony Root (白芍药, Baishaoyao) 9g
Prepared Rehmannia Root (熟地黄, Shudihuang) 9g
Fleeceflower Root (何首乌, Heshouwu) 9g
Fineleaf Schizonepeta Herb (荆芥, Jingjie) 6g
Divaricate Saposhnikovia Root (防风, Fangfeng) 6g
Tribulus Fruit (白蒺藜, Baijili) 9g
Toasted Membranous Milkvetch Root (炙黄芪, Zhi Huangqi) 6g
Prepared Licorice Root (炙甘草, Zhi Gancao) 6g

Actions: Enriching blood, expelling wind and alleviating itching.

Applied Syndrome: Cutaneous pruritus due to deficiency of blood and wind-dryness, manifested as dryness and itching of the skin, especially at night, or eczema, urticaria, red tongue with little coating, thin and rapid pulse.

Chinese Angelica Root Decoction
(Blood-Enriching and Wind-Expelling Method)

Ingredients	Effects	Combined Effects	Syndrome	Chief Symptoms
Chinese Angelica Root (当归, Danggui) 6g Szechwan Lovage Rhizome (川芎, Chuanxiong) 6g White Peong Root (白芍药, Baishaoyao) 9g Prepared Rehmannia Root (熟地黄, Shudihuang) 9g	Enriching and regulating blood	Enriching blood, expelling wind and alleviating itching	Rubella and eczema due to deficiency of blood and wind-dryness	Dryness and itching of the skin, especially at night, or eczema; urticaria, red tongue with little coating, thin and rapid pulse
Fleeceflower Root (何首乌, Heshouwu) 9g	Tonifying blood			
Fineleaf Schizonepeta Herb (荆芥, Jingjie) 6g Divaricate Saposhnikovia Root (防风, Fangfeng) 6g Tribulus Fruit (白蒺藜, Baijili) 9g	Expelling wind and alleviating itching			
Toasted Membranous Milkvetch Root (炙黄芪, Zhi Huangqi) 6g Stir-Fried Prepared Licorice Root (炙甘草, Zhi Gancao) 6g	Replenishing qi and stabilizing the exterior			

Points in Constitution: This formula is based on Four Herbs Decoction (四物汤, si wu tang) for enriching blood and regulating flow of blood. Adding Fineleaf Schizonepeta Herb (荆芥, Jingjie) and Divaricate Saposhnikovia Root (防风, Fangfeng) which have the action of expelling wind to alleviate itching. There is a saying in TCM that "itching derives from attack of wind". Thus expelling wind can alleviate itching.

Indications:
1. Senile cutaneous pruritus.
2. Eczema, allergic dermatitis.
3. Urticaria.

Precaution: This formula is indicated for cutaneous pruritus due to blood deficiency which causes attack of wind. It is forbidden for the case due to heat-dampness.

Associated Formulas:

1. Wind-Dispersing Powder (消风散, xiao feng san) *Orthodox Manual of Surgery* 《外科正宗》
This is made up of Fineleaf Schizonepeta Herb (荆芥, Jingjie), Divaricate Saposhnikovia Root (防风, Fangfeng), Chinese Angelica Root (当归, Danggui), Dried Rehmannia Root (生地黄, Shengdihuang), Lightyellow Sophora Root (苦参, Kushen), Swordlike Atractylodes Rhizome (苍术, Cangzhu), Cicada Slough (蝉蜕, Chantui), Hemp Seed (胡麻仁, Humaren), Great

Burdock Achene (牛蒡子, Niubangzi), Common Anemarrhena Rhizome (知母, Zhimu), Gypsum (石膏, Shigao), Akebia Stem (木通, Mutong) and Licorice Root (生甘草, Sheng Gancao). Its actions are expelling wind and clearing away heat, removing dampness and reducing swelling. It is indicated for eczema and rubella due to wind-heat or damp-heat.

2. Four Herbs Wind-Dispersing Decoction (四物消风饮, si wu xiao feng yin) *The Golden Mirror of Medicine* 《医宗金鉴》

This is made up of Dried Rehmannia Root (生地黄, Shengdihuang), Chinese Angelica Root (当归, Danggui), Fineleaf Schizonepeta Herb (荆芥, Jingjie), Divaricate Saposhnikovia Root (防风, Fangfeng), Red Peony Root (赤芍药, Chishaoyao), Szechwan Lovage Rhizome (川芎, Chuanxiong), Densefruit Pittany Root-Bark (白鲜皮, Baixianpi), Cicada Slough (蝉蜕, Chantui), Wild Mint Herb (薄荷, Bohe), Doubleteeth Pubescent Angelica Root (独活, Duhuo), Chinese Thorowax Root (柴胡, Chaihu) and Chinese Date (大枣, Dazao). This formula has the actions of enriching blood and expelling wind. It is indicated for urticaria and psoriasis due to endopathic wind resulting from deficiency of blood.

3. Moghania and Fleeceflower Root Decoction (千斤首乌汤, qian jin shou wu tang) *Surgery Guangzhou Traditional Chinese Medicine College* 广州中医学院《外科学》

This is made up of Moghania Root (千斤拔, Qianjinba), Fleeceflower Root (何首乌, Heshouwu), Chinese Angelica Root (当归, Danggui), Black Soya Bean Peel (乌豆衣, Wudouyi), Cicada Slough (蝉衣, Chanyi), Lightyellow Sophora Root (苦参, Kushen) and Densefruit Pittany Root-Bark (白鲜皮, Baixianpi). This formula is good at enriching blood and expelling wind. It is indicated for eczema and urticaria due to endopathic wind resulting from deficiency of blood.

4. Divaricate Saposhnikovia Miraculous Powder (防风通圣散, fang feng tong sheng san) *Formulae and Expositions* 《宣明论方》

This is made up of Divaricate Saposhnikovia Root (防风, Fangfeng), Fineleaf Schizonepeta Herb (荆芥, Jingjie), Weeping Forsythia Capsule (连翘, Lianqiao), Ephedra (麻黄, Mahuang), Wild Mint Herb (薄荷, Bohe), Szechwan Lovage Rhizome (川芎, Chuanxiong), Chinese Angelica Root (当归, Danggui), White Peony Root (白芍药, Baishaoyao), Dahurican Angelica Root (白芷, Baizhi), Cape Jasmine Fruit (山栀子, Shanzhizi), Rhubarb (生大黄, Sheng Dahuang), Mirabilite (芒硝, Mangxiao), Gypsum (石膏, Shigao), Baikal Skullcap Root (黄芩, Huangqin), Balloonflower Root (桔梗, Jiegeng), Licorice Root (生甘草, Sheng Gancao) and Talc (滑石, Huashi). Its actions are expelling the pathogenic factors from both the exterior and interior of the body, removing heat and inducing diuresis. It is indicated for eczema and urticaria due to accumulation of damp-heat in the stomach and intestines.

5. Fineleaf Schizonepeta and Ledehouriella Antiphlogistic Powder (荆防败毒散, jing fang bai du san) *Orthodox Medical Record* 《医学正传》

This is made up of Divaricate Saposhnikovia Root (防风, Fangfeng), Chinese Thorowax Root (柴胡, Chaihu), Whiteflower Hogfennel Root (前胡, Qianhu), Fineleaf Schizonepeta Herb (荆芥, Jingjie), Incised Notopterygium Rhizome or Root (羌活, Qianghuo), Doubleteeth Pubescent Angelica Root (独活, Duhuo), Bitter Orange (枳壳, Zhiqiao), Balloonflower Root (桔梗,

Jiegeng), Tuckahoe (茯苓, Fuling), Szechwan Lovage Rhizome (川芎, Chuanxiong) and Licorice Root (甘草, Gancao). Its actions are dispersing wind and expelling cold. It is indicated for urticaria due to wind-cold.

7. Lung-Clearing Loquat Powder
(清肺枇杷散, qing fei pi pa san)

Source: *A Comprehensive Summary of Surgery* 《外科大成》
Composition: Loquat Leaf (枇杷叶, Pipaye) 9g
White Mulberry Root-Bark (桑白皮, Sangbaipi) 9g
Coptis Rhizome (黄连, Huanglian) 6g
Chinese Corktree Bark (黄柏, Huangbai) 6g
Ginseng (人参, Renshen) 3g
Licorice Root (生甘草, Sheng Gancao) 3g
Actions: Clearing away lung-heat and purging fire.
Applied Syndrome: Acne due to retention of noxious heat in the skin of the face resulting from excessive heat in the lung, manifested as papular eruption in the face, chest and back which is red around the rashes and oozes white paste secretion when pressed.

Lung-Clearing Loquat Powder
(Lung Heat-Clearing and Fire-Purging Method)

Ingredients	Effects	Combined Effects	Syndrome	Chief Symptoms
Coptis Rhizome (黄连, Huanglian) 6g Chinese Corktree Bark (黄柏, Huangbai) 6g	Clearing away heat and purging fire, drying dampness and clearing toxic material	Clearing away lung heat and purging fire	Acne due to heat in the lung	Papular eruption in the face, chest and back, redness around the rashes, oozing white paste from pressed skin lesions
Loquat Leaf (枇杷叶, Pipaye) 9g White Mulberry Root-Bark (桑白皮, Sangbaipi) 9g	Purging lung and removing phlegm			
Ginseng (人参, Renshen) 3g	Replenishing lung qi and promoting pus discharge			
Licorice Root (生甘草, Sheng Gancao) 3g	Coordinating the actions of various ingredients in the prescription			

Points in Constitution: In this formula, Coptis Rhizome (黄连, Huanglian) and Chinese Corktree Bark (黄柏, Huangbai) are used to clear away heat and toxic material. White Mulberry Root-Bark (桑白皮, Sangbaipi) and Loquat Leaf (枇杷叶, Pipaye) are used to purge lung-heat. The application of Ginseng (人参, Renshen) is to support healthy qi and help promote the discharge of pathogenic factors.

Indications:

1. Acne.
2. Brandy nose.

Precaution: It should be cautiously used for the patients with insufficiency of the spleen-yang.

Associated Formulas:

1. Baikai Skullcap Lung-Clearing Decoction (黄芩清肺饮, huang qin qing fei ying) *Orthodox Manual of Surgery*《外科正宗》

This is made up of Szechwan Lovage Rhizome (川芎, Chuanxiong), Chinese Angelica Root (当归, Danggui), Red Peony Root (赤芍药, Chishaoyao), Divaricate Saposhnikovia Root (防风, Fangfeng), Dried Rehmannia Root (生地黄, Shengdihuang), Pueraria (葛根, Gegen), Snakegourd Root (天花粉, Tianhuafen), Weeping Forsythia Capsule (连翘, Lianqiao), Safflower (红花, Honghua), Baikal Skullcap Root (黄芩, Huangqin) and Wild Mint Herb (薄荷, Bohe). Its actions are clearing away heat and expelling wind, activating blood circulation and removing heat from the blood. It is indicated for acne and brandy nose due to accumulation of wind-heat in the lung meridian accompanied with blood stasis.

2. Oriental Wormwood Decoction (茵陈蒿汤, yin chen hao tang) *Treatise on Exogenous Febrile Diseases*《伤寒论》

This is made up of Oriental Wormwood Herb (茵陈, Yinchen), Cape Jasmine Fruit (山栀子, Shanzhizi) and Rhubarb (生大黄, Sheng Dahuang). Its actions are clearing away heat and inducing diuresis. It is indicated for acne, brandy nose, eczema or pemphigus and greasiness of the face due to heat-dampness in the spleen and stomach.

3. Merry Life Powder (逍遥散, xiao yao san) *Prescriptions of Peaceful Benevolent Dispensary*《和剂局方》

This is made up of Chinese Thorowax Root (柴胡, Chaihu), White Peony Root (白芍药, Baishaoyao), Chinese Angelica Root (当归, Danggui), Largehead Atractylodes Rhizome (白术, Baizhu), Tuckahoe (茯苓, Fuling), Prepared Licorice Root (炙甘草, Zhi Gancao), Fresh Ginger (生姜, Shengjiang) and Wild Mint Herb (薄荷, Bohe). Its actions are relaxing depressed liver-qi and alleviating depression, enriching blood and invigorating the spleen. It is indicated for acne and brandy nose accompanied with irregular menstruation and dysmenorrhea due to disorder of Chong and Ren Meridians and stagnation of liver-qi.

8. Great Burdock Achene Muscles-Relieving Decoction
（牛蒡解肌汤，niu bang jie ji tang）

Source: *Experience Gained in Treating Sores*《疡科心得集》
Composition: GreatBurdock Achene（牛蒡子，Niubangzi）6g
Wild Mint Herb（薄荷，Bohe）3g
Fineleaf Schizonepeta Herb（荆芥，Jingjie）3g
Weeping Forsythia Capsule（连翘，Lianqiao）6g
Cape Jasmine Fruit（山栀子，Shanzhizi）6g
Tree Peony Bark（牡丹皮，Mudanpi）6g
Dendrobium Herb（石斛，Shihu）6g
Figwort Root（玄参，Xuanshen）6g
Common Selfheal Fruit-Spike（夏枯草，Xiakucao）6g
Actions: Dispersing wind and clearing away heat, cooling the blood and removing toxic material.
Applied Syndrome: Toothache and retention of noxious heat and phlegm in the neck, manifested as local redness and swelling, unbearable itching and pain, often accompanied with chills and fever, or lump of the neck due to attack of wind-heat on the head, white or yellow tongue coating, superficial and rapid pulse.
Points in Constitution: The characteristic of this formula is to exert the expelling, clearing and tonifying actions simultaneously. Besides, it expels the evils both exteriorly and interiorly, thus, dispersing the depressed fire and clearing away the internal heat, which corresponds to the pathogenesis of disorder both the interior and exterior.
Indications:
1. Face erysipelas.
2. Cervical lymphadenitis.
3. Toothache.

Precaution: This formula is forbidden for cellulitis of yin type and is cautiously used for toothache due to fire of deficiency type.
Associated Formulas:
1. Heat-Clearing and Toxin-Removing Decoction（清热解毒汤，qing re jie du tang）*Collection of Zhao Bingnan's Experiences in Clinic*《赵炳南临床经验集》

This is composed of Dandelion（蒲公英，Pugongying）, Indian Dendranthema Flower（野菊花，Yejuhua）, indigowoad Leaf（大青叶，Daqingye）, Tokyo Violet Herb（紫花地丁，Zihuadiding）, Manyleaf Paris Rhizome（蚤休，Zaoxiu）, Snakegourd Root（天花粉，Tianhuafen）and Red·Peony Root（赤芍药，Chishaoyao）. Its action is clearing away heat and toxic material. It is indicated for erysipelas of the shank（acute erysipelas）and the beginning of all kinds of infection of the skin.

Great Burdock Achene Muscles-Relieving Decoction
(Wind-Expelling and Heat-Clearing Method)

Ingredients	Effects	Combined Effects	Syndrome	Chief Symptoms
Great Burdock Achene (牛蒡子, Niubangzi)6g Common Selfheal Fruit-Spike (夏枯草, Xiakucao)6g	Expelling wind-heat, clearing away toxic material an dissipating blockages	Expelling wind and clearing away heat, removing heat from the blood and reducing swelling	Erythema, itching and pain due to heat in the skin	Local redness and swelling, unbearable itching and pain, often accompanied with chills and fever, or lump of the neck, white or yellow tongue coating, superficial and rapid pulse
Fineleaf Schizonepeta Herb (荆芥, Jingjie)3g Wild Mint Herb (薄荷, Bohe)3g	Expelling wind and alleviating itching			
Weeping Forsythia Capsule (连翘, Lianqiao)6g Cape Jasmine Fruit (山栀子, Shanzhizi)6g	Clearing away heat and toxic material			
Tree Peony Bark (牡丹皮, Mudanpi)6g	Removing heat from the blood and dissipating blood stasis			
Dendrobium Herb (石斛, Shihu)6g Figwort Root (玄参, Xuanshen)6g	Nourishing yin and Clearing away heat			

2. Honeysuckle Flower Detoxicating Decoction (银花解毒汤, yin hua jie du tang) *Experience Gained in Treating Sores* 《疡科心得集》

This is composed of Honeysuckle Flower (金银花, Jinyinhua), Tokyo Violet Herb (紫花地丁, Zihuadiding), Weeping Forsythia Capsule (连翘, Lianqiao), Common Selfheal Fruit-Spike (夏枯草, Xiakucao), Indian Bread Pink Epidermis (赤茯苓, Chifuling), Tree Peony Bark (牡丹皮, Mudanpi), Coptis Rhizome (黄连, Huanglian) and Asiatic Rhinoceros Horn (犀角, Xijiao). Its actions are clearing away heat and toxic material, cooling blood and inducing diuresis. It is indicated for the beginning of carbuncles and sores manifested as alternate fever and chills, numbness mixed with itching, redness, swelling and hot pain due to heat-dampness and toxic fire.

Additional Formulas

Ten Herbs Antiphlogistic Decoction
(十味败毒汤, shi wei bai du tang)

Source: *Formulae of Hanaoka*《华冈青洲方》
Composition: Chinese Thorowax Root（柴胡, Chaihu）6g
Balloonflower Root（桔梗, Jiegeng）6g
Doubleteeth Pubescent Angelica Root（独活, Duhuo）3g
Szechwan Lovage Rhizome（川芎, Chuanxiong）3g
Divaricate Saposhnikovia Root（防风, Fangfeng）3g
Tuckahoe（茯苓, Fuling）6g
Japanese Cherry Bark（樱皮, Yingpi）9g
Fineleaf Schizonepeta Herb（荆芥, Jingjie）3g
Licorice Root（甘草, Gancao）3g
Fresh Ginger（生姜, Shengjiang）3g

Actions: Inducing diaphoresis and relieving the exterior syndrome, eliminating sores and alleviating pain.

Ten Herbs Antiphlogistic Decoction
(Heat-Clearing and Wind-Expelling Method)

Ingredients	Effects	Combined Effects	Syndrome	Chief Symptoms
Fineleaf Schizonepeta Herb（荆芥, Jingjie）3g Divaricate Saposhnikovia Root（防风, Fangfeng）3g Doubleteeth Pubescent Angelica Root（独活, Duhuo）3g Chinese Thorowax Root（柴胡, Chaihu）6g Szechwan Lovage Rhizome（川芎, Chuanxiong）3g	Expelling wind-heat and alleviating pain	Expelling wind-heat, detoxificating and treating sores	The beginning of sores	Local erythema, swelling, heat and pain, aversion to cold and high fever, or urticaria and eczema, red tip of tongue with thin coating, superficial pulse.
Balloonflower Root（桔梗, Jiegeng）6g	Evacuating pus			
Japanese Cherry Bark（樱皮, Yingpi）9g	Clearing away heat, alleviating pain and treating sores			
Tuckahoe（茯苓, Fuling）6g Fresh Ginger（生姜, Shengjiang）3g	Regulating the stomach			
Licorice Root（甘草, Gancao）3g	Detoxification			

Applied Syndrome:

1. The beginning of sores due to accumulation of wind-heat, manifested as local erythema, swelling, hot pain, aversion to cold and high fever, red tongue tip with thin coating, superficial or floating pulse.

2. Urticaria and eczema due to wind-heat.

Points in Constitution: The main action of this formula is expelling wind-heat, though it also has the actions of treating sores and relieving pain. Thus, it is very suitable for the initial stage of sores.

Indications:

1. The beginning of cutaneous purulent infection.
2. Acute eczema.
3. Urticaria.

Precaution: This formula is indicated for the initial stage of sores of yang syndrome. So its action of clearing away heat and toxic material is not strong enough, thus in the clinic, the drugs for clearing away heat and toxic material should be added.

Associated Formulas:

1. Everyone's Detoxicating Decoction (普济消毒饮, pu ji xiao du yin) *Dongyuan's Effective Prescriptions* 《东垣试效方》

This is composed of Baikal Skullcap Root (黄芩, Huangqin), Figwort Root (玄参, Xuanshen), Great Burdock Achene (牛蒡子, Niubangzi), Weeping Forsythia Capsule (连翘, Lianqiao), Indigowoad Root (板蓝根, Banlangen), Coptis Rhizome (黄连, Huanglian), Balloonflower Root (桔梗, Jiegeng), Chinese Thorowax Root (柴胡, Chaihu), Licorice Root (生甘草, Sheng Gancao), Tangerine Peel (橘皮, Jupi), Puff-Ball (马勃, Mabo), Silkworm with Batrytis Larva (僵蚕, Jiangcan), Wild Mint Herb (薄荷, Bohe) and Shunk Bugbane Rhizome (升麻, Shengma). Its actions are clearing away heat and toxic material, expelling wind and reducing swelling. It is indicated for infection with swollen head characterized by flushed swollen face, difficulty in opening the eyes, thirst, irritability, sore throat, aversion to cold and fever, rapid and forceful pulse.

2. Wind-Dispersing Powder (消风散, xiao feng san) *Orthodox Manual of Surgery* 《外科正宗》

This is composed of Fineleaf Schizonepeta Herb (荆芥, Jingjie), Divaricate Saposhnikovia Root (防风, Fangfeng), Chinese Angelica Root (当归, Danggui), Dried Rehmannia Root (生地黄, Shengdihuang), Lightyellow Sophora Root (苦参, Kushen), Swordlike Atractylodes Rhizome (苍术, Cangzhu), Cicada Slough (蝉蜕, Chantui), Hemp Seed (胡麻仁, Humaren), Great Burdock Achene (牛蒡子, Niubangzi), Common Anemarrhena Rhizome (知母, Zhimu), Gypsum (石膏, Shigao), Akebia Stem (木通, Mutong) and Licorice Root (生甘草, Sheng Gancao). Its actions are expelling wind and clearing away heat, removing dampness and reducing swelling. It is indicated for eczema and urticaria due to accumulation of wind and damp-heat in the skin.

Schizonepeta and Forsythia Decoction
(荆芥连翘汤, jing jie lian qiao tang)

Source: Ikando《一贯堂》

Composition: Chinese Angelica Root (当归, Danggui)9g
White Peony Root (白芍药, Baishaoyao)9g
Prepared Rehmannia Root (熟地黄, Shudihuang)9g
Szechwan Lovage Rhizome (川芎, Chuanxiong)9g
Coptis Rhizome (黄连, Huanglian)6g
Baikal Skullcap Root (黄芩, Huangqin)6g
Chinese Corktree Bark (黄柏, Huangbai)6g
Cape Jasmine Fruit (山栀子, Shanzhizi)6g
Weeping Forsythia Capsule (连翘, Lianqiao)9g
Fineleaf Schizonepeta Herb (荆芥, Jingjie)6g
Divaricate Saposhnikovia Root (防风, Fangfeng)6g
Wild Mint Herb (薄荷, Bohe)6g
Bitter Orange (枳壳, Zhiqiao)6g
Licorice Root (生甘草, Sheng Gancao)6g
Chinese Thorowax Root (柴胡, Chaihu)6g
Balloonflower Root (桔梗, Jiegeng)6g
Dahurican Angelica Root (白芷, Baizhi)6g

Actions: Clearing away heat and toxic material, expelling wind and evacuating pus, activating blood circulation and enriching blood.

Applied Syndrome: Syndrome of accumulation of heat in the interior accompanied with wind-heat in the upper-jiao, manifested as sores on the face, turbid discharge from the nose, sore throat, headache, fever, red tongue, wiry and rapid pulse.

Points in Constitution: This formula is the modification of Warming and Clearing Decoction (温清饮, wen qing yin) and Cold Limbs Powder (四逆散, si ni san) plus other drugs. The characteristic of this formula is to unite the actions of removing heat from the blood, clearing toxic material, dispersing the stagnated liver-qi and expelling wind as one and is indicated for sores, rhinorrhea and acute tonsillitis due to accumulation of heat in the interior which attacks the face and skin frequently.

Indications:
1. Inflammation of gland under the ear.
2. Parasinusitis.
3. Tonsillitis.
4. Acne.

Schizonepeta and Forsythia Decoction
(Heat-Clearing and Wind-Expelling Method)

Ingredients	Effects	Combined Effects	Syndrome	Chief Symptoms
Fineleaf Schizonepeta Herb (荆芥, Jingjie) 6g Weeping Forsythia Capsule (连翘, Lianqiao) 9g Divaricate Saposhnikovia Root (防风, Fangfeng) 6 Dahurican Angelica Root (白芷, Baizhi) 6g Wild Mint Herb (薄荷, Bohe) 6g	Expelling wind and reducing fever	Clearing away heat and toxic material, expelling wind and regulating blood	Wind-heat in the upper-jiao	Sores of the face, turbid discharge from nose, sore throat, headache, fever, red tongue, wiry and rapid pulse
Chinese Angelica Root (当归, Danggui) 9g Szechwan Lovage Rhizome (川芎, Chuanxiong) 9g White Peony Root (白芍药, Baishaoyao) 9g Prepared Rehmannia Root (熟地黄, Shudihuang) 9g Chinese Corktree Bark (黄柏, Huangbai) 6g Coptis Rhizome (黄连, Huanglian) 6g Baikal Skullcap Root (黄芩, Huangqin) 6g Cape Jasmine Fruit (山栀子, Shanzhizi) 6g	Removing heat from the blood and clearing away toxic material, enriching and regulating blood			
Chinese Thorowax Root (柴胡, Chaihu) 6g Bitter Orange (枳壳, Zhiqiao) 6g Licorice Root (生甘草, Sheng Gancao) 6g	Regulating the liver and spleen			
Balloonflower Root (桔梗, Jiegeng) 6g	Directing other herbs ascending			

Precaution: It is forbidden for the patient with insufficiency of spleen-yang.

Associated Formula:

Fineleaf Schizonepeta and Ledehouriellas Antiphlogistic Powder (荆防败毒散, jing fang bai du san) *Theory and Examples of Surgery* 《外科理例》

This is made up of Fineleaf Schizonepeta Herb (荆芥, Jingjie), Ledehouriellas (防风, Fangfeng), Ginseng (人参, Renshen), incised Notopterygium Rhizome or Root (羌活, Qianghuo), Doubleteeth Pubescent Angelica Root (独活, Duhuo), Whiteflower Hogfennel Root (前胡, Qianhu), Chinese Thorowax Root (柴胡, Chaihu), Balloonflower Root (桔梗, Jiegeng), Bitter Orange (枳壳, Zhiqiao), Tuckahoe (茯苓, Fuling), Szechwan Lovage Rhizome (川芎, Chuanxiong) and Licorice Root (生甘草, Sheng Gancao). Its actions are clearing away heat and toxic material, evacuating pus and reducing swelling. It is indicated for sores due to noxious heat characterized by swelling, pain, fever, superficial and rapid pulse.

Pueraria and Safflower Decoction
(葛根红花汤, ge gen hong hua tang)

Source: *Bank of Japanese Formulas of TCM*《方舆輗》
Composition: Pueraria(葛根, Gegen)6g
Red PeonyRroot (赤芍药, Chishaoyao)6g
Dried Rehmannia Root (生地黄, Shengdihuang)6g
Coptis Rhizome (黄连, Huanglian)3g
Cape Jasmine Fruit (山栀子, Shanzhizi)3g
Safflower (红花, Honghua)3g
Rhubarb (生大黄, Sheng Dahuang)3g
Licorice Root (生甘草, Sheng Gancao)3g

Actions: Removing heat from the blood, activating blood circulation and clearing away toxic material.

Applied Syndrome: Excessive heat of yangming which ascends along the meridian and accumulates in apex nasi, manifested as flushed apex nasi, or even dark purplish which may radiate to alae nasi, thick and uneven skin like verruca vulgaris, red tongue and rapid pulse.

Pueraria and Safflower Decoction
(Blood-Cooling and Toxin-Removing Method)

Ingredients	Effects	Combined Effects	Syndrome	Chief Symptoms
Pueraria(葛根, Gegen)6g	Expelling depressed fire of yangming	Removing heat from the blood, activating blood circulation and clearing away toxic material	Excessive heat of yangming	Red apex nasi radiating to alae nasi, rough and uneven skin, red tongue, rapid pulse
Safflower (红花, Honghua)3g	Activating blood circulation and removing blood stasis			
Dried Rehmannia Root (生地黄, Shengdihuang)6g Red Peony Root (赤芍药, Chishaoyao)6g	Removing heat from the blood, clearing away toxic material and reducing swelling			
Rhubarb (生大黄, Sheng Dahuang)3g Coptis Rhizome (黄连, Huanglian)3g Cape Jasmine Fruit (山栀子, Shanzhizi)3g	Clearing away heat and toxic material			
Licorice Root (生甘草, Sheng Gancao)3g	Coordinating the actions of various ingredients in the prescription			

Points in Constitution: Among the drugs for clearing away toxic material, removing heat from the blood and dissipating blood stasis, Pueraria(葛根, Gegen) is used for guiding other drugs to yangming meridian so as to eliminate the accumulated noxious heat in apex nasi. In this formula, Rhubarb (大黄, Dahuang) is used to remove the retention in the stomach and intestine, which is a radical treatment and a drastic measure to deal with the primary cause.

Indication: Brandy nose.

Precaution: Pungent, peppery, fat and greasy food as well as tobacco and alcohol should be avoided during the medicative period.

Associated Formulas:

1. Coptis Detoxicating Decoction (黄连解毒汤, huang lian jie du tang) *The Medical Secrets of An Offical* 《外台秘要》

This consists of Coptis Rhizome (黄连, Huanglian), Baikal Skullcap Root (黄芩, Huangqin), Chinese Corktree Bark (黄柏, Huangbai) and Cape Jasmine Fruit (山栀子, Shanzhizi). Its actions are purging fire and clearing toxic material. It is indicated for all kinds of syndromes due to fire of excess type or noxious heat, manifested as high fever, irritability, dry mouth and throat, paraphasia and insomnia; or febrile disease with hematemesis, apostaxis and skin eruptions; or fever, dysentery, jaundice due to heat and dampness; or carbuncle and nail-like boil of surgery, dark urine, red tongue with yellow coating, rapid and powerful pulse.

2. Three Huang Heart-Clearing Decoction(三黄泻心汤, san huang xie xin tang) *Source and Cause of Miscellaneous Diseases* 《杂病源流犀烛》

This consists of Rhubarb (生大黄, Sheng Dahuang), Coptis Rhizome (黄连, Huanglian) and Baikal Skullcap Root (黄芩, Huangqin). It is indicated for ulceration of throat, anus and genitals, manifested as red tongue and dark tooth, sudden change of complexion in white, red and black colour, heaviness sensation of the four limbs, lassitude, silence and somnolence, erosions in the throat with hoarseness, sores on the upper lip.

A Prescription for Treating Head Boils
(治头疮一方, zhi tou chuang yi fang)

Source: Japanese Proved Recipe (日本经验方)

Composition: Weeping Forsythia Capsule (连翘, Lianqiao)9g

Honeysuckle Flower (金银花, Jinyinhua)9g

Swordlike Atractylodes Rhizome (苍术, Cangzhu)6g

Szechwan Lovage Rhizome (川芎, Chuanxiong)6g

Divaricate Saposhnikovia Root (防风, Fangfeng)6g

Honeysuckle Stem (忍冬藤, Rendongteng)9g

Fineleaf Schizonepeta Herb (荆芥, Jingjie)6g

Licorice Root (生甘草, Sheng Gancao)6g

Safflower (红花, Honghua)6g

Rhubarb (生大黄, Sheng Dahuang) 3g

Actions: Expelling wind and activating blood circulation, clearing away heat and toxic material, expelling dampness.

Applied Syndrome: Sores and rashes due to wind-heat, manifested as eczema, redness and swelling, cutaneous pruritus, oozing, constipation, or accompanied with fever, headache, thin and white or thin and yellow tongue coating, superficial pulse.

Prescription for Treating Head Boils
(Heat-Clearing and Toxin-Removing Method)

Ingredients	Effects	Combined Effects	Syndrome	Chief Symptoms
Fineleaf Schizonepeta Herb (荆芥, Jingjie) 6g Divaricate Saposhnikovia Root (防风, Fangfeng) 6g	Expelling wind and heat	Clearing away heat and toxic material, expelling wind and removing dampness	Redness and swelling of the skin	Eczema, redness and swelling, cutaneous pruritus, oozing, constipation, or fever, headache, thin and white or yellow tongue coating, superficial pulse
Weeping Forsythia Capsule (连翘, Lianqiao) 9g Honeysuckle Flower (金银花, Jinyinhua) 9g	Clearing away heat and toxic material			
Rhubarb (生大黄, Sheng Dahuang) 3g Szechwan Lovage Rhizome (川芎, Chuanxiong) 6g Safflower (红花, Honghua) 6g	Activating blood circulation and alleviating pain			
Swordlike Atractylodes Rhizome (苍术, Cangzhu) 6g	Drying dampness			
Licorice Root (生甘草, Sheng Gancao) 6g	Coordinating the actions of various ingredients in the prescription			

Points in Constitution: This formula is comprised mainly of the drugs for expelling wind, clearing away heat, activating blood circulation and removing blood stasis. The addition of Swordlike Atractylodes Rhizome (苍术, Cangzhu) to the formula is to expel dampness and induce diuresis. Besides, it can also invigorate the spleen. The use of Rhubarb (大黄, Dahuang) and Szechwan Lovage Rhizome (川芎, Chuanxiong) lies in the fact that Szechwan Lovage Rhizome (川芎, Chuanxiong) helps the Rhubarb (大黄, Dahuang) to ascend and Rhubarb (大黄, Dahuang) aids Szechwan Lovage Rhizome (川芎, Chuanxiong) in clearing pathogenic factors. So they oppose each other but also complement each other.

Indications:
1. Eczema.
2. Redness and swelling of the face.

Precaution: This formula is only applied for eczema, local redness and swelling due to wind-heat and blood stasis. It is forbidden for eczema due to deficiency of both qi and blood.

Associated Formulas:

1. Antiphlogistic Powder with Ten Herbs(十味败毒汤, shi wei bai du tang) *Experiences of Current Dynasty* 《本朝经验》

This consists of Chinese Thorowax Root (柴胡, Chaihu), Japanese Cherry Bark(樱皮, Yingpi), Balloonflower Root (桔梗, Jiegeng), Fresh Ginger (生姜, Shengjiang), Szechwan Lovage Rhizome (川芎, Chuanxiong), Tuckahoe (茯苓, Fuling), Doubleteeth Pubescent Angelica Root (独活, Duhuo), Divaricate Saposhnikovia Root (防风, Fangfeng), Licorice Root (生甘草, Sheng Gancao) and Fineleaf Schizonepeta Herb (荆芥, Jingjie). Its actions are expelling wind, activating blood circulation, clearing away toxic material and treating sores. It is indicated for the beginning of sores manifested as redness, swelling and hot pain.

Five Herbs Detoxicating Powder
(五物解毒散, wu wu jie du san)

Source: *Experiences of Current Dynasty* 《本朝经验》
Composition: Szechwan Lovage Rhizome (川芎, Chuanxiong)9g
Honeysuckle Flower (金银花, Jinyinhua)9g
Heartleaf Houttuynia Herb (鱼腥草, Yuxingcao) 9g
Rhubarb (生大黄, Sheng Dahuang)3g
Fineleaf Schizonepeta Herb (荆芥, Jingjie)6g
Actions: Clearing away toxic material and heat, expelling wind and alleviating itching.
Applied Syndrome: Cutaneous pruritus due to accumulation of wind-heat-toxin in the skin, manifested as eczema with unbearable itching, or red eczema like cloud, thirst, constipation, yellowish urine, greasy tongue coating and rapid pulse.
Points in Constitution: The lung is related to the skin and Heartleaf Houttuynia Herb (鱼腥草, Yuxingcao) is good at clearing away heat in the lung. When it is combined with Honeysuckle Flower (金银花, Jinyinhua), the heat and toxic material can be easily removed. The combination of Rhubarb (大黄, Dahuang) with Szechwan Lovage Rhizome (川芎, Chuanxiong) has the clearing and dispersing actions and is the common recipe to treat the skin diseases due to wind-heat. Thus, this formula is very suitable for cutaneous pruritus due to attack of wind-heat.

Indications:

1. Prolonged eczema.
2. Cutaneous pruritus.
3. Congenital syphilis.

Precaution: This formula is not suitable for cutaneous pruritus and eczema due to deficiency of blood.

Associated Formula:

Five Herbs Anti-Phlogistic Drink(五味消毒饮, wu wei xiao du yin) *The Golden Mirror of*

Medicine 《医宗金鉴》

Five Herbs Detoxicating Powder
(Heat-Clearing and Toxin-Removing Method)

Ingredients	Effects	Combined Effects	Syndrome	Chief Symptoms
Honeysuckle Flower (金银花, Jinyinhua) 9g Heartleaf Houttuynia Herb (鱼腥草, Yuxingcao) 9g	Clearing away heat and toxic material	Clearing away toxic material and heat, expelling wind and alleviating itching	Wind, dampness and noxious heat accumulating in the skin	Unbearable itching, or red eczema like cloud, thirst, constipation, dark urine, greasy tongue coating, rapid pulse
Rhubarb (生大黄, Sheng Dahuang) 3g	Clearing away heat and purging fire, removing heat from the blood and clearing toxic material			
Fineleaf Schizonepeta Herb (荆芥, Jingjie) 6g Szechwan Lovage Rhizome (川芎, Chuanxiong) 9g	Expelling wind and alleviating itching			

This is composed of Honeysuckle Flower (金银花, Jinyinhua), Indian Dendranthema Flower (野菊花, Yejuhua), Dandelion (蒲公英, Pugongying), Tokyo Violet Herb (紫花地丁, Zihuadiding) and Nudicaulous Grounsel Herb (紫背天葵, Zibeitiankui). Its actions are clearing away heat and toxic material, reducing swelling and alleviating pain. It is indicated for all kinds of nail-like boils, carbuncles and sores, local redness, swelling and hot pain, or fever, red tongue and rapid pulse.

Prescription for Treating Alopecia Areata
(治斑秃方, zhi ban tu fang)

Source: Collection of Zhao Bingnan's Clinical Experiences 《赵炳南临床经验集》
Composition: Dried Rehmannia Root (生地黄, Shengdihuang) 15g
Prepared Rehmannia Root (熟地黄, Shudihuang) 15g
Fleece-Flower Stem (夜交藤, Yejiaoteng) 15g
White Peony Root (白芍药, Baishaoyao) 15g
Mulberry Seed (桑椹, Sangshen) 15g
Membranous Milkvetch Root (生黄芪, Sheng Huangqi) 30g
Szechwan Lovage Rhizome (川芎, Chuanxiong) 9g
Suberect Spatholobus Stem (鸡血藤, Jixueteng) 15g
Yerbadetajo Herb (旱莲草, Hanliancao) 9g
Gastrodia Rhizome (天麻, Tianma) 6g
Aweto (冬虫夏草, Dongchongxiacao) 6g

Common Floweringquince Fruit (木瓜, Mugua)6g

Actions: Tonifying the liver and kidney, enriching blood and promoting the growth of hair.

Applied Syndrome: Alopecia due to deficiency of essence and blood resulting from insufficiency of the liver and kidney, manifested as sudden patchy loss of hair and thin pulse.

Prescription For Treating Alopecia Areata
(Liver-Nourishing and Kidney-Invigorating Method)

Ingredients	Effects	Combined Effects	Syndrome	Chief Symptoms
Dried Rehmannia Root (生地黄, Shengdihuang)15g Prepared Rehmannia Root Root (熟地黄, Shudihuang)15g Yerbadetajo Herb (旱莲草, Hanliancao)9g Fleece-Flower Stem (夜交藤, Yejiaoteng)15g Mulberry Seed(桑椹, Sangshen)15g	Tonifying the liver and kidney, enriching blood and moistening dryness	Tonifying the liver and kidney, enriching blood and promoting the growth of hair	Alopecia due to deficiency of the liver and kidney and deficiency of essence and blood	Ellipsoidal alopecia, seborrheic alopecia, sudden patchy or speckled loss of hair and thin pulse
White Peony Root (白芍药, Baishaoyao)15g Gastrodia Rhizome (天麻, Tianma)6g Common Floweringquince Fruit (木瓜, Mugua)6g	Nourishing yin, calming the liver-wind			
Membranous Milkvetch Root (生黄芪, Sheng Huangqi)30g	Replenishing qi and promoting the production of blood			
Aweto (冬虫夏草, Dongchongxiacao)6g	Replenishing both yin and yang			
Szechwan Lovage Rhizome (川芎, Chuanxiong)9g Suberect Spatholobus Stem (鸡血藤, Jixueteng)15g	Activating blood circulation and expelling wind			

Points in Constitution: Alopecia is due to deficiency of essence and blood and the up-stirring of wind in the interior resulting from deficiency of the liver and kidney. Thus this formula is comprised of a number of drugs for replenishing the liver and kidney and nourishing essence and blood. Besides, a large dose of Membranous Milkvetch Root (黄芪, Huangqi) is used to replenish qi, promote the production of blood and ascend defensive qi so as to promote the growth of hair.

Indications:

1. Ellipsoidal alopecia.
2. Seborrheic alopecia.

Precaution: This formula should be taken for a long time to take effect.

Associated Formulas:

1. Blood-Enriching and Wind-Dispersing Decoction(养血胜风汤, yang xue sheng feng tang) *Supplement to Essence of Medicine*《医醇賸义》

This is made up of Dried Rehmannia Root(生地黄, Shengdihuang), White Peony Root(白芍药, Baishaoyao), Spine Date Seed(酸枣仁, Suanzaoren), Szechwan Lovage Rhizome(川芎, Chuanxiong), Mulberry Leaf(桑叶, Sangye), Barbary Wolfberry Fruit(枸杞子, Gouqizi), Black Sesame(黑芝麻, Heizhima), Chinese Magnoliavine Fruit(五味子, Wuweizi), Chinese Arborvitae Seed(柏子仁, Baiziren), Chrysanthemum Flower(菊花, Juhua), Chinese Angelica Root(当归, Danggui) and Chinese Date(大枣, Dazao). Its actions are enriching the blood and expelling wind. It is indicated for headache, alopecia and vertigo due to deficiency of the blood.

2. Genuine Qi-Nourishing Pellet(养真丹, yang zhen dan) *The Golden Mirror of Medicine* 《医宗金鉴》

This is made up of Incised Notopterygium Rhizome or Root(羌活, Qianghuo), Common Floweringquince Fruit(木瓜, Mugua), Gastrodia Rhizome(天麻, Tianma), Chinese Angelica Root(当归, Danggui), White Peony Root(白芍药, Baishaoyao), Chinese Dodder Seed(菟丝子, Tusizi), Prepared Rehmannia Root(熟地黄, Shudihuang) and Szechwan Lovage Rhizome(川芎, Chuanxiong). It is good at enriching blood, promoting the growth of hair, expelling wind, regulating the flow of qi and blood aand activating the meridian and collaterals. It is indicated for alopecia due to excessive wind and deficiency of blood which is unable to nourish the hair.

3. Beard and Hair-Darkening Pellet(青云独步丹, qing yun du bu dan) *Longevity and Life Prescription* 《寿世保元》

This is composed of Fleeceflower Root(何首乌, Heshouwu), Chinese Angelica Root(当归, Danggui), Indian Bread Pink Epidermis(赤茯苓, Chifuling), Tuckahoe(白茯苓, Baifuling), Malaytea Scurfpea Fruit(补骨脂, Buguzhi), Barbary Wolfberry Fruit(枸杞子, Gouqizi), Chinese Dodder Seed(菟丝子, Tusizi), Achyranthes Root(怀牛膝, Huainiuxi), Dried Rehmannia Root(生地黄, Shengdihuang) and Myrrh(没药, Moyao). Its actions are darkening both beard and hair and prolonging life. It is indicated for early graying of the beard and hair due to aging and weakness.

4. Seven Valuable Herbs Beard-improving Pellet(七宝美髯丹, qi bao mei ran dan) *Collection of Formulae with Notes* 《医方集解》

This is composed of Fleeceflower Root(何首乌, Heshouwu), Tuckahoe(白茯苓, Baifuling), Twotooth Achyranthes Root(牛膝, Niuxi), Chinese Angelica Root(当归, Danggui), Barbary Wolfberry Fruit(枸杞子, Gouqizi), Chinese Dodder Seed(菟丝子, Tusizi) and Malaytea Scurfpea Fruit(破故纸, Poguzhi). Its actions are invigorating the kidney and nourishing essence. It is indicated for early graying of the beard and hair, spermacrasia, soreness of the loins and lassitude of foot due to deficiency of kidney-yin and insufficiency of essence and blood.

5. Seven Immortals Pellet(七仙丹, qi xian dan) *Precious Mirror of Eastern Medicine* 《东医宝鉴》

This is composed of Fleeceflower Root (何首乌, Heshouwu), Ginseng (人参, Renshen), Dried Rehmannia Root (生地黄, Shengdihuang), Prepared Rehmannia Root (熟地黄, Shudihuang), Dwarf Lilyturf Root (麦门冬, Maimendong), Cochinchinese Asparagus Root (天门冬, Tianmendong), Tuckahoe (茯苓, Fuling) and Fried Fennel Fruit (炒茴香, Chao Huixiang). Its actions are nourishing the liver and kidney, enriching blood and darkening hair. It is indicated for early graying of the beard and hair.

6. Hair-Promoting Drink (生发饮, sheng fa yin) *Journal of Traditional Chinese Medicine* 《中医杂志》

This is composed of Dried Rehmannia Root (生地黄, Shengdihuang), Prepared Rehmannia Root (熟地黄, Shudihuang), Chinese Angelica Root (当归, Danggui), Chinese Arborvitae Leafy Twig (侧柏叶, Cebaiye), Black Sesame (黑芝麻, Heizhima) and Fleeceflower Root (何首乌, Heshouwu). Its actions are nourishing kidney-yin, enriching blood and supplementing essence. It is indicated for alopecia due to deficiency of kidney essence. The manifestations are alopecia, listlessness, lassitude, dizziness, soreness and weakness of the loin and knees, insomnia, red tongue with little coating, thin and rapid pulse.

7. Hair-Promoting Decoction (生发汤, sheng fa tang) *Zheng Yunxiang's Medical Records* 《邹云翔医案》

This is composed of Prepared Tuber Fleeceflower Root (制首乌, Zhishouwu), Villous Amomum Fruit (砂仁, Sharen), Prepared Rehmannia Root (熟地黄, Shudihuang), Yerbadetajo Herb (旱莲草, Hanliancao), Glossy Privet Fruit (女贞子, Nüzhenzi), Barbary Wolfberry Fruit (枸杞子, Gouqizi), Common St. Paulswort Herb (豨莶草, Xiqiancao), Black Sesame (黑芝麻, Heizhima), Pilose Asiabell Root (党参, Dangshen), Toasted Membranous Milkvetch Root (炙黄芪, Zhi Huangqi), Seed of Mulberry (桑椹子, Sangshenzi), Chinese Angelica Root (当归, Danggui), Bead of Ass-hide Glue (阿胶珠, Ejiaozhu), White Peony Root (白芍药, Baishaoyao), Longan Aril (桂圆肉, Guiyuanrou), Tangerine Peel (橘皮, Jupi), Prepared Licorice Root (炙甘草, Zhi Gancao) and Small Chinese Date (小红枣, Xiaohongzao). Its actions are benefiting the liver and kidney, replenishing qi and blood. It is indicated for alopecia due to failure of blood to nourish hair resulting from deficiency of the liver and kidney and insufficinecy of essence and blood, manifested as gradual loss of hair, yellow without lustre, vertigo, constipation, normal appetite and sleep, thin and white tongue coating, feeble and thin pulse.

Verruca-Removing Decoction
(除疣汤, chu you tang)

Source: *Journal of Traditional Chinese Medicine* 《中医杂志》
Composition: Coix Seed (薏苡仁, Yiyiren) 30g
Indigowoad Leaf (大青叶, Daqingye) 30g
Indigowoad Root (板蓝根, Banlangen) 30g
Whiteflower Patrinia Herb (败酱草, Baijiangcao) 15g

Powder of Oyster Shell（牡蛎粉，Mulifen）30g
Common Selfheal Fruit-Spike（夏枯草，Xiakucao）15g
Red Peony Root（赤芍药，Chishaoyao）10g

Actions: Clearing away heat and toxic material, softening hardness and dissipating blockages.

Applied Syndrome: Verruca vulgaris due to excessive dampness and attack of noxious heat in the interior, manifested as flat papules in the face, dorsum of hand or forearm which are the size of rice or soybean with normal colour or hazel, hard, smooth, red tongue with yellow and greasy coating, smooth and rapid pulse.

Verruca-Removing Decoction
(Heat-Clearing and Toxin-Removing Method)

Ingredients	Effects	Combined Effects	Syndrome	Chief Symptoms
Indigowoad Leaf（大青叶，Daqingye）30g indigowoad Root（板蓝根，Banlangen）30g Whiteflower Patrinia Herb（败酱草，Baijiangcao）15g	Clearing away heat and toxic material, removing heat from the blood and reducing swelling	Clearing away heat and toxic material, calming the liver and softening hardness	Accumulation of heat and toxin in the skin	Flat wart and verruca vulgaris
Coix Seed（薏苡仁，Yiyiren）30g	Clearing away heat, promoting diuresis and eliminating carbuncle			
Powder of Oyster Shell（牡蛎粉，Mulifen）30g Common Selfheal Fruit-Spike（夏枯草，Xiakucao）15g Red Peony Root（赤芍药，Chishaoyao）10g	Purging liver heat, softening hardness and dissipating blockages			

Points in Constitution: Verruca vulgaris is due to the accumulation of noxious heat in the skin, thus the main treatment for it is to clear away heat and toxic material. Coix Seed（薏苡仁，Yiyiren）is a proven drug in removing verruca vulgaris.

Indications:
1. Flat wart.
2. Acne.
3. The beginning of furuncle.

Precaution: This is a heat-clearing and toxin-removing formula. So it is forbidden for the syndrome due to deficiency of qi and blood or due to insufficiency of both the liver and kidney.

Associated Formulas:
1. Five Herbs Antiphlogistic Drink（五味消毒饮，wu wei xiao du yin）*The Golden Mirror of*

Medicine《医宗金鉴》

   This is made up of Honeysuckle Flower (金银花, Jinyinhua), Indian Dendranthema Flower (野菊花, Yejuhua), Tokyo Violet Herb (紫花地丁, Zihuadiding), Cluster Mallow Fruit (冬葵子, Dongkuizi) and Dandelion (蒲公英, Pugongying). Both this formula and Verruca-Removing Decoction (除疣汤, chu you tang) have the actions of clearing away heat, removing toxic material and eliminating nail-like boils and sores. But Verruca-Removing Decoction (除疣汤, chu you tang) is good at treating verruca vulgaris with normal colour or hazel skin due to slight noxious heat accompanied with damp-heat which fails to discharge outward while this Five Herbs Antiphlogistic Drink (五味消毒饮, wu wei xiao du yin) has a strong action of clearing away heat and toxic material and is good at treating all kinds of nail-like boils, sores, carbuncles, local redness, swelling and hot pain due to accumulation of excessive noxious heat.

Chapter Eleven
Formulas for Otorhinolaryngologic Diseases

As a branch in TCM, diseases of the ear, nose and throat or otorhinolaryngologic diseases were not separated from internal medicine until the end of the Qing Dynasty when the book Precious Works on Throat Diseases《重楼玉钥》was published which was a doctrine of throat diseases. Thus many syndromes, symptoms and treatment of the otorhinolaryngologic diseases were dealt with among the miscellaneous disease in internal medicine. According to TCM, otopathy or ear disease mainly belongs to the problem of the kidney and liver; rhinopathy or nose diseases to the lung and stomach and laryngopathy or throat diseases to the lung and kidney. Therefore, the organs mentioned above should be firstly considered and the treatment of these diseases should be based on the differentiation of the syndromes.

Diseases of allergic rhinitis, sinusitis, nasal hemorrhage, tinnitus, otitis media, Meniere's syndrome, acute laryngopharyngitis, chronic laryngopharyngitis, tonsillitis and tonsil hypertrophy are all the indications treated with Chinese drugs or by the combination of Chinese with Western medicine.

1. Miraculous Pill with Six Drugs
(六神丸, liu shen wan)

Source: *Lei Yunshang's Yongfentang Prescriptions*《雷允上涌芬堂方》
Composition: Pearl Powder (珍珠粉, Zhenzhufen)
Cow-Bezoar (牛黄, Niuhuang)
Musk (麝香, Shexiang)
Red Orpiment (雄黄, Xionghuang)
Toad Skin Secretion Cake (蟾酥, Chansu)
Borneol (冰片, Bingpian)
(It is a patent medicine. its preparation is omitted)
Actions: Clearing away heat and toxic material, diminishing inflammation and alleviating pain.
Applied Syndrome: Acute tonsillitis, acute pyogenic infection of the throat, laryngeal abscess and scarlet fever.
Points in Constitution: The drugs in this formula are all the light and effective ones so a small dose of them can take effect, which is well applicable for throat diseases. This drug should be kept in the mouth, melted by saliva and passed through the throat to exert the actions of diminishing inflammation and alleviating pain.

Miraculous Pill with Six Drugs

(Heat-Clearing and Toxin-Removing Method)

Ingredients	Effects	Combined Effects	Syndrome	Chief Symptoms
Cow-Bezoar (牛黄, Niuhuang)	Clearing away heat and toxic material	Clearing away heat and toxic material, diminishing inflammation and alleviating pain	Throat diseases due to heat-toxin	Acute tonsillitis, acute pyogenic infection of the throat, redness, swelling and pain of pharynx
Musk (麝香, Shexiang) Borneol (冰片, Bingpian)	Alleviating pain			
Toad Skin Secretion Cake (蟾酥, Chansu)	Activating the heartbeat and removing toxic material, inducing localized anesthesia			
Red Orpiment (雄黄, Xionghuang)	Detoxification			
Pearl Powder (珍珠粉, Zhenzhufen)	Protecting mucous membrane			

Indications:
1. Acute tonsillitis.
2. Pharyngitis.
3. Oral ulcer.
4. Respiratory failure.

Precautions:
1. It should be cautiously used for pregnant women.
2. Take it according to the doctor's advice. Be sure not to take it excessively.

Associated Formulas:

1. Plum Blossom Tongue-Touching Tablet(梅花点舌丹, mei hua dian she dan) *Surgery Life-Saving Collection*《外科全生集》

This is composed of Cow-Bezoar (牛黄, Niuhuang), Musk (麝香, Shexiang), Borneol (冰片, Bingpian), Toad Skin Secretion Cake (蟾酥, Chansu), Bear Gall (熊胆, Xiongdan), Chinese Eaglewood Wood (沉香, Chenxiang), Olibanum (乳香, Ruxiang), Myrrh (没药, Moyao), Pepperweed Seed or Flixweed Tansymustard Seed (葶苈子, Tinglizi), Dragon's Blood (血竭, Xuejie), Cinnabar (朱砂, Zhusha), Red Orpiment (雄黄, Xionghuang), Borax(月石, Yueshi) and Pearl (珍珠, Zhenzhu). Its actions are clearing away heat and toxic materials. It is indicated for nail-like boils, obstinate sores, inflammation of soft tissues of unknown origin, carbuncle and furuncle with redness, swelling and hot pain, acute tonsillitis and sore throat.

2. General Recipe for Sore Throat(咽炎统治方, yan yan tong zhi fang) Author's Experienced Prescription(作者经验方)

This is made up of Scrophularia Root(元参, Yuanshen), Ophiopogon Root(麦门冬, Maimendong), Bitter Orange(枳壳, Zhiqiao), Reed Rhizome(芦苇根, Luweigen), Arctium Fruit(牛蒡子, Niubangzi), Chinese Yam(山药, Shanya), Wintercherry Fruit(锦灯笼, Jindenglong) and Licorice Root(甘草, gancao). It has an action of clearing away heat and toxic materials. It is mainly applied for sore throat or folliculosis. For the case in the acute stage, Honeysuckle Flower(金银花, Jinyinhua) and Isatis Root(板蓝根, Banlangen) should be added.

2. Hoarseness-Relieving and Aphonia-Treating Pill (响声破笛丸, xiang sheng po di wan)

Source: Curative Measures for Diseases《万病回春》
Composition: Balloonflower Root (桔梗, Jiegeng)6g
Licorice Root (生甘草, Sheng Gancao)6g
Weeping Forsythia Capsule (连翘, Lianqiao)6g
Wild Mint Herb (薄荷, Bohe)9g
Rhubarb (生大黄, Sheng Dahuang)3g
Szechwan Lovage Rhizome (川芎, Chuanxiong)3g
Villous Amomum Fruit (缩砂仁, Suosharen)3g
Medicine Terminalia Fruit (诃子, Hezi)3g
Catechu (儿茶, Ercha)6g
(Grond into powder and sucked in a proper amount).

Actions: Removing intense heat from the throat and relieving sore throat.

Applied Syndrome: Sore throat and hoarseness due to laryngeal strain.

Points in Constitution: Catechu (儿茶, Ercha) is usually used externally to induce astringency and arrest bleeding. However, when it is combined with Medicine Terminalia Fruit (诃子, Hezi) and Weeping Forsythia Capsule (连翘, Lianqiao), it can be used orally to treat sore throat and hoarseness. The effectiveness of the drugs depends on the different approach of administration.

Indication: Hoarseness due to overstrain in singing or speaking.

Associated Formula:

Licorice Decoction (甘草汤, gan cao tang) *Treatise on Exogenous Febrile Diseases*《伤寒论》

This is also called Single Superb Powde(独胜散, du sheng san) or Worry-Forgetting Decoction (忘忧汤, wang you tang). This formula consists of only one drug, Licorice Root (生甘草, Sheng Gancao), which is sweet in taste, mild in nature and has the actions of alleviating pain, relieving muscular spasm and arresting cough. It is indicated for reversed flow of qi, asthma and sore throat.

Hoarseness-Relieving and Aphonia-Teating Pills
(Heat-Clearing and Sore Throat-Relieving Method)

Ingredients	Effects	Combined Effects	Syndrome	Chief Symptoms
Balloonflower Root (桔梗, Jiegeng)6g	Promoting the dispersing function of the lung, relieving sore throat and recovering from hoarseness	Clearing away heat in the throat and relieving sore throat	Heat accumulated in the throat	Sore throat, dry throat, itching of the throat, hoarseness, red tongue, thin and rapid pulse
Licorice Root (生甘草, Sheng Gancao)6g	Clearing away heat, purging fire and relieving sore throat			
Rhubarb (生大黄, Sheng Dahuang)3g Weeping Forsythia Capsule (连翘, Lianqiao)6g	Clearing away heat and toxic material			
Wild Mint Herb (薄荷, Bohe)9g	Expelling wind, clearing away heat and relieving sore throat			
Medicine Terminalia Fruit (诃子, Hezi)3g	Clearing lung-heat and descending qi, relieving sore throat and recovering from hoarseness			
Villous Amomum Fruit (缩砂仁, Suosharen)3g	Activating flow of qi and alleviating depression			
Szechwan Lovage Rhizome (川芎, Chuanxiong)3g	Activating flow of qi and activating blood circulation			
Catechu (儿茶, Ercha)6g	Relieving pain and removing phlegm of the lung			

3. Wind-Dispelling and Toxin-Removing Decoction
(驱风解毒汤, qu feng jie du tang)

Source: *Curative Measures for Diseases*《万病回春》
Composition: Great Burdock Achene (牛蒡子, Niubangzi)9g
Weeping Forsythia Capsule (连翘, Lianqiao)9g
Balloonflower Root (桔梗, Jiegeng)6g
Licorice Root (生甘草, Sheng Gancao)3g
Gypsum (生石膏, Sheng Shigao)9g
Fineleaf Schizonepeta Herb (荆芥, Jingjie)6g
Divaricate Saposhnikovia Root (防风, Fangfeng)6g
Incised Notopterygium Rhizome or Root (羌活, Qianghuo)3g
Actions: Expelling wind and clearing away heat, eliminating toxic material and relieving sore throat.
Applied Syndrome: Accumulation of noxious heat in the throat due to attack of exogenous wind-

heat, manifested as fever, redness, swelling and pain in the pharynx.

Wind-Dispelling and Toxin-Removing Decoction
(Heat-Clearing and Toxin-Removing Method)

Ingredients	Effects	Combined Effects	Syndrome	Chief Symptoms
Fineleaf Schizonepeta Herb (荆芥, Jingjie)6g Divaricate Saposhnikovia Root (防风, Fangfeng)6g incised Notopterygium Rhizome or Root (羌活, Qianghuo)3g	Expelling wind evils	Expelling wind, clearing away heat, and toxic material, relieving sore throat	Accumulation of pathogenic heat in the throat	Redness, swelling and pain of the pharynx, fever, slightly aversion to wind, dry throat and thirst, red tongue with thin and yellow coating, rapid pulse
Great Burdock Achene (牛蒡子, Niubangzi)9g Weeping Forsythia Capsule (连翘, Lianqiao)9g Balloonflower Root (桔梗, Jiegeng)6g Licorice Root (生甘草, Sheng Gancao)3g	Clearing away heat and toxic material and relieving sore throat			
Gypsum (生石膏, Sheng Shigao)9g	Clearing away heat and purging fire			

Points in Constitution: This formula pays equal attention to the relief of the exterior syndrome and removal of heat. It belongs to the prescription for expelling the pathogenic factors from both exterior and interior of the body, which should be known clearly in the clinic.

Indications:
1. Tonsillitis, peritonsillitis, laryngopharyngitis and stomatitis.
2. Inflammation of gland under the ear.

Precaution: It is cautiously used for those without the exterior syndrome.

Associated Formula:

Schizonepeta and Forsythia Decoction (荆芥连翘汤, jing jie lian qiao tang) *Curative Measures for Disease* 《万病回春》

This is composed of Fineleaf Schizonepeta Herb (荆芥, Jingjie), Weeping Forsythia Capsule (连翘, Lianqiao), Divaricate Saposhnikovia Root (防风, Fangfeng), Chinese Angelica Root (当归, Danggui), Szechwan Lovage Rhizome (川芎, Chuanxiong), White Peony Root (白芍药, Baishaoyao), Chinese Thorowax Root (柴胡, Chaihu), Bitter Orange (枳壳, Zhiqiao), Baikal Skullcap Root (黄芩, Huangqin), Cape Jasmine Fruit (山栀子, Shanzhizi), Dahurican Angelica Root (白芷, Baizhi), Balloonflower Root (桔梗, Jiegeng) and Licorice Root (生甘草, Sheng Gancao). Its actions are expelling wind and clearing away heat, reducing swelling and alleviating pain. It is indicated for swelling and pain of the ears due to wind-heat in the liver meridian or rhinorrhea due to upward attack of heat in the gallbladder upon the head.

4. Magnolia Lung-Clearing Decoction
(辛夷清肺汤, xin yi qing fei tang)

Source: *Orthodox Manual of Surgery* 《外科正宗》
Composition: Biond Magnolia Flower-Bud (辛夷, Xinyi)9g
Baikal Skullcap Root (黄芩, Huangqin)6g
Cape Jasmine Fruit (山栀子, Shanzhizi)6g
Dwarf Lilyturf Root (麦门冬, Maimendong)9g
Lily Bulb (百合, Baihe)9g
Gypsum (生石膏, Sheng Shigao)9g
Common Anemarrhena Rhizome (知母, Zhimu)9g
Licorice Root (生甘草, Sheng Gancao)3g
Loquat Leaf (枇杷叶, Pipaye)9g
Shunk Bugbane Rhizome (升麻, Shengma)9g
Actions: Clearing away lung heat, opening orifices and nourishing yin.
Applied Syndrome: Continuous turbid nasal discharge with yellow colour and odour smell, stuffy nose, aching pain of nose, headache and dizziness.

Magnolia Lung-Clearing Decoction
(Heat-Clearing and Wind-Expelling Method)

Ingredients	Effects	Combined Effects	Syndrome	Chief Symptoms
Biond Magnolia Flower-Bud (辛夷, Xinyi)9g	Expelling wind and opening the nasal passages	Clearing away lung-heat	Attack of the nose by lung-heat	Yellow turbid nasal discharge, thirst, sore throat, thin and rapid pulse thin, white and dry tongue coating
Gypsum (生石膏, Sheng Shigao)9g Common Anemarrhena Rhizome (知母, Zhimu)9g	Clearing away heat from the lung and stomach			
Cape Jasmine Fruit (山栀子, Shanzhizi)6g Baikal Skullcap Root (黄芩, Huangqin)6g	Clearing away heat and toxic material			
Dwarf Lilyturf Root (麦门冬, Maimendong)9g Lily Bulb (百合, Baihe)9g	Nourishing yin and moistening the lung			
Shunk Bugbane Rhizome (升麻, Shengma)9g Loquat Leaf (枇杷叶, Pipaye)9g	Raising clear yang and lowering turbid yin			

Points in Constitution: Rhinorrhea is caused by retention of turbid qi in the upper-jiao and failure of clear qi to descend. Thus, this lung heat-removing formula contains Shunk Bugbane Rhizome (升麻, Shengma) and Loquat Leaf (枇杷叶, Pipaye) to raise clear yang and lower turbid yin. Wind-heat is the pathogenic factor and pathogenic yang will surely impair yin fluid. The use of Dwarf Lilyturf Root (麦门冬, Maimendong) and Lily Bulb (百合, Baihe) is to protect and nourish yin and body fluid.

Indication: Parasinusitis.

Precaution: It should be cautiously used for those with deficiency of the spleen and stomach.

Associated Formula:

Pueraria Decoction plus Szechwan Lovage and Magnolia (葛根加川芎辛夷汤, ge gen jia chuan xiong xin yi tang) *Japanese Proved Recipe*《日本经验方》

This consists of Pueraria (葛根, Gegen), Ephedra (麻黄, Mahuang), Cassia Twig (桂枝, Guizhi), Fresh Ginger (生姜, Shengjiang), Prepared Licorice Root (炙甘草, Zhi Gancao), White Peony Root (白芍药, Baishaoyao), Chinese Date (大枣, Dazao), Szechwan Lovage Rhizome (川芎, Chuanxiong) and Biond Magnolia Flower-Bud (辛夷, Xinyi). Its actions are relieving the exterior syndrome and expelling cold, promoting the dispersing function of the lung and opening nasal passages. It is indicated for stuffy and running nose due to affection of exogenous wind-cold.

5. Lung-Warming and Running-Stopping Decocting
（温肺止流汤, wen fei zhi liu tang）

Source: *Complete Works for Treating Sores*《疡医大全》
Composition: Ginseng (人参, Renshen) 9g
Fineleaf Schizonepeta Herb (荆芥, Jingjie) 9g
Manchurian Wildginger Herb (细辛, Xixin) 3g
Medicine Terminalia Fruit (诃子, Hezi) 9g
Balloonflower Root (桔梗, Jiegeng) 6g
Asteriscus Pseudosciaenae (鱼脑石, Yunaoshi) 9g
Prepared Licorice Root (炙甘草, Zhi Gancao) 6g

Actions: Replenishing lung qi and expelling cold.

Applied Syndrome: Nasal obstruction. The nose is the orifice opening into the lung. Thus the deficiency of lung qi and attack of pathogenic cold result in the accumulation of exterior evils in the lung and failure of the lung qi in dispersion. It is manifested as running nose, shortness of breath, spontaneous sweating, low and faint voice, pale tongue with white coating, feeble and weak pulse.

Points in Constitution: Ginseng (人参, Renshen), combined with Fineleaf Schizonepeta Herb (荆芥, Jingjie) and Manchurian Wildginger Herb (细辛, Xixin), can expel pathogens without impairing healthy qi and replenish the lung without keeping pathogens. The combination of

Medicine Terminalia Fruit (诃子, Hezi) with Balloonflower Root (桔梗, Jiegeng) has both the expelling and astringing actions. (This method of opposing each other but also complementing each other at the same time is very suitable for the syndrome of pathogens mixed with healthy qi.)

Lung-Warming and Running-Stopping Decoction
(Qi-Replenishing and Exterior-Relieving Method)

Ingredients	Effects	Combined Effects	Syndrome	Chief Symptoms
Ginseng (人参, Renshen)9g	Tonifying the lung and replenishing qi	Replenishing qi and relieving the exterior syndrome	Deficiency of lung qi and attack of cold again	Running nose, shortness of breath and spontaneous sweating, low and feeble voice, pale tongue with white coating, feeble and weak pulse
Fineleaf Schizonepeta Herb (荆芥, Jingjie)9g Manchurian Wildginger Herb (细辛, Xixin)3g	Expelling wind and cold			
Medicine Terminalia Fruit (诃子, Hezi)9g	Astringing the lung and relieving sore throat			
Balloonflower Root (桔梗, Jiegeng)6g	Promoting the dispersing function of the lung, relieving cough and romving phlegm			
Asteriscus Pseudosciaenae (鱼脑石, Yunaoshi)9g	Clearing away heat and alleviating dizziness			
Prepared Licorice Root (炙甘草, Zhi Gancao)6g	Coordinating the actions of various ingredients in the prescription			

Indications:
1. Cold due to deficiency of lung-qi and attack of wind cold.
2. Chronic rhinitis and atrophic rhinitis.

Precaution: This formula is not suitable for a stuffy nose or running nose due to simple attack of the lung by exogenous wind-cold.

Associated Formulas:

Lung-Warming Decoction(温肺汤, wen fei tang) *Standard for Diagnosis and Treatment* 《证治准绳》

This formula consists of Shunk Bugbane Rhizome (升麻, Shengma), Toasted Membranous Milkvetch Root (炙黄芪, Zhi Huangqi), Clove Flower-Bud (丁香, Dingxiang), Pueraria(葛根, Gegen), Incised Notopterygium Rhizome or Root (羌活, Qianghuo), Divaricate Saposhnikovia Root (防风, Fangfeng), Ephedra (麻黄, Mahuang), Fistular Onion Bulb (葱白, Congbai) and Prepared Licorice Root (炙甘草, Zhi Gancao). Both of this formula and Lung-Warming and Running-Stopping Decoction (温肺止流汤, wen fei zhi liu tang) have the actions of replenishing lung-qi and dispelling wind-cold to treat stuffy nose and running nose. However, Lung-Warming and Running-Stopping Decoction (温肺止流汤, wen fei zhi liu tang) is good at treating nasal obstruction manifested as running nose, shortness of breath and spontaneous sweating and weak pulse due to obvious deficiency of lung qi with severe pathogenic cold while this Lung-Warming Decoction(温肺汤, wen fei tang) is good at treating rhinorrhea manifested as white, sticky and thick nasal discharge, severe stuffy nose, dizziness, shortness of breath and slow pulse due to slight deficiency of qi with the tendency of cold changing into heat.

Additional Formulas

Minor Bupleurum Decoction Plus Balloonflower and Gypsum
（小柴胡桔梗石膏汤，xiao chai hu jie gen shi gao tang）

Source: Japanese Proved Recipes（日本经验方）
Composition: Bupleurum（柴胡, Chaihu）9g
Baikal Skullcap Root（黄芩, Huangqin）9g
Ginseng（人参, Renshen）3g
Pinellia Rhizome（半夏, Banxia）6g
Prepared Licorice Root（炙甘草, Zhi Gancao）6g
Fresh Ginger（生姜, Shengjiang）3g
Chinese Date（大枣, Dazao）3g
Balloonflower Root（桔梗, Jiegeng）3g
Gypsum（生石膏, Sheng Shigao）9g

Actions: Harmonizing functions of shaoyang system and reducing fever, relieving sore throat and evacuating pus.

Applied Syndrome: The manifestations are redness, swelling and pain of the throat, alternative episodes of chills and fever, fullness feeling in the chest and hypochondrium, red tongue with thin and yellow coating, wiry and rapid pulse.

Minor Bupleurum Decoction Plus Balloonflower and Gypsum
(Method of Treating Shaoyang Disease by Mediation)

Ingredients	Effects	Combined Effects	Syndrome	Chief Symptoms
Bupleurum（柴胡, Chaihu）9g Baikal Skullcap Root（黄芩, Huangqin）9g Ginseng（人参, Renshen）3g Pinellia Rhizome（半夏, Banxia）6g Prepared Licorice Root（炙甘草, Zhi Gancao）6g Fresh Ginger（生姜, Shengjiang）3g Chinese Date（大枣, Dazao）3g	Treating shaoyang disease by mediation	Harmonizing functions of shaoyang system, reducing fever and relieving sore throat	Sore throat (tonsillitis)	Redness, swelling and pain of the throat, alternative episodes of chills and fever, feeling of fullness in the chest and hypochondrium, red tongue with thin and yellow coating, wiry and rapid pulse
Gypsum（生石膏, Sheng Shigao）9g	Clearing away heat of the lung and stomach			
Balloonflower Root（桔梗, Jiegeng）3g	Evacuating pus, relieving cough and sore throat			

Points in Constitution: Balloonflower Root (桔梗, Jiegeng) and Gypsum (生石膏, Sheng Shigao) are added into Minor Bupleurum Decoction (小柴胡汤, xiao chai hu tang). By doing so, the method of treating shaoyang disease by mediation, which is the indication of Minor Bupleurum Decoction(小柴胡汤, xiao chai hu tang), is changed into the one of treating both shaoyang and yangming diseases.

Indications:
1. Tonsillitis.
2. Parasinusitis.

Precaution: It should be cautiously used for those with excessive heat of yangming but without alternative episodes of chills and fever.

Associated Formula:

Wind-Dispelling and Toxin-Removing Decoction(驱风解毒汤, qu feng jie du tang) *Curative Measures for Diseases* 《万病回春》

This is made up of Great Burdock Achene (牛蒡子, Niubangzi), Weeping Forsythia Capsule (连翘, Lianqiao), Balloonflower Root (桔梗, Jiegeng), Licorice Root (甘草, Gancao), Gypsum (生石膏, Sheng Shigao), Fineleaf Schizonepeta Herb (荆芥, Jingjie), Divaricate Saposhnikovia Root (防风, Fangfeng) and Incised Notopterygium Rhizome or Root (羌活, Qianghuo). Its actions are expelling wind, clearing away heat, removing toxic material and treating sore throat. It is applied for fever, chills and sore throat due to attack of exogenous wind-heat.

Pueraria Decoction plus Szechwan Lovage and Magnolia (葛根汤加川芎辛夷汤, ge gen tang jia chuan xiong xin yi tang)

Source: Japanese Proved Recipes (日本经验方)
Composition: Pueraria(葛根, Gegen)9g
Ephedra (麻黄, Mahuang)6g
Cassia Twig (桂枝, Guizhi)6g
Fresh Ginger (生姜, Shengjiang)3g
Prepared Licorice Root (炙甘草, Zhi Gancao)6g
White Peony Root (白芍药, Baishaoyao)9g
Chinese Date (大枣, Dazao)6g
Szechwan Lovage Rhizome (川芎, Chuanxiong)9g
Biond Magnolia Flower-Bud (辛夷, Xinyi)9g

Actions: Regulating yingfen and weifen, promoting the dispersing function of the lung and dredging obstruction.

Applied Syndrome: Attack of the exterior by wind-cold, manifested as ssubjective sensation of contraction of channels, chills and fever, adiaphoresis and headache, stuffy nose and running nose, hyposmia, thin and white tongue coating, superficial and tense pulse, or accompanied with stiffness and pain of nape and back, facial spasm, deviation of the eyes and mouth.

Pueraria Decoction plus Szechwan Lovage and Magnolia
(Exterior-Relieveing Method With Drugs Pungent in Flavor and Warm in Nature)

Ingredients	Effects	Combined Effects	Syndrome	Chief Symptoms
Pueraria(葛根, Gegen)9g Ephedra(麻黄, Mahuang)6g Cassia Twig(桂枝, Guizhi)6g Fresh Ginger(生姜, Shengjiang)3g White Peony Root(白芍药, Baishaoyao)9g Chinese Date(大枣, Dazao)6g Prepared Licorice Root(炙甘草, Zhi Gancao)6g	Being acrid in flavor and warm in nature to relieve the exterior, promoting the production of body fluid and relaxing muscles and tendons	Relieving the exterior, relaxing muscles and tendons, dispersing wind-cold and opening orifices with acrid drugs	Wind-cold attacking the superficies and subjective sensation of contraction of channels	Aversion to cold and fever, adiaphoresis and headache, stuffy nose and running nose, hyposmia, thin and white tongue coating, superficial and tense pulse
Szechwan Lovage Rhizome(川芎, Chuanxiong)9g Biond Magnolia Flower-Bud(辛夷, Xinyi)9g	Expelling wind and opening orifices			

Points in Constitution: The combination of Pueraria Decoction (葛根汤, ge gen tang) with Szechwan Lovage Rhizome (川芎, Chuanxiong) increases the actions of expelling wind and activating blood circulation. The addition of Biond Magnolia Flower-Bud (辛夷, Xinyi) increases the actions of opening orifices and alleviating pain. Szechwan Lovage Rhizome (川芎, Chuanxiong) is a common drug for diseases of the head and face and has many actions. It can activate blood circulation, promote flow of wind, dispel wind, remove the obstruction, relieve pain, dredge the channels and eliminate dampness. However, it should be used cautiously for those with deficiency of yin accompanied with heat.

Indications:
1. Periarthritis of shoulder jiont.
2. Cold.
3. Rhinorrhea.

Precaution: It should be cautiously used for those without the exterior syndrome.

Associated Formula:

Pueraria Decoction(葛根汤, ge gen tang) *Synopsis of Golden Cabinet* 《金匮要略》

This is made up of Pueraria(葛根, Gegen), Ephedra(麻黄, Mahuang), Cassia Twig(桂枝, Guizhi), Fresh Ginger(生姜, Shengjiang), White Peony Root(白芍药, Baishaoyao), Chinese Date(大枣, Dazao) and Licorice Root(甘草, Gancao). Its actions are relieving exterior syndrome by dispelling cold, promoting the production of body fluid and relieving pain and spasm. It is applied for infection by wind-cold manifested as stiffiness and spasm of the nape and back.

Hoarseness-Relieving and Aphonia-Healing Tablet
(清音片, qing yin pian)

Source: *Common Chinese Patent Medicine* 《常用中成药》
Composition: Olive (橄榄, Ganlan)
Mirabilita Crystal (寒水石, Hanshuishi)
Balloonflower Root (桔梗, Jiegeng)
Indigowoad Leaf (大青叶, Daqingye)
Licorice Root (生甘草, Sheng Gancao)
Borax Refined with Water (飞硼砂, Fei Pengsha)
Menthol (薄荷脑, Bohenao)
Borneol (冰片, Bingpian)
(It is a patent medicine and its preparation is omitted)
Actions: Clearing away heat, relieving sore throat and healing aphonia.
Applied Syndrome: Aphonia and sore throat due to attack of exogenous wind-heat which is accumulated in the throat and causes failure of the lung-qi in dispersion, manifested as hoarseness, sore throat, cough, dry mouth, dysphagia, red tongue with thin and yellow coating, superficial and rapid pulse.

Hoarseness-Relieving and Aphonia-Healing Tablet
(Heat-Clearing and Toxin-Removing Method)

Ingredients	Effects	Combined Effects	Syndrome	Chief Symptoms
Olive (橄榄, Ganlan)	Clearing away heat and relieving sore throat	Clearing away heat, relieving sore throat and healing aphonia	Aphonia and sore throat due to wind-heat accumulated in the throat	Hoarseness, sore throat, dysphagia, cough, dry mouth, red tongue with thin and yellow coating, superficial and rapid pulse
Borax Refined with Water (飞硼砂, Fei Pengsha) Borneol (冰片, Bingpian)	Clearing away heat and toxic material, reducing swelling and alleviating pain			
indigowoad Leaf (大青叶, Daqingye)	Clearing away heat, cooling blood and removing toxic material			
Menthol (薄荷脑, Bohenao)	Expelling wind, Clearing away heat and relieving sore throat			
Mirabilita Crystal (寒水石, Hanshuishi)	Purging fire and clearing away toxic material			
Balloonflower Root (桔梗, Jiegeng) Licorice Root (生甘草, Sheng Gancao)	Relieving sore throat			

Points in Constitution: This formula is composed of the ingredients of Balloonflower and Licorice Decoction(桔梗甘草汤, jie geng gan cao tang) plus Powder of Borneol and Borax (冰硼散, Bingpengsan) and some other drugs for clearing toxic material and relieving sore throat.

Indications: Acute and chronic laryngopharyngitis.

Precaution: This formula is designed for aphonia and sore throat due to accumulation of wind-heat in the throat and it is not suitable for aphonia due to attack of exogenous wind-heat or dryness of the lung with yin deficiency.

Associated Formulas:

1. Decoction for Removing Heat from the Throat and Chest (清咽利膈汤, qing yan li ge tang) *Precious Collection of Throat Diseases* 《喉科紫珍集》

This is composed of Weeping Forsythia Capsule (连翘, Lianqiao), Cape Jasmine Fruit (山栀子, Shanzhizi), Baikal Skullcap Root (黄芩, Huangqin), Wild Mint Herb (薄荷, Bohe), Great Burdock Achene (牛蒡子, Niubangzi), Divaricate Saposhnikovia Root (防风, Fangfeng), Fine-leaf Schizonepeta Herb (荆芥, Jingjie), Weathered Sodium Sulfate (元明粉, Yuanmingfen), Honeysuckle Flower (金银花, Jinyinhua), Figwort Root (玄参, Xuanshen), Rhubarb (生大黄, Sheng Dahuang) and Balloonflower Root (桔梗, Jiegeng). Its actions are expelling wind and clearing away heat, purging fire and removing toxin. It is indicated for sore throat due to upward attack of the accumulated wind-heat because its wind-dispelling and heat-purging actions are better than those of Hoarseness-Relieving and Aphonia-Healing Tablet(清音片, qing yin pian).

2. Miraculous Pill with Six Drugs (六神丸, liu shen wan) *Lei Yunshang's Yongfentang Prescriptions* 《雷允上涌芬堂方》

This is made up of Pearl Powder (珍珠粉, Zhenzhufen), Cow-Bezoar (牛黄, Niuhuang), Musk (麝香, Shexiang), Red Orpiment (雄黄, Xionghuang), Toad Skin Secretion Cake (蟾酥, Chansu) and Borneol (冰片, Bingpian). Its actions are clearing away heat and toxic material, reducing swelling and alleviating pain. It is indicated for sore throat due to excessive phlegm and heat-toxin.

3. Borneol and Borax Powder (冰硼散, Bing peng san) *Orthodox Manual of Surgery* 《外科正宗》

This is made up of Borneol (冰片, Bingpian), Cinnabar (朱砂, Zhusha), Borax (硼砂, Pengsha) and Weathered Sodium Sulfate (元明粉, Yuanmingfen). Its actions are Clearing away heat and toxic material, reducing swelling and alleviating pain. By sprinkling a little of the powder over the affected areas, it can treat sore throat and erosion of mucous membrane of the oral cavity.

Chapter Twelve
Formulas for Ophthalmopathy

The first monograph on ophthalmology Essentials of Ophthalmology《银海精微》originated in Tang Dynasty and the descriptions for eye diseases are largely scattered in the books of miscelaneous diseases of internal medicine. Based on the theory of ophthalmology of TCM, the eye is regarded as five orbiculi. That is, flesh orbiculus(eyelid), blood orbiculus(canthus), qi orbiculus (the white of the eye), wind orbiculus(the black of the eye) and the water orbiculus(pupil), and they are physio-pathologically related to the five-zang(viscera) organs respectively. However, in the treatment, the eyes have a close connection with the liver and kidney. Diseases of various eye infections, chronic glaucoma, visual fatigue or asthenopia and ocular fundus illnesses are all the indications of Chinese prescriptions.

1. Four Herbs and Five Kernals Pill
（四物五子丸, si wu wu zi wan）

Source: *Standard for Diagnosis and Treatment*《证治准绳》
Composition: Chinese Angelica Root（当归, Danggui）9g
Szechwan Lovage Rhizome（川芎, Chuanxiong）9g
Prepared Rehmannia Root（熟地黄, Shudihuang）9g
White Peony Root（白芍药, Baishaoyao）9g
Barbary Wolfberry Fruit（枸杞子, Gouqizi）9g
Palmleaf Raspberry Fruit（覆盆子, Fupenzi）9g
Broom Crpress Fruit（地肤子, Difuzi）9g
Chinese Dodder Seed（菟丝子, Tusizi）9g
Plantain Seed（车前子, Cheqianzi）9g

Actions: Benefiting the kidney and supplementing essence, enriching the blood and improving acuity of sight.

Applied Syndrome: Poor vision due to deficiency of the heart and kidney, manifested as vertigo, blurred vision after a long time watching, dry mouth and throat, red tongue with little coating, thin and rapid pulse.

Points in Constitution: This formula is the Four Herbs Decoction（四物汤, si wu tang）plus some other drugs. The vision has a very close connection with yin-blood of the liver and kidney. In this formula, Four Herbs Decoction（四物汤, si wu tang）is used to enrich and regulate blood with the view to regulating the liver. The use of Barbary Wolfberry Fruit（枸杞子, Gouqizi）, Palmleaf Raspberry Fruit（覆盆子, Fupenzi）, Chinese Dodder Seed（菟丝子, Tusizi）, Broom

Crpress Fruit (地肤子, Difuzi) and Plantain Seed (车前子, Cheqianzi) is to nourish the liver and kidney, clear away liver-heat and improve acuity of sight.

Four Herbs and Five Kernels Pill
(Liver-Nourishing and Kidney-Invigorating Method)

Ingredients	Effects	Combined Effects	Syndrome	Chief Symptoms
Chinese Angelica Root (当归, Danggui) 9g Prepared Rehmannia Root (熟地黄, Shudihuang) 9g White Peony Root (白芍药, Baishaoyao) 9g Szechwan Lovage Rhizome (川芎, Chuanxiong) 9g	Enriching and regulating blood	Benefiting the kidney and supplementing essence, enriching the blood and improving acuity of sight	Deficiency of yin and blood of the liver and kidney	Blurred vision, vertigo, dry mouth and throat, red tongue with little coating, thin and rapid pulse
Barbary Wolfberry Fruit (枸杞子, Gouqizi) 9g Palmleaf Raspberry Fruit (覆盆子, Fupenzi) 9g Chinese Dodder Seed (菟丝子, Tusizi) 9g	Invigorating the kidney, supplementing essence and improving visual acuity			
Broom Crpress Fruit (地肤子, Difuzi) 9g Plantain Seed (车前子, Cheqianzi) 9g	Clearing liver heat and improving acuity of sight			

Indications:

1. Cataract.
2. Pigmentary degeneration of retina.
3. Vitreous opacity.

Associated Formulas:

1. Pill for Improving Acuity of Sight (驻景丸, zhu jing wan) *Prescriptions of Peaceful Benevolent Dispensary* 《和剂局方》

This is composed of Prepared Rehmannia Root (熟地黄, Shudihuang), Plantain Seed (车前子, Cheqianzi) and Chinese Dodder Seed (菟丝子, Tusizi). Its actions are tonifying the liver and kidney, nourishing yin and improving acuity of sight. It is indicated for blurred vision, epiphora induced by wind and thin pulse due to yin-deficiency of liver and kidney.

2. Nebula-Removing Decoction (退翳汤, tui yi tang) *Clinical Notes of Ophthalmology* 《眼科临证笔记》

This is composed of Figwort Root (玄参, Xuanshen), Common Anemarrhena Rhizome (知母, Zhimu), Dried Rehmannia Root (生地黄, Shengdihuang), Dwarf Lilyturf Root (麦门冬, Maimendong), Tribulus Fruit (白蒺藜, Baijili), Common Scouring Rush Herb (木贼, Muzei), Chrysanthemum Flower (菊花, Juhua), Feather Cockscomb Seed (青葙子, Qingxiangzi), Cicada Slough (蝉蜕, Chantui), Chinese Dodder Seed (菟丝子, Tusizi) and Licorice Root (生甘草, Sheng Gancao). Its actions are nourishing yin and removing nebula to improve the visual acuity. It is indicated for interstitial keratitis due to deficiency of liver-yin.

3. Magnetite Kidney-Tonifying Pill (补肾磁石丸, bu shen ci shi wan) *Prescriptions for Rescuing the Sick*《济生方》

This is composed of Magnetite (磁石, Cishi), Chrysanthemum Flower (菊花, Juhua), Abalone Shell (石决明, Shijueming), Desertliving Cistanche Herb (肉苁蓉, Roucongrong) and Chinese Dodder Seed (菟丝子, Tusizi). Its actions are invigorating the kidney, calming the liver, replenishing essence and improving acuity of sight. It is indicated for poor vision, hyperopia, blurred vision, lumbago, wiry pulse due to failure of essence and blood to nourish the eyes resulting from deficiency of both the liver and kidney.

4. Seven Immortals Pill (七仙丸, qi xian wan) *Prescriptions for Universal Benevolence*《普济方》

This is composed of Chinese Dodder Seed (菟丝子, Tusizi), Medicinal Indian Mulberry Root (巴戟天, Bajitian), Chrysanthemum Flower (菊花, Juhua), Prepared Rehmannia Root (熟地黄, Shudihuang), Desertliving Cistanche Herb (肉苁蓉, Roucongrong), Plantain Seed (车前子, Cheqianzi) and Barbary Wolfberry Fruit (枸杞子, Gouqizi). Its actions are benefiting the kidney and replenishing essence, enriching blood and improving acuity of sight. It is indicated for poor vision, dizziness and epiphora induced by wind due to deficiency of both the liver and kidney.

5. Rehmannia Pill with Nine Seeds (九子地黄丸, jiu zi di huang wan) *Pu Fuzhou's Medical Experience*《蒲辅周医疗经验》

This is composed of Prepared Rehmannia Root (熟地黄, Shudihuang), Asiatic Cornelian Cherry Fruit (山萸肉, Shanyurou), Common Yam Rhizome (山药, Shanyao), Tuckahoe (茯苓, Fuling), Oriental Waterplantain Rhizome (泽泻, Zexie), Tree Peony Bark (牡丹皮, Mudanpi), Chinese Magnoliavine Fruit (五味子, Wuweizi), Barbary Wolfberry Fruit (枸杞子, Gouqizi), Flatstem Milkvetch Seed (沙苑子, Shayuanzi), Cassia Seed (决明子, Juemingzi), Feather Cockscomb Seed (青葙子, Qingxiangzi), Motherwort Fruit (茺蔚子, Chongweizi), Chinese Dodder Seed (菟丝子, Tusizi), Palmleaf Raspberry Fruit (覆盆子, Fupenzi) and Plantain Seed (车前子, Cheqianzi). Its actions are nourishing the liver and kidney to improve acuity of sight. It is indicated for hypopsia, red tongue with little coating, thin and rapid pulse due to deficiency of both the liver and kidney.

2. Dendrobium Eyesight-Improving Pill
（石斛夜光丸，shi hu yin guang wan）

Source: *Mechanism and Treatment of Eye Disease*《原机启微》

Composition: Cochinchinese Asparagus Root (天门冬, Tianmendong)
Ginseng (人参, Renshen)
Tuckahoe (茯苓, Fuling)
Dried Rehmannia Root (生地黄, Shengdihuang)
Prepared Rehmannia Root (熟地黄, Shudihuang)
Dwarf lilyturf Root (麦门冬, Maimendong)
Common Yam Rhizome (山药, Shanyao)
Barbary Wolfberry Fruit (枸杞子, Gouqizi)
Twotooth Achyranthes Root (淮牛膝, Huai Niuxi)
Dendrobium Herb (石斛, Shihu)
Cassia Seed (草决明, Caojueming)
Apricot Seed (杏仁, Xingren)
Chrysanthemum Flower (菊花, Juhua)
Chinese Dodder Seed (菟丝子, Tusizi)
Antelope Horn (羚羊角, Lingyangjiao)
Desertliving Cistanche Herb (肉苁蓉, Roucongrong)
Chinese Magnoliavine Fruit (五味子, Wuweizi)
Divaricate Saposhnikovia Root (防风, Fangfeng)
Licorice Root (生甘草, Sheng Gancao)
Tribulus Fruit (白蒺藜, Baijili)
Coptis Rhizome (黄连, Huanglian)
Bitter Orange (枳壳, Zhiqiao)
Szechwan Lovage Rhizome (川芎, Chuanxiong)
Asiatic Rhinoceros Horn (犀角, Xijiao), replaced by Buffalo Horn (水牛角, Shuiniujiao)
Feather Cockscomb Seed (青葙子, Qingxiangzi)
(It is a patent medicine and its preparation is omitted)

Actions: Nourishing the liver and kidney, clearing away heat and improving acuity of sight.

Applied Syndrome: Eye diseases due to deficiency of the liver and kidney and stirring up of deficient fire, manifested as vertigo, blurred vision, photophobia and lacrimation, red tongue with little coating, thin and rapid pulse.

Points in Constitution: This formula unites the actions of benefiting the liver and kidney, clearing away liver-heat and improving acuity of sight as one. It has both the reinforcing and purging functions and is indicated for the syndrome of both deficiency and excess, thus it is a common patent medicine for all kinds of eye diseases.

Dendrobium Eyesight-Improving Pill

(Liver-Nourishing and Kindey-Invigorating Method)

Ingredients	Effects	Combined Effects	Syndrome	Chief Symptoms
Ginseng (人参, Renshen) Common Yam Rhizome (山药, Shanyao) Tuckahoe (茯苓, Fuling)	Replenishing qi and invigorating the spleen	Nourishing the liver and kidney, clearing away heat and improving acuity of sight	Deficiency of the liver and kidney and stirring up of deficient fire	Cataract or glaucoma, vertigo, blurring vision, lacrimation, visual fatigue, red tongue with little coating, thin and rapid pulse
Cochinchinese Asparagus Root (天门冬, Tianmendong) Dwarf Lilyturf Root (麦门冬, Maimendong) Dried Rehmannia Root (生地黄, Shengdihuang) Prepared Rehmannia Root Root (熟地黄, Shudihuang) Dendrobium Herb (石斛, Shihu) Barbary Wolfberry Fruit (枸杞子, Gouqizi) Chinese Dodder Seed (菟丝子, Tusizi) Chinese Magnoliavine Fruit (五味子, Wuweizi) Desertliving Cistanche Herb (肉苁蓉, Roucongrong)	Nourishing the liver and kidney			
Cassia Seed (草决明, Caojueming) Tribulus Fruit (白蒺藜, Baijili) Chrysanthemum Flower (菊花, Juhua) Antelope Horn (羚羊角, Lingyangjiao) Asiatic Rhinoceros Horn (犀角, Xijiao) Feather Cockscomb Seed (青葙子, Qingxiangzi) Coptis Rhizome (黄连, Huanglian)	Clearing away liver-heat and improving acuity of sight			
Divaricate Saposhnikovia Root (防风, Fangfeng)	Expelling wind and clearing away heat			
Apricot Seed (杏仁, Xingren) Szechwan Lovage Rhizome (川芎, Chuanxiong) Twotooth Achyranthes Root (淮牛膝, Huai Niuxi) Bitter Orange (枳壳, Zhiqiao)	Activating flow of qi and blood circulation			
Licorice Root (生甘草, Sheng Gancao)	Coordinating the actions of various ingredients in the prescription			

Indications:
1. Cataract.
2. Central retinitis.
3. Gaucoma.

Associated Formulas:

1. Abalone Shell Pill（石决明丸, shi jue ming wan）*Effective Prescriptions*《奇效良方》

This consists of Abalone Shell（石决明，Shijueming）, Chinese Magnoliavine Fruit（五味子，Wuweizi）, Chinese Dodder Seed（菟丝子，Tusizi）, Asiatic Cornelian Cherry Fruit（山萸肉，Shanyurou）, Common Anemarrhena Rhizome（知母，Zhimu）, Manchurian Wildginger Herb（细辛，Xixin）and Prepared Rehmannia Root（熟地黄，Shudihuang）. Its actions are tonifying the liver and enriching blood to improve acuity of sight. It is indicated for poor vision due to deficiency of the liver and blood.

2. Bright Pearl Decoction（明珠饮, ming zhu yin）*Journal of New Medicine*《新医药学杂志》

This consists of Nacre（珍珠母，Zhenzhumu）, Cassia Seed（决明子，Juemingzi）, Common Selfheal Fruit-Spike（夏枯草，Xiakucao）, Chinese Angelica Root（当归，Danggui）, White Peony Root（白芍药，Baishaoyao）, Fleeceflower Root（何首乌，Heshouwu）, Flatstem Milkvetch Seed（沙苑子，Shayuanzi）, Barbary Wolfberry Fruit（枸杞子，Gouqizi）and Licorice Root（生甘草，Sheng Gancao）. Its actions are enriching the blood and nourishing the liver, clearing away liver-heat and improving acuity of sight. It is indicated for hypopsia, blurred vision, pain of the eyes, thin and rapid pulse due to deficiency of liver-blood.

3. Chrysanthemum Flower Pill for Eye Diseases（菊晴丸, ju qing wan）*Prescriptions of Peaceful Benevolent Dispensary*《和剂局方》

This consists of Barbary Wolfberry Fruit（枸杞子，Gouqizi）, Medicinal Indian Mulberry Root（巴戟天，Bajitian）, Chrysanthemum Flower（菊花，Juhua）and Desertliving Cistanche Herb（肉苁蓉，Roucongrong）. Its actions are tonifying the liver and kidney, clearing away liver-heat and improving acuity of sight. It is indicated for poor vision or blurred vision characterized by black flower and cold tears in the eyes due to deficiency of the liver and kidney.

4. Szechwan Lovage and Chinese Angelica Pill for Improving Acuity of Sight（芎归明目丸, xiong gui ming mu wan）*Source and Cause of Miscellaneous Diseases*《杂病源流犀烛》

This consists of Szechwan Lovage Rhizome（川芎，Chuanxiong）, Chinese Angelica Root（当归，Danggui）, White Peony Root（白芍药，Baishaoyao）, Dried Rehmannia Root（生地黄，Shengdihuang）, Twotooth Achyranthes Root（淮牛膝，Huai Niuxi）, Licorice Root（生甘草，Sheng Gancao）, Barbary Wolfberry Fruit（枸杞子，Gouqizi）, Cochinchinese Asparagus Root（天门冬，Tianmendong）and Chrysanthemum Flower（菊花，Juhua）. Its actions are enriching blood, clearing away liver-heat and improving acuity of sight. It is indicated for photophobia, aching pain of the eyes and dysopia due to excessive loss of blood or deficiency of blood due to old age.

5. Wether Liver Pill（羊肝丸, yang gan wan）*Effective Prescriptions for Universal Relief*《普济本事方》

This is made up of Wether Liver（羯羊肝，Jieyanggan）, Chrysanthemum Flower（菊花，

Juhua), Chinese Arborvitae Seed (柏子仁, Baiziren), Incised Notopterygium Rhizome or Root (羌活, Qianghuo), Manchurian Wildginger Herb (细辛, Xixin), Cassia Bark (肉桂, Rougui), Largehead Atractylodes Rhizome (白术, Baizhu), Chinese Magnoliavine Fruit (五味子, Wuweizi) and Coptis Rhizome (黄连, Huanglian). Its actions are calming the liver and improving acuity of sight. It is indicated for cataracts.

6. Abalone Shell Yin-Nourishing Pill (决明益阴丸, ju ming yi yin wan) *Standard for Diagnosis and Treatment*《证治准绳》

This consists of Incised Notopterygium Rhizome or Root (羌活, Qianghuo), Doubleteeth Pubescent Angelica Root (独活, Duhuo), Chinese Angelica Root (当归, Danggui), Chinese Magnoliavine Fruit (五味子, Wuweizi), Prepared Licorice Root (炙甘草, Zhi Gancao), Divaricate Saposhnikovia Root (防风, Fangfeng), Calcined Abalone Shell (煅石决明, Duan Shijueming), Cassia Seed (草决明, Caojueming), Baikal Skullcap Root (黄芩, Huangqin), Coptis Rhizome (黄连, Huanglian), Chinese Corktree Bark (黄柏, Huangbai) and Common Anemarrhena Rhizome (知母, Zhimu). Its actions are nourishing yin and improving acuity of sight. It is indicated for prolonged photophobia, palpebral dryness which causes difficulty in opening the eye and excessive eye secretion and tears.

7. Antelope Horn Decoction (羚羊角饮子, ling yang jiao ying zi) *A Valuable Manual of Ophthalmology*《审视瑶函》

This is made up of Antelope Horn (羚羊角, Lingyangjiao), Divaricate Saposhnikovia Root (防风, Fangfeng), Tuckahoe (茯苓, Fuling), Baikal Skullcap Root (黄芩, Huangqin), Prepared Rehmannia Root (熟地黄, Shudihuang), Balloonflower Root (桔梗, Jiegeng), Barbary Wolfberry Fruit (枸杞子, Gouqizi), Ginseng (人参, Renshen), Plantain Seed (车前子, Cheqianzi), Manchurian Wildginger Herb (细辛, Xixin), Figwort Root (元参, Yuanshen) and Common Anemarrhena Rhizome (知母, Zhimu). Its actions are nourishing yin, clearing away liver-heat and improving acuity of sight. It is indicated for nebula due to deficiency of yin-fluid.

8. Liver-Nourishing Pill (养肝丸, yang gan wan) *Prescriptions for Rescuring the Sick*《济生方》

This is made up of Chinese Angelica Root (当归, Danggui), Plantain Seed (车前子, Cheqianzi), Divaricate Saposhnikovia Root (防风, Fangfeng), White Peony Root (白芍药, Baishaoyao), Fragrant Solomonseal Rhizome (葳蕤, Weirui), Prepared Rehmannia Root (熟地黄, Shudihuang), Szechwan Lovage Rhizome (川芎, Chuanxiong) and Pepermulberry Fruit (楮实子, Chushizi). Its actions are nourishing the liver and enriching blood. It is indicated for blurring of vision, excessive eye secretion and tears and visual fatigue due to deficiency of liver-blood.

9. Rehmannia Yin-Nourishing Pill (济阴地黄丸, ji yin di huang wan) *Standard for Diagnosis and Treatment*《证治准绳》

This is made up of Chinese Magnoliavine Fruit (五味子, Wuweizi), Dwarf Lilyturf Root (麦门冬, Maimendong), Chinese Angelica Root (当归, Danggui), Prepared Rehmannia Root (熟地黄, Shudihuang), Desertliving Cistanche Herb (肉苁蓉, Roucongrong), Asiatic Cornelian Cherry Fruit (山茱萸, Shanzhuyu), Common Yam Rhizome (山药, Shanyao), Barbary Wolfberry Fruit (枸杞子, Gouqizi), Chrysanthemum Flower (菊花, Juhua) and Medicinal Indian

Mulberry Root (巴戟天, Bajitian). Its actions are nourishing yin, clearing away heat and improving acuity of sight. It is indicated for platycoria, poor vision, dryness, uneasy feeling and pain of the eyes and photophobia due to deficiency of Three Yin Channels of Foot and stirring up of deficient fire.

10. Pupils-Benefiting Pill (益瞳丸, yi tong wan) *Records of Traditional Chinese and Western Medicine in Combination*《医学衷中参西录》

This is composed of Pilose Asiabell Root (党参, Dangshen), Asiatic Cornelian Cherry Fruit (山茱萸, Shanzhuyu), Fried Chinese Arborvitae Seed (炒柏子仁, Chao Baiziren), Figwort Root (玄参, Xuanshen), Fried Chinese Dodder Seed (炒菟丝子, Chao Tusizi) and Liver of Sheep (羊肝, Yanggan). Its actions are nourishing the liver and kidney. It is indicated for poor vision and platycoria due to deficiency of the liver and kidney.

11. Barbary Wolfberry, Chrysanthemum and Rehmannia Pill (杞菊地黄丸, qi ju di huang wan) *Medical Rank*《医级》

This is composed of Barbary Wolfberry Fruit (枸杞子, Gouqizi), Chrysanthemum Flower (菊花, Juhua), Prepared Rehmannia Root (熟地黄, Shudihuang), Asiatic Cornelian Cherry Fruit (山茱萸, Shanzhuyu), Common Yam Rhizome (山药, Shanyao), Oriental Waterplantain Rhizome (泽泻, Zexie), Tree Peony Bark (牡丹皮, Mudanpi) and Tuckahoe (茯苓, Fuling). Its actions are nourishing the liver and improving acuity of sight. It is indicated for blurring of vision, strabismal or dryness, uneasy feeling and pain of the eyes due to deficiency of liver blood.

12. Rehmannia Eyesight-Improving Pill (明目地黄丸, ming mu di huang wan) A *Valuable Manual of Ophthalmology*《审视瑶函》

This is composed of Prepared Rehmannia Root (熟地黄, Shudihuang), Dried Rehmannia Root (生地黄, Shengdihuang), Common Yam Rhizome (山药, Shanyao), Asiatic Cornelian Cherry Fruit (山茱萸, Shanzhuyu), Tree Peony Bark (牡丹皮, Mudanpi), Oriental Waterplantain Rhizome (泽泻, Zexie), Indian Bread with Hostwood (茯神, Fushen), Chinese Magnoliavine Fruit (五味子, Wuweizi) and Chinese Angelica Root (当归, Danggui). Its actions are nourishing yin and invigorating the kidney, replenishing essence and improving acuity of sight. It is indicated for blurring of vision and hypopsia due to deficiency of kidney-yin.

3. Yingzhong Powder
(应钟散, ying zhong san)

Source: *Yang's Formulae Handed Down by Family*《杨氏家藏方》
Composition: Rhubarb (生大黄, Sheng Dahuang)6g
Szechwan Lovage Rhizome (川芎, Chuanxiong)6g
Actions: Removing heat from the blood and clearing away toxic material, activating blood circulation and expelling wind.
Applied Syndrome: Various diseases of the head and face due to upward invasion of blood-heat and stagnation of noxious heat.

Yingzhong Powder
(Blood-Cooling and Toxin-Removing Method; Blood-Activating and Wind-Expelling Method)

Ingredients	Effects	Combined Effects	Syndrome	Chief Symptoms
Rhubarb (生大黄, Sheng Dahuang)6g	Purging blood stasis and heat, clearing away toxic material and activating blood circulation	Removing heat from the blood and clearing toxic material, activating blood circulation and expelling wind	Upward invasion of blood-heat and stagnation of heat-toxin in the head	Various eye diseases due to heat-toxin of the head, odontalgia and blood stasis (mixed with heat)
Szechwan Lovage Rhizome (川芎, Chuanxiong)6g	Expelling wind and heat, activating blood circulation, alleviating pain and directing the effects of other drugs ascending			

Points in Constitution: Rhubarb (生大黄, Sheng Dahuang) descends to purge the stagnated heat drastically while Szechwan Lovage Rhizome (川芎, Chuanxiong) ascends to dissipate blood stasis. Thus stagnations of qi and fire are expelled and blood stasis eliminated. Dispersing and purging the lower-jiao to treat the diseases in the upper jiao is a wonderful treatment. For those without constipation, Rhubarb (大黄, Dahuang) should be fried with wine to reduce its drastic purging action and strengthen the action of circulation of blood.

Indications:

1. Various eye diseases such as acute or chronic dacryocystitis, acute or chronic conjunctivitis, trachoma, cataract, etc.

2. Headache, dizziness, tinnitus, itching and desquamation of scurf, odontalgia accompanied with constipation.

3. Blood stasis due to trauma.

Precaution: It is forbidden for deficient syndrome.

Associated Formulas:

1. Decoction for Purging Blood Stasis (下瘀血汤, xia yu xue tang) *Synopsis of Golden Cabinet* 《金匮要略》

This is made up of Rhubarb (生大黄, Sheng Dahuang), Peach Seed (桃仁, Taoren) and Fried Ground Beetle (炒䗪虫, Chao Zhechong). Its actions are removing blood stasis drastically. It is indicated for puerperant ache in the abdomen due to blood stasis below the umbilicus. Besides, it is also indicated for irregular menstruation.

2. Resistant Decoction (抵当汤, di dang tang) *Treatise on Exogenous Febrile Diseases* 《伤寒论》

This includes Leech (水蛭, Shuizhi), Gadfly (虻虫, Mangchong), Peach Seed (桃仁, Taoren) and Rhubarb (生大黄, Sheng Dahuang). Its actions are removing blood stasis drastically. It is indicated for exogenous febrile diseases with blood retention, mania and amnestic, hardness and fullness sensation in the lower abdomen, normal urination, easy defecation with black stool, deep and knotted pulse; or irregular menstruation, hardness and fullness feeling in the lower abdomen with tenderness in woman.

4. Vision Acuity-Improving Pill
(驻景丸, zhu jing wan)

Source: *Prescriptions of Peaceful Benevolent Dispensary*《和剂局方》
Composition: Prepared Rehmannia Root (熟地黄, Shudihuang) 15g
Chinese Dodder Seed (菟丝子, Tusizi) 30g
Plantain Seed (车前子, Cheqianzi) 15g
Actions: Replenishing the liver and kidney, nourishing yin and improving acuity of sight.
Applied Syndrome: Eye diseases due to deficiency of liver-yin and kidney-yin, manifested as blurring of vision, or nebula, poor vision, epiphora induced by wind, dizziness, tinnitus, red tongue, thin and rapid pulse.

Vision Acuity-Improving Pill
(Liver-Nourishing and Kidney-Invigorating Method)

Ingredients	Effects	Combined Effects	Syndrome	Chief Symptoms
Prepared Rehmannia Root (熟地黄, Shudihuang) 15g	Nourishing yin and benefiting the kidney, enriching the blood and nourishing the liver	Strengthening the liver and kidney, replenishing the essence and improving acuity of sight	Deficiency of liver-yin and kidney yin	Blurring of vision, dryness and uneasy feeling of the eyes, dizziness and tinnitus, red tongue and rapid pulse
Chinese Dodder Seed (菟丝子, Tusizi) 30g	Replenishing the essence and improving acuity of sigh			
Plantain Seed (车前子, Cheqianzi) 15g	Improving acuity of sight, promoting urination and purging heat of the liver and kidney			

Points in Constitution: Prepared Rehmannia (熟地黄, Shudihuang) can nourish yin while Chinese Dodder Seed (菟丝子, Tusizi) can restore yang. Plantain Seed (车前子, Cheqianzi) has the actions of clearing away heat, promoting urination and improving acuity of sight. The composition of these three drugs makes the formula become a tonifying one but contains a pathogen-purging action. As a result, it exerts an invigorating effectwwithout retaining the pathogens.

Indications:
1. Central retinitis.
2. Vitreous opacity.
3. Conglutination behind sclera.
4. Optic atrophy.

Precaution: This formula is designed for blurring of vision due to deficiency of liver-yin and kidney-yin. It is not suitable for the case due to pathogenic factors of excess type and damp-heat.

Associated Formula:

Modified Vision Acuity-Improving Pill （驻景丸加减方, zhu jing wan jia jian fang） *Important Principles of Six Meridians of Ophthalmology*《眼科六经法要》

This is composed of Chinese Dodder Seed （菟丝子, Tusizi）, Pepermulberry Fruit （楮实子, Chushizi）, Barbary Wolfberry Fruit （枸杞子, Gouqizi）, Plantain Seed （车前子, Cheqianzi）, Mirabilita Crystal （寒水石, Hanshuishi）, Chinese Magnoliavine Fruit （五味子, Wuweizi）, Motherwort Fruit （茺蔚子, Chongweizi）, Sanchi Root （三七, Sanqi）, Dried Human Placenta （紫河车, Ziheche） and Common Floweringquince Fruit （木瓜, Mugua）. Its actions are nourishing the liver and kidney, activating blood circulation and improving acuity of sight. It is indicated for blurring of vision without exterior impairment of the eyes, feeling of black spots in the eyes which give muscaegenic vision, or feeling of mosquito and flies dancing in front of the eyes.

5. Qi-Replenishing, Hearing-improving and Eyesight-Acuminating Decoction （益气聪明汤, yi qi cong ming tang）

Source: *Dongyuan's Effective Prescriptions*《东垣试效方》

Composition: Toasted Membranous Milkvetch Root （炙黄芪, Zhi Huangqi）15g

Ginseng （人参, Renshen）15g

White Peony Root （白芍药, Baishaoyao）3g

Chinese Corktree Bark （黄柏, Huangbai）3g

Shunk Bugbane Rhizome （升麻, Shengma）6g

Pueraria（葛根, Gegen）6g

Threeleaf Chastertree Fruit （蔓荆子, Manjingzi）6g

Licorice Root （生甘草, Sheng Gancao）15g

Actions: Replenishing qi and lifting yang, improving faculty of hearing and acuity of sight.

Applied Syndrome: Deficiency of qi in the middle-jiao and failure of clear yang to ascend, manifested as beginning of a cataract, dim view, blurring vision, deafness and tinnitus.

Points in Constitution: This formula has the actions of replenishing qi and lifting yang simultaneously, which can raise clear yang and reduce excessive fire so that faculty of hearing and acuity of sight are improved.

Indications:
1. Senile cataract.

2. Chromatelopsia, monochromattism.
3. Hypoacusis.
4. Otogenic vertigo.

Qi-Replenishing, Hearing-improving and Eyesight-Acuminating Decoction
(Qi-Replenishing and Yang-Lifting Method)

Ingredients	Effects	Combined Effects	Syndrome	Chief Symptoms
Ginseng (人参, Renshen) 15g Toasted Membranous Milkvetch Root (炙黄芪, Zhi Huangqi) 15g Licorice Root (生甘草, Sheng Gancao) 15g	Invigorating the spleen and stomach	Replenishing qi and lifting yang, improving faculty of hearing and acuity of sight	Deficiency of middle-jiao qi and failure of clear yang to ascend	Nebula, blurring vision, deafness and tinnitus, pale tongue with thin coating, feeble and weak pulse
Shunk Bugbane Rhizome (升麻, Shengma) 6g Pueraria (葛根, Gegen) 6g	Raising clear yang and invigorating stomach-qi			
Threeleaf Chastertree Fruit (蔓荆子, Manjingzi) 6g	Clearing and benefiting the head and eyes			
White Peony Root (白芍药, Baishaoyao) 3g	Astringing yin and regulating ying			
Chinese Corktree Bark (黄柏, Huangbai) 3g	Purging ministerial fire			

Precautions:

1. Crude, cold and fat food or indigestible food should be avoided.
2. This formula is not suitable for eye disease due to deficiency of blood and hyperactivity of the liver, or tinnitus and deafness due to damp-heat in the liver and gallbladder.

Associated Formulas:

1. Threeleaf Chastertree Fruit Tang (蔓荆子汤, man jing zi tang) *Secret Record of the Chamber of Orchids* 《兰室秘藏》

2. This is made up of Threeleaf Chastertree Fruit (蔓荆子, Manjingzi), Wine-Prepared Chinese Corktree Bark (酒黄柏, Jiu Huangbai), White Peony Root (白芍药, Baishaoyao), Prepared Licorice Root (炙甘草, Zhi Gancao), Toasted Membranous Milkvetch Root (炙黄芪, Zhi Huangqi) and Ginseng (人参, Renshen). Its actions are replenishing qi and lifting yang, removing nebula and improving acuity of sight. It is indicated for cataracts due to overstrain and improper diet.

2. Qi-Replenishing, Hearing-Improving and Eyesight-Acuminating Decoction (益气聪明汤, yi

qi cong ming tang) *Comprehension of Medicine*《医学心悟》

This is made up of Toasted Membranous Milkvetch Root (炙黄芪, Zhi Huangqi), Ginseng (人参, Renshen), Largehead Atractylodes Rhizome (白术, Baizhu), Prepared Licorice Root (炙甘草, Zhi Gancao), Shunk Bugbane Rhizome (升麻, Shengma), Bupleurum (柴胡, Chaihu), Threeleaf Chastertree Fruit (蔓荆子, Manjingzi), Chinese Angelica Root (当归, Danggui), White Peony Root (白芍药, Baishaoyao), Tangerine Peel (橘皮, Jupi) and Chinese Date (大枣, Dazao). Its actions are replenishing qi and improving acuity of sight. It is indicated for poor vision due to qi deficiency.

Additional Formulas

Liver-Clearing and Kidney-Nourishing Decoction
(清肝养肾汤, qing gan yang shen tang)

Source: *Henan Journal of Traditional Chinese Medicine*《河南中医》
Composition: Common Selfheal Fruit-Spike (夏枯草, Xiakucao) 15g
Baikal Skullcap Root (黄芩, Huangqin) 9g
Cape Jasmine Fruit (山栀子, Shanzhizi) 9g
Barbary Wolfberry Fruit (枸杞子, Gouqizi) 15g
Glossy Privet Fruit (女贞子, Nüzhenzi) 15g
Siberian Solomonseal Rhizome (黄精, Huangjing) 15g
Tuckahoe (茯苓, Fuling) 9g
Chrysanthemum Flower (菊花, Juhua) 9g
Tree Peony Bark (牡丹皮, Mudanpi) 9g
Actions: Clearing and purging liver-fire and nourishing the liver and kidney.
Applied Syndrome: Hypopsia, micropsia or metamorphopsia, or even blindness.

Liver-Clearing and Kidney-Nourishing Decoction
(Liver Heat-Clearing and Eye Sight-Improving Method)

Ingredients	Effects	Combined Effects	Syndrome	Chief Symptoms
Common Selfheal Fruit-Spike (夏枯草, Xiakucao) 15g Baikal Skullcap Root (黄芩, Huangqin) 9g Cape Jasmine Fruit (山栀子, Shanzhizi) 9g Chrysanthemum Flower (菊花, Juhua) 9g Tree Peony Bark (牡丹皮, Mudanpi) 9g	Purging liver fire and improving acuity of sight	Clearing and purging liver-fire and nourishing the liver and kidney	Cataract (due to liver heat and deficiency of yin)	Cataract, central retinitis and blurring of vision
Barbary Wolfberry Fruit (枸杞子, Gouqizi) 15g Glossy Privet Fruit (女贞子, Nüzhenzi) 15g Siberian Solomonseal Rhizome (黄精, Huangjing) 15g	Nourishing yin and enriching blood, replenishing essence and improving acuity of sight			
Tuckahoe (茯苓, Fuling) 9g	Invigorating the spleen and tranquilizing the mind			

Points in Constitution: The characteristic of this formula lies in clearing liver-heat and nourishing the liver simultaneously. Most drugs in it can improve acuity of sight.

Indications:

1. Central retinitis.
2. Cataract.

Precautions: It should be cautiously used for the patient with deficiency of the spleen.

Associated Formulas:

1. Abalone Shell Pill(石决明丸, shi jue ming wan) *Effective Prescriptions* 《奇效良方》

This is composed of Abalone Shell (石决明, Shijueming), Chinese Magnoliavine Fruit (五味子, Wuweizi), Chinese Dodder Seed (菟丝子, Tusizi), Asiatic Cornelian Cherry Fruit (山茱萸, Shanzhuyu), Common Anemarrhena Rhizome (知母, Zhimu), Manchurian Wildginger Herb (细辛, Xixin) and Prepared Rehmannia Root Root (熟地黄, Shudihuang). Its actions are nourishing the liver, enriching blood and improving acuity of sight. It is indicated for poor vision due to deficiency of the liver and blood.

2. Dendrobium Eyesight-Improving Pill (石斛夜光丸, shi hu ye guang wan) *Mechanism and Treatment of Eye Disease* 《原机启微》

This is made up of Cochinchinese Asparagus Root (天门冬, Tianmendong), Ginseng (人参, Renshen), Tuckahoe (茯苓, Fuling), Chinese Magnoliavine Fruit (五味子, Wuweizi), Tribulus Fruit(白蒺藜, Baijili) Dendrobium Herb (石斛, Shihu), Desertliving Cistanche Herb (肉苁蓉, Roucongrong), Szechwan Lovage Rhizome (川芎, Chuanxiong), Prepared Licorice Root (炙甘草, Zhi Gancao), Fried Bitter Orange (炒枳壳, Chao Zhiqiao), Feather Cockscomb Seed (青葙子, Qingxiangzi), Divaricate Saposhnikovia Root (防风, Fangfeng), Coptis Rhizome (黄连, Huanglian), Asiatic Rhinoceros Horn (犀角, Xijiao), Antelope Horn (羚羊角, Lingyangjiao), Chrysanthemum Flower (菊花, Juhua), Chinese Dodder Seed (菟丝子, Tusizi), Common Yam Rhizome (山药, Shanyao), Barbary Wolfberry Fruit (枸杞子, Gouqizi), Twotooth Achyranthes Root (淮牛膝, Huai Niuxi), Apricot Seed (杏仁, Xingren), Dwarf Lilyturf Root (麦门冬, Maimendong), Prepared Rehmannia Root (熟地黄, Shudihuang), Dried Rehmannia Root (生地黄, Shengdihuang) and Cassia Seed(草决明, Caojueming). Its action is nourishing the liver and kidney. It is indicated for blurred vision, ambiopia or double vision and cataracts due to deficiency of both the liver and kidney.

3. Zhujing Kidney-Invigorating and Eyesight-Improving Pill(驻景补肾明目丸, zhu jing bu shen ming mu wan) *Essentials of Ophthalmology* 《银海精微》

This is composed of Chinese Magnoliavine Fruit (五味子, Wuweizi), Prepared Rehmannia Root (熟地黄, Shudihuang), Barbary Wolfberry Fruit (枸杞子, Gouqizi), Pepermulberry Fruit (楮实子, Chushizi), Desertliving Cistanche Herb (肉苁蓉, Roucongrong), Plantain Seed (车前子, Cheqianzi), Dendrobium Herb (石斛, Shihu), Magnetite (磁石, Cishi), Chinese Dodder Seed (菟丝子, Tusizi), Chinese Eaglewood Wood (沉香, Chenxiang) and Black Salt (青盐, Qingyan). Its actions are invigorating the kidney and improving acuity of sight. It is indicated for poor vision, which may gradually cause cataracts due to deficiency of both the liver and the kidney.

4. Rehmannia Eyesight-Improving Pill(明目地黄丸, ming mu di huang wan) *Prescriptions of Peaceful Benevolent Dispensary*《和剂局方》

This is made up of Dried Rehmannia Root(生地黄, Shengdihuang), Prepared Rehmannia Root(熟地黄, Shudihuang), Twotooth Achyranthes Root(淮牛膝, Huai Niuxi), Dendrobium Herb(石斛, Shihu), Bitter Orange(枳壳, Zhiqiao), Divaricate Saposhnikovia Root(防风, Fangfeng) and Apricot Seed(杏仁, Xingren). Its actions are tonifying the liver and the kidney, expelling wind and improving acuity of sight. It is indicated for poor vision, blurred vision and nebula due to deficient and heat of the liver and kidney.

5. Liver-Purging Decoction(泻肝汤, xie gan tang) *Long Mu's Secret Treatise on Eye Diseases*《秘传眼科龙木论》

This consists of Divaricate Saposhnikovia Root(防风, Fangfeng), White Peony Root(白芍药, Baishaoyao), Baikal Skullcap Root(黄芩, Huangqin), Balloonflower Root(桔梗, Jiegeng), Mirabilite(芒硝, Mangxiao) and Rhubarb(大黄, Dahuang). Its actions are benefiting the liver and clearing away heat. It is indicated for night blindness due to deficiency of the liver.

6. Liver-Purging Decoction(泻肝汤, xie gan tang) *Long Mu's Secret Treatise on Eye Diseases*《秘传眼科龙木论》

This is made up of Membranous Milkvetch Root(生黄芪, Sheng Huangqi), Common Anemarrhena Rhizome(知母, Zhimu), Baikal Skullcap Root(黄芩, Huangqin), Balloonflower Root(桔梗, Jiegeng), Mirabilite(芒硝, Mangxiao) and Rhubarb(生大黄, Sheng Dahuang). Its actions are replenishing qi and nourishing yin. It is indicated for nebula manifested as conjunctiva and lacrimation cuased by deficiency of liver and accumulation of heat.

7. Liver-Tonifying Pill(补肝丸, bu gan wan) A *Valuable Manual of Ophthalmology*《审视瑶函》

This consists of Swordlike Atractylodes Rhizome(苍术, Cangzhu), Prepared Rehmannia Root(熟地黄, Shudihuang), Cicada Slough(蝉蜕, Chantui), Plantain Seed(车前子, Cheqianzi), Szechwan Lovage Rhizome(川芎, Chuanxiong), Main Part of Chinese Angelica Root(当归身, Dangguishen), Weeping Forsythia Capsule(连翘, Lianqiao), Bat Dung(夜明砂, Yemingsha), Incised Notopterygium Rhizome or Root(羌活, Qianghuo), Chinese Gentian Root(龙胆草, Longdancao), Chrysanthemum Flower(菊花, Juhua) and Pig's Liver(猪肝, Zhugan). Its actions are invigorating the liver and kidney, clearing away heat and improving acuity of sight. It is indicated for nebulas which is marked by variform shapes, yellow, dim and white color or slight reddish color.

8. Liver-Nourishing Pill(养肝丸, yang gan wan) *Prescriptions for Rescuring the Sick*《济生方》

This is composed of Chinese Angelica Root(当归, Danggui), Plantain Seed(车前子, Cheqianzi), Divaricate Saposhnikovia Root(防风, Fangfeng), White Peony Root(白芍药, Baishaoyao), Fragrant Solomonseal Rhizome(玉竹, Yuzhu), Prepared Rehmannia Root(熟地黄, Shudihuang), Szechwan Lovage Rhizome(川芎, Chuanxiong) and Pepermulberry Fruit(楮实子, Chushizi). Its actions are tonifying the liver, enriching blood and improving acuity of sight. It is indicated for blurring of vision and visual fatigue due to deficiency of liver-blood.

9. Vision Acuity-Improving Pill(驻景丸, zhu jing wan) *Standard for Diagnosis and Treatment*《证治准绳》

This is made up of Prepared Rehmannia Root (熟地黄, Shudihuang), Plantain Seed (车前子, Cheqianzi), Chinese Dodder Seed (菟丝子, Tusizi), Barbary Wolfberry Fruit (枸杞子, Gouqizi) and Tuckahoe (茯苓, Fuling) or Grassleaf Sweetflag Rhizome (菖蒲, Changpu). Its actions are nourishing the liver and kidney, enriching blood and improving acuity of sight. It is indicated for blurring of vision and nebula due to deficiency of both the liver and kidney.

Chapter Thirteen
Formulas for Cancer and AIDS

There are numerous Chinese formulas which have curative effects on cancer. They may be roughly classified into five categories: 1) The formulas for clearing away heat and toxic materials; 2) The formulas for combating toxifying disease with poisonous agents; 3) Formulas for resolving phlegm and removing mass; 4) Formulas for activating the blood circulation to remove blood stasis; 5) Formulas for strengthening the body resistance to eliminate pathogenic factors. Furthermore, when they are cooperated with operation, radiotherapy or chemotherapy, vast prospects have been shown in elevating the function of the cellular and humoral immunity, regulating the ratio of CAMP to CGMP in cells, improving the metabolism and hematopoiesis of the body, decreasing side-effects of radiotherapy or chemotherapy and increasing the survival quality of the patient.

1. Cow Bezoar Pill
(犀黄丸, xi huang wan)

Source: *Surgery Life-Saving Collection* 《外科全生集》
Composition: Cow Bezoar (牛黄, Niuhuang)
Musk (麝香, Shexiang)
Olibanum (乳香, Ruxiang)
Myrrh (没药, Moyao)
(It is a patent medicine and its preparation is omitted)
Actions: Removing toxic material and reducing swelling, resolving phlegm and dissipating blockages, activating blood circulation and removing blood stasis.
Applied Syndrome: Liver cancer due to accumulation of blood stasis and phlegm in the interior, manifested as mass in the hypochondrium, pain with tenderness in the hypochondrium which may radiate to the back and aggravate in the night, distention and fullness sensation in the gastric region and abdomen, dark purplish tongue or ecchymosis, deep and thin pulse or wiry and unsmooth pulse.
Points in Constitution: Olibanum (乳香, Ruxiang) and Myrrh (没药, Moyao) have the actions of activating blood circulation and removing blood stasis. When they are combined with Cow Bezoar (牛黄, Niuhuang) which is fragrant and Musk (麝香, Shexiang) which tends to travels around the body, they can clear away toxin, resolve phlegm and remove the obstruction of the meridians and collaterals. This formula shows the characteristic of Traditional Chinese Medicine in using the animal drugs to treat the stubborn and severe diseases.

Cow Bezoar Pills
(Swelling-Reducing and Blood Stasis-Removing Method)

Ingredients	Effects	Combined Effects	Syndrome	Chief Symptoms
Cow Bezoar (牛黄, Niuhuang)	Clearing away heat and toxic material, resolving phlegm and dissipating blockages	Removing toxic material and reducing swelling, resolving phlegm and dissipating blockages, activating blood circulation and removing blood stasis	Stagnation of toxic substance in the interior due to accumulation of blood stasis and phlegm	Liver cancer, etc.
Musk (麝香, Shexiang)	Activating blood circulation, dissipating blockages and penetrating the meridians and collaterals			
Olibanum (乳香, Ruxiang) Myrrh (没药, Moyao)	Activating blood circulation and removing blood stasis, reducing swelling and alleviating pain			

Indications:
1. Liver cancer.
2. Gastric cancer.
3. Carcinoma of esophagus.
4. Mammary cancer.

Precaution: For those who are weak or have an emaciated body, it is not suitable to be taken for a long time.

Associated Formulas:

1. Modifed Cow Bezoar Pill (加味犀黄丸, jia wei xi huang wan) *Proved Recipes*《经验方》

This is made up of Olibanum (乳香, Ruxiang), Myrrh (没药, Moyao), Cow-Bezoar (牛黄, Niuhuang), Musk (麝香, Shexiang), Nux Vomica (马钱子, Maqianzi), Crumb of ivory (象牙屑, Xiangyaxie), Gecko (壁虎, Bihu), Toad Skin Secretion Cake (蟾酥, Chansu), Niter (硝仁, Xiaoren), Alum (矾石, Fanshi), Chicken Gizzard Membrane (鸡内金, Jineijin), Trogopterus Dung (五灵脂, Wulingzhi), Nux Vomica (马钱子, Maqianzi), Dead of Pangolin Scales (山甲珠, Shanjiazhu), Rhus Resin (干漆, Ganqi) and Bitter Orange (枳壳, Zhiqiao). Its actions are removing phlegm and dissipating blockages, activating blood circulation and removing blood stasis. It is indicated for late lung cancer, laryngocarcinoma, gastric cancer and carcinoma of esophagus.

2. Toxin-Clearing and Swelling-Reducing Pill (醒消丸, xing xiao wan) *Prescriptions of Peaceful Benevolent Dispensary*《和剂局方》

This is made up of Red Orpiment (雄黄, Xionghuang), Musk (麝香, Shexiang), Olibanum (乳香, Ruxiang), Myrrh (没药, Moyao) and Cooked Glutinous Millet (黄米饭, Huangmifan). Its actions are activating blood circulation, resolving phlegm, reducing swelling and relieving pain. It is indicated for liver cancer and mammary cancer.

3. Decoction for Recovery and Activating Blood Circulation (复元活血汤, fu yuan huo xue tang) *Invention of Medicine* 《医学发明》

This is composed of Bupleurum (柴胡, Chaihu), Chinese Angelica Root (当归, Danggui), Snakegourd Root (天花粉, Tianhuafen), Peach Seed (桃仁, Taoren), Safflower (红花, Honghua), Stir-Backed Pangolin Scales (炮山甲, Pao shanjia) and Prepared Rhubarb with Wine (酒大黄, Jiu Dahuang). Its actions are dispersing the stagnated liver-qi, activating channels and collaterals, promoting flow of qi and blood and removing blood stasis. It is indicated for pain in the hypochondrium due to traumatic injury. Besides, it also treats liver cancer.

4. Pizaihuang (片仔癀, pian zai huang) *Proved Recipes* 《经验方》

Since it is a patent medicine, the composition is omitted. Its actions are clearing away toxic material, dissipating blockages, alleviating pain and healing sores. It is indicated for nail-like boils and sores, insect bites and snake bite. In recent years it is applied for all kinds of cancers and chronic hepatitis.

2. Minor Panacea Pellet
(小金丹, xiao jin dan)

Source: *Surgery Life-Saving Collection* 《外科全生集》
Composition: Prepared Nux vomica (制马钱子, Zhi Maqianzi)
Musk (麝香, Shexiang)
Sweetgum Resin (白胶香, Baijiaoxiang)
Earth Worm (地龙, Dilong)
North Monkshood (草乌, Caowu)
Trogopterus Dung (五灵脂, Wulingzhi)
Chinese Angelica Root (当归, Danggui)
Olibanum (乳香, Ruxiang)
Myrrh (没药, Moyao)
Chinese Ink charcoal (墨炭, Motan)
(It is a patent medicine and its preparation is omitted.)

Actions: Activating blood circulation and removing blood stasis, reducing swelling and alleviating pain.

Applied Syndrome: Pyogenic infection of bone, scrofula and breast cancer due to blood stasis, manifested as beginning of a lump with normal skin, swelling, hardness and pain, dark purplish tongue, deep and unsmooth pulse.

Minor Panacea Pellet
(Blood Stasis-Removing and Swelling-Reducing Method)

Ingredients	Effects	Combined Effects	Syndrome	Chief Symptoms
Prepared Nux Vomica (制马钱子, Zhi Maqianzi)	Removing phlegm and toxin between the skin and the membrane	Activating blood circulation and dissolving blood stasis, reducing swelling and alleviating pain	Blood stasis in the interior	Pyogenic infection of bone, scrofula, breast cancer, beginning of lump, normal skin, swelling, hardness and pain, dark purplish tongue, deep and unsmooth pulse
Musk (麝香, Shexiang) Sweetgum Resin (白胶香, Baijiaoxiang)	Regulating flow of qi and blood, relieving carbuncle and gangrene, clearing toxic material and alleviating pain			
Trogopterus Dung (五灵脂, Wulingzhi) Chinese Angelica Root (当归, Danggui) Olibanum (乳香, Ruxiang) Myrrh (没药, Moyao) Earth Worm (地龙, Dilong)	Activating blood circulation and removing blood stasis, reducing swelling and alleviating pain			
North Monkshood (草乌, Caowu)	Warming the meridian and alleviating pain			
Chinese Ink Charcoal (墨炭, Motan)	Clearing away toxic material and reducing swelling			

Points in Constitution: In this formula, Prepared Nux Vomica (制马钱子, Zhi Maqianzi) is integrated with the drugs for activating blood circulation and dredging the collaterals. Then Musk (麝香, Shexiang) is used to dredge qi and blood in twelve channels. Thus, swelling and mass are removed.

Indications:

1. Osteosarcoma.
2. Bone tuberculosis.
3. Mammary cancer.
4. Thyroid enlargement.
5. Tuberculous lymphadenitis.

Precaution: Since Nux Vomica (马钱子, Maqianzi) is poisonous, attention should be paid to its amount. Equally, the potency of this formula is strong and drastic, thus for those with weakened bodies and deficiency of healthy qi, it can not be used internally for a long time.

3. Liver-Clearing and Stagnation-Removing Decocting
(清肝解郁汤, qing gan jie yu tang)

Source: *Orthodox Manual of Surgery* 《外科正宗》
Composition: Tangerine Peel (橘皮, Jupi)9g
White Peony Root (白芍药, Baishaoyao)9g
Szechwan Lovage Rhizome (川芎, Chuanxiong)9g
Chinese Angelica Root (当归, Danggui)9g
Dried Rehmannia Root (生地黄, Shengdihuang)9g
Pinellia Rhizome (半夏, Banxia)9g
Nutgrass Galingale Rhizome (香附, Xiangfu)9g
Green Tangerine Peel (青皮, Qingpi)9g
Thinleaf Milkwort Root (远志, Yuanzhi)9g
Indian Bread with Hostwood (茯神, Fushen)9g
Thunberg Fritillary Bulb (浙贝母, Zhe Beimu)9g
Perilla Leaf (紫苏, Zisu)6g
Balloonflower Root (桔梗, Jiegeng)9g
Licorice Root (甘草, Gancao)6g
Cape Jasmine Fruit (山栀子, Shanzhizi)9g
Akebia Stem (木通, Mutong)9g

Actions: Clearing away liver-heat and relieving the depressed qi, activating flow of qi and dissipating blockages.

Applied Syndrome: Mammary cancer due to failure of the liver in dispersion resulting from melancholy and stagnation of qi, manifested as mammary lump without pain and itching at the beginning, or discomfort of the chest, lassitude, sallow complexion, poor appetite, depression, pale tongue and wiry pulse.

Points in Constitution: This formula is similar to Merry Life Powder (逍遥散, xiao yao san). However, compared with Merry Life Powder (逍遥散, xiao yao san), the actions of activating flow of qi and dissipating blockage is powerful. This formula is not specially designed for breast cancer, but after being modified, it is suitable for breast cancer.

Indications:
1. Hyperplasia of mammary glands.
2. Fibroadenoma of breast.
3. Mammary cancer.
4. Hebephrenic mastitis.
5. Mammary tuberculosis.

Liver-Clearing and Stagnation-Removing Decocting
(Liver-Soothing and Qi-Regulating Method)

Ingredients	Effects	Combined Effects	Syndrome	Chief Symptoms
Nutgrass Galingale Rhizome (香附, Xiangfu)9g Green Tangerine Peel (青皮, Qingpi)9g Perilla Leaf (紫苏, Zisu)6g	Dispersing the stagnated liver-qi	Clearing away liver-heat and relieving the depressed qi, activating flow of qi and dissipating blockages	Mammary cancer due to stagnation of liver-qi	Mammary hard lump without pain and itching at the beginning, or discomfort of the chest, lassitude, pale tongue, wiry pulse
Tangerine Peel (橘皮, Jupi)9g Pinellia Rhizome (半夏, Banxia)9g Thunberg Fritillary Bulb (浙贝母, Zhe Beimu)9g Balloonflower Root (桔梗, Jiegeng)9g	Removing phlegm and dissipating blockages			
Chinese Angelica Root (当归, Danggui)9g White Peony Root (白芍药, Baishaoyao)9g Dried Rehmannia Root (生地黄, Shengdihuang)9g Szechwan Lovage Rhizome (川芎, Chuanxiong)9g	Enriching and regulating blood			
Thinleaf Milkwort Root (远志, Yuanzhi)9g Indian Bread with Hostwood (茯神, Fushen)9g	Tranquilizing the mind and calming the spirit			
Cape Jasmine Fruit (山栀, Shanzhi)9g Akebia Stem (木通, Mutong)9g	Clearing away heat and relieving restless			
Licorice Root (甘草, Gancao)6g	Coordinating the actions of various ingredients in the prescription			

Precaution: During the medication, the patient should pay attention to mental regulation and try to avoid worry, overthinking and anger.

Associated Formulas:

1. Merry Life Powder (逍遥散, xiao yao san) *Prescriptions of Peaceful Benevolent Dispensary* 《和剂局方》

This is made up of Bupleurum (柴胡, Chaihu), Chinese Angelica Root (当归, Danggui), White Peony Root (白芍, Baishao), Largehead Atractylodes Rhizome (白术, Baizhu), Tuckahoe (茯苓, Fuling), Prepared Licorice Root (炙甘草, Zhi Gancao), Wild Mint Herb (薄荷, Bohe) and Roasted Ginger (煨姜, Weijiang). Its actions are dispersing the stagnated liver-qi and invigorating the spleen, enriching blood and regulating menstruation. It is also indicated for irregular menstruation and distending pain of mamma due to stagnation of the liver-qi, deficiency of blood and failure of the spleen in transportation and transformation.

2. Liver-Soothing Pill (舒肝丸, shu gan wan) *Shandong Standard of Chinese Patent Medicine* 《山东中成药标准》

This consists of Szechwan Chinaberry Fruit (川楝子, Chuanlianzi), White Peony Root (白芍药, Baishaoyao), Turmeric Rhizome (姜黄, Jianghuang), Corydalis Tuber (延胡索, Yanhusuo), Fried Bitter Orange (炒枳壳, Chao Zhiqiao), Chinese Eaglewood Wood (沉香, Chenxiang), Tuckahoe (茯苓, Fuling), Common Aucklandia Root (木香, Muxiang), Tangerine Peel (橘皮, Jupi), Villous Amomum Fruit (砂仁, Sharen), Officinal Magnolia Bark (厚朴, Houpo), Round Cardamom Seed (白豆蔻, Baidoukou) and Cinnabar (朱砂, Zhusha). Its actions are dispersing the liver and relieving depression, regulating flow of qi and alleviating pain. It is indicated for mammary lumps with distending pain due to depressed liver-qi.

3. Liver-Soothing and Nodules-Eliminating Prescrioption (疏肝消核方, shu gan xiao he fang) *Huang's Prescriptions*《黄氏方》

This is composed of Bupleurum (柴胡, Chaihu), Largehead Atractylodes Rhizome (白术, Baizhu), Turmeric Root-Tuber (郁金, Yujin), Nutgrass Galingale Rhizome (香附, Xiangfu), Corydalis Tuber (延胡索, Yanhusuo), Snakegourd Peel (瓜蒌皮, Gualoupi), Chinese Angelica Root (当归, Danggui), Tangerine Seed (桔核, Juhe), Tuckahoe (茯苓, Fuling), Kwangsi Turmeric Rhizome (莪术, Ezhu) and Prepared Licorice Root (炙甘草, Zhi Gancao). Its actions are dispersing the stagnated liver-qi, dissipating blockages, activating blood circulation and alleviating pain. It is indicated for nodules of the breast (hyperplasia of mammary glands).

Additional Formulas

Lung-Strengthening and Cancer-Resisting Decoction
(固金抗癌汤, gu jin kang ai tang)

Source: *Hebei Journal of Traditional Chinese Medicine* 《河北中医》
Composition: Dried Human Placenta (紫河车, Ziheche)21g
Snakegourd Fruit (瓜蒌, Gualou)21g
Common Selfheal Fruit-Spike (夏枯草, Xiakucao)30g
Tangerine Peel (橘皮, Jupi)21g
Coix Seed (薏苡仁, Yiyiren)21g
Kwangsi Turmeric Rhizome (莪术, Ezhu)21g
Tonkin Sophora Root (山豆根, Shandougen)15g
Lily Bulb (百合, Baihe)12g
Actions: Strengthening the lung and preventing cancer, resolving phlegm and softening hardness.
Applied Syndrome: Lung cancer due to phlegm and blood stasis accumulating in the lung, manifested as cough, hemoptysis, pain in the chest, oppressing feeling in the chest, dyspnea, emanciated body and weakness, slight purple tongue or with ecchymosis, yellow and greasy tongue coating, unsmooth pulse or deep and unsmooth pulse.

Lung-Strengthening and Cancer-Resisting Decoction
(Phlegm-Resolving and Blockage-Dissipating Method)

Ingredients	Effects	Combined Effects	Syndrome	Chief Symptoms
Dried Human Placenta (紫河车, Ziheche)21g Lily Bulb (百合, Baihe)12g	Replenishing qi and enriching blood, moistening the lung and strengthening the lung	Strengthening the lung and preventing cancer, removing phlegm and softening hardness	Lung cancer due to accumulation of phlegm and blood stasis	Cough, pain in the chest, oppressing feeling in the chest and dyspnea, hemoptysis, thin and weakness, pale tongue or with ecchymosis, yellow and greasy tongue coating, unsmooth pulse or deep and unsmooth pulse
Tonkin Sophora Root (山豆根, Shandougen)15g Common Selfheal Fruit-Spike (夏枯草, Xiakucao)30g	Clearing away heat and toxic material, removing phlegm and dissipating blockages			
Snakegourd Fruit (瓜蒌, Gualou)21g Coix Seed (薏苡仁, Yiyiren)21g Tangerine Peel (橘皮, Jupi)21g	Removing phlegm and dissipating blockages			
Kwangsi Turmeric Rhizome (莪术, Ezhu)21g	Removing blood stasis and eliminating mass			

Points in Constitution: In the formula, Tonkin Sophora Root (山豆根, Shandougen), Common Selfheal Fruit-Spike (夏枯草, Xiakucao) and Kwangsi Turmeric Rhizome (莪术, Ezhu) have the cancer-resisting action. The others are used to strengthen the body resistance and resolve phlegm. This kind of composition of the formula indicates that it is a mild one.

Indications: Primary brochial lung cancer.

Associated Formulas:

1. Lung Tumor-Removing Formula (肺瘤平, fei liu ping) *Journal of Traditional Chinese Medicine* 《中医杂志》

This includes Toasted Membranous Milkvetch Root (炙黄芪, Zhi Huangqi), Pilose Asiabell Root (党参, Dangshen), Spreading Hedyotis Herb (白花蛇舌草, Baihuasheshecao), Apricot Seed (杏仁, Xingren), Balloonflower Root (桔梗, Jiegeng), Coastal Glehnia Root (北沙参, Beishashen), Whiteflower Patrinia Herb (败酱草, Baijiangcao) and Heartleaf Houttuynia Herb (鱼腥草, Yuxingcao). Its actions are replenishing qi, nourishing yin, clearing away heat and toxic material. It is indicated for late non-parvicellularl lung cancer.

Jinyan Pill
(金岩丸, jin yan wan)

Source: *Shandong Journal of Traditional Chinese Medicine* 《山东中医杂志》

Composition: Natural Cow-Bezoar (天然牛黄, Tianran Niuhuang)1g

Musk (麝香, Shexiang)2g

Powder of Antelope Horn (羚羊角粉, Lingyangjiaofen)15g

Spreading Hedyotis Herb (白花蛇舌草, Baihuasheshecao)50g

Scorpion (全蝎, Quanxie)30g

Silkworm with Batrytis Larva (僵蚕, Jiangcan)30g

Gecko (壁虎, Bihu)21g

Centipede (蜈蚣, Wugong)6g

Pangolin Scales (穿山甲, Chuanshanjia)15g

Amber (琥珀, Hupo) 15g

Red Orpiment (雄黄, Xionghuang)6g

Borneol (冰片, Bingpian)2g

Dragon's Blood (血竭, Xuejie)6g

Rhubarb (大黄, Dahuang)9g

Natural Indigo (青黛, Qingdai)9g

Prepared Nux-vomica Seed (制马钱子, Zhi Maqianzi)6g

Prepared Olibanum (制乳香, Zhi Ruxiang)6g

Prepared Myrrh (制没药, Zhi Moyao)6g

Toad Skin Secretion Cake (蟾酥, Chansu)0.5g

Cinnabar (朱砂, Zhusha)6g

Saffron Crocus Stigma (藏红花, Zanghonghua) 9g

Actions: Softening hardness and dissipating blockages, resolving phlegm and dredging the collaterals, removing blood stasis and alleviating pain, clearing away toxic material and reducing swelling.

Applied Syndrome: Lung cancer due to accumulation of phlegm and blood stasis which blocks the channels and collaterals, manifested as cough and hemoptysis, pain in the chest, dyspnea, emaciated body, anorexia, pale and dark purplish tongue, deep and unsmooth pulse.

Jinyan Pill
(Blood Stasis-Removing and Blockage-Dissipating Method)

Ingredients	Effects	Combined Effects	Syndrome	Chief Symptoms
Cow-Bezoar (牛黄, Niuhuang) 1g Musk (麝香, Shexiang) 2g Powder of Antelope Horn (羚羊角粉, Lingyangjiaofen) 15g Borneol (冰片, Bingpian) 2g Toad Skin Secretion Cake (蟾酥, Chansu) 0.5g	Inducing resuscitation, relieving pain and penetrating the meridians and collaterals	Softening hardness and dissipating blockages, removing phlegm and dredging the collaterals, activating blood circulation and alleviating pain, clearing toxic material and reducing swelling	Lung cancer due to accumulation of phlegm and blood stasis which blocks the collaterals	Cough or hemoptysis, pain in the chest and dyspnea, emaciated body, poor appetite, anorexia, pale and dark purplish tongue, deep and unsmooth pulse
Spreading Hedyotis Herb (白花蛇舌草, Baihuasheshecao) 50g Cow-Bezoar (牛黄, Niuhuang) Natural indigo (青黛, Qingdai) 9g Rhubarb (大黄, Dahuang) 9g Red Orpiment (雄黄, Xionghuang) 6g Cinnabar (朱砂, Zhusha) Toad Skin Secretion Cake (蟾酥, Chansu) Prepared Nux Vomica (制马钱子, Zhi Maqianzi) 6g	Clearing toxic material and reducing swelling			
Silkworm with Batrytis Larva (僵蚕, Jiangcan) 30g Scorpion (全蝎, Quanxie) 30g Centipede (蜈蚣, Wugong) 6g Gecko (壁虎, Bihu) 21g Pangolin Scales (穿山甲, Chuanshanjia) 15g	Being insects and animal drugs and inclined to remove obstruction in the meridians, soften hardness and dissipate blockages, combating toxifying disease with poisons			
Prepared Myrrh (制没药, Zhi Moyao) 6g Prepared Olibanum (制乳香, Zhi Ruxiang) 6g Saffron Crocus Stigma (藏红花, Zanghonghua) 9g Dragon's Blood (血竭, Xuejie) 6g	Activating blood circulation and dissipating blood stasis, removing blood stasis and alleviating pain			
Amber (琥珀, Hupo) 15g Cinnabar (朱砂, Zhusha) 6g	Calming the heart and tranquilizing the mind			

· 383 ·

Points in Constitution: This formula is actually the combination of the three "toxin-removing" prescriptions of Peaceful Palace Bovine-Gallstone Pill (安宫牛黄丸, an gong niu huang wan), Miraculous Pill with Six Drugs (六神丸, liu shen wan) and Cow Bezoar Pill (犀黄丸, xi huang wan) plus other drugs. In this formula, the drugs of Rhubarb (大黄, Dahuang), Toad Skin Secretion Cake (蟾酥, Chansu), Scorpion (全蝎, Quanxie), Centipede (蜈蚣, Wugong) and Spreading Hedyotis Herb (白花蛇舌草, Baihuasheshecao) all have a powerful action of restraining tumor cells. They are often combined with a number of drugs for activating blood circulation, removing blood stasis, reducing swelling, alleviating pain, calming the convulsion and tranquilizing the mind to adapt to the condition of cancer in late stage.

Indication: Terminal lung cancer.

Precautions:

1. This formula should be used at least for more than three courses, one month constituting a course. Between two courses, one week's interval is needed.

2. This formula emphasizes expelling pathogens. Thus, for the weak patient, some drugs for strengthening the body resistance and consolidating the origin should be added.

Associated Formulas:

1. Cow Bezoar Pill (犀黄丸, xi huang wan) *Surgery Life-Saving Collection* 《外科全生集》

This is composed of Cow-Bezoar (牛黄, Niuhuang), Musk (麝香, Shexiang), Myrrh (没药, Moyao) and Olibanum (乳香, Ruxiang). Its actions are clearing away toxic material, reducing swelling, activating blood circulation and removing blockages. It is indicated for cancer and scrofula.

2. Miraculous Pill with Six Drugs (六神丸, liu shen wan) *Proved Recipes* 《验方》

This is made up of Musk (麝香, Shexiang), Cow-Bezoar (牛黄, Niuhuang), Borneol (冰片, Bingpian), Toad Skin Secretion Cake (蟾酥, Chansu), Pearl (珍珠, Zhenzhu), Red Orpiment (雄黄, Xionghuang) and Soot (百草霜, Baicaoshuang). Its actions are clearing toxic material and reducing swelling. It is indicated for inflammation of soft tissues of unknown origin, carbuncle and gangrenenail-like boil and sore, acute pyogenic infection of the throat and acute tonsillitis.

2. Toxin-Clearing and Swelling-Reducing Pill (醒消丸, xing xiao wan) *Prescriptions of Peaceful Benevolent Dispensary* 《和剂局方》

This is made up of Olibanum (乳香, Ruxiang), Myrrh (没药, Moyao), Musk (麝香, Shexiang) and Red Orpiment (雄黄, Xionghuang). Its actions are regulating ying, dredging the collaterals, reducing swelling and alleviating pain. It is indicated for carbuncle, gangrene and multiple abscess.

Dwarf Lilyturf, Cochinchinese Asparagus and Tonkin Sophora Decoction (双冬豆根汤, shuang dong dou gen tang)

Source: *Treatment of Cancer by Strengthening Body Resistance and Consolidating the Origin* 《癌的扶正培本治疗》

Composition: Dwarf Lilyturf Root (麦门冬, Maimendong)12g
Cochinchinese Asparagus Root (天门冬, Tianmendong)12g
Cape Jasmine Fruit (山栀子, Shanzhizi)9g
Thunberg Fritillary Bulb (浙贝母, Zhe Beimu)9g
Coastal Glehnia Root and Fourleaf Ladybell Root (沙参, Shashen)12g
Baikal Skullcap Root (黄芩, Huangqin)9g
Heterophylly Falsestarwort Root (太子参, Taizishen)9g
Figwort Root (玄参, Xuanshen)9g
Tonkin Sophora Root (山豆根, Shandougen)12g
Largehead Atractylodes Rhizome (白术, Baizhu)9g
Honeysuckle Flower (金银花, Jinyinhua)9g
Licorice Root (生甘草, Sheng Gancao)12g
Tuckahoe (茯苓, Fuling)12g
Spreading Hedyotis Herb (白花蛇舌草, Baihuasheshecao)21g

Actions: Nourishing yin, removing heat from the blood and clearing away heat and toxic material.

Applied Syndrome: Laryngocarcinoma due to accumulation of dry-heat in the interior resulting from deficiency of yin-fluid, manifested as dry throat, blocked throat and hoarseness.

Dwarf Lilyturf, Cochinchinese Asparagust and Tonkin Sophora Decoction
(Yin-Nourishing and Heat-Clearing Method)

Ingredients	Effects	Combined Effects	Syndrome	Chief Symptoms
Dwarf Lilyturf Root (麦门冬, Maimendong)12g Cochinchinese Asparagus Root (天门冬, Tianmendong)12g Figwort Root (玄参, Xuanshen)9g Coastal Glehnia Root and Fourleaf Ladybell Root (沙参, Shashen)12g	Nourishing yin, moistening the lung	Nourishing yin and removing heat from the blood and Clearing away heat and toxic material	Laryngocarcinoma due to deficiency of yin and dry-heat	Dry throat, blocked throat, hoarseness, etc.
Heterophylly Falsestarwort Root (太子参, Taizishen)9g Largehead Atractylodes Rhizome (白术, Baizhu)9g Tuckahoe (茯苓, Fuling)12g Licorice Root (生甘草, Sheng Gancao)12g	Replenishing qi, invigorating the spleen and removing phlegm			
Cape Jasmine Fruit (山栀子, Shanzhizi)9g Baikal Skullcap Root (黄芩, Huangqin)9g Spreading Hedyotis Herb (白花蛇舌草, Baihuasheshecao)21g Honeysuckle Flower (金银花, Jinyinhua)9g Thunberg Fritillary Bulb (浙贝母, Zhe Beimu)9g	Clearing away heat and toxic material			

Points in Constitution: Tonkin Sophora Root (山豆根, Shandougen) can clear away heat and toxic material and is the key drug for relieving sore throat. When it is combined with Cochinchinese Asparagus Root (天门冬, Tianmendong) and Spreading Hedyotis Herb (白花蛇舌草, Baihuasheshecao), it can exert the effect of resisting tumor. This formula also contains lots of qi-replenishinng and yin-nourishing drugs to support the healthy qi and remove phlegm. Thus, it is a prescription for treating both the primary and secondary aspects of the disease at the same time.

Indications:
1. Laryngocarcinoma.
2. Nasopharyngeal carcinoma.

Precautions:
1. If the patient has no obvious symptoms of deficiency of qi, Heterophylly Falsestarwort Root (太子参, Taizishen), Tuckahoe (茯苓, Fuling), Largehead Atractylodes Rhizome (白术, Baizhu) and Licorice Root (生甘草, Sheng Gancao) can be removed.
2. Tonkin Sophora Root (山豆根, Shandougen) has a toxic reaction and can cause headache, dizziness, nausea, vomiting, atony of limbs, tremble, pain in the abdomen and diarrhea. Thus, attention should be paid to the dose and the medicative term of it.

Associated Formula:

Sore Throat-Relieving and Lung-Clearing Decoction (利咽清金汤, li yan qing jin tang) Treatment of *Cancer by Strengthening Body Resistance and Consolidating the Origin* 《癌的扶正培本治疗》

This is made up of Balloonflower Root (桔梗, Jiegeng), Baikal Skullcap Root (黄芩, Huangqin), Thunberg Fritillary Bulb (浙贝母, Zhe Beimu), Dwarf Lilyturf Root (麦门冬, Maimendong), Cape Jasmine Fruit (山栀子, Shanzhizi), Wild Mint Herb (薄荷, Bohe), Tonkin Sophora Root (山豆根, Shandougen), Bistort(草河车, Caoheche), Great Burdock Achene (牛蒡子, Niubangzi), Indigowoad Root (板蓝根, Banlangen), Perilla Leaf (紫苏, Zisu) and Tinospori Root(金果榄, Jinguolan). It can exert the effects of nourishing yin, removing heat from the blood and clearing away heat and toxic material. It is indicated for laryngocarcinoma due to retention of phlegm resulting from deficicency of yin and dry-heat.

Silkworm with Batrytis Larva and Wasps Nest Decoction
(僵蚕蜂房汤, jiang can feng fang tang)

Source: *Prevention and Treatment of Cancer by Traditional Chinese Medicine* 《中医药防治肿瘤》

Composition: Figwort Root (玄参, Xuanshen)12g

Cochinchinese Asparagus Root (天门冬, Tianmendong)15g

Dwarf Lilyturf Root (麦冬, Maidong)15g

Tonkin Sophora Root (山豆根, Shandougen)12g

Puff-Ball (马勃, Mabo)10g

Silkworm with Batrytis Larva (僵蚕, Jiangcan)12g

Wasps Nest (露蜂房, Lufengfang)15g

Honeysuckle Flower (金银花, Jinyinhua)15g

Barbed Skullcap Herb (半枝莲, Banzhilian)30g

Spreading Hedyotis Herb (白花蛇舌草, Baihuasheshecao)30g

Actions: Clearing away heat and toxic material, relieving sore throat, nourishing yin, resolving phlegm and dissipating blockages.

Applied Syndrome: Laryngocarcinoma due to retention of phlegm resulting from noxious heat and deficiency of yin, manifested as swelling of the throat and hoarseness, dry mouth, constipation, yellow tongue coating, smooth and rapid pulse.

Silkworm with Batrytis Larva and Wasps Nest Decoction
(Heat-Clearing and Toxin-Removing Method)

Ingredients	Effects	Combined Effects	Syndrome	Chief Symptoms
Wasps Nest (露蜂房, Lufengfang)15g	Combating toxifying disease with poisons, reducing swelling and dissipating blockages	Expelling wind, clearing away heat, relieving sore throat, nourishing yin, removing phlegm and dissipating blockages	Laryngocarcinoma (due to heat-toxin accumulated in the interior and deficiency of yin and retention of phlegm)	Swelling of the throat and hoarseness, dry mouth, yellow tongue coating, smooth and rapid pulse
Silkworm with Batrytis Larva (僵蚕, Jiangcan)12g	Removing phlegm and dissipating blockages			
Tonkin Sophora Root (山豆根, Shandougen)12g Puff-Ball (马勃, Mabo)10g Honeysuckle Flower (金银花, Jinyinhua)15g Barbed Skullcap Herb (半枝莲, Banzhilian)30g Spreading Hedyotis Herb (白花蛇舌草, Baihuasheshecao)30g	Clearing away heat and toxic material			
Figwort Root (玄参, Xuanshen)12g Cochinchinese Asparagus Root (天门冬, Tianmendong)15g Dwarf Lilyturf Root (麦冬, Maidong)15g	Nourishing yin and moistening dryness			

Points in Constitution: This formula is comprised of heat-clearing and toxin-removing drugs plus yin-nourishing and dryness-moistening drugs, but it emphasizes detoxifying and dissipating blockages. It is recorded in Prescriptions for Universal Benevolence《普济方》that the ash of Wasps Nest (露蜂房, Lufengfang), when it is combined with Silkworm with Batrytis Larva (白僵蚕, Baijiangcan), is good at clearing away toxic material and dissipating blockages, and is indicated for sore throat with swelling and pain. Wasps Nest (露蜂房, Lufengfang), Tonkin Sophora Root (山豆根, Shandougen), Barbed Skullcap Herb (半枝莲, Banzhilian) and Spreading

Hedyotis Herb (白花蛇舌草, Baihuasheshecao) are the common Chinese drugs for preventing and resisting cancer in the clinic.

Indications:

1. Laryngocarcinoma.
2. Nasopharyngeal carcinoma.

Precaution: Since Wasps Nest (露蜂房, Lufengfang) is poisonous, it should be cautiously used for those with deficiency of qi and blood.

Associated Formula:

Dwarf Lilyturft, Cochinchinese Asparagus and Tonkin Sophora Decoction (双冬豆根汤, shuang dong dou gen tang) *Treatment of Cancer by Strengthening Body Resistance and Consolidating the Origin* 《癌的扶正培本治疗》

This is made up of Dwarf Lilyturf Root (麦门冬, Maimendong), Cochinchinese Asparagus Root (天门冬, Tianmendong), Cape Jasmine Fruit (山栀子, Shanzhizi), Thunberg Fritillary Bulb (浙贝母, Zhe Beimu), Coastal Glehnia Root and Fourleaf Ladybell Root (沙参, Shashen), Baikal Skullcap Root (黄芩, Huangqin), Heterophylly Falsestarwort Root (太子参, Taizishen), Figwort Root (玄参, Xuanshen), Tonkin Sophora Root (山豆根, Shandougen), Largehead Atractylodes Rhizome (白术, Baizhu), Honeysuckle Flower (金银花, Jinyinhua), Licorice Root (生甘草, Sheng Gancao), Tuckahoe (茯苓, Fuling) and Spreading Hedyotis Herb (白花蛇舌草, Baihuasheshecao). The basic actions of this formula are clearing away heat and toxic material, nourishing yin and moistening the dryness. Besides, it also has the actions of replenishing qi, invigorating the spleen and strengthening body resistance. It is suitable to laryngocarcinoma due to deficiency of yin and dryness-heat accompanied with insufficiency of healthy qi.

Dysphagia-Treating Powder
(治膈散, zhi ge san)

Source: *Zhejiang Journal of Traditional Chinese Medicine* 《浙江中医杂志》
Composition: Appendiculate Cremastra Pseudobulb (山慈姑, Shancigu)

Borax (硼砂, Pengsha)

Sal-Ammoniac (硇砂, Naosha)

Sanchi Root (三七, Sanqi)

Borneol (冰片, Bingpian)

Chinese Eaglewood Wood (沉香, Chenxiang)

(Taking equal amount of the above drugs and grinding them into fine powder for oral use. 10g each time, 4 times a day).

Actions: Activating blood circulation and removing blood stasis, removing phlegm and relieving dysphagia.

Applied Syndrome: Dysphagia due to accumulation of phlegm and blood stasis in the esophagus, manifested as difficulty in swallowing food, pain in the chest and hypochondrium, inability to swallow food or a drop of water, vomiting immediately after eating, dark complexion, dry and withered skin, emanciated body, or hematochezia, dark purplish tongue, thin and unsmooth pulse.

Dysphagia-Treating Powder
(Blood Stasis-Resolving and Phlegm-Removing Method)

Ingredients	Effects	Combined Effects	Syndrome	Chief Symptoms
Appendiculate Cremastra Pseudobulb (山慈姑, Shancigu)	Clearing away heat and toxic material, reducing swelling and dissipating blockages	Activating blood circulation and removing blood stasis and treating dysphagia	Dysphagia (due to accumulation of phlegm and blood stasis)	Difficulty in swallowing food, pain in the chest, dark complexion, dry and withered skin, dark purplish tongue, thin and unsmooth pulse
Borax (硼砂, Pengsha) Sal-Ammoniac (硇砂, Naosha)	Clearing away heat and toxic material and removing phlegm			
Sanchi Root (三七, Sanqi)	Removing blood stasis, activating blood circulation and reducing swelling			
Borneol (冰片, Bingpian)	Inducing resuscitation and treating dysphagia			
Chinese Eaglewood Wood (沉香, Chenxiang)	Keeping the adverse qi downwards and regulating the middle-jiao			

Points in Constitution: Appendiculate Cremastra Pseudobulb (山慈姑, Shancigu) which is pungent in flavor, cold in nature and slight poisonous, is good at treating nail-like boils, cellulites and obstinate sores. Of the Appendiculate Cremastra Pseudobulb (山慈姑, Shancigu), the one produced in Lijiang area contains colchicines which has the anti-tumor action. Sal-Ammoniac (硇砂, Naosha) has the actions of drastically removing blood stasis, dissipating blockages, eliminating retention and softening hardness while Borax (硼砂, Pengsha) has the actions of clearing away toxic material, reducing swelling, removing heat and resolving phlegm. The combination of these two can treat dysphagia and regurgitation.

Indications:
1. Esophageal cancer.
2. Gastric cancer.

Precaution: Appendiculate Cremastra Pseudobulb (山慈姑, Shancigu) and Sal-Ammoniac (硇砂, Naosha) are poisonous drugs. Thus, attention should be paid to the dose of them in the clinic.

Associated Formulas:

1. Pylorus-Dredging Decoction (通幽汤, tong you tang) *Treatise on the Spleen and the Stomach* 《脾胃论》

This is composed of Dried Rehmannia Root (生地黄, Shengdihuang), Prepared Rehmannia

Root (熟地黄, Shudihuang), Peach Seed (桃仁, Taoren), Safflower (红花, Honghua), Chinese Angelica Root (当归, Danggui), Prepared Licorice Root (炙甘草, Zhi Gancao) and Shunk Bugbane Rhizome (升麻, Shengma). Its actions are nourishing yin and activating blood circulation. It is indicated for dysphagia due to interior blockage of blood stasis accompanied with deficiency of yin-fluid.

2. Dysphagia-Opening Powder (启膈散, qi ge san) *Comprehension of Medicine* 《医学心悟》

This is composed of Coastal Glehnia Root and Fourleaf Ladybell Root (沙参, Shashen), Tuckahoe (茯苓, Fuling), Dan-Shen Root (丹参, Danshen), Tendrilleaf Fritillary Bulb (川贝母, Chuan Beimu), Turmeric Root-Tuber (郁金, Yujin), Villous Amomum Fruit (砂仁, Sharen) and Lotus Leaf (荷叶, Heye). Its actions are resolving phlegm, relieving the depressed qi, moistening dryness and keeping the adverse qi downwards. It is indicated for dysphagia due to accumulation of phlegm and qi.

3. Borneol and Borax Powder (冰硼散, bing peng san) *Orthodox Manual of Surgery* 《外科正宗》

This is made up of Borax (硼砂, Pengsha), Weathered Sodium Sulfate (玄明粉, Yuanmingfen), Borneol (冰片, Bingpian) and Cinnabar (朱砂, Zhusha). Its actions are clearing away heat and removing toxic material. It is indicated for aphtha and sore throat. It is also indicated for hoarseness and pain due to phlegm-fire.

Liver-Recuperating Prescription
(肝复方, gan fu fang)

Source: *Beijing Journal of Traditional Chinese Medicine* 《北京中医杂志》

Composition: Toasted Membranous Milkvetch Root (炙黄芪, Zhi Huangqi)9g

Pilose Asiabell Root (党参, Dangshen)9g

Largehead Atractylodes Rhizome (白术, Baizhu)9g

Tuckahoe (茯苓, Fuling)9g

Bupleurum (柴胡, Chaihu)9g

Pangolin Scales (穿山甲, Chuanshanjia)9g

Peach Seed (桃仁, Taoren)9g

Dan-Shen Root (丹参, Danshen)9g

Sappan Wood (苏木, Sumu)9g

Manyleaf Paris Rhizome (蚤休, Zaoxiu)9g

Oyster Shell (生牡蛎, Sheng Muli)15g

Pillb Driedug(鼠妇, Shufu)6g

Actions: Replenishing qi and invigorating the spleen, activating blood circulation and removing blood stasis.

Applied Syndrome: Liver cancer due to obstruction of qi and blood stasis resulting from deficiency of spleen-qi, manifested as mass in the hypochondrium, pain with tenderness in the hypochondrium which radiates to the back and aggravates in the night, distention and fullness sensation in the gastric and abdominal region, poor appetite, irregular defecation, lassitude, dark purplish tongue with petechia and ecchymosis, deep and thready pulse or wiry and unsmooth pulse.

Liver-Recuperating Prescription
(Qi-Replenishing and Blood-Activating Method)

Ingredients	Effects	Combined Effects	Syndrome	Chief Symptoms
Bupleurum (柴胡, Chaihu)9g	Dispersing the stagnated liver-qi and alleviating pain	Replenishing qi and invigorating the spleen, activating blood circulation and removing blood stasis	Blood stasis and deficiency of spleen-qi	Mass in the hypochondrium, pain with tenderness in the hypochondrium which may radiate to the back and aggravate in the night, distention and fullness feeling in the gastric and abdominal area, poor appetite, irregular defecation, lassitude, dark purplish tongue, deep and thin pulse or wiry and unsmooth pulse
Toasted Membranous Milkvetch Root (炙黄芪, Zhi Huangqi)9g Pilose Asiabell Root (党参, Dangshen)9g Largehead Atractylodes Rhizome (白术, Baizhu)9g Tuckahoe (茯苓, Fuling)9g	Replenishing qi and invigorating the spleen			
Peach Seed (桃仁, Taoren)9g Dan-Shen Root (丹参, Danshen)9g Sappan Wood (苏木, Sumu)9g	Activating blood circulation and removing blood stasis			
Manyleaf Paris Rhizome (蚤休, Zaoxiu)9g	Clearing away heat and toxic material, activating blood circulation and reducing swelling			
Pillb Driedug(鼠妇, Shufu)6g	Removing blood stasis drastically and alleviating pain			
Oyster Shell (生牡蛎, Sheng Muli)15g	Softening hardness and dissipating blockages			
Pangolin Scales (穿山甲, Chuanshanjia)9g	Activating blood circulation and dredging the collaterals, reducing swelling and dissipating blockages			

Points in Constitution: This formula is actually the modification of Turtle Carapace Pill(鳖甲丸, bie jia wan) recorded in *Synopsis of Golden Cabinet*《金匮要略》. It emphasizes replenishing qi, strengthening body resistance, removing blood stasis and softening hardness simultaneously. It is a method of both reinforcement and elimination, i.e. strenthening the body resistance and removing pathogens in combination.

Indication: Midtrimester and terminal liver cancer.

Precaution: This is a prescription for gradually eliminating masses in the hypochondrium and is suitable to be taken for a long time.

Associated Formulas:

1. Bitter Orange and Officinal Magnolia Bark Six Gentlemen Decoction(枳朴六君子汤, zhi po liu jun zi tang)*Shanxi Journal of Traditional Chinese Medicine*《陕西中医》

This is composed of Pilose Asiabell Root(党参, Dangshen), Tuckahoe(茯苓, Fuling), Dan-Shen Root(丹参, Danshen), Largehead Atractylodes Rhizome(白术, Baizhu), Tangerine Peel(橘皮, Jupi), Pinellia Rhizome(半夏, Banxia), Bitter Orange(枳壳, Zhiqiao), Officinal Magnolia Bark(厚朴, Houpo), Garter Snake(乌梢蛇, Wushaoshe), Ground Bettle(䗪虫, Zhechong), Centipede(蜈蚣, Wugong) and Licorice Root(生甘草, Sheng Gancao). Its actions are replenishing qi, invigorating the spleen, regulating flow of qi, removing phlegm, activating blood circulation and removing blood stasis. It is indicated for liver cancer due to stagnation of qi and retention of phlegm resulting from blood stasis in the interior and deficiency of the spleen-qi.

2. Decoction for Recovery and Activating Blood Circulation(复元活血汤, fu yuan huo xue tang)*Invention of Medicine*《医学发明》

This is made up of Bupleurum(柴胡, Chaihu), Snakegourd Root(瓜蒌根, Gualougen), Chinese Angelica Root(当归, Danggui), Safflower(红花, Honghua), Licorice Root(生甘草, Sheng Gancao), Pangolin Scales(穿山甲, Chuanshanjia), Rhubarb(生大黄, Sheng Dahuang) and Peach Seed(桃仁, Taoren). Its actions are activating blood circulation and flow of qi. It is indicated for liver cancer due to blood stasis and qi stagnation.

Modified Tuckahoe Powder With Five Herbs
(加味五苓散, jia wei wu ling san)

Source: *Sichuan Journal of Traditional Chinese Medicine*《四川中医》

Composition: Umbellate Pore Fungus(猪苓, Zhuling)15g

Tuckahoe(茯苓, Fuling)15g

Largehead Atractylodes Rhizome(白术, Baizhu)15g

Membranous Milkvetch Root(黄芪, Huangqi)15g

Oriental Waterplantain Rhizome(泽泻, Zexie)18g

Climbing Fern Spore(海金沙, Haijinsha)18g

Seaweed(海藻, Haizao)18g

Cassia Twig(桂枝, Guizhi)9g

Sanguisorba Root(地榆, Diyu)30g

Coix Seed(薏苡仁, Yiyiren)30g

Spreading Hedyotis Herb(白花蛇舌草, Baihuasheshecao)30g

Actions: Invigorating the spleen and expelling dampness, promoting diuresis and activating flow of qi, supporting the healthy qi and preventing cancer.

Applied Syndrome: Cancer of the urinary bladder due to deficiency of the healthy qi and retention of dampness in the interior, manifested as hematuria with large or small amount of blood, or even with blood clots, often accompanied with frequency of urination, urgency of micturition, urodynia, dysuria, pain in the loins and abdomen, lassitude, pallor of complexion, pale tongue or with ecchymosis, white and greasy tongue coating, thin and weak pulse.

Modified Tuckahoe Powder With Five Herbs
(Qi-Replenishing and Diuresis-Inducing Method)

Ingredients	Effects	Combined Effects	Syndrome	Chief Symptoms
Umbellate Pore Fungus (猪苓, Zhuling)15g Tuckahoe (茯苓, Fuling)15g Oriental Waterplantain Rhizome (泽泻, Zexie)18g Coix Seed (薏苡仁, Yiyiren)30g	Promoting urination and removing dampness	Invigorating the spleen and expelling dampness, activating low of qi and promoting diuresis, supporting the healthy qi and resisting cancer	Cancer of urinary bladder due to deficiency of the healthy qi and retention of dampness in the interior	Hematuria, frequency of urination, urgency of micturition, urodynia, dysuria, pain in the loins and abdomen, lassitude, pallor, pale tongue with ecchymosis, deep pulse
Membranous Milkvetch Root (生黄芪, Sheng Huangqi)15g Largehead Atractylodes Rhizome (白术, Baizhu)15g	Replenishing qi and invigorating the spleen			
Cassia Twig (桂枝, Guizhi)9g	Warming yang and improving qi transformation			
Sanguisorba Root (地榆, Diyu)30g Spreading Hedyotis Herb (白花蛇舌草, Baihuasheshecao)30g	Clearing away heat and removing heat from the blood, clearing away toxic material and resisting cancer			
Seaweed (海藻, Haizao)18g	Softening hardness and dissipating blockages			
Climbing Fern Spore (海金沙, Haijinsha)18g	Clearing away heat and treating stranguria			

Points in Constitution: This formula is based on Poria Powder with Five Herbs(五苓散, wu ling san) plus addditional drugs for clearing away heat and relieving stranguria. It has the actions of supporting the healthy qi or strengthening the body resistace, eliminating pathogenic factors, invigorating the spleen, removing blood stasis and promoting urination.

Indications:
1. Terminal cancer of urinary bladder.
2. Prostatic cancer.

Precaution: For the case with deficiency of yin, this formula should be modified before it is used.
Associated Formulas:

1. Poria Powder with Five Herbs(五苓散, wu ling san) *Treatise on Exogenous Febrile Diseases* 《伤寒论》

This is composed of Tuckahoe (茯苓, Fuling), Umbellate Pore Fungus (猪苓, Zhuling), Oriental Waterplantain Rhizome (泽泻, Zexie), Cassia Twig (桂枝, Guizhi) and Largehead Atractylodes Rhizome (白术, Baizhu). Its actions are warming yang, improving qi transformation, promoting urination and removing dampness. It is indicated for dysuria due to retention of water-dampness in urinary bladder of lower-jiao.

2. Umbellate Pore Fungus Decoction (猪苓汤, zhu ling tang) *Treatise on Exogenous Febrile Diseases* 《伤寒论》

This is made up of Tuckahoe (茯苓, Fuling), Umbellate Pore Fungus (猪苓, Zhuling), Oriental Waterplantain Rhizome (泽泻, Zexie), Ass-hide Glue (阿胶, Ejiao) and Talc (滑石, Huashi). Its actions are inducing diuresis, removing dampness, clearing away heat and nourishing yin. It is indicated for dysuria or stranguria complicated by hematuria, hematuria due to water and heat accumulating in the lower-jiao.

Pilose Asiabell, Membranous Milkvetch, Desertliving Cistanche and Shorthorned Epimedium Decoction (参芪蓉仙汤, shen qi rong xian tang)

Source: *A Complete Work of Secret Recipes of Traditional Chinese Medicine* 《中国中医秘方大全》

Composition: Membranous Milkvetch Root (生黄芪, Sheng Huangqi)15g
Pilose Asiabell Root (党参, Dangshen)12g
Shorthorned Epimedium Herb (淫羊藿, Yinyanghuo)12g
Desertliving Cistanche Herb (肉苁蓉, Roucongrong)6g
Medicinal Indian Mulberry Root (巴戟天, Bajitian)6g
Barbary Wolfberry Fruit (枸杞子, Gouqizi)12g
Prepared Tuber Fleeceflower Root (制首乌, Zhishouwu)12g
Pangolin Scales (穿山甲, Chuanshanjia)15g
Medicinal Achyranthes Root (川牛膝, Chuan Niuxi)12g
Prepared Rhubarb (制大黄, Zhi Dahuang)6g
Fried Chinese Corktree Bark (炒黄柏, Chao Huangbai)9g
Common Anemarrhena Rhizome (知母, Zhimu)6g
Glabrous Greenbrier Rhizome (土茯苓, Tufuling)15g
Manyleaf Paris Rhizome (七叶一枝花, Qiyeyizhihua)12g
Spreading Hedyotis Herb (白花蛇舌草, Baihuasheshecao)15g
White Peony Root (白芍药, Baishaoyao)12g

Prepared Licorice Root (炙甘草, Zhi Gancao)6g

Actions: Replenishing qi and invigorating the kidney, clearing away heat and dissipating blockages.

Pilose Asiabell, Membranous Milkvetch, Desertliving Cistanche and Shorthorned Epimedium Decoction
(Kidney-Invigorating and Heat-Clearing Method)

Ingredients	Effects	Combined Effects	Syndrome	Chief Symptoms
Barbary Wolfberry Fruit (枸杞子, Gouqizi)12g Prepared Tuber Fleeceflower Root (制首乌, Zhishouwu)12g Membranous Milkvetch Root (生黄芪, Sheng Huangqi)15g Pilose Asiabell Root (党参, Dangshen)12g White Peony Root (白芍药, Baishaoyao)12g Shorthorned Epimedium Herb (淫羊藿, Yinyanghuo)12g Desertliving Cistanche Herb (肉苁蓉, Roucongrong)6g Medicinal Indian Mulberry Root (巴戟天, Bajitian)6g	Replenishing qi, blood, yin and yang uniformly	Replenishing qi and invigorating the kidney, clearing away heat and dissipating blockages	Prostatic cancer due to deficiency of both the spleen and the kidney and accumulation of heat and dampness in the interior	Dripping of urination, or like filament, or even anuria, feeling of distention, fullness and pain in the lower abdomen, soreness of loins, shortness of breath and lassitude, thirst, pale and reddissh tongue with yellow coating, smooth and rapid pulse
Prepared Rhubarb (制大黄, Zhi Dahuang)6g Fried Chinese Corktree Bark (炒黄柏, Chao Huangbai)9g Common Anemarrhena Rhizome (知母, Zhimu)6g Glabrous Greenbrier Rhizome (土茯苓, Tufuling)15g Manyleaf Paris Rhizome (七叶一枝花, Qiyeyizhihua)12g Spreading Hedyotis Herb (白花蛇舌草, Baihuasheshecao)15g	Clearing away heat and toxic material			
Pangolin Scales (穿山甲, Chuanshanjia)15g	Activating blood circulation and dredging the collaterals, dissipating blockages and promoting lumps to be broken			
Medicinal Achyranthes Root (川牛膝, Chuan Niuxi)12g	Conducting blood or fire going downward and opening orifices			
Prepared Licorice Root (炙甘草, Zhi Gancao)6g	Coordinating the actions of various ingredients in the prescription			

Applied Syndrome: Prostatic cancer due to deficiency of both the spleen and the kidney and accumulation of heat and dampness in the interior, manifested as dripping of urination, or micturition like filament, or even anuria, feeling of distention, fullness and pain in the lower abdomen, soreness of the loins, shortness of breath, lassitude, thirst, pale and reddissh tongue with yellow coating, smooth and rapid pulse.

Points in Constitution: In this formula, the drugs for benefiting the kidney and invigorating the spleen are used together with those for clearing away heat, drying dampness and removing toxins. In addition, the drugs for removing blood stasis and dissipating blockages are included. In the formula, Glabrous Greenbrier Rhizome (土茯苓, Tufuling), Manyleaf Paris Rhizome (七叶一枝花, Qiyeyizhihua, also called Zaoxiu 蚤休) and Spreading Hedyotis Herb (白花蛇舌草, Baihuasheshecao) have the action of resisting against tumor. The combined use of a large number of nourishing and replenishing drugs is to enhance and improve the immunity of the human body.

Indications:
1. Prostatic cancer.
2. Cancer of urinary bladder.

Precaution: It should be cautiously used to those with loose stool.

Associated Formulas:

1. Eight Corrections Powder(八正散, ba zheng san) *Prescriptions of Peaceful Benevolent Dispensary* 《和剂局方》

This is made up of Common Knotgrass Herb (萹蓄, Bianxu), Lilac Pink Herb (瞿麦, Qumai), Plantain Seed (车前子, Cheqianzi), Talc (滑石, Huashi), Cape Jasmine Fruit (山栀子, Shanzhizi), Rhubarb (生大黄, Sheng Dahuang), Akebia Stem (木通, Mutong) and Ending Part of Licorice Root (甘草梢, Gancaoshao). Its actions are clearing away heat, purging fire, promoting urination and treating stranguria. It is indicated for urodynia or retention of urine due to heat-dampness accumulated in urinary bladder of the lower-jiao.

2. Cold Natured Stranguria-Treating Decoction (寒通汤, han tong tang) *Records of Traditional Chinese and Western Medicine in Combination* 《医学衷中参西录》

This is composed of Talc (滑石, Huashi), White Peony Root (白芍药, Baishaoyao), Common Anemarrhena Rhizome (知母, Zhimu) and Chinese Corktree Bark (黄柏, Huangbai). Its actions are clearing away heat and dampness, promoting urination and relieving stranguria. It is indicated for distention of the urinary bladder, dripping of urination or anuria due to excessive heat in the lower-jiao.

3. Modified Peach Kernel and Safflower Decoction (加味桃红汤, jia wei tao hong tang) *Surgery* by Guangzhou Traditional Chinese Medicine College 广州中医学院《外科学》

This is composed of Peach Seed (桃仁, Taoren), Safflower (红花, Honghua), Amber (琥珀, Hupo), Medicinal Achyranthes Root (川牛膝, Chuan Niuxi), Cassia Bark (肉桂, Rougui) and Rhubarb (生大黄, Sheng Dahuang). Its actions are activating blood circulation, removing blood stasis and dredging the water passage. It is indicated for dripping urination, anuria with pain, unbearable acute pain in the lower abdomen due to blood stasis in the urinary bladder.

Modified Toxin-Removing Fairy Decoction
(解毒玉女煎加减方, jie du yu nü jian jia jian fang)

Source: *Hebei Journal of Traditional Chinese Medicine*《河北中医》

Composition: Powder of Antelope Horn（羚羊角粉, Lingyangjiaofen）1g（taking it separately with water）

Figwort Root（玄参, Xuanshen）15g

Honeysuckle Flower（金银花, Jinyinhua）21g

Weeping Forsythia Capsule（连翘, Lianqiao）15g

Dandelion（蒲公英, Pugongying）15g

Gypsum（生石膏, Sheng Shigao）30g

Common Anemarrhena Rhizome（知母, Zhimu）9g

Dried Rehmannia Root（生地黄, Shengdihuang）15g

Dwarf Lilyturf Root（麦门冬, Maimendong）15g

Indigowoad Root（板蓝根, Banlangen）15g

Hairyvein Agrimonia Herb（仙鹤草, Xianhecao）15g

Sanguisorba Root（地榆, Diyu）15g

Actions: Clearing away heat and toxic material, nourishing yin and removing heat from the blood.

Applied Syndrome: Acute non-lymphocytic leukemia due to retention of heat-toxin in the interior, deficiency of yin and heat in the blood, manifested as fever, headache, irritability, mucocutaneous hemorrhage, ecchymosis, epistaxis, bleeding from the gum, unconsciousness, crimson tongue, thin and rapid pulse.

Points in Constitution: This formula pays equal attention to the drugs for removing heat from the blood, clearing away heat in qifen and eliminating heat and toxic material, and aims at clearing away noxious heat and nourishing yin-fluid. It is mainly applied for fever and hemorrhage due to leukemia.

Indications:

1. Acute non lymphocytic leukemia.
2. Acute leukemia.

Precaution: It is forbidden for the case of hemorrhage due to deficiency of qi which faills to control blood.

Associated Formulas:

1. Modified Orifice-Opening and Blood-Activating Prescription(通窍活血加减方, tong qiao huo xue jia jian fang) *Information of Traditional Chinese Medicine*《中医药信息》

This is made up of Musk（麝香, Shexiang）, Dragon's Blood（血竭, Xuejie）, Peach Seed（桃仁, Taoren）, Safflower（红花, Honghua）, Red Peony Root（赤芍药, Chishaoyao）, Szechwan Lovage Rhizome（川芎, Chuanxiong）, Corydalis Tuber（延胡索, Yanhusuo）, Turmeric Root-Tuber（郁金, Yujin）and Dan-Shen Root（丹参, Danshen）. Its actions are activating blood circulation to open orifices, removing blood stasis, dredging the collaterals, regulating flow of qi and alleviating pain. It is indicated for acute leukemia with severe pain.

Modified Toxin-Removing Fairy Decoction
(Heat-Removing and Blood-Cooling Method)

Ingredients	Effects	Combined Effects	Syndrome	Chief Symptoms
Powder of Antelope Horn (羚羊角粉, Lingyangjiaofen)1g Dried Rehmannia Root (生地黄, Shengdihuang)15g Figwort Root (玄参, Xuanshen)15g Sanguisorba Root (地榆, Diyu)15g	Removing heat from the blood	Clearing away heat and toxic material, nourishing yin and removing heat from the blood	Leukemia due to retention of heat-toxin in the interior, deficiency of yin and blood heat	Fever, headache and irritability, mucocutaneous hemorrhage, or epistaxis, bleeding from the gum, unconsciousness, crimson tongue, thin and rapid pulse
Gypsum (生石膏, Sheng Shigao)30g Common Anemarrhena Rhizome (知母, Zhimu)9g Dwarf Lilyturf Root (麦门冬, Maimendong)15g	Clearing away heat and promoting the production of body fluid			
Honeysuckle Flower (金银花, Jinyinhua)21g Weeping Forsythia Capsule (连翘, Lianqiao)15g Dandelion (蒲公英, Pugongying)15g indigowoad Root (板蓝根, Banlangen)15g	Clearing away heat and toxic material			
Hairyvein Agrimonia Herb (仙鹤草, Xianhecao)15g	Removing heat from the blood and arresting bleeding			

2. Anti-pyretic and Anti-toxic Decoction(清瘟败毒饮, qing wen bai du yin) *An Experience on Pestieent Rashes*《疫疹一得》

This consists of Gypsum (生石膏, Sheng Shigao), Dried Rehmannia Root (生地黄, Shengdihuang), Baikal Skullcap Root (黄芩, Huangqin), Cape Jasmine Fruit (山栀子, Shanzhizi), Common Anemarrhena Rhizome (知母, Zhimu), Red Peony Root (赤芍药, Chishaoyao), Figwort Root (玄参, Xuanshen), Weeping Forsythia Capsule (连翘, Lianqiao), Tree Peony Bark (牡丹皮, Mudanpi), Balloonflower Root (桔梗, Jiegeng), Tophatherum Leaf (竹叶, Zhuye), Asiatic Rhinoceros Horn (犀角, Xijiao), Coptis Rhizome (黄连, Huanglian) and Licorice Root (生甘草, Sheng Gancao). Its actions are clearing away heat and toxic material, removing heat from the blood and nourishing yin. It is indicated for high fever, irritability, haematemesis, apostaxis and skin eruptions due to epidemic pestilence which causes intense heat in both qifen and xuefen.

3. Modified Anti-pyretic and Anti-toxic Decoction (加减清瘟败毒饮, jia jian qing wen bai du yin) *Practical Formulae-ology* by Zhou Fengwu 周凤梧《实用方剂学》

This is composed of Gypsum (生石膏, Sheng Shigao), Honeysuckle Flower (金银花, Jinyinhua), Weeping Forsythia Capsule (连翘, Lianqiao), Dried Rehmannia Root (生地黄, Shengdihuang), Gambirplant Hooked Stem and Branch (钩藤, Gouteng), Common Anemarrhena Rhizome (知母, Zhimu), Figwort Root (玄参, Xuanshen), Cape Jasmine Fruit (山栀子, Shanzhizi), Sinkiang Arnebia Root or Redroot Gromwell Root (紫草, Zicao) and Grassleaf Sweetflag Rhizome (石菖蒲, Shichangpu). Its actions are clearing away heat and toxic material and cooling blood. It is indicated for seasonal febrile disease manifested as high fever and headache, vomiting and irritability, coma and convulsion, dry and crimson tongue, thin and rapid pulse.

Pathogen-Clearing and Mass-Resolving Decoction
(清消汤, qing xiao tang)

Source: *Hebei Journal of Traditional Chinese Medicine* 《河北中医》
Composition: Tonkin Sophora Root (山豆根, Shandougen) 9g
Appendiculate Cremastra Pseudobulb (山慈姑, Shancigu) 9g
Glabrous Greenbrier Rhizome (土茯苓, Tufuling) 9g
Honeysuckle Flower (金银花, Jinyinhua) 9g
Weeping Forsythia Capsule (连翘, Lianqiao) 9g
Giant Knotweed Rhizome (虎杖, Huzhang) 9g
Charred Cape Jasmine Fruit (焦栀子, Jiao Zhizi) 9g
Barbed Skullcap Herb (半枝莲, Banzhilian) 9g
Thunberg Fritillary Bulb (浙贝母, Zhe Beimu) 9g
Common Burreed Rhizome (三棱, Sanleng) 9g
Kwangsi Turmeric Rhizome (莪术, Ezhu) 9g
Dan-Shen Root (丹参, Danshen) 9g
Red Peony Root (赤芍药, Chishaoyao) 9g
Pangolin Scales (穿山甲, Chuanshanjia) 9g
Turtle Carapace (鳖甲, Biejia) 9g
Pilose Asiabell Root (党参, Dangshen) 9g
Roasted Membranous Milkvetch Root (炙黄芪, Zhi Huangqi) 9g
Charred Hawthorn Fruit (焦山楂, Jiaoshanzha) 9g
Charred Medicated Leaven (焦神曲, Jiaoshenqu) 9g
Charred Malt (焦麦芽, Jiaomaiya) 9g

Actions: Clearing away heat and toxic material, reducing swelling and strengthening body resistance.

Applied Syndrome: All kinds of cancers due to stagnation of heat-toxin.

Pathogen-Clearing and Mass-Resolving Decoction
(Heat-Clearing and Blood Stasis-Removing Method)

Ingredients	Effects	Combined Effects	Syndrome
Tonkin Sophora Root (山豆根, Shandougen)9g Appendiculate Cremastra Pseudobulb (山慈姑, Shancigu)9g Glabrous Greenbrier Rhizome (土茯苓, Tufuling)9g Honeysuckle Flower (金银花, Jinyinhua)9g Weeping Forsythia Capsule (连翘, Lianqiao)9g Giant Knotweed Rhizome (虎杖, Huzhang)9g Charred Cape Jasmine Fruit (焦栀子, Jiao Zhizi)9g Barbed Skullcap Herb (半枝莲, Banzhilian)9g Thunberg Fritillary Bulb (浙贝母, Zhe Beimu)9g	Clearing away heat and toxic material	Clearing away heat and toxic material, reducing swelling and supporting the healthy qi	All kinds of cancer due to stagnation of heat-toxin
Common Burreed Rhizome (三棱, Sanleng)9g Kwangsi Turmeric Rhizome (莪术, Ezhu)9g Dan-Shen Root (丹参, Danshen)9g Red Peony Root (赤芍药, Chishaoyao)9g	Activating blood circulation and removing blood stasis		
Pangolin Scales (穿山甲, Chuanshanjia)9g Turtle Carapace (鳖甲, Biejia)9g	Removing blood stasis, dredging the collaterals and dissipating blockages		
Pilose Asiabell Root (党参, Dangshen)9g Toasted Membranous Milkvetch Root (炙黄芪, Zhi Huangqi)9g	Replenishing qi and supporting the healthy qi		
Charred Hawthorn Fruit, Charred Medicated Leaven and Charred Malt (焦三仙, Jiaosanxian) 9g	Promoting digestion and regulating the stomach qi		

Points in Constitution: This formula contains many kinds of drugs for clearing away heat and toxic material and emphasizes resisting cancer. Meanwhile, it also contains various drugs for activating blood circulation and dissipating blockages to eliminate mass. Thus it is called Pathogen-Clearing and Mass-Resolving Decoction(清消汤, qing xiao tang). In addition, this formula also contains Pilose Asiabell Root (党参, Dangshen) and Toasted Membranous Milkvetch Root (炙黄芪, Zhi Huangqi) to strengthen the body resiatance with the view to expelling pathogens without impairing healthy qi.

Indications:

1. Gastric cancer.

2. Skin carcinoma.
3. Ovarian cancer.
4. Cancer of urinary bladder.
5. Cancer of pancreas.
6. Mammary cancer.

Precaution: The main action of this prescription is to expel pathogens. Thus, for the case with a weakened body, some replenishing and nourishing drugs should be added or alternately used with this formula. Associated Formulas:

1. Minor Panacea Pellet (小金丹, xiao jin dan) *Surgery Life-Saving Collection*《外科全生集》 This is made up of Sweetgum Resin (白胶香, Baijiaoxiang), North Monkshood (草乌, Caowu), Trogopterus Dung (五灵脂, Wulingzhi), Earth Worm (地龙, Dilong), Semen Momordicae (木鳖子, Mubiezi), Olibanum (乳香, Ruxiang), Myrrh (没药, Moyao), Chinese Angelica Root (当归, Danggui), Musk (麝香, Shexiang) and Fragrant Black Charcoal (香墨炭, Xiangmotan). Its actions are activating blood circulation and dissolving blood stasis, reducing swelling and alleviating pain. It is indicated for all kinds of cancers due to blood stasis.

Jackinthepulpit, Pinellia, Common Selfheal Fruit-Spike, GrassleafSweetflag and Two Pieces of Centipedes Decoction (星夏草菖双龙汤, xing xia cao chang shuang long tang)

Source: *Journal of Traditional Chinese Medicine*《中医杂志》
Composition: Pinellia Rhizome (半夏, Banxia) 9g
Jackinthepulpit Tuber (天南星, Tiannanxing) 6g
Common Selfheal Fruit-Spike (夏枯草, Xiakucao) 9g
Grassleaf Sweetflag Rhizome (石菖蒲, Shichangpu) 6g
Silkworm with Batrytis Larva (僵蚕, Jiangcan) 6g
Oyster Shell (生牡蛎, Sheng Muli) 15g
Earth Worm (地龙, Dilong) 6g
Gecko (壁虎, Bihu) 6g
Centipede (蜈蚣, Wugong) 2 Pieces
Umbellate Pore Fungus (猪苓, Zhuling) 9g
Tuckahoe (茯苓, Fuling) 9g
Toad Skin Secretion Cake (蟾酥, Chansu) 0.01g (taking it with water)
Ground Bettle (䗪虫, Zhechong) 9g

Actions: Removing phlegm and stopping the wind, eliminating toxin and resisting against cancer.

Applied Syndrome: Primary tumor of central nervous system, caused by turbid phlegm accumulating in the interior and up-stirring of the liver. The manifestations are severe headache, blurred vision, continuous vomiting, vertigo, insomnia, convulsion, hemiplegia, pale tongue with white and greasy coating, wiry and smooth pulse.

Jackinthepulpit, Pinellia, Common Selfheal Fruit-Spike, Grassleaf Sweetflag and Two Pieces of Centipedes Decoction
(Phlegm-Resolving and Wind-Stopping Method)

Ingredients	Effects	Combined Effects	Syndrome	Chief Symptoms
Jackinthepulpit Tuber (天南星, Tiannanxing)6g Earth Worm (地龙, Dilong)6g Silkworm with Batrytis Larva (僵蚕, Jiangcan)6g Gecko (壁虎, Bihu)6g Centipede (蜈蚣, Wugong)2 pieces	Stopping the wind and relieving convulsion	Removing phlegm and stopping the wind, detoxification and resisting cancer	Turbid phlegm accumulated in the interior and up-stirring of the liver	Severe headache, blurred vision, continuous vomiting, vertigo, insomnia, convulsion, hemiplegia, pale tongue with white and greasy coating, wiry and smooth pulse
Pinellia Rhizome (半夏, Banxia)9g Tuckahoe (茯苓, Fuling)9g Umbellate Pore Fungus (猪苓, Zhuling)9g	Expelling dampness and removing phlegm			
Common Selfheal Fruit-Spike (夏枯草, Xiakucao)9g Oyster Shell (生牡蛎, Sheng Muli) 15g	Softening hardness and dissipating blockages			
Ground Bettle (䗪虫, Zhechong)9g	Removing blood stasis drastically and dissipating blockages			
Toad Skin Secretion Cake (蟾酥, Chansu)0.01g	Detoxification and alleviating pain			

Points in Constitution: Encephalopathy usually belongs to wind-phlegm syndrome. This formula is designed for stopping the wind and removing phlegm, thus five kinds of insect and animal drugs are used. In the prescription, Toad Skin Secretion Cake (蟾酥, Chansu), Common Selfheal Fruit-Spike (夏枯草, Xiakucao), Umbellate Pore Fungus (猪苓, Zhuling) and Gecko (壁虎, Bihu) are the common drugs for treating cancer.

Indications: Brain glioma.

Precaution: Toad Skin Secretion Cake (蟾酥, Chansu) is poisonous and the dose should be carefully controlled.

Associated Formula:

Pinellia, Largehead Atractylodes and Gastordia Decoction(半夏白术天麻汤, ban xia bai zhu tian ma tang) *Comprehension of Medicine*《医学心悟》

This is made up of Pinellia Rhizome (半夏, Banxia), Tangerine Peel (橘皮, Jupi), Tuckahoe (茯苓, Fuling), Licorice Root (生甘草, Sheng Gancao), Largehead Atractylodes Rhizome (白

术, Baizhu) and Tall Gastrodia Rhizome (天麻, Tianma). Its actions are removing phlegm and stopping the wind. It is indicated for headache and vertigo due to upward attack of wind-phlegm upon the head.

Bupleurum, Snakegourd Fruit and Appendiculate Cremastra Pseudobulb Decoction(柴胡蒌姑汤, chai hu lou gu tang)

Source: Oncology of Traditional Chinese Medicine《中医肿瘤学》
Composition: Bupleurum (柴胡, Chaihu)9g
Green Tangerine Peel (青皮, Qingpi)9g
Turmeric Root-Tuber (郁金, Yujin)9g
Tangerine Leaf (橘叶, Juye)9g
Chinese Angelica Root (当归, Danggui)9g
White Peony Root (白芍药, Baishaoyao)9g
Tuckahoe (茯苓, Fuling)9g
Largehead Atractylodes Rhizome (白术, Baizhu)9g
Dahurican Angelica Root (白芷, Baizhi)9g
Appendiculate Cremastra Pseudobulb (山慈姑, Shancigu)15g
Snakegourd Fruit (全瓜蒌, Quangualou)30g

Actions: Dispersing the stagnated liver-qi, removing phlegm and dissipating blockages.

Applied Syndrome: Mammary cancer due to stagnation of the liver-qi and retention of phlegm, manifested as uneven mammary lumps which is unable to move about, often without obvious boundary, feeling of distention, fullness and pain in the chest and hypochondrium, restlessness or irritability, pale tongue with greasy coating, wiry pulse.

Points in Constitution: This formula is the modification of Merry Life Powder(逍遥散, xiao yao san) whose basic actions are dispersing the stagnated liver-qi and invigorating the spleen. The added drugs of Green Tangerine Peel (青皮, Qingpi), Tangerine Leaf (桔叶, Juye), Snakegourd Fruit (瓜蒌, Gualou), Dahurican Angelica Root (白芷, Baizhi) and Turmeric Root-Tuber (郁金, Yujin), which have the actions of activating flow of qi and dissipating blockages, are all the common drugs for diseases of the breast. Appendiculate Cremastra Pseudobulb (山慈姑, Shancigu) has the cancer-resisting action.

Indications:
1. Mammary cancer.
2. Hyperplasia of lobules of mammary gland.

Precaution: Appendiculate Cremastra Pseudobulb (山慈姑, Shancigu) has good actions of resisting cancer, removing phlegm and dissipating blockages, but it also has a comparatively powerful toxin. So attention should be paid to its dosage.

Bupleurum, Snakegourd Fruit and Appendiculate Cremastra Pseudobulb Decoction
(Qi-Activating and Phlegm-Resolving Method)

Ingredients	Effects	Combined Effects	Syndrome	Chief Symptoms
Bupleurum (柴胡, Chaihu) 9g Green Tangerine Peel (青皮, Qingpi) 9g Tangerine Leaf (橘叶, Juye) 9g Turmeric Root-Tuber (郁金, Yujin) 9g	Relieving the depressed liver and activating flow of qi	Dispersing the stagnated liver-qi, removing phlegm and dissipating blockages	Mammary cancer due to stagnation of qi and retention of phlegm	Uneven mammary lumps which are uneasy to move about, often without obvious boundary, feeling of distention and fullness and pain in the chest and hypochondrium, irritability, pale tongue with greasy coating, wiry pulse
Chinese Angelica Root (当归, Danggui) 9g White Peony Root (白芍药, Baishaoyao) 9g	Enriching blood and activating blood circulation			
Tuckahoe (茯苓, Fuling) 9g Largehead Atractylodes Rhizome (白术, Baizhu) 9g	Replenishing qi and invigorating the spleen			
Appendiculate Cremastra Pseudobulb (山慈姑, Shancigu) 15g	Removing phlegm, dissipating blockages and anticancer			
Snakegourd Fruit (全瓜蒌, Quangualou) 30g	Regulating flow of qi, removing phlegm and dissipating blockages			
Dahurican Angelica Root (白芷, Baizhi) 9g	Alleviating pain and reducing swelling			

Associated Formulas:

1. Turmeric Root-Tuber Merry Life Powder (郁金逍遥散, yu jin xiao yao san) *Intermediate Journal of Medical Publication* 《中级医刊》

This is made up of Bupleurum (柴胡, Chaihu), Chinese Angelica Root (当归, Danggui), White Peony Root (白芍药, Baishaoyao), Largehead Atractylodes Rhizome (白术, Baizhu), Tuckahoe (茯苓, Fuling), Tangerine Peel (橘皮, Jupi), Turmeric Root-Tuber (郁金, Yujin) and Common Selfheal Fruit-Spike (夏枯草, Xiakucao). Its actions are soothing the liver, regulating flow of qi, invigorating the spleen and regulating the stomach-qi. It is indicated for mammary cancer due to stagnation of the liver-qi.

2. A Prescription for Breast Nodule (乳一方, ru yi fang, also called 乳核内消片, ru he nei xiao pian) *Famous Prescriptions of the Ancient and Present times* 《古今名方》

This is composed of Bupleurum (柴胡, Chaihu), Chinese Angelica Root (当归, Danggui), Turmeric Root-Tuber (郁金, Yujin), Tangerine Seed (橘核, Juhe), Appendiculate Cremastra Pseudobulb (山慈姑, Shancigu), Nutgrass Galingale Rhizome (香附, Xiangfu), Globethistle (漏芦, Loulu), Common Selfheal Fruit-Spike (夏枯草, Xiakucao), Madder Root (茜草, Qiancao), Red Peony Root (赤芍药, Chishaoyao), Green Tangerine Peel (青皮, Qingpi), Towel Gourd Vegetable Sponge (丝瓜络, Sigualuo) and Licorice Root (生甘草, Sheng Gancao). Its actions are dispersing the stagnated liver-qi, activating blood circulation, softening hardness and dissipating blockages. It is indicated for hyperplasia of lobules of mammary gland.

Prescription for Ovarian Cancer
(治卵巢癌方, zhi luan cao ai fang)

Source: Gynecology 《妇产科学》
Composition: Spreading Hedyotis Herb (白花蛇舌草, Baihuasheshecao) 15g
Solamum Lyratum (白英, Baiying) 15g
Barbed Skullcap Herb (半枝莲, Banzhilian) 15g
Turtle Carapace (鳖甲, Biejia) 12g
Tangerine Seed (橘核, Juhe) 9g
Kwangsi Turmeric Rhizome (莪术, Ezhu) 9g
Peach Seed (桃仁, Taoren) 9g
Safflower (红花, Honghua) 9g
Ground Bettle (䗪虫, Zhechong) 15g
Kelp (昆布, Kunbu) 9g
Fennel Fruit (小茴香, Xiaohuixiang) 9g
Coix Seed (薏苡仁, Yiyiren) 30g
Pilose Asiabell Root (党参, Dangshen) 9g

Actions: Activating flow of qi and clearing away toxic material, breaking blood stasis and eliminating hardness.

Applied Syndrome: Ovarian cancer, caused by blood stasis in the interior and accumulation of blood stasis and stagnant heat, manifested as lump in the abdomen, discomfort, distention or pain in the abdomen, or irregular menstruation, or postmenopause hemorrhage, red tongue with petechia or ecchymosis, deep and unsmooth pulse.

Points in Constitution: In this formula Solamum Lyratum (白英, Baiying), which is also called shu yang quan (蜀羊泉), is often used together with Black Nightshade Herb (龙葵, Longkui), Duchesnea (蛇莓, Shemei) and Spreading Hedyotis Herb (白花蛇舌草, Baihuasheshecao) to treat malignant tumors.

Indications:
1. Ovarian cancer.
2. Ovarian cyst.
3. Cancer of uterine tube.

Precaution: For the patients who have a weak body accompanied with continuous uterine bleeding, the drugs for removing blood stasis and arresting bleeding, or the drugs for restoring qi to control blood should be added.

Prescription for Ovarian Cancer
(Blood-Activating And Stasis-Removing Method)

Ingredients	Effects	Combined Effects	Syndrome	Chief Symptoms
Kwangsi Turmeric Rhizome (莪术, Ezhu)9g Peach Seed (桃仁, Taoren)9g Safflower (红花, Honghua)9g Ground Bettle (䗪虫, Zhechong)15g	Activating blood circulation and removing blood stasis drastically	Activating flow of qi and clearing toxic material, removing blood stasis drastically and eliminating hardness	Ovarian cancer (due to accumulation of blood stasis and stagnant heat)	Lump in the abdomen, distention and pain in the abdomen, irregular menstruation, or postmenopause hemorrhage, red tongue with petechia or ecchymosis, deep and unsmooth pulse.
Kelp (昆布, Kunbu)9g Turtle Carapace (鳖甲, Biejia)12g	Softening hardness and dissipating blockages			
Fennel Fruit (小茴香, Xiaohuixiang)9g Tangerine Seed (橘核, Juhe)9g	Activating flow of qi and alleviating pain			
Spreading Hedyotis Herb (白花蛇舌草, Baihuasheshecao)15g Solamum Lyratum (白英, Baiying)15g Barbed Skullcap Herb (半枝莲, Banzhilian)15g	Clearing away heat and toxic material			
Coix Seed (薏苡仁, Yiyiren)30g	Clearing away heat and promoting diuresis			
Pilose Asiabell Root (党参, Dangshen)9g	Replenishing qi and strengthening body resistance			

Associated Formulas:

1. Amber Pill (琥珀丸, hu po wan) *The Complete Effective Prescriptions for Diseases of Women* 《妇人大全良方》

This is made up of Amber (琥珀, Hupo), Cassia Bark (桂心, Guixin), Medicinal Achyranthes Root (川牛膝, Chuan Niuxi), Lilac Daphne Flower-Bud (芫花, Yuanhua), Areca Seed (槟榔, Binglang), Peach Seed (桃仁, Taoren), Dried Rehmannia Root (生地黄, Shengdihuang), Corydalis Tuber (延胡索, Yanhusuo), Chinese Angelica Root (当归, Danggui), Turtle Carapace (鳖甲, Biejia), Common Burreed Rhizome (三棱, Sanleng), Ture Lacquertree Dried Lacquer (干漆, Ganqi), Sal-Ammoniac (硇砂, Naosha), Rhubarb (生大黄, Sheng Dahuang), Gadfly (虻虫, Mangchong) and Leech (水蛭, Shuizhi). Its actions are activating blood circulation and removing blood stasis. It is indicated for prolonged abdominal mass formed by blood stasis in woman which is like hydatidiform mole(hysteromyoma).

2. Compound Decoction of Wasps Nest (复方蜂房汤, fu fang feng fang tang) *New Medicine* 《新医学》

This is composed of Wasps Nest (露蜂房, Lufengfang), Dead of Pangolin Scales (山甲珠, Shanjiazhu), Hawthorn Fruit (山楂, Shanzha), Hirsute Shiny Bugleweed Herb (泽兰, Zelan),

Dan-Shen Root (丹参, Danshen), Chinese Angelica Root (当归, Danggui) and Tuckahoe (茯苓, Fuling). Its actions are activating blood circulation, removing blood stasis, softening hardness and dissipating blockages. It is applied for chorionic somatotropin and primary vaginal cancer.

Associated Formulas:

1. Sweet Dew Detoxication Pill (甘露消毒丹, gan lu xiao du dan) *Secretly Handed Down Effective Remedy*《医效秘传》

This consists of Talc Refined with Water (飞滑石, Fei Huashi), Baikal Skullcap Root (黄芩, Huangqin), Capillary Wormwood Herb (茵陈, Yinchen), Wrinkled Gianthyssop Herb (藿香, Huoxiang), Weeping Forsythia Capsule (连翘, Lianqiao), Grassleaf Sweetflag Rhizome (石菖蒲, Shichangpu), Round Cardamon Seed (白豆蔻, Baidoukou), Wild Mint Herb (薄荷, Bohe), Akebia Stem (木通, Mutong), Musk (麝香, Shexiang) and Tendrilleaf Fritillary Bulb (川贝母, Chuan Beimu). Its actions are clearing away heat and toxic material, eliminating turbid evils and promoting diuresis. It is indicated for AIDS due to interior accumulation of turbid-dampness and noxious heat.

Compound Jade Spring Pill
(复方玉泉丸, fu fang yu quan wan)

Source: *Practical Prescriptions for the Diseases of Urogenital System*《泌尿生殖系病实用方》
Composition: Snakegourd Root (天花粉, Tianhuafen)30g
Pueraria(葛根, Gegen)9g
Dried Rehmannia Root (生地黄, Shengdihuang)15g
Chinese Magnoliavine fruit (五味子, Wuweizi)9g
Licorice Root (生甘草, Sheng Gancao)9g
Hypericumm Perfora(Guanyejinsitao, 贯叶金丝桃)15g
Lucid Ganoderma (灵芝, Lingzhi)15g
Glabrous Greenbrier Rhizome (土茯苓, Tufuling)15g

Actions: Clearing away heat, promoting the production of body fluid, eliminating pathogenic factors and toxin.

Applied Syndrome: AIDS or HIV infector, caused by excessive toxin and impairment of body fluid, manifested as fever, hidrosis, irritability, sore or ulcer of mouth and tongue, dry throat and mouth, dry cough with little sputum, or hectic fever and night sweating, flushed face or even coma, macular eruption, red tongue with yellow coating, rapid pulse.

Points in Constitution: This formula emphasizes strengthening body resistance, promoting the production of body fluid and clearing away heat and toxic material. Snakegourd Root (天花粉, Tianhuafen) and Lucid Ganoderma (灵芝, Lingzhi) are the main drugs in the formula. Since AIDS is subject to change, the prescription for this disease can be modified based on the different syndrome in the clinic.

Indications: It is applied for both AIDS or HIV infection due to excessive heat which impairs body fluid.

Precaution: This formula is designed for AIDS due to noxious heat in the interior and impairment of body fluid. Thus for AIDS with deficiency of healthy qi, this formula should be used with other drugs.

Compound Jade Spring Pill
(Heat-Clearing and Toxin-Removing Method)

Ingredients	Effects	Combined Effects	Syndrome	Chief Symptoms
Snakegourd Root (天花粉, Tianhuafen)30g Hypericumm Perfora (Guanyejinsitao, 贯叶金丝桃)15g Glabrous Greenbrier Rhizome (土茯苓, Tufuling)15g	Clearing away heat and toxic material	Clearing away heat and toxic material, nourishing yin and promoting the production of body fluid	AIDS (due to excessive heat impairing body fluid)	Fever, hidrosis, irritability, ulcer of mouth and tongue, dry throat and mouth, dry cough with little sputum, or hectic fever and night sweating, red complexion or coma, macular eruption, red tongue, yellow tongue coating, rapid pulse
Dried Rehmannia Root (生地黄, Shengdihuang)15g Chinese Magnoliavine Fruit (五味子, Wuweizi)9g Pueraria(葛根, Gegen)9g	Nourishing yin and promoting the production of body fluid			
Lucid Ganoderma (灵芝, Lingzhi)15g	Supporting the healthy qi			
Licorice Root (生甘草, Sheng Gancao)9g	Clearing away heat and toxic material			

2. Anjilike (安吉利克, an ji li ke) *Practical Prescriptions for the Diseases of Urogenital System* 《泌尿生殖系病实用方》

This is made up of Ginseng (人参, Renshen), Chinese Angelica Root (当归, Danggui) and Glossy Privet Fruit (女贞子, Nüzhenzi). Its actions are restoring qi, enriching blood, strengthening body resistance and eliminating pathogenic factors. It is indicated for AIDS due to deficiency of the healthy qi and insufficiency of both qi and blood.

3. Proven AIDS-Resisting Formula (抗艾滋病经验方, kang ai zi bing jing yan fang) *Proved Recipes* 《验方》

This is made up of Hypericumm Perfora(Guanyejinsitao, 贯叶金丝桃) and Snakegourd Root (天花粉, Tianhuafen). The main action of this formula is clearing away heat and toxic material. It has a certain effect on AIDS but a better effect on anti-HIV infection.

Chapter Fourteen
Formulas for External Use and Others

In TCM, there has been a great variety of drugs and therepies for external use since ancient times which include herb paste, ointment, powder, lotion, fumigant, eye or nose drops, suppository, plaster, medicated roll(or thread) and hot medicated compress. They have proved extremely effective for both the internal and external diseases. Thus, it is necessary to make a further reseach and expand their utilization in the clinic.

1. Golden Powder
（金黄散，jin huang san）

Source: *Golden Mirror of Medicine* 《医宗金鉴》
Composition: Rhubarb（生大黄，Sheng Dahuang）25g
Chinese Corktree Bark（黄柏，Huangbai）25g
Turmeric Rhizome（姜黄，Jianghuang）25g
Dahurican Angelica Root（白芷，Baizhi）25g
Jackinthepulpit Tuber（天南星，Tiannanxing）10g
Tangerine Peel（橘皮，Jupi）10g
Swordlike Atractylodes Rhizome（苍术，Cangzhu）10g
Officinal Magnolia Bark（厚朴，Houpo）10g
Licorice Root（生甘草，Sheng Gancao）10g
Snakegourd Root（天花粉，Tianhuafen）50g
(Ground into powder, mixed with wine and applied for external use.)

Actions: Clearing away heat and toxic material, reducing swelling and alleviating pain.

Applied Syndrome: Sores of yang syndrome manifested as local redness, swelling and hot pain with no formation of pus or pus without perforation.

Points in Constitution: Sores due to heat-toxin is, in fact, the result of local accumulation of qi, blood and phlegm. On the basis of the application of Rhubarb（大黄，Dahuang）and Chinese Corktree Bark（黄柏，Huangbai）which have the actions of clearing away heat and toxic material, this formula uses the ingredients of Stomach-Calming Powder（平胃散，ping wei san）to eliminate turbid evils and Turmeric Rhizome（姜黄，Jianghuang）, Dahurican Angelica Root（白芷，Baizhi）and Jackinthepulpit Tuber（天南星，Tiannanxing）to warm and activate flow of qi and circulation of blood to dissipate blockages, which rightly correspond to the pathogenesis. Snakegourd Root（天花粉，Tianhuafen）is the key drug for sores, and it can reduce the swelling if the pus has not been formed and evacuate pus if the swelling has suppurated. This formula can both clear away heat and nourish yin, therefore it treats every aspect of the disease.

Golden Powder
(Heat-Clearing, Toxin-Removing, Swelling-Reducing and Blockage-Dissipating Method)

Ingredients	Effects	Combined Effects	Syndrome	Chief Symptoms
Rhubarb (生大黄, Sheng Dahuang)25g Chinese Corktree Bark (黄柏, Huangbai)25g	Clearing away heat and toxic material	Clearing away heat and toxic material, reducing swelling and alleviating pain	Sores of yang syndrome	Local redness, swellingt and hot pain, or with aversion to cold and fever, red tongue with yellow and greasy coating, smooth and rapid pulse
Snakegourd Root (天花粉, Tianhuafen)50g	Reducing swelling and evacuating pus			
Turmeric Rhizome (姜黄, Jianghuang)25g Dahurican Angelica Root (白芷, Baizhi)25g Jackinthepulpit Tuber (天南星, Tiannanxing)10g	Dissipating blockage and alleviating pain			
Swordlike Atractylodes Rhizome (苍术, Cangzhu)10g Officinal Magnolia Bark (厚朴, Houpo)10g Tangerine Peel (橘皮, Jupi)10g Licorice Root (生甘草, Sheng Gancao)10g	Clearing dampness-turbid by fragrant drugs			

Indication: Initial stage of all kinds of skin and sofe tissue infection without suppuration.
Precaution: It is forbidden for those with suppurative pus or ulceration.

2. Yang-Harmonizing and Stagnation-Removing Plaster
(阳和解凝膏, yang he jie ning gao)

Source: *Surgery Life-Saving Collection* 《外科全生集》
Composition: Root and Leaf of Great Burdock Achene (牛蒡根叶, Niubanggenye)
Impatiens Stem (白凤仙梗, Baifengxiangeng)
Common Monkshood's Mother Root (生川乌, Sheng Chuanwu)
North Monkshood (生草乌, Sheng Caowu)
Prepared Aconite Root (附子, Fuzi)
Cassia Bark (肉桂, Rougui)
Cassia Twig (桂枝, Guizhi)
Rhubarb (大黄, Dahuang)

Chinese Angelica Root (当归, Danggui)
Red Peony Root (赤芍药, Chishaoyao)
Olibanum (乳香, Ruxiang)
Myrrh (没药, Moyao)
Earth Worm (地龙, Dilong)
Silkworm with Batrytis Larva (僵蚕, Jiangcan)
Dahurican Angelica Root (白芷, Baizhi)
Japanese Ampelopsis Root (白蔹, Bailian)
Bletilla Tuber (白及, Baiji)
Szechwan Lovage Rhizome (川芎, Chuanxiong)
Himalayan Teasel Root (续断, Xuduan)
Divaricate Saposhnikovia Root (防风, Fangfeng)
Fineleaf Schizonepeta Herb (荆芥, Jingjie)
Trogopterus Dung (五灵脂, Wulingzhi)
Common Acklandia Root (木香, Muxiang)
Citron Fruit (香橼, Xiangyuan)
Tangerine Peel (橘皮, Jupi)
Storesin Oil (苏合油, Suheyou)
Musk (麝香, Shexiang)
Marijuana Oil (大麻油, Damayou)
Huangda Powder (黄丹, Huangdan)
(Prepared into plaster and applied to the affected part after it is heated and softened. It is a patent medicine and its detailed preparation is omitted.).

Actions: Warming the meridian and expelling cold, activating flow of qi and circulation of blood, dredging the collaterals and alleviating pain.

Applied Syndrome: Sores of yin type such as cellulitis, phlegmon, multiple abscess, scrofula, subcutaneous nodule and frostbite due to stagnation of cold-dampness, or arthralgia and aching pain of bones and muscels due to wind-cold.

Indications:

1. Pyogenic inflammation of various skin and subcutaneous or deep tissue with normal colour which belongs to yin syndrome.
2. The period of sclerosis or induration of lymph tuberculosis and thoracic tuberculosis.
3. Frostbite of Ⅰ~Ⅱ degree.
4. The beginning of bone and joint tuberculosis.
5. Dysentery due to cold-dampness.
6. Rheumatic arthralgia.

Precautions:

1. This formula is hot in nature and it is suitable for sores of yin type. It can not be used for febrile disease of yang syndrome.
2. It is forbidden to be applied on the abdominal region of pregnant woman.

Associated Formulas:

1. Jade and Dragon Ointment for Restoring Yang(回阳玉龙膏, hui yang yu long gao) *Orthodox Manual of Surgery*《外科正宗》

This is made up of Fried North Monkshood（炒草乌，Chao Caowu）, Dried Ginger（干姜，Ganjiang）, Fried Red Peony Root（炒赤芍药，Chao Chishaoyao）, Dahurican Angelica Root（白芷，Baizhi）, Fried Jackinthepulpit Tuber（制南星，Zhi Nanxing）and Cassia Bark（肉桂，Rougui）, which are ground into fine powder, mixed with hot wine and applied to the affected area. It can also be mixed into a plaster for application. Its actions are warming the meridian, activating blood circulation and dissipating cellulitis of yin type. It is indicated for cellulitis of yin-type with swelling and pain.

Cassia Bark and Musk Powder（桂麝散，gui she san）*Revealment of the Collection of Prescriptions*《药蔹启秘》

This is made up of Ephedra（麻黄，Mahuang）, Manchurian Wildginger Herb（细辛，Xixin）, Cassia Bark（肉桂，Rougui）, Clove Flower-Bud（丁香，Dingxiang）, Chinese Honeylocust Abnormal Fruit（猪牙皂，Zhuyazao）, Pinellia Rhizome（生半夏，Sheng Banxia）, Jackinthepulpit Tuber（生天南星，Sheng Tiannanxing）, Musk（麝香，Shexiang）and Borneol（冰片，Bingpian）which are ground into powder and Prepared into plaster for topical application. Its actions are warming and removing phlegm-dampness, reducing swelling and alleviating pain. It is indicatd for cellulitis of yin type with swelling and pain, or nodules of breast.

3. Sores-Treating Medicated Thread
（三品一条枪，san pin yi tiao qiang）

Source: *Orthodox Manual of Surgery*《外科正宗》
Composition: Alum（明矾，Mingfan）
Arsenolite Ore（白砒，Baipi）
Red Orpiment（雄黄，Xionghuang）
Olibanum（乳香，Ruxiang）
(Ground into fine powder, made into thick paste, rubbed into thready shape, dried in the shade and inserted into the hole of the sore for treatment. It is a patent medicine and its detailed preparation is omitted.)

Actions: Eroding bad or slough flesh.
Applied Syndrome: Hemorrhoid, anal fistula, scrofula, goiter, nail-like boil and lumbodorsal cellulitis.
Indications:

1. The midtrimester and late internal hemorrhoid.
2. Paronychia.
3. Carbuncles

4. Tuberculosis of bone and joint with multiple fistula.

5. Yellow and pink atheroma.

Precaution: It has the actions of eliminating slough and eroding fistula. When applied, it should be inserted into the hole of the sore. For those without a hole, the sore should be first stabbed by a needle.

Associated Formula:

Seven Immortal Rolls (七仙条, qi xian tiao) *Surgery* 《外科学》

This is made up of the ingredients of Baijiang Powder(白降丹, bai jiang dan) and Hongsheng Powder (红升丹, hong sheng dan) plus Calcined Gypsum (熟石膏, Shu Shigao) and Borneol (冰片, Bingpian). They are prepared into medicated rolls and have the actions of eroding fistula. It is indicated for hemorrhoids and pyogenic infection of bone.

4. Nine to One Powder
(九一丹, jiu yi dan)

Source: *The Golden Mirror of Medicine* 《医宗金鉴》
Composition: Calcined Gypsum (煅石膏, Duan Shigao) 9g
Hongsheng Powder (红升丹, hong sheng dan) 1g

The two drugs are ground into fine powder, spread on the sore and covered with a piece of plaster topically. The powder and plaster are to be changed once a day or every other a day; or inserting the powdered rolls into the hole of the sore and covering it with a plaster, once or twice a day.

Note: Hongsheng Powder (红升丹, hong sheng dan) is a patent medicine which is prepared with Mercury (水银, Shuiyin)30g, Nitrum (火硝, Huoxiao)120g, Alum (白矾, Baifan)30g, Malachite Ore (皂矾, Zaofan)18g, Cinnabar (朱砂, Zhusha)15g and Red Orpiment (雄黄, Xionghuang)15g.

Actions: Evacuating pus and detoxification, removing slough and promoting regeneration of tissues.

Applied Syndrome: Sores which are resistant to healing after suppuration due to incomplete elimination of purulence and toxin.

Indications:

1. All kinds of sores without complete elimination of pus.

2. Perianorectal abscess and anal fistula.

3. Infectious soft wart.

4. Acute lymphadenitis, ulcerated thromboangiitis obliterans.

Precautions:

1. The dose ratio of Calcined Gypsum (煅石膏, Duan Shigao) and Hongsheng Powder(红升丹, hong sheng dan) is nine to one. That is why it is named Nine to One Powder(九一丹, jiu yi dan).

2. It is for external use only.

Associated Formulas:

1. Baijiang Powder (白降丹, bai jiang dan) *The Golden Mirror of Medicine* 《医宗金鉴》

This is made up of Cinnabar (朱砂, Zhusha), Red Orpiment (雄黄, Xionghuang), Mercury (水银, Shuiyin), Borax (硼砂, Pengsha), Nitrum (火硝, Huoxiao), Salt (食盐, Shiyan), Alum (白矾, Baifan) and Malachite Ore (皂矾, Zaofan). It is prepared with the method of sublimation. Its actions are removing slough, eliminating pterygium, detoxifying and evacuating pus. It is applied for sores with stubborn slough, verruca vulgaris and scrofula.

5. Yuhong Ointment for Promoting Tissue Regeneration (生肌玉红膏, sheng ji yu hong gao)

Source: *Orthodox Manual of Surgery* 《外科正宗》
Composition: Sinkiang Arnebia Root or Redroot Gromwell Root (紫草, Zicao)
Dahurican Angelica Root (白芷, Baizhi)
Licorice Root (甘草, Gancao)
Chinese Angelica Root (当归, Danggui)
Dragon's Blood (血竭, Xuejie)
Mercuros Chloride (轻粉, Qingfen)
Cera Chinensis (白蜡, Baila)
Sesame Oil (麻油, Mayou)
(Prepared into ointment and applied externally to the affected area. It is a patent medicine and its detailed preparation is omitted.)

Actions: Removing slough and promoting regeneration of tissue, activating blood circulation and easing pain.

Applied Syndrome: Suppurated carbuncle, gangrene and sores characterized by inclined healing of the sores but with a slow regeraration of new tissues.

Points in Constitution: In the formula, Mercuros Chloride (轻粉, Qingfen) is the main drug which can remove and erode the slough. This is because that after the sores have been suppurated, the slow regeneration of new tissues is mostly due to the incomplete elimination of slough. In order to promote the regenration of the new tissues, it is essential to remove the slough. The other drugs in the formula are to aid the Mercuros Chloride (轻粉, Qingfen) in activating blood flow, relieving pain, evacuating pus and promoting regeneration of tissues.

Indications:
1. Ulcerated or suppurated sores.
2. Scald by hot water or fire.
3. Fracture and broken tendons due to incised wound.

Precautions:
1. It is not suitable to the beginning of sores with excessive toxin-fire.
2. Since this formula is poisonous, attention should be paid to the dosage, term and sensitive reaction of the drugs when they are used.
3. It is contraindicated in those who suffer from hepato-renal incompetence.

Yuhong Ointment for Promoting Tissue Regeneration
(Slough-Removing and Tissue-Generatiog Method)

Ingredients	Effects	Combined Effects	Syndrome	Chief Symptoms
Sinkiang Arnebia Root or Redroot Gromwell Root (紫草, Zicao) Chinese Angelica Root (当归, Danggui) Dragon's Blood (血竭, Xuejie)	Activating blood circulation and alleviating pain	Removing slough and promoting regeneration of tissue, removing toxic material and alleviating pain	Carbuncle, gangrene and sores, which are just going to heal	Suppurated carbuncle, gangrene and sores characterized by inclined healing of the sores but with a slow regeraration of new tissues
Mercuros Chloride (轻粉, Qingfen)	Removing slough, promoting regeneration of tissue and removing toxic material			
Dahurican Angelica Root (白芷, Baizhi)	Evacuating pus and alleviating pain			
Licorice Root (甘草, Gancao)	Detoxification and mediating the actions of other herbs			
Sesame Oil (麻油, Mayou) Cera Chinensis (白蜡, Baila)	Excipient for protecting skin			

Associated Formulas:

1. Eight Treasures Powder (八宝丹, ba bao dan) *Complete Works for Treating Sores* 《疡医大全》

This consists of Pearl (珍珠, Zhenzhu), Cow-Bezoar (牛黄, Niuhuang), Elephant Hide (象皮, Xiangpi), Amber (琥珀, Hupo), Calcined Dragon's Bone (煅龙骨, Duan Longgu), Mercuros Chloride (轻粉, Qingfen), Borneol (冰片, Bingpian) and Calcined Calamine (煅炉甘石, Duan Luganshi), which are made into powder and applied externally on the sores. Its actions are promoting regeneration of tissue and astringing sore. It is indicated for all kinds of sores without any slough and pus.

2. Tissue-Rregeneration Powder (生肌散, sheng ji san) *Experienced Prescriptions* 《经验方》

This consists of Calcined Calamine (炉甘石, Luganshi), Stalactite (乳石, Rushi), Talc (滑石, Huashi), Amber (琥珀, Hupo), Cinnabar (朱砂, Zhusha) and Borneol (冰片, Bingpian), which are ground into fine powder and spread externally on the affected area. Its actions are promoting regeneration of tissue and healing of the sores. It is indicated for suppurated carbuncle and gangrene without pus.

6. Itching-Stopping Decoction
(㭎痒汤, ta yang tang)

Source: *Orthodox Manual of Surgery* 《外科正宗》
Composition: Lightyellow Sophora Root (苦参, Kushen) 15g

Common Cnidium Fruit (蛇床子, Shechuangzi)15g

Fischer Euphorbia Root (狼毒, Langdu)15g

Ending Part of Chinese Angelica Root (当归尾, Dangguiwei)15g

Chinese Clematis Root (威灵仙, Weilingxian)15g

Common Carpesium Fruit (鹤虱, Heshi)30g

(Decocted in the 2000ml of water and use the steam and hot decoction to fumigate and wash the affected part.)

Actions: Clearing away heat and drying dampness, destrroying parasites and arresting itching.

Applied Syndrome: Pruritus of vulvae and sores inside and outside the vagina due to downward attack of damp-heat on the lower-jiao.

Itching-Stopping Decoction
(Heat-Clearing and Dampness-Drying Method)

Ingredients	Effects	Combined Effects	Syndrome	Chief Symptoms
Lightyellow Sophora Root (苦参, Kushen)15g Common Cnidium Fruit (蛇床子, Shechuangzi)15g Fischer Euphorbia Root (狼毒, Langdu)15g Common Carpesium Fruit (鹤虱, Heshi)30g	Clearing away heat and removing dampness, destroying parasites and alleviating itching	Clearing away heat and drying dampness, destrroying parasites and stopping itching	Pruritus of vulvae and sores inside and outside the vagina due to downward attack of damp-heat on the lower-jiao	Unbearable itching of vulvae and vagina, profuse yellow sticky or spumescent leucorrhea, yellow, white, thick and greasy tongue coating, soft and rapid pulse or smooth and rapid pulse
Chinese Clematis Root (威灵仙, Weilingxian)15g	Expelling wind and drying dampness			
Ending Part of Chinese Angelica Root (当归尾, Dangguiwei)15g	Activating blood circulation and removing blood stasis			

Points in Constitution: Common Cnidium Fruit (蛇床子, Shechuangzi) is warm, potent and violent in nature and is indicated for pain and sweeling of valva in woman, impotence of man and damp-itching caused by deficiency of kidney-yang and excessiveness of cold water. When it is combined with Lightyellow Sophora Root (苦参, Kushen) and Fischer Euphorbia Root (狼毒, Langdu) it can remove damp-heat; when it is combined with Common Carpesium Fruit (鹤虱, Heshi), it can destroy parasites. The ending part of Chinese Angelica Root (当归尾, Dangguiwei) and Chinese Clematis Root (威灵仙, Weilingxian) have the actions of regulating blood and expelling wind. Itching is usually caused by damp-heat, parasites and wind. When they are removed by this formula, the itching is of course eliminated.

Indications:

1. Pruritus of vulva.
2. Trichomonal vaginitis.

Precaution: It is forbidden for those with deficiency of yin and dryness of blood.

Associated Formulas:

1. Common Cnidium Powder(蛇床子散, she chuang zi san) *Synopsis of Golden Cabinet*《金匮要略》

This is made up of Common Cnidium Fruit (蛇床子, Shechuangzi) and Power of Minium (铅粉, Qianfen), which are made into a vaginal suppository. Its actions are warming uterus and expelling cold, removing dampness and destroying parasites. It is indicated for prolonged pruritus of vulva and leucorrhea with clear and thin discharge, soreness, heaviness and sinking sensation in the loins.

2. Tiandi Pill (天滴丸, tian di wan) *Experienced Prescriptions*《经验方》

This is composed of Common Cnidium Fruit (蛇床子, Shechuangzi) and Alum (白矾, Baifan), which are made into a vaginal suppository. Its actions are removing dampness and destroying parasites and it is used for pruritus of vulva and leucorrhea which is white or yellow, thick and greasy like spumescence with a foul smell.

Associated Formula:

Itching-Stopping Decoction (塌痒汤, ta yang tang) *Orthodox Manual of Surgery*《外科正宗》

This is made up of Common Carpesium Fruit (鹤虱, Heshi), Lightyellow Sophora Root (苦参, Kushen), Chinese Clematis Root (威灵仙, Weilingxian), Common Cnidium Fruit (蛇床子, Shechuangzi), Ending Part of Chinese Angelica Root (当归尾, Dangguiwei) and Fischer Euphorbia Root (狼毒, Langdu). A better effect can be got if proper amount of pig's bile(猪胆汁, Zhudanzhi) is added to them. Its actions are destroying parasites and arresting itching. It is indicated for itching of women's vagina and sores inside and outside the vagina due to downward attack of damp-heat on the lower-jiao. At present, it is usually used for vaginal trichomoniasis.

7. Common Cnidium Powder
(蛇床子散, she chuang zi san)

Source: *Gynecology*《妇产科学》

Composition: Common Cnidium Fruit (蛇床子, Shechuangzi) 9~15g

Lightyellow Sophora Root (苦参, Kushen) 9~15g

Bunge Pricklysh (花椒, Huajiao) 9~15g

Sessile Stemona Root (百部, Baibu) 9~15g

Baked Alum (枯矾, Kufan) 9~15g

(Decoct the drugs with water, use the steam of hot decoction to fumigate the external genitalia, then wash it twice a day, ten days constituting a single course).

Actions: Removing dampness, destroying parasites and arresting itching.

Applied Syndrome: Pruritus of vulvae manifested as itching of the external genitalia, restlessness, leucorrhea with yellow and white or red and white discharge, or like broken bits of bean curd, or accompanied with irritability, bitter taste in the mouth, dry throat, red tongue with yellow coating.

Points in Constitution: This formula emphasizes destroying parasites and removing dampness to stop itching.

Indications:

1. Trichomonal vaginitis, colpomycosis.
2. Eczema of external genitalia, eczema of scrotum, scrotal itching.
3. Leukoplakia vulvae.

Common Cnidium Powder

(Dampness-Drying and Itching-Arresting Method)

Ingredients	Effects	Combined Effects	Syndrome	Chief Symptoms
Common Cnidium Fruit (蛇床子, Shechuangzi) 9~15g Bunge Pricklysh (花椒, Huajiao) 9~15g Sessile Stemona Root (百部, Baibu) 9~15g	Destroying parasites and alleviating itching	Removing dampness, destroying parasites and alleviating itching	Pruritus of vulva	Itching of external genitalia, restlessness, profuse and foul leucorrhea with white or yellow and red discharge, or like broken bits of bean curd
Baked Alum (枯矾, Kufan) 9~15g	Destrroying parasites, alleviating itching and drying dampness			
Lightyellow Sophora Root (苦参, Kushen) 9~15g	Clearing away heat, removing dampness and alleviating itching			

8. Borneol and Borax Powder
(冰硼散, bing peng san)

Source: *Orthodox Manual of Surgery* 《外科正宗》

Composition: Borneol (冰片, Bingpian) 1.5g

Cinnabar (朱砂, Zhusha) 1.8g

Weathered Sodium Sulfate (玄明粉, Yuanmingfen) 15g

Borax (硼砂, Pengsha) 15g

(Ground into fine powder. Firstly gargle the throat with cold tea, then blow a little of the powder to the affected part and rub it.)

Actions: Clearing away heat and dissipating blockages, reducing swelling and alleviating pain.

Applied Syndrome: Upward attack on throat and tongue along the meridians by accumulated noxious heat, manifested as sore throat, toothache, alveolar abscess, aphtha, laryngeal abscess, acute aphonia, hoarseness and laryngalgia.

Indications:
1. Acute tonsillitis, pharyngitis, laryngitis.
2. Stomatitis, oral ulcer, esophagitis.
3. Pulptis, gingivitis.
4. Hypoglossiadentis, mumps.
5. Acute or chronic otitis externa, tympanitis.
6. Neonatal omphalitis.

Precaution: This formula is designed for heat syndrom of excessive type characterized by upward attack along the meridian by accumulated noxious heat, thus it is not suitable to those with yin deficiency and hyperactivity of fire.

Borneol and Borax Powder
(Heat-Clearing and Toxin-Removing Method)

Ingredients	Effects	Combined Effects	Syndrome	Chief Symptoms
Borneol (冰片, Bingpian) 1.5g	Reducing swelling and alleviating pain	Clearing away heat and toxic material, reducing swelling and alleviating pain	Upward attack on throat and tongue along the meridians by accumulated noxious heat	Sore throat, erosion of mucous membrane of the oral cavity, hoarseness and laryngalgia
Cinnabar (朱砂, Zhusha) 1.8g	Clearing away heat and toxic material			
Weathered Sodium Sulfate (玄明粉, Yuanmingfen) 15g	Softening hardness and purging fire			
Borax (硼砂, Pengsha) 15g	Removing toxic material and reducing swelling			

Associated Formula:

Natural indigo, Borneol and Borax Powder(青黛冰硼散, qing dai bing peng san) *National Selected Prescriptions of Chinese Patent Medicine*, *Fuzhou Volume*《全国中药成药处方集·福州方》

This consists of Borneol (冰片, Bingpian), Natural indigo (青黛, Qingdai), Borax (硼砂, Pengsha)(Calcined), Coptis Rhizome (黄连, Huanglian), Urine of Boy Under 12(人中白, Renzhongbai), Licorice Root (生甘草, Sheng Gancao) and Calcined Gypsum (石膏, Shigao) which are ground into fine powder and blow it to the affected part. Its actions are clearing away heat and toxic material, reducing swelling and alleviating pain. It is indicated for infantile erosion of mucous membrane of the oral cavity due to excessive fetal fire and adult laryngalgia.

9. Instant Effective Powder
(立效散, li xiao san)

Source: *Secret Record of the Chamber of Orchids* 《兰室秘藏》
Composition: Manchurian Wildginger Herb (细辛, Xixin) 3g
Prepared Licorice Root (炙甘草, Zhi Gancao) 6g
Shunk Bugbane Rhizome (升麻, Shengma) 6g
Divaricate Saposhnikovia Root (防风, Fangfeng) 9g
Chinese Gentian Root (龙胆草, Longdancao) 9g
(Decocting the drugs with water and gargling the mouth with it)
Actions: Expelling wind and alleviating pain.
Applied Syndrome: Odontalgia due to wind-fire manifested as unbearable pain which radiates to the head, neck and back, slightly aversion to cold drink and severe aversion to hot drink.

Instant Effective Powder
(Wind-Expelling and Pain-Alleviating Method)

Ingredients	Effects	Combined Effects	Syndrome	Chief Symptoms
Manchurian Wildginger Herb (细辛, Xixin) 3g	Alleviating pain	Dispelling wind, clearing away heat and alleviating pain	Odontalgia due to wind-heat	Odontalgia, gingivitis, headache, thin and white or thin and yellow tongue coating, floating, wiry and rapid pulse
Shunk Bugbane Rhizome (升麻, Shengma) 6g	Removing toxic material			
Divaricate Saposhnikovia Root (防风, Fangfeng) 9g	Dispelling wind			
Chinese Gentian Root (龙胆草, Longdancao) 9g	Clearing away heat			
Prepared Licorice Root (炙甘草, Zhi Gancao) 6g	Coordinating the actions of various ingredients in the prescription			

Points in Constitution: The combination of Chinese Gentian Root (龙胆草, Longdancao) and Manchurian Wildginger Herb (细辛, Xixin) is a method of using cold-natured and heat-natured drugs together. When Manchurian Wildginger Herb (细辛, Xixin) is combined with Chinese Gentian Root (龙胆草, Longdancao), the pungent flavor and warm nature of Manchurian Wildginger Herb (细辛, Xixin) can be inhibited and has got an obvious pain-alleviating action. When Chinese Gentian Root (龙胆草, Longdancao) is combined with Manchurian Wildginger Herb (细辛, Xixin), heat can be removed without impairing the stomach by cold.

Indications:
1. Odontalgia.
2. Gingivitis.
3. Headache due to wind-heat.

Precaution: This formula can be used both for a gargle and oral medication.

Associated Formulas:

1. Yellow-Purging Powder(泻黄散, xie huang san) *Key to Therapeutics of Children's Diseases* 《小儿药证直诀》

This is made up of Wrinkled Gianthyssop Herb (藿香, Huoxiang), Cape Jasmine Fruit (山栀子, Shanzhizi), Gypsum (生石膏, Sheng Shigao), Licorice Root (生甘草, Sheng Gancao) and Divaricate Saposhnikovia Root (防风, Fangfeng). Its action is clearing and purging stagnated fire of the spleen and stomach. It is indicated for dry mouth and lips, aphtha, halitosis, dysphoria with smothery sensation, polyrexia and frequent playing with the tongue due to spleen-heat.

2. Stomach-Clearing Powder(清胃散, qing wei san) *Secret Record of the Chamber of Orchids* 《兰室秘藏》

This is composed of Chinese Angelica Root (当归身, Dangguishen), Coptis Rhizome (黄连, Huanglian), Dried Rehmannia Root (生地黄, Shengdihuang), Tree Peony Bark (牡丹皮, Mudanpi) and Shunk Bugbane Rhizome (升麻, Shengma). Its action is clearing away heat of yangming channel. It is indicated for unbearable toothache which may radiates to the head and whole of the face, fever, headache, desire for cold and aversion to heat and toothache which can be relieved by cold and aggravated by heat.

3. General Recope for Treating Toothache (牙痛统治方, ya tong tong zhi fang) Author's Experienced Prescription (作者经验方)

This consists of Ephedra(麻黄, Mahuang), Cassia Twig(桂枝, guizhi), Bitter Apricot Seed(杏仁, xingren), Gypsum(石膏, Shigao), Asarum Herb(细辛, Xixin) and Licorice Root(甘草, Gancao). It has the effect of dredging the channels to alleviate pain. It is applicable for unbearable toothache which can not be relieved with other therapies.

Additional Formulas

Zhonghuang Ointment
(中黄膏, zhong huang gao)

Source: *Formulae of Hanaoka*《华冈青洲方》

Composition: Balm (香油, Xiangyou) 10g

Yellow Wax (黄蜡, huangla) 38g

Turmeric Root-Tuber (郁金, Yujin) 4g

Chinese Corktree Bark (黄柏, Huangbai) 2g

Coptis Rhizome (黄连, Huanglian) 2g

〔Heating the balm up, adding yellow wax, then, after the wax melted, putting the powder of Turmeric Root-Tuber (郁金, Yujin), Chinese Corktree Bark (黄柏, Huangbai) and Coptis Rhizome (黄连, Huanglian) into it, mixing them up for use.〕

Actions: Clearing away heat and toxic material and alleviating pain.

Applied Syndrome: Sores of yang type manifested as redness, swelling, hot pain, hardness with deep root, thick and yellow pus, red tongue with yellow and greasy coating, forceful pulse.

Zhonghuang Ointment
(Heat-Clearing and Toxin-Removing Method)

Ingredients	Effects	Combined Effects	Syndrome	Chief Symptoms
Coptis Rhizome (黄连, Huanglian) 2g Chinese Corktree Bark (黄柏, Huangbai) 2g	Clearing away heat and toxic material, drying dampness and restraining bacterium	Clearing away heat and toxic material, dissipating blood stasis and alleviating pain	Sores of yang type due to traumatic injury	Local redness and swelling, hardness with deep root, yellow and thick pus, red tongue with yellow coating, forceful pulse
Turmeric Root-Tuber (郁金, Yujin) 4g	Dissipating blood stasis and alleviating pain			
Balm (香油, Xiangyou) 10g Yellow Wax (黄蜡, Huangla) 38g	Clearing away heat, protecting the skin, used as excipient			

Indications:

1. The beginning of acute pyogenic dermatosis.

2. All kinds of trauma such as traumatic injury, contusion, bruise, strain and sprain.

3. Frostbite, bite by insect or mosquito.

Precaution: This formula is forbidden for sores due to cold of insufficiency type.

Associated Formulas:

1. Purple Cloud Ointment (紫云膏, zi yun gao) *Brief Letters of Prescriptions frrom Chunxingxuan*《春杏轩撮要方函》

This is made up of the ingredients of Skin-Moistening Ointment(润肤膏, run fu gao) recorded in *Orthodox Manual of Surgery*《外科正宗》, i. e, Chinese Angelica Root（当归, Danggui）, Sinkiang Arnebia Root or Redroot Gromwell Root（紫草根, Zicaogen）, Benne Oil（胡麻油, Humayou）, Yellow Wax(黄腊, Huangla) plus Lard（猪油, Zhuyou）. Its actions are moistening the skin and promoting regeneration of tissues. It is used topically to treat the skin diseases due to deficiency of blood resulting from wind and dryness such as chronic eczema, dry tinea, keratodermia, rhagas, bed sore, skin ulcer and pigmentation.

Sovereign Wart-Eliminating Liniment
(疣灵搽剂, you ling cha ji)

Source: *Jiangsu Journnal of Traditional Chinese Medicine*《江苏中医》

Composition: Indigowoad Root（板蓝根, Banlangen）250g

Lightyellow Sophora Root（苦参, Kushen）250g

Nutgrass Galingale Rhizome（生香附, Sheng Xiangfu）250g

Common Scouring Rush Herb（木贼草, Muzeicao）250g

Wasps Nest（露蜂房, Lufengfang）250g

Mature Vinegar（陈醋, Chencu）500ml

(Decocting the first five drugs with 5000ml of water for 1 hour until the decoction remains to 2000ml, adding mature vinegar, then applying it on the affected part 3~5 times a day, 2 weeks constituting a treating course).

Actions: Clearing away heat and toxic material, removing dampness and eliminating wart.

Applied Syndrome:

Wart due to downward attack of damp-heat which accumulates and transforms into toxin. The manifestations are soft neoplasm on the male vaginal orifice, vaginal mucous membrane and cervix, or female urethral orifice, coronary sulcus, inner side of foreskin, common boundary of the skin and mucous membrane.

Points in Constitution: In recent years, it has been reported that Nutgrass Galingale Rhizome (香附, Xiangfu) can be used to treat flat wart. The other drugs in this formula are the detoxifying drugs. If Coix seed(薏苡仁, Yiyiren) is added, an obvious effect can be gained.

Indications:

1. Acuate condyloma.
2. Genital herpes.

Precaution: In clinic, for acuate condyloma and genital herpes, the combined use of internal and external drugs can obtain the best curative effect.

Sovereign Wart-Eliminating Liniment
(Heat-Clearing and Dampness-Drying Method)

Ingredients	Effects	Combined Effects	Syndrome	Chief Symptoms
Lightyellow Sophora Root (苦参, Kushen)	Clearing away heat and drying dampness, expelling wind and destroying parasites	Clearing away heat and toxic material, removing dampness and eliminating wart	Damp-heat and noxious heat accumulating in the lower-jiao	Wart in the pudendum
Indigowoad Root (板蓝根, Banlangen)	Clearing away heat and toxic material, removing heat from the blood and reducing swelling			
Common Scouring Rush Herb (木贼草, Muzicao) Wasps Nest (露蜂房, Lufengfang)	Expelling wind and removing toxic material			
Nutgrass Galingale Rhizome (生香附, Sheng Xiangfu)	Regulating flow of qi and dissipating blockages			
Mature Vinegar (陈醋, Chencu)	Detoxifying and alleviating itching			

Associated Formulas:

1. Eczema Powder (湿疹散, shi zhen san) *Yunnan Journal of Traditional Chinese Medicine* 《云南中医杂志》

This is composed of Hematite (代赭石, Daizheshi), Baked Alum (枯矾, Kufan) and Borneol (冰片, Bingpian). Its actions are drying dampness and detoxification. It is used externally and indicated for acute condyloma and genital herpes due to accumulation of heat-dampness and toxin.

2. Wart-Eliminating Decoction (消疣汤, xiao you tang) *Hunan Journal of Traditional Chinese Medicine* 《湖南中医》

This is composed of Purslane Herb (马齿苋, Machixian), Whiteflower Patrinia Herb (败酱草, Baijiangcao), Mirabilite (芒硝, Mangxiao), Glabrous Greenbrier Rhizome (土茯苓, Tufuling), Indigowoad Root (板蓝根, Banlangen) and Common Knotgrass Herb (萹蓄, Bianxu). Its actions are clearing away heat and toxic material, inducing diuresis and eliminating warts. It is indicated for acuate condyloma.

Three Huang Lotion
(三黄洗剂, san huang xi ji)

Source: *Surgery of Traditional Chinese Medicine* 《中医外科学》
Composition: Rhubarb (大黄, Dahuang),
Chinese Corktree Bark (黄柏, Huangbai),
Baikal Skullcap Root (黄芩, Huangqin),
Lightyellow Sophora Root (苦参, Kushen)
(Ground into fine powder, mixed with proper amount of distilled water and medical phenol, prepared into a lotion and applied on affected part, 4~5 times a day).

Actions: Clearing away heat and drying dampness, detoxifying and alleviating itching.

Applied Syndrome: Sores of yang type manifested as redness and swelling of the skin with burning pain, ulceration and oozing, furuncle and boils.

Three Huang Lotion
(Heat-Clearing and Dampness-Drying Method)

Ingredients	Effects	Combined Effects	Syndrome	Chief Symptoms
Rhubarb (大黄, Dahuang) Chinese Corktree Bark (黄柏, Huangbai) Baikal Skullcap Root (黄芩, Huangqin)	Purging fire and clearing away toxic material, drying dampness and reducing swelling	Clearing away heat and drying dampness, removing toxic material and alleviating itching	Sores of yang type	Local redness, swelling and burning pain, ulceration, oozing, furuncle and boils
Lightyellow Sophora Root (苦参, Kushen)	Clearing away toxic material and destroying parasites, removing dampness and alleviating itching			

Points in Constitution: These four drugs are all bitter in taste and cold in nature. They have the actions of clearing away heat and toxic materil and are good at treating sore syndrome due to fire-toxin. They can be used both internally and externally.

Indications:
1. Eczema.
2. Contact dermatitis.
3. Rice-field dermatitis.
4. The beginning of skin infection with redness and swelling.

Associated Formulas:

1. Three Wonderful Herbs Powder（三妙散, san miao san）*The Golden Mirror of Medicine*《医宗金鉴》

This is made up of Chinese Corktree Bark（黄柏, Huangbai）, Swordlike Atractylodes Rhizome（苍术, Cangzhu）and Areca Seed（槟榔, Binglang）which are ground into fine powder and sprinkled drily on the umbilicus. Its actions are clearing away heat, drying dampness and alleviating itching. it is indicated for itching of umbilicus accompanied with frequent discharge of yellow liquid, sores and tinea due to wetness.

2. Reversion Powder（颠倒散, dian dao san）*The Golden Mirror of Medicine*《医宗金鉴》

This is made up of Rhubarb（大黄, Dahuang）and Sulfur（硫黄, Liuhuang）which are ground into powder, mixed with cool boiled water or tea and applied or sprinkled on the affected part. Its actions are clearing away heat and dissipating blood stasis. It is applied for acne due to lung affection or acne rosacea with redness, swelling and pain.

Pain-Alleviating and Swelling-Reducing Plaster
（镇痛消肿膏, zhen tong xiao zhong gao）

Source: *Transaction of Traditional Chinese Medicine*《中医药学报》

Composition: Toad Skin Secretion Cake（蟾酥, Chansu）

Nux-Vomica Seed（马钱子, Maqianzi）

Common Monkshood's Mother Root（生川乌, Sheng Chuanwu）

Jackinthepulpit Tuber（生天南星, Sheng Tiannanxing）

Dahurican Angelica Root（白芷, Baizhi）

Turmeric Rhizome（姜黄, Jianghuang）

Borneol（冰片, Bingpian）

（Prepared into medicated fabric plaster for use. It is a patent medicine and its detailed preparation is omitted.）

Actions: Alleviating pain and reducing swelling.

Applied Syndrome: Pain of late cancer due to accumulation of phlegm and blood stasis which causes blockage of meridians and collaterals, manifested as unbearable pain with tenderness, dark purplish tongue or with ecchymosis, deep and unsmooth pulse.

Points in Constitution: Though the drugs in this formula are different in machanism and action, all of them have the characteristics of being fragrant and inclined to travel about and penetrate. They may exert the action of penetrating skin and alleviating pain.

Indications:

1. All kinds of late cancer (gastric cancer, liver cancer, mammary cancer, intestinal cancer, cancer of bone, lymphosarcoma, etc).

2. Pain of benign tumour.

Precaution: Remove the plaster after applied for 12 hours. The applicaton can only be done three times at most with a 12 hours' interval. Stop usage immediately if the skin is diabrotic.

Pain-Alleviating and Swelling-Reducing Plaster
(Blood Stasis-Removing and Pain-Alleviating Method)

Ingredients	Effects	Combined Effects	Syndrome	Chief Symptoms
Toad Skin Secretion Cake (蟾酥, Chansu)	Detoxifying and resisting cancer, reducing swelling and relieving pain	Alleviating pain and reducing swelling	Pain of late cancer	Late cancer with obvious lump, unbearable pain, dark purplish tongue or with ecchymosis, deep and unsmooth pulse
Nux Vomica (马钱子, Maqianzi)	Activating blood circulation and alleviating pain			
Common Monkshood's Mother Root (生川乌, Sheng Chuanwu)	Warming the meridian and alleviating pain			
Jackinthepulpit Tuber (生天南星, Sheng Tiannanxing)	Resolving phlegm and reducing swelling, dissipating blockages and alleviating pain			
Dahurican Angelica Root (白芷, Baizhi)	Dredging the collaterals, reducing swelling and alleviating pain			
Turmeric Rhizome (姜黄, Jianghuang)	Activating blood circulation and flow of qi, alleviating pain			
Borneol (冰片, Bingpian)	Dredging the collaterals and inducing resuscitation, alleviating pain and reducing swelling			

Associated Formulas:

1. Cassia Bark and Musk Powder (桂麝散 gui she san) *Revealment of the Collection of Prescriptions*《药蔹启秘》

This is composed of Ephedra (生麻黄, Sheng Mahuang), Manchurian Wildginger Herb (细辛, Xixin), Pinellia Rhizome (生半夏, Sheng Banxia), Jackinthepulpit Tuber (生南星, Sheng Nanxing), Cassia Bark (肉桂, Rougui), Clove Flower-Bud (丁香, Dingxiang), Chinese Honeylocust Abnormal Fruit (猪牙皂, Zhuyazao), Musk (麝香, Shexiang) and Borneol (冰片, Bingpian). Its actions are warming and removing phlegm-dampness, reducing swelling and alleviating pain. By local application it is indicated for cellulitis and multiple abscess without suppuration.

2. Internal Eliminating Powder for Yin-Toxin (阴毒内消散, yin du nei xiao san) *Revealment of the Collection of Prescriptions*《药蔹启秘》

This is made up of Olibanum (乳香, Ruxiang), Myrrh (没药, Moyao), Chinese Honeylocust Abnormal Fruit (猪牙皂, Zhuyazao), Clove Flower-Bud (丁香, Dingxiang), Derynaria Rhizome (生姜, Shengjiang), Camphor (樟冰, Zhangbing), Red Orpiment (雄黄, Xionghuang), Stir-

Backed Pangolin Scales (炮山甲, Paoshanjia), Prepared Common Monkshood's Mother Root (制川乌, Zhi Chuanwu), Mercuros Chloride (轻粉, Qingfen), Chinese Asafetida (阿魏, Awei), Cassia Bark (肉桂, Rougui), Pepper (胡椒, Hujiao) and Musk (麝香, Shexiang). Its actions are warming the meridian and expelling cold, removing phlegm and softening hardness. By applying it topically, it is indicated for swelling and sores of yin-syndrome or cancer.

Applied Syndrome: Carcinoma of uterine cervix due to internal accumulation of heat-toxin and mutual blockage of blood stasis and heat stagnation, manifested as contact hemorrhage or irregular hemorrhage, leucorrhagia with yellow watery or bloody discharge and a foul odour, lower abdominal pain or accompanied with frequency of urination, dysuria, hematuria etc, reddish tongue with yellow and greasy coating, deep pulse.

Centipede Powder
(蜈蚣粉, wu gong fen)

Source: *Tianjin Medicine* 《天津医药》

Composition: Mercuros Chloride (轻粉, Qingfen) 9g

Borneol (冰片, Bingpian) 1.5g

Red Orpiment (雄黄, Xionghuang) 9g

Centipede (蜈蚣, Wugong) 3 Pieces

Chinese Corktree Bark (黄柏, Huangbai) 30g

Musk (麝香, Shexiang) 1g

(Ground into powder and used topically).

Actions: Clearing away heat and toxic material, softening hardness and dissipating blockages.

Points in Constitution: Mercuros Chloride (轻粉, Qingfen), Red Orpiment (雄黄, Xionghuang) and Centipede (蜈蚣, Wugong) have the actions of clearing away toxic material and dissipating blockages. The use of these three drugs is to treating the toxifying disease with poisonous agents. The addition of Borneol (冰片, Bingpian) and Musk (麝香, Shexiang) is to reduce swelling and alleviate pain.

Indications:

1. Carcinoma of uterine cervix.
2. Vaginal cancer.

Precaution: Both Mercuros Chloride (轻粉, Qingfen) and Red Orpiment (雄黄, Xionghuang) are poisonous, so special attention should be paid to the dose of them. Besides, they can not be used for a long time.

Associated Formula:

Cancer-Treating Powder (治癌散, zhi ai san) *Research on Prevention and Cure of Tumor* 《肿瘤防治研究》

Centipede Powder
(Method of Combating Poison with Poison)

Ingredients	Effects	Combined Effects	Syndrome	Chief Symptoms
Mercuros Chloride (轻粉, Qingfen) 9g	Detoxifying and destroying parasites	Clearing away heat and toxic material, softening hardness and dissipating blockages	Carcinoma of uterine cervix due to accumulation of blood stasis and heat stagnation in the interior	Contact hemorrhage or irregular hemorrhage, leucorrhagia with discharge of yellow liquid, lower abdominal pain or accompanied with frequency of urination and dysuria, pale tongue, yellow and greasy tongue coating, smooth pulse
Red Orpiment (雄黄, Xionghuang) 9g	Clearing away toxic material and poisoning parasites			
Centipede (蜈蚣, Wugong) 3 pieces	Clearing toxic material and dissipating blockages, dredging the collaterals and alleviating pain			
Borneol (冰片, Bingpian) 1.5g Musk (麝香, Shexiang) 1g	Activating blood circulation and dissipating blockages, reducing swelling and alleviating pain			
Chinese Corktree Bark (黄柏, Huangbai) 30g	Clearing away heat and drying dampness			

    This is made up of Arsenolite Ore (砒石, Pishi), Sal-Ammoniac (硇砂, Naosha), Baked Alum (枯矾, Kufan), Iodoform (碘仿, Dianfang) and Borneol (冰片, Bingpian). Its actions are detoxifying and resisting cancer, elimination slough and promoting regeneration of tissue. Used topically, it is indicated for carcinoma of the uterine cervix.

Appendix
Index of Formula Names (English)

A

A Prescription for Breast Nodule (乳一方, ru yi fang) .... (404)
A Prescription for Treating Head Boils (治头疮一方, zhi tou chuang yi fang) .... (334)
Abalone Shell Pill (石决明丸, shi jue ming wan) .... (362)
Abalone Shell Yin-Nourishing Pill (决明益阴丸, jue ming yi yin wan) .... (363)
Abdominal Mass-Removing Pill (化积丸, hua ji wan) .... (96)
Aconite and Rhubarb Decoction (附子大黄汤, fu zi da huang tang) .... (153)
Amber Embracing Dragon Pill (琥珀抱龙丸, hu po bao long wan) .... (273)
Amber Pill (琥珀丸, hu po wan) .... (406)
An Obesity-Reducing Formula (轻身一方, qing shen yi fang) .... (214)
Anemarrhena, Phellodendron and Rehmannia Pill
 (知柏地黄丸, zhi bai di huang wan) .... (212)
Anjilike (安吉利克, an ji li ke) .... (363)
Antelop's Horn and Gambirplant Hooked Stem and Branch Decoction
 (羚角钩藤汤, ling jiao gou teng tang) .... (178)
Antelope Horn Decoction (羚羊角饮子, ling yang jiao yin zi) .... (363)
Anti-Bruise Powder (七厘散, qi li san) .... (302)
Antiphlogistic Powder with Ten Herbs (十味败毒汤, shi wei bai du tang) .... (329)
Arctium Muscles-Relieving Decoction (牛蒡解肌汤, niu bang jie ji tang) .... (171)
Arthralgia-Relieving Decoction (蠲痹汤, juan bi tang) .... (294)
Ascaris-Expelling Decoction Number One (驱蛔汤一号, qu hui tang yi hao) .... (103)
Ascaris-Expelling Decoction Number Three (驱蛔汤三号, qu hui tang san hao) .... (103)
Ascaris-Expelling Decoction Number Two (驱蛔汤二号, qu hui tang er hao) .... (103)
Cow Bezoar Pill (犀黄丸, xi huang wan) .... (374)
Ass-Hide Glue and Yolk Decoction (阿胶鸡子黄汤, e jiao ji zi huang tang) .... (49)
Ass-Hide Glue plus Four Herbs Decoction (阿胶四物汤, e jiao si wu tang) .... (17)
Aucklandia, Amomum Fruit, Immature Bitter Orange and
 Largehead Atractylodes Pill (香砂枳术丸, xiang sha zhi zhu wan) .... (82)

B

"B" Character Decoction (乙字汤, yi zi tang) .... (91)
Baby-Nourishing Pill (肥儿丸, fei er wan) .... (266)
Back to the Left Pill (左归丸, zuo gui wan) .... (55)

Back to the Spleen Decoction (归脾汤, gui pi tang) ······················· (206)
Baijiang Powder (白降丹, bai jiang dan) ······························· (413)
Baikai Skullcap Decoction (黄芩汤, huang qin tang) ······················ (89)
Baikal Skullcap Lung-Clearing Decoction (黄芩清肺饮, huang qin qing fei yin) ········ (326)
Bamboo Shavings Gallbladder-Warming Decoction
　(竹茹温胆汤, zhu ru wen dan tang) ································ (174)
Bank-Consolidating Pill (巩堤丸, gong di wan) ························· (142)
Barbary Wolfberry, Chrysanthemum and Rehmannia Pill
　(杞菊地黄丸, qi ju di huang wan) ································· (364)
Beard and Hair-Darkening Pellet (青云独步丹, qing yun du bu dan) ·············· (339)
Bitter Apricot and Pepperweed Pill (苦葶苈丸, ku ting li wan) ·················· (62)
Bitter Orange and Officinal Magnolia Bark Six
　Gentlemen Decoction (枳朴六君子汤, zhi po liu jun zi tang) ················· (392)
Bleeding-Arresting Panacea (止血灵, zhi xue ling) ························ (252)
Blood Pressure-Reducing Decoction (降压汤, jiang ya tang) ··················· (49)
Blood Stasis-Removing and Bleeding-Arresting Decoction
　(逐瘀止血汤, zhu yu zhi xue tang) ································· (250)
Blood Stasis-Removing and Metrorrhagia-Stopping Decoction
　(逐瘀止崩汤, zhu yu zhi beng tang) ································ (251)
Blood Stasis-Removing Decoction (通瘀煎, tong yu jian) ··················· (241)
Blood Stasis-Removing Decoction for Acute Appendicitis
　(阑尾化瘀汤, lan wei hua yu tang) ································· (99)
Heat-Clearing and Stasis-Removing Decoction for Acute Appendicitis
　(阑尾清化汤, Lan wei qing hua tang) ······························· (100)
Blood Stasis-Resolving and Metrorrhagia-Stopping Decoction
　(化瘀止崩汤, hua yu zhi beng tang) ································ (252)
Blood Sugar-Reducing Decoction (降糖汤, jiang tang tang) ·················· (210)
Blood Sugar-Reducing Formula (降糖方, jiang tang fang) ··················· (212)
Blood-Activating and Hardness-Removing Decoction
　(活血化坚汤, huo xue hua jian tang) ································ (304)
Minor Gold Tablet (小金片, xiao jin pian) ····························· (306)
Blood-Activating and Pain-Alleviating Decoction
　(活血止痛汤, huo xue zhi tong tang) ································ (300)
Blood-Activating Decoction (活血汤, huo xue tang) ······················· (301)
Blood-Enriching and Heart-Replenishing Decoction
　(养血补心汤, yang xue bu xin tang) ································ (235)
Blood-Enriching and Wind-Dispersing Decoction
　(养血胜风汤, yang xue sheng feng tang) ····························· (339)
Blood-House Blood Stasis-Dispelling Decoction (血府逐瘀汤, xue fu zhu yu tang) ······ (57)
Blood-Producing Powder (生血散, shen xue san) ························ (219)

Blue-Purging Pill（泻青丸, xie qing wan） ……………………………………… (47)
Boat and Cart Pill（舟车丸, zhou che wan） …………………………………… (129)
Borneol and Borax Powder（冰硼散, bing peng san） ………………………… (418)
Brain-Benefiting and Blood-Activating Formula
　　（益脑活血方, yi nao huo xue fang） ……………………………………… (195)
Brain-Benefiting and Spirit-Invigorating Pill（益脑强神丸, yi nao qian shen wan）…… (184)
Bright Pearl Decoction（明珠饮, ming zhu yin） ……………………………… (362)
Bupleurum Liver-Clearing Decoction（柴胡清肝饮, chai hu qing gan yin） ………… (313)
Bupleurum Liver-Soothing Powder（柴胡舒肝散, chai hu shu gan san） …………… (229)
Bupleurum, Snakegourd Fruit and Appendiculate Cremastra
　　Pseudobulb Decoction（柴胡蒌姑汤, chai hu lou gu tang）……………… (403)

C

Caloglossa Leprieurii Decoction（鹧鸪菜汤, zhe gu cai tang） ……………… (279)
Cancer-Treating Powder（治癌散, zhi ai san） ………………………………… (428)
Capillary Wormwood Decoction（茵陈蒿汤, yin chen hao tang） ……………… (102)
Capillary Wormwood Herb Fat-Lowering Formula
　　（茵陈降脂方, yin chen jiang zhi fang）…………………………………… (197)
Capillary Wormwood Lipid-Reducing Formula
　　（茵陈降脂方, yin chen jiang zhi fang）…………………………………… (216)
Capillary Wormwood, Chinese Thorowax Gallbladder-Clearing Decoction
　　（茵柴清胆汤, yin chai qing dan tang） …………………………………… (103)
Cassia Bark and Musk Powder（桂麝散, gui she san） ………………………… (412)
Cassia Twig and Aconite Decoction（桂枝附子汤, gui zhi fu zi tang） ……… (289)
Cassia Twig and Licorice Decoction
　　（桂枝甘草汤, gui zhi gan cao tang） ……………………………………… (60)
Cassia Twig and Tuckahoe Pill（桂枝茯苓丸, gui zhi fu ling wan） ………… (227)
Cassia Twig plus White Tiger Decoction（白虎加桂枝汤, bai hu jia gui zhi tang）…… (291)
Cassia Twig, Licorice, Dragon's Bone and Oyster Shell Decoction
　　（桂枝甘草龙骨牡蛎汤, gui zhi gan cao long gu mu li tang） …………… (60)
Cassia Twig, White Peony and Common Anemarrhena Decoction
　　（桂枝芍药知母汤, gui zhi shao yao zhi mu tang） ……………………… (289)
Centipede Powder（蜈蚣粉, wu gong fen） ……………………………………… (428)
Channels-Dredging and Blood-Activating Decoction
　　（疏经活血汤, shu jin huo xue tang） ……………………………………… (295)
Charred Fortune Windmillpalm Petiole and Charred Cattail Pollen Powder
　　（棕蒲散, zong pu san） ……………………………………………………… (250)
Chicken's Liver Powder（鸡肝散, ji gan san） ………………………………… (266)
Chinese Angelica Blood-Tonifying Decoction（当归补血汤, dang gui bu xue tang）…… (60)
Chinese Angelica Decoction（当归汤, dang gui tang） ………………………… (70)

Chinese Angelica Decoction (当归饮子, dang gui yin zi) ······ (322)
Chinese Angelica, Gentian and Aloes Pill (当归龙荟丸, dang gui long hui wan) ······ (45)
Chinese Eaglewood Powder (沉香散, chen xiang san) ······ (125)
Chinese Gentian, Earth Worm, Impotence-Treating Decoction
　(龙胆地龙起痿汤, long dan di long qi wei tang) ······ (138)
Chinese Pulsatilla Decoction (白头翁汤, bai tou weng tang) ······ (89)
Chinese Pulsatilla Decoction plus Ass-hide Glue
　(白头翁加阿胶汤, bai tou weng jia e jiao tang) ······ (90)
Chinese Taxillus Twig Miscarriage-Preventing Decoction
　(安胎寄生汤, an tai ji sheng tang) ······ (238)
Chinese Thorowax Liver-Clearing Decoction (柴胡清肝饮, chai hu qing gan yin) ······ (313)
Chinese Thorowax Liver-Soothing Powder (柴胡疏肝散, chai hu shu gan san) ······ (106)
Chrysanthemum Flower Pill for Eye Diseases (菊晴丸, ju qing wan) ······ (362)
Coastal Glehnia and Ophiopogon Decoction
　(沙参麦门冬汤, sha shen mai Meng dong tang) ······ (115)
Cochinchinese Asparagus Decoction (门冬饮子, men dong yin zi) ······ (8)
Coix Seed Decoction (薏苡仁汤, yi yi ren tang) ······ (286)
Coix Seed, Prepared Aconite and Whiteflower Patrinia Powder
　(薏苡附子败酱散, yi yi fu zi bai jiang san) ······ (100)
Cold Natured Stranguria-Treating Decoction (寒通汤, han tong tang) ······ (396)
Cold-Expelling and Convulsion-Relieving Decoction
　(逐寒荡惊汤, zhu han dang jing tang) ······ (260)
Combined Spicebush Root Powder (天台乌药散, tian tai wu yao san) ······ (142)
Common Anemarrhena, Chinese Corktree Bark and Motherwort Decoction
　(知柏坤草汤, zhi bai kun cao tang) ······ (157)
Common Aucklandia and Areca Seed Pill (木香槟榔丸, mu xiang bing lang wan) ······ (76)
Common Aucklandia and Coptis Decoction
　(木香黄连汤, mu xiang huang lian tang) ······ (90)
Common Aucklandia Qi-Soothing Powder (木香顺气散, mu xiang shun qi san) ······ (79)
Common Aucklandia Stagnation-Removing Pill
　(木香导滞丸, mu xiang dao zhi wan) ······ (79)
Common Burreed and Kwangsi Turmeric Decoction (荆蓬煎丸, jing peng jian wan) ······ (94)
Common Cnidium Powder (蛇床子散, she chuang zi san) ······ (417)
Compound Decoction of Wasps Nest (复方蜂房汤, fu fang feng fang tang) ······ (406)
Compound Jade Spring Pill (复方玉泉丸, fu fang yu quan wan) ······ (407)
Compound Tablet of Extract of Tendrilleaf Fritillary Bulb
　(复方川贝精片, fu fang chuan bei jing pian) ······ (31)
Convulsion-Relieving Powder (止痉散, zhi jing san) ······ (188)
Coptis Decoction (黄连汤, huang lian tang) ······ (86)
Coptis Detoxicating Decoction (黄连解毒汤, huang lian jie du tang) ······ (270)

Coptis Gallbladder-Warming Decoction (黄连温胆汤, huang lian wen dan tang) ...... (176)
Cormorant Saliva Pill (鸬鹚涎丸, lu ci xian wan) .... (273)
Coronary Heart Disease Tablet (冠心片, guan xin pian) .... (56)
Coronary Heart Disease Tablet Number Two (冠心Ⅱ号, guan xin er hao) ...... (56)
Cough-Relieving and Phlegm-Resolving Decoction
   (宁嗽化痰汤, ning sou hua tan tang) .... (2)
Cough-Relieving Decoction (宁嗽汤, ning sou tang) .... (3)
Cough-Stopping Powder (止嗽散, zhi sou san) .... (1)
Cow Bezoar Embracing Dragon Pill (牛黄抱龙丸, niu huang bao long wan) ...... (273)
Cow Bezoar Toxin-Removing and Swelling-Reducing Pill
   (牛黄醒消丸, niu huang xin xiao wan) .... (319)
Cowherb Seed Powder (王不留行散, wang bu liu xing san) .... (150)

D

Dampness-Removing and Arthralgia-Relieving Decoction
   (除湿蠲痹汤, chu shi juan bi tang) .... (294)
Dampness-Removing Decoction (胜湿汤, shen shi tang) .... (288)
Dan-Shen and Tuber Fleeceflower Blood-Producing Panacea
   (丹首生血灵, dan shou sheng xue ling) .... (219)
Dan-Shen Decoction (丹参饮, dan shen yin) .... (72)
Dawn Formula for Vascular Headache
   (曙光血管头痛方, shu guang xue guan tou tong fang) .... (193)
Decoction for Dispersing the Stagnated Qi and Recuperating the Middle-jiao
   (达郁宽中汤, da yu kuan zhong tang) .... (111)
Decoction for Diuresis (疏凿饮子, shu zao yin zi) .... (127)
Decoction for Nourishing the Lung and Removing Heat
   (补肺清金饮, bu fei qing jin yin) .... (17)
Decoction for Purging Blood Stasis (下瘀血汤, xia yu xue tang) .... (365)
Decoction for Recovery and Activating Blood Circulation
   (复元活血汤, fu yuan huo xue tang) .... (376)
Decoction for Removing Heat from the Throat and Chest
   (清咽利膈汤, qing yan li ge tang) .... (356)
Decoction for Renal Colic (肾绞痛汤, shen jiao tong tang) .... (150)
Decoction for Stranguria due to Overstrain (劳淋汤, lao lin tang) .... (147)
Decoction for Wind-Cold-Dampness Arthralgia (三痹汤, san bi tang) .... (286)
Decoction with Ginseng for Lung Disorders and Puerperal Blood Stasis
   (加参安肺生化汤, jia shen an fei sheng hua tang) .... (3)
Decoction Worth A Thousand Copper Coins (一贯煎, yi guan jian) .... (114)
Dementia-Curing Pill (转呆丹, zhuan dai dan) .... (181)
Dendrobium Eyesight-Improving Pill (石斛夜光丸, shi hu ye guang wan) .... (360)

Devine Black Bird Decoction (真武汤, zhen wu tang) ·········· (60/62)
Diabete-Relieving Formula (消渴方, xiao ke fang) ·········· (199)
Diabetes-Relieving Formula (消渴方, xiao ke fang) ·········· (211)
Diaphragm-Cooling Powder (凉膈散, liang ge san) ·········· (270)
Digestion-Promoting Pill for Five Infantile Malnutrition
　(五疳消食丸, wu gan xiao shi wan) ·········· (30)
Divaricate Saposhnikovia Miraculous Powder
　(防风通圣散, fang feng tong sheng san) ·········· (25)
Divine Black Bird Decoction (真武汤, zhen wu tang) ·········· (131/155)
Double Expelling Powder (双解散, shuang jie san) ·········· (27)
Doubleteeth Pubescent Angelica Decoction (独活汤, du huo tang) ·········· (294)
Doubleteeth Pubescent Angelica and Chinese Taxillus Twig Decoction
　(独活寄生汤, du huo ji sheng tang) ·········· (292)
Doubleteeth Pubescent Angelica and Largeleaf Gentian Decoction
　(独活秦艽汤, du huo qin jiao tang) ·········· (293)
Dreging and Dissipating Powder (通导散, tong dao san) ·········· (298)
Dryness-Moistening and Stomach-Nourishing Decoction
　(润燥养胃汤, run zao yang wei tang) ·········· (113)
Dwarf Lilyturf Decoction (麦门冬汤, mai men dong tang) ·········· (16/20)
Dwarf Lilyturf, Cochinchinese Asparagus and Tonkin Sophora Decoction
　(双冬豆根汤, shuang dong dou gen tang) ·········· (384)
Dysentery-Stopping Pill (驻车丸, zhu che wan) ·········· (88)
Dysphagia-Treating Powder (治膈, zhi ge san) ·········· (388)

E

Eagle Wood Qi-Lowering Powder (沉香降气散 chen xiang jiang qi san) ·········· (35)
Eaglewood Indigestion-Relieving Pill (沉香化滞丸, chen xiang hua zhi wan) ·········· (81)
Eaglewood Qi Stagnation-Dissipating Pill (沉香化气丸, chen xiang hua qi wan) ·········· (81)
Eczema Powder (湿疹散, shi zhen san) ·········· (424)
Effective Formula for Impotence (亢痿灵, kang wei ling) ·········· (159)
Effective Formula for Kidney Recuperation (肾康灵, shen kang ling) ·········· (148)
Efficacious Vessels-Softening Formula (软脉灵, ruan mai ling) ·········· (197)
Eight Corrections Powder (八正散, ba zheng san) ·········· (120)
Eight Treasures Decoction (八珍汤, ba zhen tang) ·········· (53)
Eight Treasures Motherwort Pill (八珍益母丸, ba zhen yi mu wan) ·········· (236)
Eight Treasures Powder (八宝丹, ba bao dan) ·········· (415)
Emission-Condolidating Pill (固精丸, gu jing wan) ·········· (136)
Ephedra, Aconite and Manchurian Wildginger Decoction
　(麻黄附子细辛汤, ma huang fu zi xi xin tang) ·········· (28)
Epilepsy-Relieving Pill (定痫丸 ding xian wan) ·········· (186)

Esophagitis Pill (食道炎丸, shi dao yan wan) ……………………………… (111)
Essence-Astringing Pill (固精丸, gu jing wan) ……………………………… (247)
Essence-Astringing Pill (约精丸, yue jing wan) ……………………………… (136)
Essence-Nourishing and Pregnancy-Promoting Decoction
    (养精种玉汤, yang jing zhong yu tang) ……………………………… (236)
Essence-Supplementing and Infertility-Treating Pill
    (填精嗣续丸, tian jing ci xu wan) ……………………………… (163)
Essence-Supplementing, Kidney-Invigorating and Breeding Decoction
    (填精补肾育种汤, tian jing bu shen yu zhong tang) ……………… (162)
Everyone's Detoxicating Decoction (普济消毒饮, pu ji xiao du yin) …… (330)
Evodia, Fresh Ginger plus Chinese Angelica Cold Limbs Decoction
    (当归四逆加吴茱萸生姜汤, dang gui si ni jia wu zhu yu sheng jiang tang)… (69)

F

Face Distortion-Treating Powder (牵正散, qian zheng san) ……………… (187)
Fairy Gelatin Containing Tortoise Shell and Plastron and Antler
    (龟鹿二仙胶, gui lu er xian jiao) ……………………………… (163)
Field Thistle Decoction (小蓟饮子, xiao ji yin zi) ……………………… (116)
Fineleaf Schizonepeta and Ledehouriella Antiphlogistic Powder
    (荆防败毒散, jin fang bai du san) ……………………………… (316)
Five Herbs Anti-Phlogistic Drink (五味消毒饮, wu wei xiao du yin) …… (336)
Five Herbs Detoxicating Powder (五物解毒散, wu wu jie du san) ……… (336)
Five Kinds of Kernels Pills (五仁丸, wu ren wan) ……………………… (85)
Five kinds of Peels Decoction (五皮饮, wu pi yin) ……………………… (131)
Five Kinds of Seeds Pill for Sterility (五子衍宗丸, wu zi yan zong wan) …… (160)
Five Miraculous Drugs Decoction (五神汤, wu shen tang) ……………… (322)
Five Retentions Powder (五积散, wu ji san) ……………………………… (27)
Five Seafoods Goiter-Dissolving Pill (消瘿五海丸, xiao ying wu hai wan) …… (204)
Five Treasures Powder (五宝散, wu bao san) …………………………… (320)
Foot-Minding Decoction (顾步汤, gu bu tang) …………………………… (307)
Formula for Cervicitis Number Two (宫颈炎Ⅱ号, gong jing yan er hao) …… (244)
Formula for Craniocerebral Contusion Number Two (头伤Ⅱ号, tou shang er hao) … (311)
Formula for Exfetation Number One (宫外孕Ⅰ号方, gong wai yun yi hao fang) …… (253)
Formula for Exfetation Number Two (宫外孕Ⅱ号方, gong wai yun er hao fang) … (252)
Formula for Immune Infertility Number One
    (免疫性不育Ⅰ号方, mian yi xing bu yu yi hao fang) …………… (165)
Formula for Immune Infertility Number Three
    (免疫性不育Ⅲ号方, mian yi xing bu yu san hao fang) ………… (166)
Formula for Immune Infertility Number Two
    (免疫性不育Ⅱ号方, mian yi xing bu yu er hao fang) …………… (166)

Formula for Qi and Fire of the Liver Meridian
   (肝经气火方, gan jing qi huo fang) ·· (194)
Four Fresh Herbs pill (四生丸, si sheng wan)··· (24)
Four Herbs and Five Kernals Pill (四物五子丸, si wu wu zi wan) ················ (357)
Four Herbs Decoction (四物汤, si wu tang) ·· (53)
Four Herbs Stasis-Dissolving Decoction (四物化郁汤, si wu hua yu tang) ········ (73)
Four Herbs Wind-Dispersing Decoction (四物消风饮, si wu xiao feng yin) ·········· (324)
Four Herbs with Corydalis Tuber Decoction (四物延胡汤, si wu yan hu tang) ········ (73)
Four Herbs with Rubia Root and Inula Flower Decoction
   (四物绛覆汤, si wu jiang fu tang) ·· (76)
Four Miraculous Herbs Pill (四神丸, si shen wan) ····································· (76)
Four Powerful Herbs Decoction (四妙勇安汤, si miao yong an tang)·············· (306)
Four-Process Nutgrass Galingale Pill (四制香附丸, si zhi xiang fu wan) ·········· (231)
Fourstamen Stephania and Membranous Milkvetch Decoction
   (防己黄芪汤, fang ji huang qi tang) ··· (151)
Fourstamen Stephania and Tuckahoe Decoction (防己茯苓汤, fang ji fu ling tang) ··· (152)
Fresh Ginger Heart-Purging Decoction (生姜泻心汤, sheng jiang xie xin tang) ·········· (87)

G

Gallbladder-Calming Decoction (安胆汤, an dan tang) ······························ (102)
Gallbladder-Warming Decoction (温胆汤, wen dan tang) ··························· (171)
Gallstones-Removing Decoction (胆道排石汤, dan dao pai shi tang) ··············· (101)
Gambirplant Hooked Stem and Branch Decoction (钩藤饮, gou teng yin) ············· (44)
Gambirplant Hooked Stem and Branch Powder (钩藤散, gou teng san) ·············· (43)
Gastrodian and Uncaria Decoction (天麻钩藤饮, tian ma gou teng yin) ············· (194)
General Recipe for Sore Throat(咽炎统治方, yan yan tong zhi fang) ················· (345)
General Recipe for Treating Toothache (牙痛统治方, ya tong tong zhi fang) ········· (421)
General Recipe for Treating Asthma (哮喘统治方, xiao chuan tong zhi fang) ········· (5)
General Recipe for Treating Climacterium
   (更年期统治方, geng nian qi tong zhi fang) ····································· (255)
General Recipe for Treating Cough (咳嗽统治方, ke sou tong zhi fang) ············· (4)
General Recipe for Treating Epilepsy (癫痫统治方, dian xian tong zhi fang) ······· (186)
General Recipe for Treating Fatigue (疲劳统治方, pi lao tong zhi fang) ············ (216)
General Recipe for Treating Headache (头痛统治方, tou tong tong zhi fang) ········· (171)
General Recipe for Treating Metrorrhagia and Metrostaxis
   (血崩统治方, xue beng tong zhi fang) ·· (252)
General Recipe for Treating Mogratory Arthralgia
   (痛风统治方, tong feng tong zhi fang) ·· (291)
General Recipe for Treating Sciatica
   (坐骨神经统治方, zuo gu shen jing tong zhi fang) ···························· (295)

General Recite for Treating Prosopagia
　　（三叉神经统治方，san cha shen jing tong zhi fang） ·················· (188)
Gentian Liver-Purging Decoction（龙胆泻肝汤，long dan xie gan tang） ············· (46)
Genuine Qi-Nourishing Pellet（养真丹，yang zhen dan） ························· (339)
Ginseng and Giant Gecko Powder（人参蛤蚧散，ren shen ge jie san） ············· (20)
Ginseng Blood-tonitfying Decoction（人参养血汤，ren shen yang xue tang） ······· (217)
Ginseng Decoction（人参汤，ren shen tang） ·································· (217)
Ginseng Nutrition Decoction（人参养荣汤，ren shen yang rong tang） ······ (206/218)
Goddess Powder（女神散，nu sheng san） ····································· (231)
Goiter-Curing Decoction（平甲汤，ping jia tang） ······························· (212)
Golden Lock Pill for Solidating Essence（金锁固精丸，jin shuo gu jing wan） ······· (134)
Golden Powder（金黄散，jin huang san） ······································ (409)
Grassleaf Sweetflag Rhizome Pill（菖蒲丸，chang pu wan） ······················ (265)
Great Burdock Achene Muscles-Removing Decoction
　　（牛蒡解肌汤，niu bang jie ji tang） ·· (327)

H

Hair-Promoting Decoction（生发汤，sheng fa tang） ···························· (340)
Hair-Promoting Drink（生发饮，sheng fa yin） ································· (340)
Hairy Antler Pill（鹿茸丸，lu rong wan） ······································· (143)
Hang Xie Pellet（沆瀣丹，hang xie dan） ······································ (268)
Hardness-Removing Decoction（化坚汤，hua jian tang） ························ (111)
Harmony-Preserving Decoction（保和汤，bao he tang） ························· (17)
Harmony-Preserving Pill（保和丸，bao he wan） ······························· (81)
Head-Clearing and Pain-Alleviating Decoction
　　（清上蠲痛汤，qing shang juan tong tang） ································ (167)
Head-Clearing Divaricate Saposhnikovia Decoction
　　（清上防风汤，qing shang fang feng tang） ································ (315)
Heart Failure Mixture（心衰合剂，xin shuai he ji） ······························ (60)
Heart Rhythm-Adjusting Mixture（整律合剂，zheng lu he ji） ···················· (63)
Heart Rhythm-Regulating Decoction（调律汤，tiao lu tang） ····················· (66)
Heart -Washing Decoction（洗心汤，xi xin tang） ······························· (180)
Heart-Clearing Lotus Seed Decoction（清心莲子饮，qing xin lian zi yin） ········· (122)
Heart-Stimulating Decoction（强心饮，qiang xin yin） ··························· (59)
Heat-Clearing and Toxin-Relieving Decoction（清热解毒汤，qing re jie du tang） ··· (327)
Heat-Removing Decoction for Acute Pancreatitis
　　（胰腺清化汤，yi xian qing hua tang） ····································· (97)
Hemiplegia-Treating and Stroke-Healing Decoction
　　（补偏愈风汤，bu pian yu feng tang） ····································· (40)
Hemocyte-Increasing Mixtur（升血合剂，sheng xue he ji） ······················ (217)

Hemp Seed Pill (麻子仁丸, ma zi ren wan) ·················· (85)
Himalayan Teasel Decoction (续断饮, xu duan yin) ·················· (62)
Hoarseness-Relieving and Aphonia-Healing Tablet (清音片, qing yin pian) ·················· (355)
Hoarseness-Relieving andAphonia-Treating Pill
 (响声破笛丸, xiang sheng po di wan) ·················· (345)
Holy Disease-Curing Decoction (圣愈汤, sheng yu tang) ·················· (209)
Honeysuckle Flower Detoxicating Decoction (银花解毒汤, yin hua jie du tang) ·················· (328)
Honeysuckle, Weeping Forsythia and Dendrobium Decoction
 (银翘石斛汤, yin qiao shi hu tang) ·················· (148)
Human Placenta Marrow-Sealing Pellets (河车封髓丹, he che feng sui dan) ·················· (163)
Hundred Flowers Pill (百花丸, bai hua wan) ·················· (16)
Hyperparathyroidism-Treating Decoction with Five Methods
 (五法合一甲亢汤, wu fa he yi jia kang tang) ·················· (214)

I

Immature Bitter Orange Stagnation-Dispelling Pill
 (枳实导滞丸, zhi shi dao zhi wan) ·················· (79)
Immature Bitter Orange Stagnation-Removing Decoction
 (枳实化滞汤, zhi shi hua zhi tang) ·················· (82)
Immature Bitter Orange, Longstamen Onion and Cassia Twig Decoction
 (枳实薤白桂枝汤, zhu shi xie bai gui zhi tang) ·················· (58)
Immatures Bitter Orange Stuffiness-Removing Pill
 (枳实消痞丸, zhi shi xiao pi wan) ·················· (82)
Immortal Viscera-Nourishing Decoction (真人养脏汤, zhen ren yang zang tang) ·················· (74)
Infantile Convulsion-Relieving Pill (小儿回春丹, xiao er hui chun dan) ·················· (271)
Infantile Cough-Relieving Pallet (小儿止咳金丹, xiao er zhi ke jin dan) ·················· (7)
Infantile Four Symptoms Pill (小儿四症丸, xiao er si zhen wan) ·················· (275)
Inflammation-Diminishing and Membrane-Protecting Formula
 (消炎护膜方, xiao yan hu mo fang) ·················· (113)
Innateness-Tonifying and Breeding Pill (补天育麟丹, bu tian yu lin dan) ·················· (164)
Instant Effective Powder (立效散, li xiao san) ·················· (420)
Interior-Replenishing Hairy Antler Pill (内补鹿茸丸, nei bu lu rong wan) ·················· (163)
Interior-Replenishing Pill (内补丸, nei bu wan) ·················· (245)
Internal Eliminating Powder for Yin-Toxin (阴毒内消散, yin du nei xiao san) ·················· (427)
Internally Scrofula-Eliminating Pill (内消瘰疬丸, nei xiao lei li wan) ·················· (202)
Internally Tumour-Relieving Pill (内消肿瘤丸, nei xiao zhong liu wan) ·················· (201)
Intestines-Calming Decoction (肠宁汤, chang ning tang) ·················· (242)
Intestines-Moistening Pill (润肠丸, run chang wan) ·················· (84)
Inula Herb Powder (金沸草散, jin fei cao san) ·················· (32)
Iron Scales Decoction (生铁落饮, sheng tie luo yin) ·················· (190)

Itching-Stopping Decoction (塌痒汤, ta yang tang) ……………………… (415)

J

Jackinthepulpit, Pinellia, Common Selfheal Fruit-Spike,
　　Grassleaf Sweetflag and Two Pieces of Centipedes Decoction
　　(星夏草菖双龙汤, xing xia cao chang shuang long tang) ………… (401)
Jade and Dragon Ointment for Restoring Yang
　　(回阳玉龙膏, hui yang yu long gao) ……………………………… (412)
Jade Liquid Decoction (玉液汤, yu ye tang) ………………………… (198)
Jade Maid Decoction (玉女煎, yu nu jian) …………………………… (211)
Japanese Felt Fern Powder (石韦散, shi wei san) …………………… (120)
Jinyan Pill (金岩丸, jin yan wan) …………………………………… (382)

K

Kidney Yang-Strengthening Pill (壮阳丹, zhang yang dan) ………… (136)
Kidney-Benefiting Decoction (益肾汤, yi shen tang) ………………… (154)
Kidney-Invigorating and Chong Meridian-Consolidating Pill
　　(补肾固冲丸, bu shen gu chong wan) …………………………… (238)
Kidney-Invigorating and Essence-Supplementing Decoction
　　(益肾填精汤, yi shen tian jing tang) ……………………………… (161)
Kidney-Invigorating and Stone-Removing Decoction
　　(补肾通石汤, bu shen tong shi tang) …………………………… (150)
Kidney-Invigorating, Cold-Expelling and Arthralgia-Relieving Decoction
　　(补肾祛寒治痹汤, bu shen qu han zhi bi tang) ………………… (439)
Kidney-Replenishing Rehmannia Pill (补益地黄丸, bu yi di huang wan) ………… (161)
Kidney-Warming and Toxin-Clearing Decoction
　　(温肾排毒汤, wen shen pai du tang) …………………………… (155)

L

Lactation-Inducing Pill (通乳丹, tong ru dan) ……………………… (249)
Land and Water Two Fairies Pellet (水陆二仙丹, shui lu er xian dan) ………… (135)
Largehead Atractylodes Miscarriage-Preventing Powder
　　(安胎白术散, an tai bai zhu san) ………………………………… (238)
Largehead Atractylodes Powder with Seven Herbs
　　(七味白术散, qi wei bai zhu san) ………………………………… (258)
Largehead Atractylodes, Chinese Angelica, Cassia Bark and
　　Licorice Decoction (术归桂草汤, zhu gui gui cao tang) ………… (243)
Laughing Powder (失笑散, shi xiao san) ……………………………… (73)
Left Golden Pill (左金丸, zuo jin wan) ……………………………… (47)
Licorice Decoction (甘草汤 gan cao tang) …………………………… (345)

Licorice Heart-Purging Decoction (甘草泻心汤, gan cao xie xin tang) ············ (88)
Licorice, Dried Ginger, Tuckahoe and Largehead Atractylodes Decoction
　（甘草干姜茯苓白术汤, gan cao gan jiang fu ling bai zhu tang) ············ (131)
Life-Preserving Kidney-Qi Pill (济生肾气丸, ji sheng shen qi wan) ············ (156)
Lily Bubus Decoction for Strengthening the Lung (百合固金汤, bai he gu jin tang) ··· (14)
Lipide-Lowering and Vessels-Dredging Decoction
　（降脂通脉饮, jiang zhi tong mai yin) ············ (53)
Liver-Calming and Wind-Stopping Decoction (镇肝息风汤, zhen gan xi feng tang) ······ (51)
Liver-Clearing and Depression-Alleviating Decoction
　（清肝达郁饮, qing gan da yu yin) ············ (228)
Liver-Clearing and Kidney-Nourishing Decoction
　（清肝养肾汤, qing gan yang shen tang) ············ (370)
Liver-Clearing and Stagnation-Removing Decocting
　（清肝解郁汤, qing gan jie yu tang) ············ (381)
Liver-Clearing and Stranguria-Treating Decoction
　（清肝止淋汤, qin gan zhi lin tang) ············ (243)
Liver-Dispersing and Gallbladder-Bene fiting Decoction
　（疏肝利胆汤, shu gan li dan tang) ············ (101)
Liver-Inhibiting Powder (抑肝散, yi gan san) ············ (176)
Liver-Nourishing Pill (养肝丸, yang gan wan) ············ (363)
Liver-Purging Decoction (泻肝汤, xie gan tang) ············ (372)
Liver-Recuperating Pill (复肝丸, fu gan wan) ············ (107)
Liver-Recuperating Prescription (肝复方, gan fu fang) ············ (390)
Liver-Soothing and Nodules-Eliminating Prescrioption
　（疏肝消核方, shu gan xiao he fang) ············ (380)
Liver-Soothing and Spleen-Regulating Pill (舒肝理脾丸, shu gan li pi wan) ············ (101)
Liver-Soothing Decoction (舒肝饮, shu gan yin) ············ (104)
Liver-Soothing Four Drugs Powder (疏肝四味散, shu gan si wei san) ············ (138)
Liver-Soothing Pill (舒肝丸, shu gan wan) ············ (110)
Liver-Strengthening and Hardness-Softening Decoction
　（强肝软坚汤, qiang gan ruan jian tang) ············ (109)
Liver-Strengthening and Hardness-Softening Decoction Number Five
　（强肝软坚汤五号, qiang gan ruan jian tang wu hao) ············ (110)
Liver-Strengthening and Hardness-Softening Decoction Number Four
　（强肝软坚汤四号, qiang gan ruan jian tang si hao) ············ (110)
Liver-Strengthening and Hardness-Softening Decoction Number Six
　（强肝软坚汤六号, qiang gan ruan jian tang liu hao) ············ (110)
Liver-Strengthening and Hardness-Softening Decoction Number Three
　（强肝软坚汤三号, qiang gan ruan jian tang san hao) ············ (109)
Liver-Strengthening and Hardness-Softening Decoction Number Two

（强肝软坚汤二号, qiang gan ruan jian tang er hao） ················· (109)
Liver-Subduing and Wind-Stopping Decoction（镇肝息风汤, zhen gan xi feng tang） ··· (38)
Liver-Tonifying Pill（补肝丸, bu gan wan） ··························· (372)
Liver-Warming Decoction（暖肝煎, nuan gan jian） ····················· (138)
Lobed Kudzuvine, Baikal Skullcap and Coptis Decoction
    （葛根黄芩黄连汤, ge gen huang qin huang lian tang） ············· (89)
Longevity Pill（寿星丸, shou xing wan） ······························ (182)
Lower Abdomen Blood Stasis-Dispelling Decoction
    （少腹逐瘀汤, shao fu zhu yu tang） ····························· (227)
Lower-Warming and Upper-Clearing Decoction
    （温下清上汤, wen xia qing shang tang） ························· (278)
Lucid Yang-Generating Decoction（滋生清阳汤, zi sheng qing yang tang） ··· (182)
Lunar Corona Pill（月华丸, yue hua wan） ····························· (20)
Lung Tumor-Removing Formula（肺瘤平, fei liu ping） ················· (382)
Lung-Clearing and Phlegm-Resolving Decoction
    （清金化痰汤, qing jin hua tan tang） ···························· (10)
Lung-Clearing Decoction（清肺汤, qing fei tang） ····················· (8)
Lung-Clearing Drink（清肺饮, qing fei yin） ·························· (123)
Lung-Clearing Loquat Powder（清肺枇杷散, qing fei pi pa san） ········ (325)
Lung-Invigorating Ass-hide Glue Decoction（补肺阿胶汤, bu fei e jiao tang） ··· (21)
Lung-Nourishing Decoction（养金汤, yang jin tang） ··················· (16)
Lung-Rising Decoction（举肺汤, ju fei tang） ························· (20)
Lung-Strengthening and Cancer-Resisting Decoction
    （固金抗癌汤, gu jin kang ai tang） ····························· (381)
Lung-Warming and Running-Stopping Decocting
    （温肺止流汤, wen fei zhi liu tang） ···························· (349)
Lung-Warming Decoction（温肺汤, wen fei tang） ······················ (350)

M

Magnetite and Cinnabar Pill（磁朱丸, ci zhu wan） ···················· (185)
Magnetite Kidney-Tonifying Pill（补肾磁石丸, bu shen ci shi wan） ····· (359)
Magnolia Lung-Clearing Decoction（辛夷清肺汤, xin yi qing fei tang） ··· (348)
Major Divaricate Saposhnikovia Decoction（大防风汤, da fang feng tang） ··· (283)
Major Gentian Decoction（大秦艽汤 da qin jiao tang） ················· (190)
Major Middle-Strengthening Decoction（大建中汤, da jian zhong tang） ··· (69)
Major Miscarriage-Preventing Decoction（大安胎如胜饮, da an tai ru sheng yin） ··· (238)
Major Weeping Forsythia Capsule Decoction（大连翘汤, da lian qiao tang） ··· (317)
Major Yin-Replenishing Pill（大补阴丸, da bu yin wan） ··············· (12)
Mantis Egg-Case Powder（桑螵蛸散, sang piao xiao san） ··············· (136)
Mass-Eliminating Powder（消癥散, xiao zheng san） ···················· (253)

Membranous Milkvetch and Largehead Atractylodes Powder for
　Regulating Menstruation (芪术调经散 qi zhu tiao jing san) ……………… (245)
Membranous Milkvetch Decoction (黄芪汤, huang qi tang) ……………… (148)
Membranous Milkvetch Kidney-Benefiting Decoction
　(黄芪益肾汤, huang qi yi shen tang) ………………………………… (154)
Menstruation-Normalizing Decoction (顺经汤, shun jing tang) …………… (232)
Mental Depression-Alleviating Decoction (达郁汤, da yu tang) …………… (161)
Meridian-Warming Decoction (温经汤, wen jing tang) …………………… (232)
Merry Life Powder (逍遥散, xiao yao san) ……………………………… (106/326)
Middle-Jiao- Soothing Powder (安中散, an zhong san) ……………………… (67)
Middle-Regulating Pill (理中丸, li zhong wan) ……………………………… (69)
Mind-Tranquilizing and Heart-Easing Pill (安神定心丸, an shen ding xin wan) … (180)
Minor Bupleurum Decoction Plus Balloonflower and Gypsum
　(小柴胡桔梗石膏汤, xiao chai hu jie gen shi gao tang) ……………… (352)
Minor Chinese Thorowax Decoction (小柴胡汤, xiao chai hu tang) ………… (98)
Minor Life-prolonging Decoction (小续命汤, xiao xu ming tang) …………… (188)
Minor Panacea Pellet (小金丹, xiao jin dan) ………………………………… (376)
Miraculous Collateral-Activating Pill (活络效灵丹, huo luo xiao ling dan) …… (300)
Miraculous Musk Powder (妙香散, miao xiang san) ………………………… (178)
Miraculous Pill with Six Drugs (六神丸, liu shen wan) …………………… (343)
Miscarriage-Preventing Decoction (安胎饮, an tai yin) …………………… (237)
Miscarriage-Preventing Pi (寿胎丸, shou tai wan) ………………………… (236)
Modifed Asiatic Rhinoceros Bezoar Pill (加味犀黄丸, jia wei xi huang wan) … (375)
Modified Anti-pyretic and Anti-toxic Decoction
　(加减清瘟败毒饮, jia jian qing wen bai du yin) ……………………… (398)
Modified Chinese Thorowax Decoction (加味柴胡汤, jia wei chai hu tang) … (98)
Modified coction of Three Miraculous Drugs (加减三奇汤, jia jian san qi tang) … (3)
Modified Cold Limbs Powder (加减四逆散, jia jian si ni san) ……………… (33)
Modified Incised Notopterygium Decoction (加味羌活汤, jia wei jiang huo tang) … (283)
Modified Magnetite and Cinnabar Pill (加味磁朱丸, jia wei ci zhu wan) …… (186)
Modified Merry Life Powder (加味逍遥散, jia wei xiao yao san) …………… (14)
Modified Orifice-Opening and Blood-Activating Prescription
　(通窍活血加减方, tong qiao huo xue jia jian fang) …………………… (397)
Modified Peach Kernel and Safflower Decoction
　(加味桃红汤, jia wei tao hong tang) ………………………………… (396)
Modified Pulse-Restoring Decoction (加减复脉汤, jia jian fu mai tang) …… (64)
Modified Snakegourd Fruit and Great Burdock Achene Decoction
　(加减瓜蒌牛蒡汤, jia jian gua lou niu bang tang) …………………… (308)
Modified Toxin-Removing Fairy Decoction
　(解毒玉女煎加减方, jie du yu nu jian jia jian fang) ………………… (397)

Modified Tuckahoe Powder With Five Herbs (加味五苓散, jia wei wu ling san) …… (392)
Modified Vision Acuity-Improving Pill (驻景丸加减方, zhu jing wan jia jian fang) … (367)
Moghania Root and Fleeceflower Root Decoction
　　(千斤首乌汤, qian jin shou wu tang) ……………………………………… (324)
Motherwort Gold-Exceeding Pill (益母胜金丹, yi mu sheng jin dan) ………… (230)
Motherwort Herb Ointment (益母草膏, yi mu cao gao) ………………………… (230)
Mulbery and Chrysanthemum Decoction (桑菊饮, sang ju yin) …………………… (3)
Mysterious Red Pellet (秘红丹, mi hong dan) ……………………………………… (25)
Mystery Decoction (神秘汤, shen mi tang) ………………………………………… (4)

N

Natural indigo, Borneol and Borax Powder (青黛冰硼散, qing dai bing peng san) …… (419)
Nature Pill (天真丹, tian zhen dan) ………………………………………………… (154)
Nebula-Removing Decoction (退翳汤, tui yi tang) ……………………………… (358)
Nephritis Decoction (肾炎汤, shen yang tang) ………………………………… (151)
Nine to One Powder (九一丹, jiu yi dan) ……………………………………… (413)
Notopterygium Dampness-Expelling Decoction
　　(羌活胜湿汤, qiang huo sheng shi tang) ……………………………… (281)

O

Ophiopogon Decoction (麦门冬汤, mai men dong tang) ………………………… (115)
Oriental Wormwood Decoction (茵陈蒿汤, yin chen hao tang) ……………… (326)
Origin-Reinforcing and Essence-Locking Pill (固本锁精丸, gu ben suo jing wan) …… (135)

P

Pain-Alleviating and Swelling-Reducing Plaster
　　(镇痛消肿膏, zhen tong xiao zhong gao) ……………………………… (426)
Palpitation-Relieving Decoction (宁心汤, ning xin tang) ……………………… (65)
Pantalgia-Relieving and Blood Stasis-Dispelling Decoction
　　(身痛逐瘀汤, shen tong zhu yu tang) ………………………………… (302)
Parasite-Eliminating Pill (化虫丸, hua chong wan) …………………………… (267)
Pathogen-Clearing and Mass-Resolving Decoction (清消汤, qing xiao tang) ……… (399)
Peach Blossom Decoction (桃花汤, tao hua tang) ……………………………… (76)
Peach Kernel and Chinese Angelica Decoction
　　(桃仁当归汤, tao ren dang gui tang) ………………………………… (242)
Peach Kernel Purgative Decoction (桃核承气汤, tao he cheng qi tang) ……… (299)
Perilla Decoction for Keeping Qi Downward (苏子降气汤, su zi jiang qi tang) ………… (5)
Perilla Seed and Apricot Seed Decoction (苏子杏汤, su zi xing tang) ……………… (7)
Phlegm-Conducting Decoction (导痰汤 dao tan tang) ………………………… (173)
Phlegm-Dispelling Decoction (涤痰汤 di tan tang) …………………………… (173)

Phlegm-Removing and Brain-Activating Pill (化痰透脑丸, hua tan tou nao wan) …… (184)
Pill for Balancing the Heart and the Kidney (交泰丸, jiao tai wan) …………… (254)
Pill for Clearing Away Heat at Qifen and Resolving Phlegm
　(清气化痰丸, qing qi hua tan wan) ……………………………………………… (3)
Pill for Improving Acuity of Sight (驻景丸, zhu jing wan) …………………… (358)
Pill for Stranguria from Urolithiasis (沙淋丸, sha lin wan) ………………… (150)
Pilose Asiabell, Membranous Milkvetch Decoction for
　Stranguria due to Overstrain (参芪劳淋汤, shen qi lao lin tang) ………… (146)
Pilose Asiabell, Membranous Milkvetch, Desertliving Cistanche and
　Shorthorned Epimedium Decoction (参芪蓉仙汤, shen qi rong xian tang) … (394)
Pinellia and Sulfur Pill (半硫丸, ban liu wan) ………………………………… (84)
Pinellia Heart-Purging Decoction (半夏泻心汤, ban xia xie xin tang) ……… (86)
Pinellia, Largehead Atractylodes and Tall Gastordia Decoction
　(半夏白术天麻汤, ban xia bai zhu tian ma tang) …………………………… (55)
Pizaihuang (片仔癀, pian zai huang) …………………………………………… (376)
Pleurisy Decoction Number One (胸膜炎Ⅰ汤号, xiong mo yan tang yi hao) ……… (33)
Peurisy Decoction Number Two (胸膜炎汤Ⅱ号, xiong mo yan tang er hao) ……… (35)
Plum Blossom Tongue-Touching Tablet (梅花点舌丹, mei hua dian she dan) ……… (344)
Poria Powder with Five Herbs (五苓散, wu ling san) …………………………… (394)
Postmenopausal Bleeding-Preventing Decoction (安老汤, an lao tang) ……… (244)
Powder for Five Kinds of Stranguria (五淋散, wu lin san) …………………… (118)
Powder for Sallow Complexion (益黄散, yi huang san) ……………………… (258)
Powder for Urine Retention (癃闭散, long bi san) …………………………… (155)
Powder of Ending Part of Chinese Angelica Root (当归须散, dang gui xu san) ……… (74)
Pregnancy-Promoting Pearl (毓麟珠, yu lin zhu) ……………………………… (234)
Prepared Aconite Decoction (附子汤, fu zi tang) …………………………… (131)
Prepared Licorice Decoction (炙甘草汤, zhi gan cao tang) ………………… (20)
Prescription for Ovarian Cancer (治卵巢癌方, zhi luan chao ai fang) ……… (405)
Prescription for Treating Alopecia Areata (治斑秃方, zhi ban tu fang) …… (337)
Primary Qi-Regulating Powder (调元散, tiao yuan san) ……………………… (263)
Procreation-Helping Pellet (赞育丹, zan yu dan) …………………………… (138)
Proven AIDS-Resisting Formula (抗艾滋病经验方, kang ai zi bing jing yan fang) … (408)
Proven Recipes for Arthralgia of Damp type (着痹验方, zhuo bi yan fang) … (288)
Pueraria and Safflower Decoction (葛根红花汤, ge gen hong hua tang) …… (333)
Pueraria Decoction Plus Szechwan Lovage and Magnolia
　(葛根汤加川芎辛夷汤, ge gen tang jia chuan xiong xin yi tang) ………… (353)
Pueraria Decoction (葛根汤, ge gen tang) …………………………………… (354)
Pulse-Activating Powder (生脉散, sheng mai san) …………………………… (208)
Pupils-Benefiting pill (益瞳丸, yi tong wan) ………………………………… (364)
Purple Cloud Ointment (紫云膏, zi yun gao) ………………………………… (423)

Purpura-Relieving Decoction (消癜汤, xiao dian tang) ……………………… (222)
Pylorus-Dredging Decoction (通幽汤, tong you tang) ………………………… (389)

Q

Qi-Clearing and Phlegm-Resolving Pill (清气化痰丸, qing qi hua tan wan) ………… (10)
Qi-Dispersing and Lung-Regulating Pill (通宣理肺丸, tong xuan li fei wan) ……… (31)
Qi-Invigorating, Blood-Replenishing and Tendons-Nourishing Decoction
　(气血并补荣筋汤, qi xue bing bu rong jin tang) ……………………………… (284)
Qi-Replenishing and Rash-Dissipating Decoction (益气化斑汤, yi qi hua ban tang) … (220)
Qi-Replenishing and Vertigo-Relieving Decoction
　(补气解晕汤, bu qi jie yun tang) ……………………………………………… (312)
Qi-Replenishing and Yin-Nourishing Decoction (益气养阴汤, yi qi yang yin tang) …… (51)
Qi-Replenishing, Hearing-improving and Eyesight-Acuminating Decoction
　(益气聪明汤, yi qi cong ming tang) …………………………………………… (367)
Qi-Replenishing, Retention-Removing and Poison-Clearing Decoction
　(益气化积解毒汤, yi qi hua ji jie du tang) …………………………………… (106)
Qi-Restoration and Blood-Activating Decoction
　(复元活血汤, fu yuan huo xue tang) …………………………………………… (35)

R

Red Halloysite and Limonite Decoction
　(赤石脂禹余粮汤, chi shi zhi yu yu liang tang) ………………………………… (76)
Rehmannia Eyesight-Improving Pill (明目地黄丸, ming mu di huang wan) ………… (364)
Rehmannia Pill with Nine Seeds (九子地黄丸, jiu zi di huang wan) ……………… (359)
Rehmannia Yin-Nourishing Pill (济阴地黄丸, ji yin di huang wan) ……………… (363)
Renal Colic Decoction (肾绞痛汤, shen jiao tong tang) …………………………… (157)
Resistant Decoction (抵当汤, di tang tang) …………………………………………… (365)
Reversion Powder (颠倒散, dian dao san) …………………………………………… (426)
Rhubarb and Prepared Aconite Decoction (大黄附子汤, da huang fu zi tang) ……… (84)
Rong-Sooth Decoction (安荣汤, an rong tang) ……………………………………… (238)

S

Saliva-Controlling Pill (控涎丹, kong xian dan) …………………………………… (37)
Sancai Marrow-Preserving Pill Containing Cochinchinese Asparagus,
　Rehmannia and Ginsen (三才封髓丹, san cai feng sui dan) ………………… (144)
Schizonepeta and Forsythia Decoction (荆芥连翘汤, jing jie lian qiao tang) ……… (331)
Scrofula-Dispelling Pill (消瘰丸, xiao lei wan) …………………………………… (204)
Seaweed Jade Kettle Decoction (海藻玉壶汤, hai zao yu hu tang) ……………… (200)
Sessile Stemona Syrup for Relieving Cough
　(百部止咳糖浆, bai bu zhi ke tang jiang) …………………………………… (275)

Seven Immortals Roll (七仙条, qi xian tiao) ·········· (413)
Seven Immortals Pellet (七仙丹, qi xian dan) ·········· (339)
Seven Immortals Pill (七仙丸, qi xian wan) ·········· (359)
Seven Valuable Herbs Beard-Improving Pellet (七宝美髯丹, qi bao mei ran dan) ····· (339)
Sevenlobed Yam Decoction (萆薢饮, bi xie yin) ·········· (121)
Sevenlobed Yam Decoction for Clearing Turbid Urine
　(萆薢分清饮, bi xie fen qing yin) ·········· (120)
Sevenlobed Yam Diuresis-Inducing Decoction (萆薢渗湿汤, bi xie shen shi tang) ··· (321)
Shen's Pill for Decreasing Urination (沈氏闷泉丸, shen shi men quan wan) ·········· (267)
Silk Pouch Pill (布袋丸, bu dai wan) ·········· (265)
Silkworm with Batrytis Larva and Wasps Nest Decoction
　(僵蚕蜂房汤, jiang can feng fang tang) ·········· (386)
Silky Fowl Black-Bone Chicken Bolus (乌鸡丸, wu ji wan) ·········· (236)
Snake Gallbladder and Tendrilleaf Fritillary Bulb Powder
　(蛇胆川贝散, she dan chuan bei san) ·········· (8)
Snakegourd and Great Burdock Achene Decoction
　(瓜蒌牛蒡汤, gua lou niu bang tang) ·········· (308)
Snakegourd Fruit Powder (瓜蒌散, gua lou san) ·········· (310)
Snakegourd, Longstamen Onion and Pinellia Decoction
　(瓜蒌薤白半夏汤, gua lou xie bai ban xia tang) ·········· (58)
Sophora Flower Powder (槐花散, huai hua san) ·········· (92)
Sore Throat-Relieving and Lung-Clearing Decoction
　(利咽清金汤, li yan qing jin tang) ·········· (386)
Sores-Treating Medicated Thread (三品一条枪, san pin yi tiao qiang) ·········· (412)
Sovereign Wart-Eliminating Liniment (疣灵搽剂, you ling cha ji) ·········· (423)
Spleen-Invigorating Body-Nourishing Powder (健脾肥儿散, jian pi fei er san) ·········· (258)
Spleen-Invigorating Pill (启脾丸, qi pi wan) ·········· (256)
Spleen-Reinforcing Decoction (实脾饮, shi pi yin) ·········· (129)
Spleen-Strengthening Pill (健脾丸, jian pi wan) ·········· (257)
Spleen-Warming Decoction (温脾汤, wen pi tang) ·········· (82)
Springing like Lactation-Promoting Powder (下乳涌泉散, xia ru yong quan san) ····· (247)
Stagnation-Relieving Pill (越鞠丸, yue ju wan) ·········· (29)
Stomach-Clearing and Ascaris-Calming Decoction
　(清肌安蛔汤, qing ji an hui tang) ·········· (280)
Stomach-Clearing Powder (清胃散, qing wei san) ·········· (421)
Storesin Pill (苏合香丸, su he xiang wan) ·········· (58)
Storesin Pill for Coronary Heart Disease (冠心苏合丸, guan xin su he wan) ·········· (58)
Substitutive Resistant Pill (代抵当丸, dai di dang wan) ·········· (126)
Summer heat-Clearing and Qi-Benefiting Decoction
　(清暑益气汤, qing shu yi qi tang) ·········· (278)

Sweeping Down Decoction for Tension Hypertension (建瓴汤, jian ling tang) ……… (41)
Sweet Dew Detoxication Pill (甘露消毒丹, gan lu xiao du dan) …………… (407)
Swelling-Reducing and Detoxicificating Decoction
　　(消肿解毒汤, xiao zhong jie du tang) …………………………………… (308)
Swordlike Atractylodes and Largehead Atractylodes Decoction
　　(二术汤, er zhu tang) ……………………………………………………… (288)
Szechwan Chinaberry Powder (金铃子散, jin ling zi san) ………………… (159)
Szechwan Lovage and Chinese Angelica Decoction for Regulating Blood Flow
　　(芎归调血饮, xiong gui tiao xue yin) …………………………………… (223)
Szechwan Lovage and Chinese Angelica Pill for Improving Acuity of Sight
　　(芎归明目丸, xiong gui ming mu wan) ………………………………… (362)
Szechwan Lovage Rhizome and Manchurian Wildginger Herb Powder
　　(芎辛散, xiong xin san) …………………………………………………… (195)
Szechwan Lovage Rhizome, Chinese Angelica Root, Ass-hide Glue and
　　Argy Wormwood Leaf Decoction (芎归胶艾汤, xiong gui jiao ai tang) …… (225)

T

Taishan Rock Powder (泰山盘石散, tai shan pan shi san) ………………… (239)
Tall Gastrodia and Gambirplant Hooked Stem and Branch Decoction
　　(天麻钩藤饮, tian ma gou teng yin) …………………………………… (51/55)
Tangerine Leaf, Bitter Orange, Dragon's Bone and Oyster Shell Decoction
　　(桔枳龙牡汤, jiu zhi long mu tang) ……………………………………… (192)
Tangerine Seed Pill (橘核丸, ju he wan) …………………………………… (140)
Tea-Blended Chrysanthemum Flower Powder (菊花茶调散, jiu hua cha tiao san) …… (171)
Tea-Blended Szechwan Lovage Powder (川芎茶调散, chuan xiong cha tiao san) …… (169)
Ten Charred Herbs Powder (十灰散, shi hui san) ………………………… (23)
Ten Chinese Dates Decoction (十枣汤, shi zao tang) ……………………… (37)
Ten Drugs Decoction for Warming Gallbladder
　　(十味温胆汤, shi wei wen dan tang) …………………………………… (176)
Ten Herbs Antiphlogistic Decoction (十味败毒汤, shi wei bai du tang) … (329)
Ten Strong Tonic Herbs Decoction (十全大补汤, shi quan da bu tang) …… (225)
Ten Strong Tonic Herbs Wan (十全大补丸, shi quan da bu wan) ………… (204)
Ten Treasures Powder (十宝散, shi bao san) ……………………………… (304)
Tendrilleaf Fritillary Bulb and Snakegourd Fruit Powder
　　(贝母瓜蒌散, bei mu gua lou san) ……………………………………… (6)
Tendrilleaf Fritillary Bulb Powder (贝母散, bei mu san) ………………… (7)
Three Herbs Baikal Skullcap Decoction (三物黄芩汤, san wu huang qin tang) …… (228)
Three Herbs Emergency Pill (三物备急丸, san wu bei ji wan) …………… (84)
Three Huang Heart-Clearing Decoction (三黄泻心汤, san huang xie xin tang) …… (334)
Three Huang Lotion (三黄洗剂, san huang xi ji) …………………………… (425)

Three Wonderful Herbs Powder (三妙散, san miao san) ………………………… (426)
Threeleaf Chastertree Fruit Tang (蔓荆子汤, man jing zi tang) ……………… (368)
Tiandi Pill (天滴丸, tian di wan) ……………………………………………… (417)
Tiantai Combined Spicebush Powder (天台乌药散, tian tai wu yao san) ……… (140)
Tissue-Rregeneration Powder (生肌散, sheng ji san) ………………………… (415)
Toxin-Clearing and Swelling-Reducing Pill (醒消丸, xing xiao wan) ………… (320)
Tree Peony Bark and Cape Jasmine Merry Life Power
　(丹栀逍遥散, dan zhi xiao yao san) ………………………………………… (314)
Tuckahoe and Oriental Waterplantain Decoction (茯苓泽泻汤, fu ling ze xie tang) … (134)
Tuckahoe Water-Removing Decoction (茯苓导水汤, fu ling dao shui tang) …… (131)
Tuckahoe, Cassia Twig, Largehead Atractylodes and Licorice Decoction
　(苓桂术甘汤, ling gui zhu gan tang) ………………………………………… (131)
Turbid Urine-Clearing Decoction (分清饮, fen qing yin) ……………………… (121)
Turmeric Root-Tuber Merry Life Powder (郁金逍遥散, yu jin xiao yao san) …… (404)
Two Fresh Herbs Decoction (二鲜饮, er xian yin) …………………………… (24)
Two Immortals Powder (二仙汤, er xian tang) ……………………………… (254)
Two Organs-Replenishing Decoction (双补汤, shuang bu tang) ……………… (222)
Two Vintage Herbs Decoction (二陈汤 er chen tang) ………………………… (173)
Twotooth Achyranthes Root Powder (牛膝散, niu qi san) …………………… (227)

U

Umbellate Pore Fungus Decoction (猪苓汤, zhu ling tang) …………………… (394)
Urination-Decreasing Pill (缩泉丸, suo quan wan) …………………………… (267)
Ursine Seal Kidney-Benefiting Decoction (海狗益肾饮, hai gou yi shen yin) …… (160)
Uterus-Warming Powder (温胞散, wen bao san) ……………………………… (234)

V

Verruca-Removing Decoction (除疣汤, chu you tang) ………………………… (340)
Viscera-Benefiting and Consciousness-Restoring Decoction
　(可保立苏汤, ke bao li su tang) ……………………………………………… (263)
Vision Acuity-Improving Pill (驻景丸, zhu jing wan) ………………………… (366)
Vital Qi-Consolidating Decoction (固真汤, gu zhen tang) …………………… (263)

W

Wart-Eliminating Decoction (消疣汤, xiao you tang) ………………………… (424)
Water Retention-Removing Decoction (分消汤, fen xiao tang) ……………… (132)
Wether Liver Pill (羊肝丸, yang gan wan) …………………………………… (362)
White Peony and Coptis Decoction (芍药黄连汤, shao yao huang lian tang) …… (90)
White Peony Decoction (芍药汤, shao yao tang) ……………………………… (89)
Wind-Calming Decoction (镇风汤, zhen feng tang) …………………………… (40)

Wind-Dispelling and Toxin-Removing Decoction
  (驱风解毒汤, qu feng jie du tang) ·················· (346)
Wind-Dispersing Powder(消风散, xiao feng san) ·················· (171)
Wounds-Healing and Pain-Relieving Pill(和伤拈痛丹, he shang nian tong dan) ······ (300)
Wrinkled Gianthyssop Health-Restoring Decoction
  (藿香正气散, huo xiang zheng qi san) ·················· (276)

Y

Yang Hyperactivity-Checking Decoction with Seven Drugs
  (七物降下汤, qi wu jiang xia tang) ·················· (48)
Yang-Lifting Decoction (升阳汤, sheng yang tang) ·················· (94)
Yang-Harmonizing and Stagnation-Removing Plaster
  (阳和解凝膏, yang he jie ning gao) ·················· (410)
Yang-Lifting and Stomach-Benefiting Decoction
  (升阳益胃汤, sheng yang yi wei tang) ·················· (92)
Yellow-Purging Powder (泻黄散, xie huang san) ·················· (421)
Yingzhong Powder (应钟散, ying zhong san) ·················· (364)
Yin-Nourishing and Fire-Eliminating Decoction
  (滋阴降火汤, zi yin jiang huo tang) ·················· (10)
Yin-Nourishing and Wind-Calming Decoction (滋阴息风汤, zi yin xi feng tang) ········ (42)
Yin-Nourishing Real Treasure Decoction (滋阴至宝汤, zi yin zhi bao tang) ·········· (12)
Yuhong Ointment for Promoting Tissue Regeneration
  (生肌玉红膏, sheng ji yu hong gao) ·················· (414)

Z

Zhechong Decoction (折冲饮, zhe chong yin) ·················· (225)
Zhonghuang Ointment (中黄膏, zhong huang gao) ·················· (422)
Zhujing Kidney-Invigorating and Eyesight-Improving Pill
  (驻景补肾明目丸, zhu jing bu shen ming mu wan) ·················· (371)

Appendix
Index of Formula Names (Chinese with Pingin)

A

安胆汤, an dan tang (Gallbladder-Calming Decoction) ················· (102)
安吉利克, an ji li ke (Anjilike) ·························· (363)
安老汤, an lao tang (Postmenopausal Bleeding-Preventing Decoction) ········ (244)
安荣汤, an rong tang (Rong-Sooth Decoction) ················· (238)
安神定心丸, an shen ding xin wan (Mind-Tranquilizing and Heart-Easing Pill) ······ (180)
安胎白术散, an tai bai zhu san
  (Largehead Atractylodes Miscarriage-Preventing Powder) ··············· (238)
安胎寄生汤, an tai ji sheng tang
  (Chinese Taxillus Twig Miscarriage-Preventing Decoction) ············ (238)
安胎饮, an tai yin (Miscarriage-Preventing Decoction) ················· (237)
安中散, an zhong san (Middle-Soothing Powder) ················· (67)

B

八宝丹, ba bao dan (Eight Treasures Powder) ·················· (415)
八珍汤, ba zhen tang (Eight Treasures Decoction) ·················· (53)
八珍益母丸, ba zhen yi mu wan (Eight Treasures Motherwort Pill) ············ (236)
八正散, ba zheng san (Eight Corrections Powder) ················· (120)
百部止咳糖浆, bai bu zhi ke tang jiang
  (Sessile Stemona Syrup for Relieving Cough) ················· (275)
百合固金汤, bai he gu jin tang (Lily Bubus Decoction for Strengthening the Lung) ··· (14)
白虎加桂枝汤, bai hu jia gui zhi tang (Cassia Twig plus White Tiger Decoction) ······ (291)
百花丸, bai hua wan (Hundred Flowers Pill) ·················· (16)
白降丹, bai jiang dan (Baijiang Powder) ·················· (413)
白头翁汤, bai tou weng tang (Chinese Pulsatilla Decoction) ··············· (89)
白头翁加阿胶汤, bai tou weng jia e jiao tang
  (Chinese Pulsatilla Decoction plus Ass-hide Glue) ················ (90)
半硫丸, ban liu wan (Pinellia and Sulfur Pill) ·················· (84)
半夏白术天麻汤, ban xia bai zhu tian ma tang
  (Pinellia, Largehead Atractylodes and Tall Gastordia Decoction) ············ (55)
半夏泻心汤, ban xia xie xin tang (Pinellia Heart-Purging Decoction) ············ (86)
保和汤, bao he tang (Harmony-Preserving Decoction) ············· (17)
保和丸, bao he wan (Harmony-Preserving Pill) ················· (81)

贝母瓜蒌散，bei mu gua lou san
  (Tendrilleaf Fritillary Bulb and Snakegourd Fruit Powder) ……………… (6)
贝母散，bei mu san (Tendrilleaf Fritillary Bulb Powder) ……………………… (7)
萆薢饮，bi xie yin (Sevenlobed Yam Decoction) ………………………………… (121)
萆薢分清饮，bi xie fen qing yin
  (Sevenlobed Yam Decoction for Clearing Turbid Urine) ………………… (120)
萆薢渗湿汤，bi xie shen shi tang (Sevenlobed Yam Diuresis-Inducing Decoction) …… (321)
冰硼散，bing peng san (Borneol and Borax Powder) ………………………… (418)
布袋丸，bu dai wan (Silk Pouch Pill) ………………………………………… (265)
补肺阿胶汤，bu fei e jiao tang (Lung-Invigorating Ass-hide Glue Decoction) ……… (21)
补肺清金饮，bu fei qing jin yin
  (Decoction for Nourishing the Lung and Removing Heat) ………………… (17)
补肝丸，bu gan wan (Liver-Tonifying Pill) …………………………………… (372)
补偏愈风汤，bu pian yu feng tang
  (Hemiplegia-Treating and Stroke-Healing Decoction) …………………… (40)
补气解晕汤，bu qi jie yun tang
  (Qi-Replenishing and Vertigo-Relieving Decoction) …………………… (312)
补肾磁石丸，bu shen ci shi wan (Magnetite Kidney-Tonifying Pill) ………… (359)
补肾固冲丸，bu shen gu chong wan
  (Kidney-Invigorating and Chong Meridian-Consolidating Pill) ………… (238)
补肾祛寒治痹汤，bu shen qu han zhi bi tang
  (Kidney-Invigorating, Cold-Expelling and Arthralgia-Relieving Decoction) …… (439)
补肾通石汤，bu shen tong shi tang
  (Kidney-Invigorating and Stone-Removing Decoction) …………………… (150)
补天育麟丹，bu tian yu lin dan (Innateness-Tonifying and Breeding Pill) …… (164)
补益地黄丸，bu yi di huang wan (Kidney-Replenishing Rehmannia Pill) …… (161)

C

磁朱丸，ci zhu wan (Magnetite and Cinnabar Pill) …………………………… (185)
柴胡蒌姑汤，chai hu lou gu tang (Bupleurum,
  Snakegourd Fruit and Appendiculate Cremastra Pseudobulb Decoction) …… (403)
柴胡清肝饮，chai hu qing gan yin (Bupleurum Liver-Clearing Decoction) …… (313)
柴胡清肝饮，chai hu qing gan yin (Chinese Thorowax Liver-Clearing Decoction) …… (313)
柴胡舒肝散，chai hu shu gan san (Bupleurum Liver-Soothing Powder) ……… (229)
柴胡疏肝散，chai hu shu gan san (Chinese Thorowax Liver-Soothing Powder) …… (106)
肠宁汤，chang ning tang (Intestines-Calming Decoction) …………………… (242)
菖蒲丸，chang pu wan (Grassleaf Sweetflag Rhizome Pill) ………………… (265)
沉香化气丸，chen xiang hua qi wan (Eaglewood Qi Stagnation-Dissipating Pill) …… (81)
沉香化滞丸，chen xiang hua zhi wan (Eaglewood Indigestion-Relieving Pill) …… (81)
沉香降气散，chen xiang jiang qi san (Eaglewood Qi-Lowering Powder) ……… (35)

沉香散, chen xiang san (Chinese Eaglewood Powder) ········· (125)
赤石脂禹余粮汤, chi shi zhi yu yu liang tang
  (Red Halloysite and Limonite Decoction) ········· (76)
除湿蠲痹汤, chu shi juan bi tang (Dampness-Removing and
  Arthralgia-Relieving Decoction) ········· (294)
除疣汤, chu you tang (Verruca-Removing Decoction) ········· (340)
川芎茶调散, chuan xiong cha tiao san (Tea-Blended Szechwan Lovage Powder) ······ (169)

D

大安胎如胜饮, da an tai ru sheng yin (Major Miscarriage-Preventing Decoction) ······ (238)
大补阴丸, da bu yin wan (Major Yin-Replenishing Pill) ········· (12)
大防风汤, da fang feng tang (Major Divaricate Saposhuikovia Decoction) ········· (283)
大黄附子汤, da huang fu zi tang (Rhubarb and Prepared Aconite Decoction) ········· (84)
大建中汤, da jian zhong tang (Major Middle-Strengthening Decoction) ········· (69)
大连翘汤, da lian qiao tang (Major Weeping Forsythia Capsule Decoction) ········· (317)
大秦艽汤, da qin jiao tang (Major Gentian Decoction) ········· (190)
达郁宽中汤, da yu kuan zhong tang
  (Decoction for Dispersing the Stagnated Qi and Recuperating the Middle-jiao) ······ (111)
达郁汤, da yu tang (Mental Depression-Alleviating Decoction) ········· (161)
代抵当丸, dai di dang wan (Substitutive Resistant Pill) ········· (126)
胆道排石汤, dan dao pai shi tang (Gallstones-Removing Decoction) ········· (101)
丹参饮, dan shen yin (Dan-Shen Decoction) ········· (72)
丹首生血灵, dan shou sheng xue ling
  (Dan-Shen and Tuber Fleeceflower Blood-Producing Panacea) ········· (219)
丹栀逍遥散, dan zhi xiao yao san
  (Tree Peony Bark and Cape Jasmine Merry Life Power) ········· (314)
导痰汤, dao tan tang (Phlegm-Conducting Decoction) ········· (173)
当归补血汤, dang gui bu xue tang (Chinese Angelica Blood-Tonifying Decoction) ······ (60)
当归四逆加吴茱萸生姜汤, dang gui si ni jia wu zhu yu sheng jiang tang
  (Evodia, Fresh Ginger plus Chinese Angelica Cold Limbs Decoction) ········· (69)
当归汤, dang gui tang (Chinese Angelica Decoction) ········· (70)
当归饮子, dang gui yin zi (Chinese Angelica Decoction) ········· (322)
当归须散, dang gui xu san (Powder of Ending Part of Chinese Angelica Root) ········· (74)
独活汤, du huo tang (Doubleteeth Pubescent Angelica Decoction) ········· (294)
独活寄生汤, du huo ji sheng tang
  (Doubleteeth Pubescent Angelica and Chinese Taxillus Twig Decoction) ········· (292)
独活秦艽汤, du huo qin jiao tang
  (Doubleteeth Pubescent Angelica and Largeleaf Gentian Decoction) ········· (293)
涤痰汤, di tan tang (Phlegm-Dispelling Decoction) ········· (173)
抵当汤, di dang tang (Resistant Decoction) ········· (365)

颠倒散, dian dao san (Reversion Powder) ……… (426)
癫痫统治方, dian xian tong zhi fang (General Recipe for Treating Epilepsy) ……… (186)
定痫丸, ding xian wan (Epilepsy-Relieving Pill) ……… (186)

E

二陈汤, er chen tang (Two Vintage Herbs Decoction) ……… (173)
二仙汤, er xian tang (Two Immortals Powder) ……… (254)
二鲜饮, er xian yin (Two Fresh Herbs Decoction) ……… (24)
阿胶四物汤, e jiao si wu tang (Ass-hide Glue plus Four Herbs Decoction) ……… (17)
阿胶鸡子黄汤, e jiao ji zi huang tang (Ass-Hide Glue and Yolk Decoction) ……… (49)
二术汤, er zhu tang (Swordlike Atractylodes and
　　Largehead Atractylodes Decoction) ……… (288)

F

防风通圣散, fang feng tong sheng san
　　(Divaricate Saposhnikovia Miraculous Powder) ……… (25)
防己茯苓汤, fang ji fu ling tang (Fourstamen Stephania and Tuckahoe Decoction) ……… (152)
防己黄芪汤, fang ji huang qi tang
　　(Fourstamen Stephania and Membranous Milkvetch Decoction) ……… (151)
肥儿丸, fei er wan (Baby-Nourishing Pill) ……… (266)
肺瘤平, fei liu ping (Lung Tumor-Removing Formula) ……… (382)
分清饮, fen qing yin (Turbid Urine-Clearing Decoction) ……… (121)
分消汤, fen xiao tang (Water Retention-Removing Decoction) ……… (132)
复方川贝精片, fu fang chuan bei jing pian
　　(Compound Tablet of Extract of Tendrilleaf Fritillary Bulb) ……… (31)
复方蜂房汤, fu fang feng fang tang (Compound Decoction of Wasps Nest) ……… (406)
复元活血汤, fu yuan huo xue tang
　　(Decoction for Recovery and Activating Blood Circulation) ……… (376)
复方玉泉丸, fu fang yu quan wan (Compound Jade Spring Pill) ……… (407)
复肝丸, fu gan wan (Liver-Recuperating Pill) ……… (107)
茯苓导水汤, fu ling dao shui tang (Tuckahoe Water-Removing Decoction) ……… (131)
茯苓泽泻汤, fu ling ze xie tang (Tuckahoe and Oriental Waterplantain Decoction) ……… (134)
复元活血汤, fu yuan huo xue tang
　　(Qi-Restoration and Blood-Activating Decoction) ……… (35)
附子大黄汤, fu zi da huang tang (Aconite and Rhubarb Decoction) ……… (153)
附子汤, fu zi tang (Prepared Aconite Decoction) ……… (131)

G

甘草干姜茯苓白术汤, gan cao gan jiang fu ling bai zhu tang
　　(Licorice, Dried Ginger, Tuckahoe and Largehead Atractylodes Decoction) ……… (131)

甘草汤，gan cao tang (Licorice Decoction) ······ (345)
甘草泻心汤，gan cao xie xin tang (Licorice Heart-Purging Decoction) ······ (88)
肝复方，gan fu fang (Liver-Recuperating Prescription) ······ (390)
肝经气火方，gan jing qi huo fang
　(Formula for Qi and Fire of the Liver Meridian) ······ (194)
甘露消毒丹，gan lu xiao du dan (Sweet Dew Detoxication Pill) ······ (407)
葛根红花汤，ge gen hong hua tang (Pueraria and Safflower Decoction) ······ (333)
葛根汤加川芎辛夷汤，ge gen tang jia chuan xiong xin yi tang
　(Pueraria Decoction Plus Szechwan Lovage and Magnolia) ······ (353)
葛根汤，ge gen tang (Pueraria Decoction) ······ (354)
葛根黄芩黄连汤，ge gen huang qin huang lian tang
　(Lobed Kudzuvine, Baikal Skullcap and Coptis Decoction) ······ (89)
更年期统治方，geng nian qi tong zhi fang
　(General Recipe for Treating Climacterium) ······ (255)
钩藤散，gou teng san (Gambirplant Hooked Stem and Branch Powder) ······ (43)
钩藤饮，gou teng yin (Gambirplant Hooked Stem and Branch Decoction) ······ (44)
巩堤丸，gong di wan (Bank-Consolidating Pill) ······ (142)
宫颈炎Ⅱ号，gong jing yan er hao (Formula for Cervicitis Number Two) ······ (244)
宫外孕Ⅰ号方，gong wai yun yi hao fang (Formula for Exfetation Number One) ······ (253)
宫外孕Ⅱ号方，gong wai yun er hao fang (Formula for Exfetation Number Two) ······ (252)
顾步汤，gu bu tang (Foot-Minding Decoction) ······ (307)
固本锁精丸，gu ben suo jing wan (Origin-Reinforcing and Essence-Locking Pill) ······ (135)
固金抗癌汤，gu jin kang ai tang
　(Lung-Strengthening and Cancer-Resisting Decoction) ······ (381)
固精丸，gu jing wan (Emission-Condolidating Pill) ······ (136)
固精丸，gu jing wan (Essence-Astringing Pill) ······ (247)
固真汤，gu zhen tang (Vital Qi-Consolidating Decoction) ······ (263)
瓜蒌牛蒡汤，gua lou niu bang tang
　(Snakegourd and Great Burdock Achene Decoction) ······ (308)
瓜蒌散，gua lou san (Snakegourd Fruit Powder) ······ (310)
瓜蒌薤白白酒汤，gua lou xie bai bai jiu tang
　(Snakegourd, Longstamen Onion and Liquor Decoction) ······ (58)
瓜蒌薤白半夏汤，gua lou xie bai ban xia tang
　(Snakegourd, Longstamen Onion and Pinellia Decoction) ······ (58)
冠心Ⅱ号，guan xin er hao (Coronary Heart Disease Tablet Number Two) ······ (56)
冠心片，guan xin pian (Coronary Heart Disease Tablet) ······ (56)
冠心苏合丸，guan xin su he wan (Storesin Pill for Coronary Heart Disease) ······ (58)
龟鹿二仙胶，gui lu er xian jiao
　(Fairy Gelatin Containing Tortoise Shell and Plastron and Antler) ······ (163)
归脾汤，gui pi tang (Back to the Spleen Decoction) ······ (206)

桂麝散，gui she san (Cassia Bark and Musk Powder) ……………………………… (412)
桂枝茯苓丸，gui zhi fu ling wan (Cassia Twig and Tuckahoe Pill) ……………… (227)
桂枝附子汤，gui zhi fu zi tang (Cassia Twig and Aconite Decoction) …………… (289)
桂枝甘草汤，gui zhi gan cao tang (Cassia Twig and Licorice Decoction) ……… (60)
桂枝甘草龙骨牡蛎汤，gui zhi gan cao long gu mu li tang
　(Cassia Twig, Licorice, Dragon's Bone and Oyster Shell Decoction) ………… (60)
桂枝芍药知母汤，gui zhi shao yao zhi mu tang
　(Cassia Twig, White Peony and Common Anemarrhena Decoction) ………… (289)

H

海狗益肾饮，hai gou yi shen yin (Ursine Seal Kidney-Benefiting Decoction) ………… (160)
海藻玉壶汤，hai zao yu hu tang (Seaweed Jade Kettle Decoction) ……………… (200)
寒通汤，han tong tang (Cold Natured Stranguria-Treating Decoction) ………… (396)
沆瀣丹，hang xie dan (Hang Xie Pellet) ………………………………………… (268)
河车封髓丹，he che feng sui dan (Human Placenta Marrow-Sealing Pellets) ………… (163)
和伤拈痛丹，he shang nian tong dan (Wounds-Healing and Pain-Relieving Pill) ……… (300)
琥珀抱龙丸，hu po bao long wan (Amber Embracing Dragon Pill) ……………… (273)
琥珀丸，hu po wan (Amber Pill) ………………………………………………… (406)
化虫丸，hua chong wan (Parasite-Eliminating Pill) ……………………………… (267)
化积丸，hua ji wan (Abdominal Mass-Removing Pill) …………………………… (96)
化坚汤，hua jian tang (Hardness-Removing Decoction) ………………………… (111)
化痰透脑丸，hua tan tou nao wan (Phlegm-Removing and Brain-Activating Pill) …… (184)
化瘀止崩汤，hua yu zhi beng tang
　(Blood Stasis-Resolving and Metrorrhagia-Stopping Decoction) ……………… (252)
槐花散，huai hua san (Sophora Flower Powder) ………………………………… (92)
黄连解毒汤，huang lian jie du tang (Coptis Detoxificating Decoction) …………… (270)
黄芪汤，huang qi tang (Membranous Milkvetch Decoction) ……………………… (148)
黄芪益肾汤，huang qi yi shen tang
　(Membranous Milkvetch Kidney-Benefiting Decoction) ……………………… (154)
黄连汤，huang lian tang (Coptis Decoction) …………………………………… (86)
黄连温胆汤，huang lian wen dan tang (Coptis Gallbladder-Warming Decoction) …… (176)
黄芩汤，huang qin tang (Baikal Skullcap Decoction) …………………………… (89)
黄芩清肺饮，huang qin qing fei yin (Baikal Skullcap Lung-Clearing Decoction) ……… (326)
回阳玉龙膏，hui yang yu long gao
　(Jade and Dragon Ointment for Restoring Yang) ……………………………… (412)
活络效灵丹，huo luo xiao ling dan (Miraculous Collateral-Activating Pill) …………… (300)
藿香正气散，huo xiang zheng qi san
　(Wrinkled Gianthyssop Health-Restoring Decoction) ………………………… (276)
活血化坚汤，huo xue hua jian tang
　(Blood-Activating and Hardness-Removing Decoction) ……………………… (300)

活血汤, huo xue tang (Blood-Activating Decoction) ……………………………… (301)
活血止痛汤, huo xue zhi tong tang
　(Blood-Activating and Pain-Alleviating Decoction) ……………………… (300)

J

鸡肝散, ji gan san (Chicken's Liver Powder) ………………………………… (266)
济生肾气丸, ji sheng shen qi wan (Life-Preserving Kidney-Qi Pill) ……… (156)
济阴地黄丸, ji yin di huang wan (Rehmannia Yin-Nourishing Pill) ……… (363)
加减清瘟败毒饮, jia jian qing wen bai du yin
　(Modified Anti-pyretic and Anti-toxic Decoction) ……………………… (398)
加减复脉汤, jia jian fu mai tang (Modified Pulse-Restoring Decoction) …… (64)
加减瓜蒌牛蒡汤, jia jian gua lou niu bang tang
　(Modified Snakegourd Fruit and Great Burdock Achene Decoction) …… (308)
加减三奇汤, jia jian san qi tang (Modified Decoction of Three Miraculous Drugs) ……… (3)
加减四逆散, jia jian si ni san (Modified Cold Limbs Powder) …………… (33)
加参安肺生化汤, jia shen an fei sheng hua tang
　(Decoction with Ginseng for Lung Disorders and Puerperal Blood Stasis) …… (3)
加味磁朱丸, jia wei ci zhu wan (Modified Magnetite and Cinnabar Pill) …… (186)
加味柴胡汤, jia wei chai hu tang (Modified Chinese Thorowax Decoction) …… (98)
加味羌活汤, jia wei jiang huo tang (Modified Incised Notopterygium Decoction) …… (283)
加味桃红汤, jia wei tao hong tang
　(Modified Peach Kernel and Safflower Decoction) ……………………… (396)
加味五苓散, jia wei wu ling san (Modified Tuckahoe Powder With Five Herbs) …… (392)
加味犀黄丸, jia wei xi huang wan (Modified Asiatic Rhinoceros Bezoar Pill) …… (375)
加味逍遥散, jia wei xiao yao san (Modified Merry Life Powder) ………… (14)
建瓴汤, jian ling tang (Sweeping Down Decoction for Tension Hypertension) …… (41)
健脾肥儿散, jian pi fei er san (Spleen-Invigorating Body-Nouirishing Powder) …… (258)
健脾丸, jian pi wan (Spleen-Strengthening Pill) ……………………………… (257)
僵蚕蜂房汤, jiang can feng fang tang
　(Silkworm with Batrytis Larva and Wasps Nest Decoction) …………… (386)
羌活胜湿汤, jiang huo sheng shi tang
　(Notopterygium Dampness-Expelling Decoction) ……………………… (281)
降糖方, jiang tang fang (Blood Sugar-Reducing Formula) ………………… (212)
降糖汤, jiang tang tang (Blood Sugar-Reducing Decoction) ……………… (210)
降压汤, jiang ya tang (Blood Pressure-Reducing Decoction) ……………… (49)
降脂通脉饮, jiang zhi tong mai yin
　(Lipide-Lowering and Vessels-Dredging Decoction) …………………… (53)
交泰丸, jiao tai wan (Pill for Balancing the Heart and the Kidney) ……… (254)
解毒玉女煎加减方, jie du yu nü jian jia jian fang
　(Modified Toxin-Removing Fairy Decoction) …………………………… (397)

荆防败毒散, jin fang bai du san
　　(Fineleaf Schizonepeta and Ledehouriella Antiphlogistic Powder) ········· (316)
金沸草散, jin fei cao san (Inula Herb Powder) ·· (32)
金黄散, jin huang san (Golden Powder) ··· (409)
金铃子散, jin ling zi san (Szechwan Chinaberry Powder) ······························ (159)
金锁固精丸, jin shuo gu jing wan (Golden Lock Pill for Solidating Essence) ········ (134)
金岩丸, jin yan wan (Jinyan Pill) ··· (382)
菊花茶调散, jiu hua cha tiao san (Tea-Blended Chrysanthemum Flower Powder) ····· (171)
荆芥连翘汤, jing jie lian qiao tang (Schizonepeta and Forsythia Decoction) ········· (331)
荆蓬煎丸, jing peng jian wan (Common Burreed and Kwangsi Turmeric Pill) ········· (94)
九一丹, jiu yi dan (Nine to One Powder) ·· (413)
九子地黄丸, jiu zi di huang wan (Rehmannia Pill with Nine Seeds) ··················· (359)
桔枳龙牡汤, jiu zhi long mu tang
　　(Tangerine Leaf, Bitter Orange, Dragon's Bone and Oyster Shell Decoction) ····· (192)
举肺汤, ju fei tang (Lung-Rising Decoction) ·· (20)
橘核丸, ju he wan (Tangerine Seed Pill) ··· (140)
菊晴丸, ju qing wan (Chrysanthemum Flower Pill for Eye Diseases) ··················· (362)
蠲痹汤, juan bi tang (Arthralgia-Relieving Decoction) ································· (294)
决明益阴丸, jue ming yi yin wan (Abalone Shell Yin-Nourishing Pill) ················ (363)

K

抗艾滋病经验方, kang ai zi bing jing yan fang (Proven AIDS-Resisting Formula) ··· (408)
亢痿灵, kang wei ling (Effective Formula for Impotence) ······························ (159)
可保立苏汤, ke bao li su tang
　　(Viscera-Benefiting and Consciousness-Restoring Decoction) ······················ (263)
咳嗽统治方, ke sou tong zhi fang (General Recipe for Treating Cough) ················ (4)
控涎丹, kong xian dan (Saliva-Controlling Pill) ··· (37)
苦葶苈丸, ku ting li wan (Bitter Apricot and Pepperweed Pill) ························· (62)

L

阑尾化瘀汤, lan wei hua yu tang
　　(Blood Stasis-Removing Decoction for Acute Appendicitis) ························ (99)
阑尾清化汤, lan wei qing hua tang
　　(Heat-Clearing and Stasis-Removing Decoction for Acute Appendicitis) ········· (100)
劳淋汤, lao lin tang (Decoction for Stranguria due to Overstrain) ····················· (147)
立效散, li xiao san (Instant Effective Powder) ·· (420)
利咽清金汤, li yan qing jin tang
　　(Sore Throat-Relieving and Lung-Clearing Decoction) ···························· (386)
理中丸, li zhong wan (Middle-Regulating Pill) ·· (69)
良附丸, liang fu wan (Galangal and Cyperus Pill) ································· (69/159)

凉膈散，liang ge san (Diaphiagm-Cooling Powder) ·················· (270)
苓桂术甘汤，ling gui zhu gan tang
    (Tuckahoe, Cassia Twig, Largehead Atractylodes and Licorice Decoction) ·········· (131)
羚角钩藤汤，ling jiao gou teng tang
    (Antelop's Horn and Gambirplant Hooked Stem and Branch Decoction) ·········· (178)
羚羊角饮子，ling yang jiao yin zi (Antelope Horn Decoction) ·················· (363)
六神丸，liu shen wan (Miraculous Pill with Six Drugs) ·················· (343)
癃闭散，long bi san (Powder for Urine Retention) ·················· (155)
龙胆地龙起痿汤，long dan di long qi wei tang
    (Chinese Gentian, Earth Worm, Impotence-Treating Decoction) ·················· (138)
龙胆泻肝汤，long dan xie gan tang (Gentian Liver-Purging Decoction) ·········· (46)
鸬鹚涎丸，lu ci xian wan (Cormorant Saliva Pill) ·················· (273)
鹿茸丸，lu rong wan (Hairy Antler Pill) ·················· (143)

M

麻黄附子细辛汤，ma huang fu zi xi xin tang
    (Ephedra, Aconite and Manchurian Wildginger Decoction) ·················· (28)
麻子仁丸，ma zi ren wan (Hemp Seed Pill) ·················· (85)
麦门冬汤，mai men dong tang (Dwarf Lilyturf Decoction) ·················· (16/20)
麦门冬汤，mai men dong tang (Ophiopogon Decoction) ·················· (115)
蔓荆子汤，man jing zi tang (Threeleaf Chastertree Fruit Decoction) ·········· (368)
门冬饮子，men dong yin zi (Cochinchinese Asparagus Decoction) ·················· (8)
梅花点舌丹，mei hua dian she dan (Plum Blossom Tongue-Touching Tablet) ·········· (344)
秘红丹，mi hong dan (Mysterious Red Pellet) ·················· (25)
免疫性不育Ⅱ号方，mian yi xing bu yu er hao fang
    (Formula for Immune Infertility Number Two) ·················· (166)
免疫性不育Ⅲ号方，mian yi xing bu yu san hao fang
    (Formula for Immune Infertility Number Three) ·················· (166)
免疫性不育Ⅰ号方，mian yi xing bu yu yi hao fang
    (Formula for Immune Infertility Number One) ·················· (165)
妙香散，miao xiang san (Miraculous Musk Powder) ·················· (178)
明目地黄丸，ming mu di huang wan (Rehmannia Eyesight-Improving Pill) ·········· (364)
明珠饮，ming zhu yin (Bright Pearl Decoction) ·················· (362)
木香槟榔丸，mu xiang bing lang wan (Common Aucklandia and Areca Seed Pill) ······ (76)
木香导滞丸，mu xiang dao zhi wan
    (Common Aucklandia Stagnation-Removing Pill) ·················· (79)
木香黄连汤，mu xiang huang lian tang
    (Common Aucklandia and Coptis Decoction) ·················· (90)
木香顺气散，mu xiang shun qi san (Common Aucklandia Qi-Soothing Powder) ·········· (79)

N

内补鹿茸丸, nei bu lu rong wan (Interior-Replenishing Hairy Antler Pill) ……… (163)
内补丸, nei bu wan (Interior-Replenishing Pill) ……… (245)
内消瘰疬丸, nei xiao lei li wan (Internally Scrofula-Eliminating Pill) ……… (202)
内消肿瘤丸, nei xiao zhong liu wan (Internally Tumour-Relieving Pill) ……… (201)
宁嗽化痰汤, ning sou hua tan tang
　(Cough-Relieving and Phlegm-Resolving Decoction) ……… (2)
宁嗽汤, ning sou tang (Cough-Relieving Decoction) ……… (2)
宁心汤, ning xin tang (Palpitation-Relieving Decoction) ……… (65)
牛蒡解肌汤, niu bang jie ji tang (Arctium Muscles-Relieving Decoction) ……… (171)
牛黄抱龙丸, niu huang bao long wan (Cow Bezoar Embracing Dragon Pill) ……… (273)
牛蒡解肌汤, niu bang jie ji tang
　(Great Burdock Achene Muscles-Removing Decoction) ……… (327)
牛黄醒消丸, niu huang xin xiao wan
　(Cow Bezoar Toxin-Removing and Swelling-Reducing Pill) ……… (319)
牛膝散, niu qi san (Twotooth Achyranthes Root Powder) ……… (227)
暖肝煎, nuan gan jian (Liver-Warming Decoction) ……… (138)
女神散, nü shen san (Goddess Powde) ……… (231)

P

疲劳统治方, pi lao tong zhi fang (General Recipe for Treating Fatigue) ……… (216)
片仔癀, pian zai huang (Pizaihuang) ……… (376)
平甲汤, ping jia tang (Goiter-Curing Decoction) ……… (212)
普济消毒饮, pu ji xiao du yin (Everyone's Detoxicating Decoction) ……… (330)

Q

七宝美髯丹, qi bao mei ran dan (Seven Valuable Herbs Beard-Improving Pellet) …… (339)
启膈散, qi ge san (Dysphagia-Opening Powder) ……… (390)
杞菊地黄丸, qi ju di huang wan
　(Barbary Wolfberry, Chrysanthemum and Rehmannia Pill) ……… (364)
七厘散, qi li san (Anti-Bruise Powder) ……… (302)
启脾丸, qi pi wan (Spleen-Invigorating Pill) ……… (256)
七味白术散, qi wei bai zhu san
　(Largehead Atractylodes Powder with Seven Herbs) ……… (258)
七物降下汤, qi wu jiang xia tang
　(Yang Hyperactivity-Checking Decoction with Seven Drugs) ……… (48)
七仙丹, qi xian dan (Seven Immortals Pellet) ……… (339)
七仙条, qi xian tiao (Seven Immortals Roll) ……… (413)
七仙丸, qi xian wan (Seven Immortals Pill) ……… (359)

气血并补荣筋汤, qi xue bing bu rong jin tang
（Qi-Invigorating, Blood-Replenishing and Tendons-Nourishing Decoction） ………… (284)

芪术调经散, qi zhu tiao jing san (Membranous Milkvetch and
Largehead Atractylodes Powder for Regulating Menstruation) …………………… (245)

千斤首乌汤, qian jin shou wu tang
（Moghania Root and Fleeceflower Root Decoction）……………………………………… (324)

牵正散, qian zheng san (Face Distortion-Treating Powder) …………………… (187)

强肝软坚汤二号, qiang gan ruan jian tang er hao
（Liver-Strengthening and Hardness-Softening Decoction Number Two） ………… (109)

强肝软坚汤六号, qiang gan ruan jian tang liu hao
（Liver-Strengthening and Hardness-Softening Decoction Number Six）………… (110)

强肝软坚汤三号, qiang gan ruan jian tang san hao
（Liver-Strengthening and Hardness-Softening Decoction Number Three）……… (109)

强肝软坚汤四号, qiang gan ruan jian tang si hao
（Liver-Strengthening and Hardness-Softening Decoction Number Four） ………… (110)

强肝软坚汤五号, qiang gan ruan jian tang wu hao
（Liver-Strengthening and Hardness-Softening Decoction Number Five） ………… (110)

强肝软坚汤, qiang gan ruan jian tang
（Liver-Strengthening and Hardness-Softening Decoction） ……………………… (109)

强心饮, qiang xin yin (Heart-Stimulating Decoction) …………………………… (59)

青黛冰硼散, qing dai bing peng san (Natural Indigo, Borneol and Borax Powder) … (419)

清肺饮, qing fei yin (Lung-Clearing Drink) ……………………………………… (123)

清肺汤, qing fei tang (Lung-Clearing Decoction) ………………………………… (8)

清肺枇杷散, qing fei pi pa san (Lung-Clearing Loquat Powder) ……………… (325)

清肝达郁饮, qing gan da yu yin
（Liver-Clearing and Depression-Alleviating Decoction） ……………………… (228)

清肝解郁汤, qing gan jie yu tang
（Liver-Clearing and Stagnation-Removing Decocting）……………………………… (381)

清肝养肾汤, qing gan yang shen tang
（Liver-Clearing and Kidney-Nourishing Decoction）……………………………… (370)

清肝止淋汤, qing gan zhi lin tang
（Liver-Clearing and Stranguria-Treating Decoction） ……………………………… (243)

清肌安蛔汤, qing ji an hui tang
（Stomach-Clearing and Ascaris-Calming Decoction） …………………………… (280)

清金化痰汤, qing jin hua tan tang
（Lung-Clearing and Phlegm-Resolving Decoction） ……………………………… (10)

清气化痰丸, qing qi hua tan wan
（Pill for Clearing Away Heat at Qifen and Resolving Phlegm） ………………… (3)

清气化痰丸, qing qi hua tan wan (Qi-Clearing and Phlegm-Resolving Pill) ………… (10)

清热解毒汤, qing re jie du tang (Heat-Clearing and Toxin-Relieving Decoction) …… (327)

清上蠲痛汤, qing shang juan tong tang
　　(Head-Clearing and Pain-Alleviating Decoction) ……………………… (167)
清上防风汤, qing shang fang feng tang
　　(Head-Clearing Divaricate Saposhnikovia Decoction) ………………… (315)
轻身一方, qing shen yi fang (An Obesity-Reducing Formula) …………… (214)
清暑益气汤, qing shu yi qi tang
　　(Summer Heat-Clearing and Qi-Benefiting Decoction) ………………… (278)
清胃散, qing wei san (Stomach-Clearing Powder) ………………………… (421)
清瘟败毒饮, qing wen bai du yin (Anti-pyretic and Anti-toxic Decoction) … (398)
清消汤, qing xiao tang (Pathogen-Clearing and Mass-Resolving Decoction) … (399)
清心莲子饮, qing xin lian zi yin (Heart-Clearing Lotus Seed Decoction) …… (122)
清咽利膈汤, qing yan li ge tang
　　(Decoction for Removing Heat from the Throat and Chest) …………… (356)
清音片, qing yin pian (Hoarseness-Relieving and Aphonia-Healing Tablet) … (355)
青云独步丹, qing yun du bu dan (Beard and Hair-Darkening Pellet) ……… (339)
驱风解毒汤, qu feng jie du san (Wind-Dispelling and Toxin-Removing Decoction) … (346)
驱蛔汤二号, qu hui tang er hao (Ascaris-Expelling Decoction Number Two) … (103)
驱蛔汤三号, qu hui tang san hao (Ascaris-Expelling Decoction Number Three) …… (103)
驱蛔汤一号, qu hui tang yi hao (Ascaris-Expelling Decoction Number One) … (103)

R

人参蛤蚧散, ren shen ge jie san (Ginseng and Giant Gecko Powder) ………… (20)
人参汤, ren shen tang (Ginseng Decoction) …………………………………… (217)
人参养荣汤, ren shen yang rong tang (Ginseng Nutrition Decoction) ……… (206/218)
人参养血汤, ren shen yang xue tang (Ginseng Blood-tonitfying Decoction) …… (217)
乳一方, ru yi fang (A Prescription for Breast Nodule) …………………………… (404)
软脉灵, ruan mai ling (Efficacious Vessels-Softening Formula) ……………… (197)
润肠丸, run chang wan (Intestines-Moistening Pill) …………………………… (84)
润燥养胃汤, run zao yang wei tang
　　(Dryness-Moistening and Stomach-Nourishing Decoction) ……………… (113)

S

三痹汤, san bi tang (Decoction for Wind-Cold-Dampness Arthralgia) ………… (286)
三才封髓丹, san cai feng sui dan (Sancai Marrow-Preserving Pill
　　Containing Cochinchinese Asparagus, Rehmannia and Ginseng) ……… (144)
三叉神经统治方, san cha shen jing tong zhi fang
　　(General Recite for Treating Prosopagia) ………………………………… (188)
三黄洗剂, san huang xi ji (Three Huang Lotion) ……………………………… (425)
三黄泻心汤, san huang xie xin tang (Three Huang Heart-Clearing Decoction) ……… (334)
三妙散, san miao san (Three Wonderful Herbs Powder) ……………………… (426)

三品一条枪，san pin yi tiao qiang (Sores-Treating Medicated Thread) ………… (412)
三物备急丸，san wu bei ji wan (Three Herbs Emergency Pill) ………………… (84)
三物黄芩汤，san wu huang qin tang (Three Herbs Baikal Skullcap Decoction) ……… (228)
桑菊饮，sang ju yin (Mulbery and Chrysanthemum Decoction) ……………… (3)
桑螵蛸散，sang piao xiao san (Mantis Egg-Case Powder) ……………………… (136)
四妙勇安汤，si miao yong an tang (Four Powerful Herbs Decoction) ………… (306)
四神丸，si shen wan (Four Miraculous Herbs Pill) ……………………………… (76)
四生丸，si sheng wan (Four Fresh Herbs Pill) …………………………………… (24)
四物化郁汤，si wu hua yu tang (Four Herbs Stasis-Dissolving Decoction) ………… (73)
四物绛覆汤，si wu jiang fu tang
　(Four Herbs with Rubia Root and Inula Flower Decoction) ………………… (76)
四物汤，si wu tang (Four Herbs Decoction) ……………………………………… (53)
四物五子丸，si wu wu zi wan (Four Herbs and Five Kernals Pill) ……………… (357)
四物消风饮，si wu xiao feng yin (Four Herbs Wind-Dispersing Decoction) …… (324)
四物延胡汤，si wu yan hu tang (Four Herbs with Corydalis Tuber Decoction) ……… (73)
四制香附丸，si zhi xiang fu wan (Four-Process Nutgrass Galingale Pill) ……… (231)
苏合香丸，su he xiang wan (Storesin Pill) ……………………………………… (58)
苏子降气汤，su zi jiang qi tang (Perilla Decoction for Keeping Qi Downward) …… (5)
苏子杏汤，su zi xing tang (Perilla Seed and Apricot Seed Decoction) ………… (7)
缩泉丸，suo quan wan (Urination-Decreasing Pill) ……………………………… (267)
沙淋丸，sha lin wan (Pill for Stranguria from Urolithiasis) …………………… (150)
沙参麦门冬汤，sha shen mai men dong tang
　(Coastal Glehnia and Ophiopogon Decoction) ……………………………… (115)
少腹逐瘀汤，shao fu zhu yu tang
　(Lower Abdomen Blood Stasis-Dispelling Decoction) ……………………… (227)
芍药黄连汤，shao yao huang lian tang (White Peony and Coptis Decoction) ……… (90)
芍药汤，shao yao tang (White Peony Decoction) ………………………………… (89)
蛇床子散，she chuang zi san (Common Cnidium Powder) ……………………… (417)
蛇胆川贝散，she dan chuan bei san
　(Snake Gallbladder and Tendrilleaf Fritillary Bulb Powder) ………………… (8)
肾绞痛汤，shen jiao tong tang (Decoction for Renal Colic) …………………… (150)
肾绞痛汤，shen jiao tong tang (Renal Colic Decoction) ………………………… (157)
肾康灵，shen kang ling (Effective Formula for Kidney Recuperation) ………… (148)
神秘汤，shen mi tang (Mystery Decoction) ……………………………………… (4)
参芪劳淋汤，shen qi lao lin tang (Pilose Asiabell, Membranous Milkvetch
　Decoction for Stranguria due to Overstrain) ………………………………… (146)
参芪蓉仙汤，shen qi rong xian tang (Pilose Asiabell, Membranous Milkvetch,
　Desertliving Cistanche and Shorthorned Epimedium Decoction) ………… (394)
沈氏闷泉丸，shen shi men quan wan (Shen's Pill for Decreasing Urination) …… (267)
胜湿汤，shen shi tang (Dampness-Removing Decoction) ……………………… (288)

身痛逐瘀汤, shen tong zhu yu tang
　　(Pantalgia-Relieving and Blood Stasis-Dispelling Decoction) …………… (302)
生血散, shen xue san (Blood-Producing Powder) …………………………… (219)
肾炎汤, shen yan tang (Nephritis Decoction) ……………………………… (151)
生发汤, sheng fa tang (Hair-Promoting Decoction) …………………………… (340)
生发饮, sheng fa yin (Hair-Promoting Drink) ………………………………… (340)
生肌散, sheng ji san (Tissue-Rregeneration Powder) ………………………… (415)
生肌玉红膏, sheng ji yu hong gao
　　(Yuhong Ointment for Promoting Tissue Regeneration) ……………… (414)
生姜泻心汤, sheng jiang xie xin tang (Fresh Ginger Heart-Purging Decoction) ……… (87)
生脉散, sheng mai san (Pulse-Activating Powder) …………………………… (208)
生铁落饮, sheng tie luo yin (Iron Scales Decoction) ………………………… (190)
升血合剂, sheng xue he ji (Hemocyte-Increasing Mixture) ………………… (217)
圣愈汤, sheng yu tang (Holy Disease-Curing Decoction) …………………… (209)
升阳汤, sheng yang tang (Yang-Lifting Decoction) ………………………… (94)
升阳益胃汤, sheng yang yi wei tang
　　(Yang-Lifting and Stomach-Benefiting Decoction) …………………… (92)
十宝散, shi bao san (Ten Treasures Powder) ………………………………… (304)
食道炎丸, shi dao yan wan (Esophagitis Pill) ………………………………… (111)
石斛夜光丸, shi hu ye guang wan (Dendrobium Eyesight-Improving Pill) … (360)
十灰散, shi hui san (Ten Charred Herbs Powder) …………………………… (23)
石决明丸, shi jue ming wan (Abalone Shell Pill) …………………………… (362)
实脾饮, shi pi yin (Spleen-Reinforcing Decoction) ………………………… (129)
十全大补汤, shi quan da bu tang (Ten Strong Tonic Herbs Decoction) …… (225)
十全大补丸, shi quan da bu wan (Ten Strong Tonic Herbs Pill) …………… (204)
十味败毒汤, shi wei bai du tang (Antiphlogistic Powder with Ten Herbs) … (329)
十味败毒汤, shi wei bai du tang (Ten Herbs Antiphlogistic Decoction) …… (329)
石韦散, shi wei san (Japanese Felt Fern Powder) …………………………… (120)
十味温胆汤, shi wei wen dan tang
　　(Ten Drugs Decoction for Warming Gallbladder) …………………… (176)
失笑散, shi xiao san (Laughing Powder) ……………………………………… (73)
十枣汤, shi zao tang (Ten Chinese Dates Decoction) ………………………… (37)
湿疹散, shi zhen san (Eczema Powder) ……………………………………… (424)
寿胎丸, shou tai wan (Miscarriage-Preventing Pill) ………………………… (236)
寿星丸, shou xing wan (Longevity Pill) ……………………………………… (182)
疏肝利胆汤, shu gan li dan tang
　　(Liver-Dispersing and Gallbladder-Benefiting Decoction) …………… (101)
舒肝理脾丸, shu gan li pi wan (Liver-Soothing and Spleen-Regulating Pill) …… (101)
疏肝四味散, shu gan si wei san (Liver-Soothing Four Drugs Powder) ……… (138)
疏肝消核方, shu gan xiao he fang

（Liver-Soothing and Nodules-Eliminating Prescrioption） ……… （380）
舒肝丸，shu gan wan（Liver-Soothing Pill）……… （110）
舒肝饮，shu gan yin（Liver-Soothing Decoction）……… （104）
疏经活血汤，shu jin huo xue tang
　　（Channels-Dredging and Blood-Activating Decoction）……… （295）
曙光血管头痛方，shu guang xue guan tou tong fang
　　（Dawn Formula for Vascular Headache）……… （193）
疏凿饮子，shu zao yin zi（Decoction for Diuresis）……… （127）
双补汤，shuang bu tang（Two Organs-Replenishing Decoction）……… （222）
双冬豆根汤，shuang dong dou gen tang
　　（Dwarf Lilyturf, Cochinchinese Asparagus and Tonkin Sophora Decoction） ……… （384）
双解散，shuang jie san（Double Expelling Powder）……… （27）
水陆二仙丹，shui lu er xian dan（Land and Water Two Fairies Pellet）……… （135）
顺经汤，shun jing tang（Menstruation-Normalizing Decoction）……… （232）

T

塌痒汤，ta yang tang（Itching-Stopping Decoction）……… （415）
泰山盘石散，tai shan pan shi san（Taishan Rock Powder）……… （239）
桃核承气汤，tao he cheng qi tang（Peach Kernel Purgative Decoction）……… （299）
桃花汤，tao hua tang（Peach Blossom Decoction）……… （76）
桃仁当归汤，tao ren dang gui tang
　　（Peach Kernel and Chinese Angelica Decoction）……… （242）
天滴丸，tian di wan（Tiandi Pill）……… （417）
填精补肾育种汤，tian jing bu shen yu zhong tang
　　（Essence-Supplementing, Kidney-Invigorating and Breeding Decoction）……… （162）
填精嗣续丸，tian jing ci xu wan
　　（Essence-Supplementing and Infertility-Treating Pill）……… （163）
天麻钩藤饮，tian ma gou teng yin（Gastrodian and Uncaria Decoction）……… （194）
天麻钩藤饮，tian ma gou teng yin
　　（Tall Gastrodia and Gambirplant Hooked Stem and Branch Decoction）……… （51/55）
天台乌药散，tian tai wu yao san（Combined Spicebush Root Powder）……… （142）
天台乌药散，tian tai wu yao san（Tiantai Combined Spicebush Powder）……… （140）
天真丹，tian zhen dan（Nature Pill）……… （154）
调律汤，tiao lu tang（Heart Rhythm-Regulating Decoction）……… （66）
调元散，tiao yuan san（Primary Qi-Regulating Powder）……… （263）
通导散，tong dao san（Dreging and Dissipating Powder）……… （298）
痛风统治方，tong feng tong zhi fang
　　（General Recipe for Treating Mogratory Arthralgia）……… （291）
通窍活血加减方，tong qiao huo xue jia jian fang
　　（Modified Orifice-Opening and Blood-Activating Prescription）……… （397）

通乳丹, tong ru dan (Lactation-Inducing Pill) ……………………………… (249)
通宣理肺丸, tong xuan li fei wan (Qi-Dispersing and Lung-Regulating Pill) ……… (31)
通幽汤, tong you tang (Pylorus-Dredging Decoction) ……………………… (389)
通瘀煎, tong yu jian (Blood Stasis-Removing Decoction) ………………… (241)
头伤 II 号, tou shang er hao
　　(Formula for Craniocerebral Contusion Number Two) ……………… (311)
头痛统治方, tou tong tong zhi fang (General Recipe for Treating Headache) ……… (171)
退翳汤, tui yi tang (Nebula-Removing Decoction) ………………………… (358)

W

王不留行散, wang bu liu xing san (Cowherb Seed Powder) ………………… (150)
温胞散, wen bao san (Uterus-Warming Powder) …………………………… (234)
温胆汤, wen dan tang (Gallbladder-Warming Decoction) ………………… (171)
温肺汤, wen fei tang (Lung-Warming Decoction) ………………………… (350)
温肺止流汤, wen fei zhi liu tang
　　(Lung-Warming and Running-Stopping Decocting) ………………… (349)
温经汤, wen jing tang (Meridian-Warming Decoction) …………………… (232)
温脾汤, wen pi tang (Spleen-Warming Decoction) ………………………… (82)
温肾排毒汤, wen shen pai du tang
　　(Kidney-Warming and Toxin-Clearing Decoction) ………………… (155)
温下清上汤, wen xia qing shang tang
　　(Lower-Warming and Upper-Clearing Decoction) ………………… (278)
五宝散, wu bao san (Five Treasures Powder) ……………………………… (320)
五法合一甲亢汤, wu fa he yi jia kang tang
　　(Hyperparathyroidism-Treating Decoction with Five Methods) ……… (214)
五疳消食丸, wu gan xiao shi wan
　　(Digestion-Promoting Pill for Five Infantile Malnutrition) …………… (30)
蜈蚣粉, wu gong fen (Centipede Powder) ………………………………… (428)
五积散, wu ji san (Five Retentions Powder) ……………………………… (27)
乌鸡丸, wu ji wan (Silky Fowl Black-Bone Chicken Bolus) ……………… (236)
五淋散, wu lin san (Powder for Five Kinds of Stranguria) ……………… (118)
五苓散, wu ling san (Poria Powder with Five Herbs) …………………… (394)
五皮饮, wu pi yin (Five kinds of Peels Decoction) ………………………… (131)
五仁丸, wu ren wan (Five Kinds of Kernels Pills) ………………………… (85)
五神汤, wu shen tang (Five Miraculous Drugs Decoction) ……………… (322)
五味消毒饮, wu wei xiao du yin (Five Herbs Antiphlogistic Drink) ……… (336)
五物解毒散, wu wu jie du san (Five Herbs Detoxicating Powder) ……… (336)
五子衍宗丸, wu zi yan zong wan (Five Kinds of Seeds Pill for Sterility) ……… (160)

X

犀黄丸，xi huang wan（Cow Bezoar Pill） ………………………………………（374）
洗心汤，xi xin tang（Heart-Washing Decoction）……………………………（180）
下乳涌泉散，xia ru yong quan san（Springing like Lactation-Promoting Powder）……（247）
下瘀血汤，xia yu xue tang（Decoction for Purging Blood Stasis）……………（365）
香砂枳术丸，xiang sha zhi zhu wan（Aucklandia, Amomum Fruit,
　　Immature Bitter Orange and Largehead Atractylodes Pill）……………（82）
响声破笛丸，xiang sheng po di wan
　　（Hoarseness-Relieving and Aphonia-Treating Pill）………………………（345）
小柴胡桔梗石膏汤，xiao chai hu jie gen shi gao tang
　　（Minor Bupleurum Decoction Plus Balloonflower and Gypsum）…………（352）
小柴胡汤，xiao chai hu tang（Minor Chinese Thorowax Decoction）…………（98）
哮喘统治方，xiao chuan tong zhi fang（General Recipe for Treating Asthma）……（5）
消癜汤，xiao dian tang（Purpura-Relieving Decoction）………………………（222）
小儿回春丹，xiao er hui chun dan（Infantile Convulsion-Relieving Pill）……（271）
小儿四症丸，xiao er si zhen wan（Infantile Four Symptoms Pill）……………（275）
小儿止咳金丹，xiao er zhi ke jin dan（Infantile Cough-Relieving Pellet）……（7）
消风散，xiao feng san（Wind-Dispersing Powder）……………………………（171）
小蓟饮子，xiao ji yin zi（Field Thistle Decoction）……………………………（116）
小金丹，xiao jin dan（Minor Panacea Pellet）…………………………………（376）
小金片，xiao jin pian（Minor Gold Tablet）……………………………………（306）
消渴方，xiao ke fang（Diabetes-Relieving Formula）…………………………（211）
消瘰丸，xiao lei wan（Scrofula-Dispelling Pill）………………………………（204）
消炎护膜方，xiao yan hu mo fang
　　（Inflammation-Diminishing and Membrane-Protecting Formula）………（113）
逍遥散，xiao yao san（Merry Life Powder）……………………………（106/326）
消瘿五海丸，xiao ying wu hai wan（Five Seafoods Goiter-Dissolving Pill）……（204）
消疣汤，xiao you tang（Wart-Eliminating Decoction）………………………（424）
消癥散，xiao zheng san（Mass-Eliminating Powder）…………………………（253）
消肿解毒汤，xiao zhong jie du tang
　　（Swelling-Reducing and Detoxificating Decoction）………………………（308）
泻肝汤，xie gan tang（Liver-Purging Decoction）……………………………（372）
泻黄散，xie huang san（Yellow-Purging Powder）……………………………（421）
泻青丸，xie qing wan（Blue-Purging Pill）………………………………………（47）
心衰合剂，xin shuai he ji（Heart Failure Mixture）……………………………（60）
醒消丸，xin xiao wan（Toxin-Clearing and Swelling-Reducing Pill）…………（320）
辛夷清肺汤，xin yi qing fei tang（Magnolia Lung-Clearing Decoction）……（348）
星夏草菖双龙汤，xing xia cao chang shuang long tang
　　（Jackinthepulpit, Pinellia, Common Selfheal Fruit-Spike,

Grassleaf Sweetflag and Two Pieces of Centipedes Decoction) ……………… (401)
芎归胶艾汤, xiong gui jiao ai tang (Szechwan Lovage Rhizome,
　Chinese Angelica Root, Ass-hide Glue and Argy Wormwood Leaf Decoction) ……… (225)
芎归明目丸, xiong gui ming mu wan (Szechwan Lovage and
　Chinese Angelica Pill for Improving Acuity of Sight) ……………………………… (362)
芎归调血饮, xiong gui tiao xue yin (Szechwan Lovage and
　Chinese Angelica Decoction for Regulating Blood Flow) …………………………… (223)
胸膜炎汤Ⅱ号, xiong mo yan tang er hao (Pleurisy Decoction Number Two) ………… (35)
胸膜炎汤Ⅰ号, xiong mo yan tang yi hao (Pleurisy Decoction Number One) ………… (33)
芎辛散, xiong xin san (Szechwan Lovage Rhizome and
　Manchurian Wildginger Herb Powder) ………………………………………………… (195)
续断饮, xu duan yin (Himalayan Teasel Decoction) ……………………………………… (62)
血崩统治方, xue beng tong zhi fang
　(General Recipe for Treating Metrorrhagia and Metrostaxis) ……………………… (252)
血府逐瘀汤, xue fu zhu yu tang (Blood-House Blood Stasis-Dispelling Decoction) …… (57)

Y

牙痛统治方, ya tong tong zhi fang (General Recipe for Treating Toothache) ………… (421)
咽炎统治方, yan yan tong zhi fang (General Recipe for Sore Throat) ………………… (345)
养肝丸, yang gan wan (Liver-Nourishing Pill) …………………………………………… (363)
羊肝丸, yang gan wan (Wether Liver Pill) ………………………………………………… (362)
阳和解凝膏, yang he jie ning gao
　(Yang-Harmonizing and Stagnation-Removing Plaster) ……………………………… (410)
养金汤, yang jin tang (Lung-Nourishing Decoction) ……………………………………… (16)
养精种玉汤, yang jing zhong yu tang
　(Essence-Nourishing and Pregnancy-Promoting Decoction) ………………………… (236)
养血补心汤, yang xue bu xin tang
　(Blood-Enriching and Heart-Replenishing Decoction) ………………………………… (235)
养血胜风汤, yang xue sheng feng tang
　(Blood-Enriching and Wind-Dispersing Decoction) …………………………………… (339)
养真丹, yang zhen dan (Genuine Qi-Nourishing Pellet) ………………………………… (339)
一贯煎, yi guan jian (Decoction Worth A Thousand Copper Coins) …………………… (114)
益黄散, yi huang san (Powder for Sallow Complexion) ………………………………… (258)
益母草膏, yi mu cao gao (Motherwort Herb Ointment) ………………………………… (230)
益母胜金丹, yi mu sheng jin dan (Motherwort Gold-Exceeding Pill) ………………… (230)
益脑活血方, yi nao huo xue fang
　(Brain-Benefiting and Blood-Activating Formula) …………………………………… (195)
益脑强神丸, yi nao qiang shen wan
　(Brain-Benefiting and Spirit-Invigorating Pill) ………………………………………… (184)
益肾汤, yi shen tang (Kidney-Benefiting Decoction) …………………………………… (154)

益肾填精汤, yi shen tian jing tang
（Kidney-Invigorating and Essence-Supplementing Decoction） …… （161）
胰腺清化汤, yi xian qing hua tang
（Heat-Removing Decoction for Acute Pancreatitis） ……………… （97）
玉液汤, yu ye tang (Jade Liquid Decoction (Yuye Decoction)) ……… （198）
薏苡附子败酱散, yi yi fu zi bai jiang san
（Coix Seed, Prepared Aconite and Whiteflower Patrinia Powder） …… （100）
薏苡仁汤, yi yi ren tang (Coix Seed Decoction) ………………… （286）
乙字汤, yi zi tang ("B" Character Decoction) ………………… （91）
抑肝散, yi gan san (Liver-Inhibiting Powder) ………………… （176）
益气聪明汤, yi qi cong ming tang
（Qi-Replenishing, Hearing-improving and Eyesight-Acuminating Decoction） ……… （367）
益气化斑汤, yi qi hua ban tang
（Qi-Replenishing and Rash-Dissipating Decoction） ………………… （220）
益气化积解毒汤, yi qi hua ji jie du tang
（Qi-Replenishing, Retention-Removing and Poison-Clearing Decoction） ……… （106）
益气养阴汤, yi qi yang yin tang
（Qi-Replenishing and Yin-Nourishing Decoction） ………………… （51）
益瞳丸, yi tong wan (Pupils-Benefiting Pill) ………………… （364）
茵柴清胆汤, yin chai qing dan tang
（Capillary Wormwood, Chinese Thorowax Gallbladder-Clearing Decoction） ……… （103）
茵陈蒿汤, yin chen hao tang (Capillary Wormwood Decoction) ……… （102）
茵陈蒿汤, yin chen hao tang (Oriental Wormwood Decoction) ……… （326）
茵陈降脂方, yin chen jiang zhi fang
（Capillary Wormwood Lipid-Reducing Formula） ………………… （197）
阴毒内消散, yin du nei xiao san (Internal Eliminating Powder for Yin-Toxin) ……… （427）
银花解毒汤, yin hua jie du tang (Honeysuckle Flower Detoxicating Decoction) …… （328）
银翘石斛汤, yin qiao shi hu tang
（Honeysuckle, Weeping Forsythia and Dendrobium Decoction） ……… （148）
应钟散, ying zhong san (Yingzhong Powder) ………………… （364）
疣灵搽剂, you ling cha ji (Sovereign Wart-Eliminating Liniment) ……… （423）
郁金逍遥散, yu jin xiao yao san (Turmeric Root-Tuber Merry Life Powder) …… （404）
毓麟珠, yu lin zhu (Pregnancy-Promoting Pearl) ………………… （234）
玉女煎, yu nü jian (Jade Maid Decoction) ………………… （211）
月华丸, yue hua wan (Lunar Corona Pill) ………………… （20）
约精丸, yue jing wan (Essence-Astringing Pill) ………………… （136）
越鞠丸, yue ju wan (Stagnation-Relieving Pill) ………………… （29）

Z

赞育丹, zan yu dan (Procreation-Helping Pellet) ………………… （138）

滋生清阳汤, zi sheng qing yang tang (Lucid Yang-Generating Decoction) ……………… (182)
滋阴降火汤, zi yin jiang huo tang
　(Yin-Nourishing and Fire-Eliminating Decoction) ……………………………… (10)
滋阴至宝汤, zi yin zhi bao tang (Yin-Nourishing Real Treasure Decoction) ………… (12)
紫云膏, zi yun gao (Purple Cloud Ointment) ……………………………………… (423)
棕蒲散, zong pu san (Charred Fortune Windmillpalm Petiole and
　Charred Cattail Pollen Powder) ……………………………………………… (250)
坐骨神经统治方, zuo gu shen jing tong zhi fang
　(General Recipe for Treating Sciatica) ………………………………………… (295)
左归丸, zuo gui wan (Back to the Left Pill) ……………………………………… (55)
左金丸, zuo jin wan (Left Golden Pill) …………………………………………… (47)
壮阳丹, zhang yang dan (Kidney Yang-Strengthening Pill) ……………………… (136)
折冲饮, zhe chong yin (Zhechong Decoction) …………………………………… (225)
鹧鸪菜汤, zhe gu cai tang (Caloglossa Leprieurii Decoction) …………………… (279)
镇风汤, zhen feng tang (Wind-Calming Decoction) ……………………………… (40)
镇肝息风汤, zhen gan xi feng tang (Liver-Calming and Wind-Stopping Decoction) …… (51)
镇肝息风汤, zhen gan xi feng tang (Liver-Subduing and Wind-Stopping Decoction) … (38)
整律合剂, zheng lu he ji (Heart Rhythm-Adjusting Mixture) ……………………… (63)
真人养脏汤, zhen ren yang zang tang (Immortal Viscera-Nourishing Decoction) …… (74)
镇痛消肿膏, zhen tong xiao zhong gao
　(Pain-Alleviating and Swelling-Reducing Plaster) ……………………………… (426)
真武汤, zhen wu tang (Devine Black Bird Decoction) ………………………… (60/62)
真武汤, zhen wu tang (Divine Black Bird Decoction) ……………………… (131/155)
治癌散, zhi ai san (Cancer-Treating Powder) …………………………………… (428)
知柏地黄丸, zhi bai di huang wan
　(Anemarrhena, Phellodendron and Rehmannia Pill) …………………………… (212)
知柏坤草汤, zhi bai kun cao tang
　(Common Anemarrhena, Chinese Corktree Bark and Motherwort Decoction) …… (157)
治斑秃方, zhi ban tu fang (Prescription for Treating Alopecia Areata) …………… (337)
炙甘草汤, zhi gan cao tang (Prepared Licorice Decoction) ……………………… (20)
止痉散, zhi jing san (Convulsion-Relieving Powder) …………………………… (188)
治卵巢癌方, zhi luan chao ai fang (Prescription for Ovarian Cancer) …………… (405)
枳朴六君子汤, zhi po liu jun zi tang
　(Bitter Orange and Officinal Magnolia Bark Six Gentlemen Decoction) ………… (392)
止嗽散, zhi suo san (Cough-Stopping Powder) …………………………………… (1)
枳实导滞丸, zhi shi dao zhi wan
　(Immature Bitter Orange Stagnation-Dispelling Pill) …………………………… (79)
枳实化滞汤, zhi shi hua zhi tang
　(Immature Bitter Orange Stagnation-Removing Decoction) …………………… (82)
枳实消痞丸, zhi shi xiao pi wan

（Immatures Bitter Orange Stuffiness-Removing Pill） ……………… (82)
治头疮一方，zhi tou chuang yi fang (A Prescription for Treating Head Boils) ……… (334)
止血灵，zhi xue ling (Bleeding-Arresting Panacea) ……………………… (252)
滋阴息风汤，zhi yin xi feng tang (Yin-Nourishing and Wind-Calming Decoction) …… (42)
舟车丸，zhou che wan (Boat and Cart Pill) ……………………………… (129)
中黄膏，zhong huang gao (Zhonghuang Ointment) ……………………… (422)
驻车丸，zhu che wan (Dysentery-Stopping Pill) ………………………… (88)
术归桂草汤，zhu gui gui cao tang (Largehead Atractylodes,
　　Chinese Angelica, Cassia Bark and Licorice Decoction) ……………… (243)
逐寒荡惊汤，zhu han dang jing tang (Cold-Expelling and
　　Convulsion-Relieving Decoction) ………………………………… (260)
驻景补肾明目丸，zhu jing bu shen ming mu wan
　　(Zhujing Kidney-Invigorating and Eyesight-Improving Pill) …………… (371)
驻景丸，zhu jing wan (Vision Acuity-Improving Pill) …………………… (366)
驻景丸，zhu jing wan (Pill for Improving Acuity of Sight) ……………… (358)
驻景丸加减方，zhu jing wan jia jian fang
　　(Modified Vision Acuity-Improving Pill) ………………………… (367)
猪苓汤，zhu ling tang (Umbellate Pore Fungus Decoction) ……………… (394)
竹茹温胆汤，zhu ru wen dan tang
　　(Bamboo Shavings Gallbladder-Warming Decoction) ……………… (174)
枳实薤白桂枝汤，zhu shi xie bai gui zhi tang
　　(Immature Bitter Orange, Longstamen Onion and Cassia Twig Decoction) ……… (58)
逐瘀止崩汤，zhu yu zhi beng tang
　　(Blood Stasis-Removing and Metrorrhagia-Stopping Decoction) ……… (251)
逐瘀止血汤，zhu yu zhi xue tang
　　(Blood Stasis-Removing and Bleeding-Arresting Decoction) ………… (250)
转呆丹，zhuan dai dan (Dementia-Curing Pill) …………………………… (181)
着痹验方，zhuo bi yan fang (Proven Recipes for Arthralgia of Damp Type) …… (288)

图书在版编目(CIP)数据

方剂学发挥/刘公望主编;刘长林译. —北京:华夏出版社,2002.9
ISBN 7-5080-2797-3

Ⅰ.方… Ⅱ.①刘…②刘… Ⅲ.方剂学-英文 Ⅳ.R289

中国版本图书馆 CIP 数据核字(2002)第 074523 号

华 夏 出 版 社 出 版 发 行
(北京东直门外香河园北里4号 邮编:100028)
新 华 书 店 经 销
北京中科印刷有限公司印刷
787×1092 1/16开本 30.75印张 754千字 插页1
2002年9月北京第1版 2002年9月北京第1次印刷
定价:128.00元

本版图书凡印刷、装订错误,可及时向我社发行部调换